PHARMACO EPIDEMIOLOGY

An Introduction

3rd Edition

EDITED BY

Abraham G Hartzema, Miquel Porta, and Hugh H Tilson

Harvey Whitney Books

First Edition, copyright © 1988
Second Edition, copyright © 1991
Third Edition, copyright © 1998

Copyright © 1998 by HARVEY WHITNEY BOOKS COMPANY
Printed in the United States of America

Pharmacoepidemiology: an introduction / edited by Abraham G. Hartzema, Miquel S. Porta, and Hugh H. Tilson. -- 3rd ed.
    p.   cm.
  Includes bibliographical references and index.
  ISBN 0-929375-18-1 (alk. paper)
  1. Pharmacoepidemiology. I. Hartzema, Abraham G.   II. Porta, Miquel S.   III. Tilson, Hugh Hanna.
  [DNLM: 1. Drug Therapy--adverse effects. 2. Epidemiologic Methods. 3. Product Surveillance, Postmarketing .
4. Pharmacoepidemiology--methods. QZ 42 P537 1997]
RM302.5.P54   1997
615'.704--DC21
DNLM/DLC
for Library of Congress   97-34219
                                                CIP

HARVEY WHITNEY BOOKS COMPANY
4906 Cooper Rd., P.O. Box 42696, Cincinnati, OH 45242 USA

Table of Contents

Foreword

We all face disease as part of life, but the sadness it brings is all the more poignant when the disease results from drugs intended to promote health rather than to impair it. Drugs are developed and used to prevent or mitigate disease and pain, and our continued reliance on them is a testament to their wondrous efficacy and safety. But agents that have the power to alter some biological processes to our benefit can alter other biological processes to our detriment, sometimes in occult and surprising ways. To live up to the dictum that we should first of all do no harm, or at least less harm than good, we must bring our best evaluative alternative methods to bear on the measurement of drug effects, both beneficial and adverse.

Pharmacoepidemiology is a natural crossing of scientific paths. Epidemiology is the study of disease occurrence, and pharmacology aims to reduce disease incidence and prevalence through biochemical intervention. The heavy reliance on epidemiologic methods — I include among these the clinical trial — in modern drug development has been instrumental in producing a pharmacopoeia of highly effective and reliable medicines that are among the major contributors to a better quality of life. Epidemiologic methods also have provided crucial insights into modern iatrogenic epidemics, such as adenocarcinoma of the vagina caused by diethylstilbestrol, endometrial cancer caused by exogenous estrogens, and toxic shock caused by the use of tampons.

The escalating health consciousness of our society guarantees an even broader role in the future for pharmacoepidemiologic research. Drug trials for efficacy usually have been clinical trials, aimed at improving the prognosis or symptoms of patients with active disease. Field trials, which evaluate the efficacy of primary preventives, are much more ambitious undertakings. They ordinarily require many thousands of subjects to be followed for long periods, presenting difficult logistical problems. Because these subjects are not ill, recruiting them and maintaining contact is more of a problem than in clinical trials, in which the clinic can be used for both recruitment and follow-up. For these reasons field trials of pharmaceutical agents for primary prevention have been conducted only rarely, usually for vaccines. With growing interest in the primary prevention of disease, however, field trials of disease preventives may become more common.

We shall also see more studies that evaluate adverse drug effects, many of which will be case–control studies. Unintended drug effects (UDEs) that occur soon after the administration of a drug are usually discovered early in clinical testing, provided that they occur frequently enough. When UDEs are rare or occur only with a lengthy induction time, however, they may easily go undetected. Case–control studies provide an opportunity to investigate rare or delayed

UDEs without undertaking cumbersome follow-up studies of awesome cost and logistical complexity. One big obstacle to case–control studies of drug use has been ascertaining the drug history. Information about drug use recorded in medical records varies in quality and completeness, often being little better or even worse than the information about drug use stored in the cerebral cortex of users. Obtaining valid information on drug use is aided greatly by systems that automatically record drug information in computer-readable form as it is prescribed or dispensed. (Of course, even this information differs from actual use.) Automated databases that include drug information and the capability to link it with medical records are increasing in number, and with passing time accumulating data become more valuable as resources for pharmacoepidemiologic research.

Even with the best data resources, there remains a crucial epidemiologic problem in the study of many UDEs: confounding stemming from the indication for drug use. The causal association between illness and drugs employed to treat the illness can make it difficult or impossible to distinguish whether it is the drug or its therapeutic indication that is responsible for subsequent disease occurrence. Even when people with the same disease are treated with different therapies, there are usually important biologic differences among these groups. Confounding from other drugs and the possibility of drug interactions further complicate research of this type. Except in randomized trials, these problems will challenge pharmacoepidemiologists to the limits of their ingenuity and knowledge, making pharmacoepidemiology a proving ground for advances in epidemiologic methods.

Nevertheless, the basic tools to deal with these problems exist, and will inevitably become more refined as researchers gain experience, but the application of currently accepted epidemiologic principles could improve the understanding of many drug effects. For example, a disease such as "analgesic nephropathy" might cease to exist under the scrutiny of epidemiologic principles. This disease is defined as kidney disease following analgesic use. Because the definition includes the presence of the hypothesized cause, it is impossible to determine whether analgesic use is associated with kidney disease, much less whether a causal relation exists that would merit the term analgesic nephropathy. Even if an association were shown to exist using a proper disease definition that was independent of exposure, confounding by the indication for the analgesic use might account for it. To address such questions requires an epidemiologic perspective. This book will help introduce this perspective to all researchers concerned with the evaluation of drug effects.

Kenneth J Rothman

Preface to the First Edition

The reasons for this book will be immediately clear to readers who, like us, have been waiting for an overview of pharmacoepidemiology to be compiled in a single place. Such a single source of information can serve different purposes: personal or professional reference; a textbook in pharmacy, pharmacology, or epidemiology; a reference for operating pharmacoepidemiology programs in academia, government, and industry; for drug information units or product surveillance programs; or for rigorous structured pharmacoepidemiologic study.

We became keenly aware of the need for a compendium on pharmacoepidemiology because, wearing one hat or another, we were searching for a reference to accomplish one or more purposes when this happy collaboration began in 1985. At that time, we were developing a short course in pharmacoepidemiology to be offered in the Department of Epidemiology at the School of Public Health at the University of North Carolina. Having canvassed the educational opportunities in and around the area, we found no course offerings suitable for the audience needing to know more about the rapidly evolving field of pharmacoepidemiology. Therefore, we undertook to implement the course designs of Audrey Smith Rogers, a postdoctoral fellow at that time; a contribution of hers appears in this book.

In preparing the syllabus for the course in May 1985, we once again became aware of the lack of good teaching materials, especially those capturing the progress in the field during the 1980s. This was a time period in which new questions were formulated, new approaches taken, new technologies developed, new policies set, and new expectations raised providing for a state of flux in pharmacoepidemiology.

We were somewhat daunted by the complexity of the tasks of designing the course, compiling the materials, and providing expertise in a complex and multidisciplinary area, and particularly by the realization that we — like most workers in this relatively new field — lacked the experience (and, some of our friends even observed, the skills) to do it all ourselves. How did we start?

One of us (H.T.) had recently put together a set of "house rules" for the practicing epidemiologist at a workshop on pharmacoepidemiology, in Minister Lovell, England, sponsored by Dr. Hershel Jick, distinguished pharmacoepidemiologist and one of the founders of the field. Among these "house rules" the cardinal principle was: "In this complex field, don't wait for something to go wrong before you get help!" As the reader can surely judge, the editors succeeded in following this golden rule and established happy and fruitful collaboration with a series of first-rate colleagues who clearly do have claim to expertise, competence, and accomplishment in their chosen disciplinary areas and are highly motivated to contribute to the further development of pharmacoepidemiology.

The materials we have elected to include derive from that early course outline but were, in fact, solicited as a nine-part series in the journal *Drug Intelligence and Clinical Pharmacy*. Those materials were solicited to follow in a logical sequence that now works as this textbook. Still, no journal series, however complete, can cover the entire length and breadth of a field, much less its depth. Therefore, this book includes significant new material.

This new material includes a chapter on risk assessment providing an international perspective, and an extensive glossary on terms used in the field. The new chapter addresses the international dimensions in pharmacoepidemiology that relate to risk assessment. Further, we determined that, as in any specialized field, the field of pharmacoepidemiology had developed both a jargon and a lore of its own. This language was often needlessly confusing to the neophyte, even to the extent of discouraging excellent scientists with specialty in one, but not the other, of the disciplines that form the basis of pharmacoepidemiology from undertaking work for which they are well qualified. Therefore, we have appended the requisite glossary.

Perhaps it goes without saying (except in a preface like this) that the real reason for this endeavor is the conviction of the three of us that the activities of pharmacoepidemiology are important. It is important for therapeutics, for medicine, for public health, and, hopefully, for the public's health. It is probably necessary to underscore that verity here, because there will be readers or their superiors who date back to the era before the watershed report of the Melmon Commission in January 1980 and remember a time when the contributions of the field were less respected because they were less respectable. Long-term follow-up of large numbers of people is neither easy or cheap; controlling the multiple biases of observational methodology, without knowing the tricks of the trade of the experimentalist, is likewise no easy task. Also, performing the sleuthing tasks of the epidemiologist in an arena dominated by clinicians — nurses, pharmacists, and physicians — is not always either understood or appreciated! Further, some of our predecessors have used manipulative approaches and unobtrusive methods motivated by a desire to co-opt collaborators in the quest for promotion or to distort data in the search for a good image for a drug product. Nor would we assert that the field was wholly purged itself of technical problems, attitudinal barriers, or ethical dilemmas. Most importantly, we suspect that while the potential contributions of epidemiology to pharmacology, and vice versa, are reasonably well established, a proper scientific evaluation of the actual contributions and accomplishments has been only partially undertaken. The valuable trends in the field are presented throughout the book. Chapters 7, 8, and 10 describe the emergence of affordable and powerful technologies using automated data sets. Chapters 1, 14, and 16 describe the development of meaningful products to improve medical practice and public policy and, in the process, protect people who are taking medications.

Finally, we have many people to thank for bringing this book into reality. Each of the contributors will be known by his or her works, but we would like to thank them for the energy and enthusiasm which they brought to these labors. We also thank Barbara Hulka, and the students of "Methods and Issues in Pharmacoepi-demiology" for their valuable comments. Most especially, we thank Burroughs Wellcome Co. and the University of North Carolina, whose generosity of spirit provided encouragement to undertake this task and the setting in which this endeavor can grow. Finally, we thank friends and families for understanding the importance of this effort and supporting our preoccupation with it.

Abraham G Hartzema
Miquel Porta
Hugh H Tilson

Preface to the Second Edition

Pharmacoepidemiology: An Introduction enjoyed a splendid reception: the first edition sold out in one year's time. We have heard from colleagues from Australia to Zimbabwe who are using the book to increase their knowledge in the field; in classes as the primary or sole text, or in combination with reprints; and as the basis for continuing education and professional seminars. That the book partly filled a need in the profession became instantly clear. We are grateful for the comments, suggestions, and encouragement we received to enhance and update the book and are pleased now to offer this second edition.

We have taken all the suggestions we received to heart and, with the help of our prior collaborators and more authors, have compiled a more complete, somewhat more didactic, and up-to-date textbook on pharmacoepidemiology without compromising the immediacy and pragmatism of the first edition. Our first book was an attempt to define the boundaries and content of pharmacoepidemiology as a field. Although we were told we were successful through our own work in the field and our experience using the book in our own classes, we have learned a lot in the time period between the publication of the first edition and the start of the preparation of the second edition and have gained a deeper understanding of what pharmacoepidemiology is. The second edition reflects this understanding.

We have expanded the second edition in areas that readers considered important, broadening the scope by providing a more in-depth discussion, for example, of causality assessment; increasing the didactic value of the book by adding chapters about the statistical analyses used in pharmacoepidemiologic studies; and because of the increased political relevance of pharmacoepidemiology, adding chapters that discuss the implications of and standards for pharmacoepidemiologic research. In addition, all chapters of our first edition are included here, and all but two (which have stood the test of time) have been substantially revised and updated. Further, to increase the value as a reference, we have added an annotated bibliography of selected pharmacoepidemiologic studies.

In summary, the second edition will provide readers with a detailed overview of pharmacoepidemiology. As always, we are open to suggestions and comments from our readers. Please let us know your needs so they can be incorporated into the next edition.

Abraham G Hartzema
Miquel Porta
Hugh H Tilson

Preface to the Third Edition

We are pleased to present the third edition of *Pharmacoepidemiology: An Introduction*. The text has maintained its original outline, an outline proven useful by previous readers. The third edition has been expanded to keep up with the needs of our colleagues who are using the book in teaching and applied work and those who may need an "introduction and more" in the field. We have provided more depth to the discussion in methods sections and expanded the discussion of specific applications of pharmacoepidemiology.

Pharmacoepidemiology has significantly evolved over the 5 years since the last edition, becoming more diverse in its applications. For some health disciplines it has matured as a true clinical science, providing important contributions in the preapproval drug development process. Clearly, its role has greatly evolved to a discipline involved in all aspects of drug development (Phases I–III), postmarketing surveillance (Phase IV), and outcomes research, as in the preparation of evidence-based medicine tables for practice guideline development. Pharmacoepidemiology has become deeply involved in all aspects of pharmacotherapy through its role in the study of actual drug effectiveness, safety, and pharmacoeconomics.

Congruent with these developments, most chapters have been significantly updated. We have added new chapters, including one discussing observational study methodologies and others focused on approaches to data collection and outcomes research. Another new chapter outlines the latest methodology underlying the US Food and Drug Administration (FDA) drug safety monitoring program. The intervening 5 years have also brought substantial scientific contributions to our understanding of actual drug experience. Some of these findings are reported in four problem-focused chapters: cardiovascular pharmacoepidemiology, psychopharmacoepidemiology, pharmacoepidemiology of asthma treatments, and actual case studies from the FDA.

Pharmacoepidemiology: An Introduction was the first text to define pharmacoepidemiology. We hope the third edition will continue to lead the way in further defining pharmacoepidemiology and exploring the frontiers of application for this discipline. The book has never claimed to be a complete and detailed analysis of the topic, but rather has used a series of pragmatic approaches to pharmacoepidemiology.

As always we are deeply indebted to the contributors of each of the chapters of this and prior editions. Special thanks for great skill and infinite patience are due to our publishers at Harvey Whitney Books Company, especially our co-editor in spirit Timothy E Welty PharmD. We also appreciate the hundreds of readers who provided considerable suggestions for this edition. As you use this book in teaching, practice, or research, we hope you will share your suggestions and comments for future editions with us.

Abraham G Hartzema
Miquel Porta
Hugh H Tilson
February 1998

Contributing Authors

H Michael Arrighi PhD
Director of Epidemiology, Amgen Inc.
Thousand Oaks, California
Chapter 13

Olav M Bakke MD
Visiting Professor, Department of Pharmacology and Toxicology
Institut Municipal d'Investigacio Medica
Barcelona, Spain
Chapter 18

Richard Beasley MD
Professor, Wellington Asthma Research Group
Department of Medicine, Wellington School of Medicine
Wellington, New Zealand
Chapter 20

Darrel C Bjornson PhD
Associate Professor, Social and Administrative Sciences
Department of Pharmacy Practice, College of Pharmacy and Health Sciences
Drake University, Des Moines, Iowa
Chapter 6

J Gregory Boyer PhD
International Director, Pharmacoeconomic Research–Development
Glaxo Wellcome Research and Development
Greenford, Middlesex, United Kingdom
Chapter 13

Carl Burgess FRACP
Associate Professor, Wellington Asthma Research Group
Department of Medicine, Wellington School of Medicine
Wellington, New Zealand
Chapter 20

Laurie B Burke RPh MPH
Senior Regulatory Research Officer, Division of Drug Marketing
Advertising and Communications, Center for Drug Evaluation and Research
Food and Drug Administration, Rockville, Maryland
Chapter 9

Thomas J Craig MD MPH
Clinical Manager VISN 3, Veterans Health Administration
Bronx, New York
Chapter 21

Julian Crane FRACP
Associate Professor, Wellington Asthma Research Group
Department of Medicine, Wellington School of Medicine
Wellington, New Zealand
Chapter 20

Stanley A Edlavitch PhD MA

Professor of Preventive Medicine, Director of Masters of Public Health Program
Department of of Preventive Medicine, University of Kansas Medical Center
Kansas City, Kansas
Chapter 4

Thomas R Einarson PhD

Associate Professor, Faculty of Pharmacy, University of Toronto
Toronto, Ontario, Canada
Chapter 12

Robert S Epstein MD MS

Vice President, Merck-Medco Managed Care
Columbus, Ohio
Chapter 8

Jacqueline S Gardner PhD

Associate Professor, Department of Pharmacy, School of Pharmacy
University of Washington, Seattle, Washington
Chapter 14

Denis M Grant PhD

Assistant Professor of Pediatrics and Pharmacology, University of Toronto, Division of
Clinical Pharmacology and Toxicology, Hospital for Sick Children
Toronto, Ontario, Canada
Chapter 7

Thaddeus H Grasela Jr PharmD

President, Pharmaceutical Outcomes Research, Inc.
Williamsville, New York
Chapter 15

Abraham G Hartzema PhD MSPH

Professor, Division of Pharmacy Policy and Evaluative Sciences, School of Pharmacy
Clinical Professor, Epidemiology, Director, Center for Pharmaceutical Outcomes Research,
School of Public Health
University of North Carolina, Chapel Hill, North Carolina
Preface, Chapters 1,6,11,23,24

Ron MC Herings PhD

Department of Pharmacoepidemiology and Pharmacotherapy
Utrecht University, Utrecht, Netherlands
Chapter 16

James R Hunter RPh MPH

Associate Director for Science, Office of Special Investigations
Department of Health and Human Services, Food and Drug Administration
Rockville, Maryland
Chapters 2, 9

Dianne L Kennedy RPh MPH

Director, MedWatch, Office of the Commissioner
Food and Drug Administration, Rockville, Maryland
Chapter 9

Kate L Lapane PhD

Assistant Professor (Research), Department of Community Health
Co-Director, SAGE Study Group
Center for Gerontology and Health Care Research, Brown University
Providence, Rhode Island
Chapter 10

Hubert G Leufkens PhD
Department of Pharmacoepidemiology and Pharmacotherapy
Utrecht University, Utrecht, Netherlands
Chapter 16

Michael A Lewis MD BSc DTM Dipl Epi
Director, EPES Epidemiology, Pharmacoepidemiology and Systems Research GmbH,
Berlin, Germany
Senior Lecturer, University of Potsdam, Potsdam, Germany
Chapter 22

Donald C McLeod MSPharm FCCP
Director, McLeod Pharma, Ltd., Chapel Hill, North Carolina
Chapter 23

Steven R Moore BSPharm MPH
Assistant Chief of Staff, Office of the Assistant Surgeon General
US Public Health Service, Rockville, Maryland
Chapter 2

Lisa Stockwell Morris RPh PhD
Director, Disease Treatment and Outcomes Information Services
IMS America Ltd., Pharmaceutical Division, Plymouth Meeting, Pennsylvania
Chapter 8

Ann Myers BSPharm MPH
Chief, Document Management and Reporting Branch
Center for Drug Evaluation and Research
Food and Drug Administration, Rockville, Maryland
Chapter 2

Robert C Nelson PhD
Associate Director (Epidemiology), Office of Epidemiology and Biostatistics
Center for Drug Evaluation and Research
Food and Drug Administration, Rockville, Maryland
Chapter 17

Byung Joo Park MD PhD
Associate Professor, Department of Preventive Medicine, College of Medicine
Seoul National University, Seoul, Korea
Chapter 14

Neil Pearce PhD
Associate Professor, Wellington Asthma Research Group
Department of Medicine, Wellington School of Medicine
Wellington, New Zealand
Chapter 20

Eleanor Perfetto PhD RPh
CEO, MEDTAP Systems, LLC, Bethesda, Maryland
Chapters 8,11

Miquel Porta MD MPH
Adjunct Associate Professor, Department of Epidemiology
School of Public Health, University of North Carolina, Chapel Hill
Associate Professor, Institut Municipal d'Investigacio Medica
Universitat Autonoma de Barcelona, Barcelona, Spain
Preface, Chapters 1,24

Audrey Smith Rogers PhD MPH
Pediatric, Adolescent, and Maternal AIDS Branch
Center for Research for Mothers and Children
National Institute of Child Health and Human Development
Bethesda, Maryland
Chapter 5

Kenneth J Rothman DrPH
Professor of Public Health, Boston University Medical Center
Boston, Massachusetts
Foreword

Joaquima Serradell PhD MPH
Serradel Consultants, Blue Bell, Pennsylvania
Chapter 6

Stephen P Spielberg MD PhD FRCPC
Executive Director, Exploratory Biochemical Toxicology & Strategic Operations
Merck Research Laboratories, Blue Bell, Pennsylvania
Chapter 7

Bert Spilker MD PhD
President, Orphan Medical, Minnetonka, Minnesota
Chapters 3,19

Paul E Stang PhD Pa-C
Director, Worldwide Epidemiology, SmithKline Beecham
Collegeville, Pennsylvania
Chapter 13

Andy S Stergachis PhD
Professor and Chairman, Department of Pharmacy, School of Pharmacy
Department of Epidemiology, University of Washington
School of Public Health and Community Medicine
Scientific Investigator, Center for Health Studies
Group Health Cooperative of Puget Sound, Seattle, Washington
Chapter 14

Hugh H Tilson MD DrPH
Clinical Professor of Epidemiology and Health Policy, Center for Public Health Practice
School of Public Health, and Adjunct Professor, School of Medicine and School of
Pharmacy, University of North Carolina, Chapel Hill, North Carolina
Senior Medical Advisor for Health Affairs, Glaxo Wellcome, Inc.
Research Triangle Park, North Carolina
Preface, Chapters 1,24

Raymond J Townsend PharmD
President, RJ Townsend & Company
Chapel Hill, North Carolina
Chapter 13

Julie Magno Zito PhD
Associate Professor of Pharmacy and Medicine
Director of Graduate Studies, University of Maryland, Baltimore
Baltimore, Maryland
Chapter 21

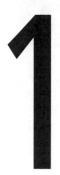

The Contribution of Epidemiology to the Study of Drug Uses and Effects

Miquel Porta
Abraham G Hartzema
Hugh H Tilson

Abstract

This chapter is an introduction to the contributions of epidemiology to the study of drug uses and effects. Epidemiology is concerned with the distribution of disease and health in human populations. Drugs and vaccines are among the factors that influence such a distribution. Pharmacoepidemiology is defined as the application of the epidemiologic knowledge, methods, and reasoning to the study of the uses and effects (beneficial and adverse) of drugs in human populations. Pharmacoepidemiology aims to describe, explain, control, and predict the uses and effects of drugs and vaccines in a defined time, space, and population. In addition to the traditional role in pharmacovigilance, pharmacoepidemiology supports the drug development process, provides for the assessment of drug effectiveness/efficacy, and contributes to summarize the scientific evidence (meta-analysis of efficacy) in the development, evaluation, and maintenance of practice guidelines. Pharmacoepidemiology supports pharmaceutical outcomes research in health-related quality-of-life outcome evaluations and in establishing outcome probabilities for pharmacoeconomic analysis. The actual contribution of epidemiology to the study of drug uses and effects has been only partially assessed. However, because the health of our society benefits from the dynamic cross-fertilization of pharmacology, epidemiology, economics, and clinical medicine, the field of pharmacoepidemiology is full of promise and potential.

Outline

1. Introduction
2. Definition and aims
3. The rationale for postmarketing surveillance and the role of pharmacoepidemiology
   Limitations of premarketing clinical trials
   Beyond Phase III

   Strengths of randomized, clinical trials
   Drugs pose unique research problems
4. Further issues, further opportunities
5. Summary
6. References

M edications have become an essential therapeutic tool in the hands of healthcare professionals. With the aging of Western populations and, consequently, a higher prevalence of medical problems, increasingly large numbers of people are exposed to multiple drugs for longer periods of time. Pharmacoepidemiology offers a way of reasoning, a rich set of methods, and a body of substantive knowledge that can both expand the health benefits of drugs and reduce their risks.

Although drug studies historically were the prerogative of biologists, medicinal chemists, pharmacologists, and clinicians, epidemiologic methods also have for many years been applied to the study of vaccines and drugs.[1,2] Today, a significant number of medical, pharmacy, and public health schools have established programs in pharmacoepidemiology.[3] Also, major pharmaceutical firms have launched medical surveillance and research programs based on epidemiologic methods. Thus, the value of epidemiology in drug research and development is gaining widespread recognition.

The purpose of this chapter is to provide the reader with an introduction to the potential contributions of pharmacoepidemiology to the study of drug uses and effects, as well as to indicate the common grounds that pharmacoepidemiology shares with other health disciplines. In fact, because the relationship between epidemiology and pharmacology is synergistic, as illustrated in this chapter, the study of drugs with epidemiologic methods furthers our understanding of the etiology of human illness. According to this view, pharmacoepidemiology becomes not only a subspecialty in epidemiology but also, in some respects, an extension of epidemiology.

Definition and Aims

Pharmacoepidemiology can be defined as the application of epidemiologic reasoning, methods, and knowledge to the study of the uses and effects (beneficial and adverse) of drugs in human populations. It aims to describe, explain, control, and predict the uses and effects of pharmacologic treatments in a defined time, space, and population. Its core lies at the intersection of two subspecialties: clinical pharmacology and clinical epidemiology.[1-3]

Outlining questions that pharmacoepidemiology attempts to answer or that it poses to other disciplines can help define the interests and boundaries of this fledgling field. Thus, examples of the problems addressed within the realm of pharmacoepidemiology include the following:

1. Are there differences in the number of people with hypertension diagnosed and treated among different populations in a given geographic area? What is the impact on cardiocerebrovascular morbidity of such differences? How much of the past years' decline in coronary

heart disease can be accounted for by the effects of cardiovascular drugs? What are the most common uses of beta-blockers? Why is it that some of those uses do not agree with the academic recommendations? Will the treatment of hypertension be influenced by changes in the healthcare system in the next 10 years?

2. What is the effectiveness of psychotropic drugs in defined populations? Does the effectiveness of psychotropic drugs depend on age, gender, and sociocultural level? What changes can we predict in the prevalence of mental illness based on current drug consumption trends? How can new therapeutic developments improve the long-term outcome of psychiatric patients? Is therapeutic information a determinant of the quality of psychotropic drug prescriptions? What can we learn about our culture from the way mental illness is treated?

3. In the evaluation of practice guidelines, what is the effectiveness rate under general medical conditions or practice for the different antimicrobials indicated for the treatment of uncomplicated urinary tract infection? What is the effectiveness rate of conventional versus short-term treatment lengths? What is the cost of a treatment episode including physician visit, laboratory costs, and drug costs? Based on this information, what is the cost-effectiveness ratio for each of the antimicrobials under general medical practice conditions?

While these clusters of questions relate to antihypertensive, psychotropic, and antimicrobial drugs, similar questions can be developed for other therapeutic categories. Pharmacoepidemiology provides the key to answering many questions that arise in the process of drug development, prescribing, and use. More examples are presented in Table 1 to illustrate the scope of the discipline and common research questions that pharmacoepidemiology shares with other professions and disciplines, such as medicine, pharmacy, health economics, the social sciences, and the laboratory sciences.

Beyond specialty labels, one crucial set of questions expands throughout this book: How can different professional and scientific traditions, cultures, routines, reasonings, methodologies, techniques, and substantive bits of knowledge be *integrated* with each other so that we can increase our clinical and community impact, intervene more effectively upon risk groups and individuals, and implement preventive and therapeutic strategies at both the population and individual levels?[4-16] With respect to the integration of genetics, pharmacology, and epidemiology, examples are provided in Chapter 7.

Three fundamental questions flow from the previous discussion: Can epidemiology help to improve the development and use of drugs? Can pharmacology help to expand our knowledge of the causes of illness? Is the health status of individuals and communities going to benefit from the

Table 1 Examples of Questions Addressed by Pharmacoepidemiology	How can we accelerate the process of discovery of new, clinically relevant, intended, and unintended drug effects?
	What factors in the physician–patient encounter influence treatment compliance and continuity of care?
	How clinically relevant is it to compare the effectiveness of an angiotensin-converting enzyme inhibitor with methyldopa for the treatment of mild hypertension?
	What is the most appropriate control group for a hospital-based case-control study of drug-related congenital malformations?
	How should the validation of large clinical databases be approached?
	What factors should guide the decision to conduct formal postmarketing epidemiologic studies?
	What is a good design for studying the factors that influence clinical decision-making, including prescribing?
	What is the relative effectiveness of nonsteroidal antiinflammatory drugs, acetaminophen, weight reduction, and exercise in osteoarthritis?
	What is the cost–effectiveness of hepatitis B vaccine, oral hypoglycemic agents, cerebrovascular vasodilators, hypolipidemic agents, estrogens, or cephalosporins for selected indications?
	What can be done by the pharmaceutical industry, government, and third-party payers to alleviate the burden of disease in older populations?
	In what type of clinical trials is it desirable to incorporate economic analysis?
	How does cancer chemotherapy interact with the natural course of the disease?
	What can be done to prevent the development of resistance to antibiotics in the general population?
	What algorithms are most useful to validate unintended drug effect reports?
	Is end-stage renal disease caused by regular analgesic use?
	Can we use a composite measure of health status in epidemiologic studies to evaluate patient outcomes?
	Can we learn something about the prognostic factors for juvenile arthritis from the way it is treated by primary care physicians?
	What psychological factors and sociocultural values influence risk perception?

interrelationship of medicine, pharmacy, epidemiology, and economics? Because the answer to these three questions is a resounding "yes," the field of pharmacoepidemiology is full of promise and potential. This potential and the actual accomplishments are what this book is all about.

The fundamental rationale for epidemiologists being interested in drugs stems from the following: (1) epidemiology studies the distribution of health and disease in human populations, and (2) drugs and vaccines are among the factors that influence such distribution. Hence, from a public health perspective, it is of utmost importance that pharmacoepidemiologists assess the impact that vaccines and drugs have on the overall patterns of diseases, that is, on morbidity and mortality patterns in well-defined populations.[17-23]

Because of the complexities involved in evaluating therapeutic outcomes, specific epidemiologic techniques must be used in the study of drugs. This chapter briefly discusses these techniques. The quantitative techniques available to the pharmacoepidemiologist are discussed in more detail in Chapters 4, 10, and 12.

The Rationale for Postmarketing Surveillance and the Role of Pharmacoepidemiology

The term *pharmacoepidemiology* emphasizes the use of epidemiologic thinking and methods regardless of the phase of drug development. Postmarketing surveillance (PMS) refers to a specific time in the life of a drug: the time span that begins when a drug enters the general market (also known as Phase IV). At present, PMS is one of the most common activities of pharmacoepidemiologists.[2,24]

PMS is important because, at the time a drug is approved for marketing, the answers to a number of questions—vital for patients, professionals, and the healthcare system—are only partially known. Premarketing studies, for example, assess the efficacy of hypoglycemic agents in controlling diabetic symptoms (so-called primary efficacy), but they rarely assess their usefulness in preventing the cardiovascular or renal complications of diabetes (secondary efficacy); the effectiveness and efficiency are also seldom analyzed in premarketing studies. Although hypoglycemic agents were originally approved solely for their primary effects, they are widely used for both.[25] The possible role of aspirin and other nonsteroidal antiinflammatory drugs (NSAIDs) in preventing colorectal cancer[26-28] and selected cardiovascular diseases[29-32] provides another set of examples. Indeed, the long-term effects of drugs in the prevention of disease or its complications are among the numerous questions unknown at the time of marketing. These questions must be addressed by postmarketing studies. Table 2 summarizes the major steps in the process of drug development, and Table 3 gives the basic types of questions addressed in PMS studies.[33]

When marketing approval of a new drug is granted by the appropriate regulatory agency, thousands of individuals become exposed to the drug in a variety of sociocultural and clinical settings. Furthermore, the therapeu-

Table 2
Major Steps in the Process of Drug Development[a]

Preclinical testing. A potentially therapeutic agent is first subjected to extensive chemical, toxicologic, and animal testing. Answers are sought to two main questions: Is the substance biologically active? Is it safe? Testing in humans will proceed only if the answers to both questions appear to be affirmative.

Clinical testing. This is conventionally divided into four phases:

Phase I. *Safety and pharmacologic profiles.* During this phase, researchers attempt to determine the drug's pharmacologic actions, its safe dosage range, absorption, distribution, metabolism and excretion, and the duration of its action. Tests involve a small number of healthy volunteers.

Phase II. *Pilot efficacy studies.* Controlled studies are conducted to assess the drug's efficacy. Up to 300 volunteer patients are typically involved. Phase II studies may raise questions that trigger new animal and healthy volunteer studies to improve the determination of safety.

Phase III. *Extensive clinical trials.* The drug is administered by practicing physicians to patients actually diagnosed with the condition the drug is intended to treat. The aims are to confirm earlier efficacy studies and to identify less common adverse effects. Trials may last up to 3 years (although individual follow-up may be <1 y) and involve 500–3000 patients.

Phase IV. *Postmarketing surveillance.* Once approval to market the drug has been granted, several methods (generally observational) exist to monitor its use and effects. To the extent that studies have an epidemiologic dimension, this is properly where pharmacoepidemiology can be said to begin (i.e., the study includes a population well defined in terms of space and time, and the epidemiologic reasoning is applied to select subjects, collect information, and account for confounding factors). Nonetheless, the nature of some Phase IV methods is typically clinical (e.g., case-series and spontaneous reporting of adverse drug events). Additional Phase III studies may be conducted if, during the postmarketing phase, evidence appears of a potential new therapeutic indication; however, few such studies can properly be considered epidemiologic. In contrast, many large clinical trials studying the drug's role in secondary prevention have a strong epidemiologic component.

[a]See also Chapter 2.

tic use of drugs is often extended to population subgroups not included in premarketing studies, to new indications emerging in clinical practice, and for periods of time much longer than those covered in most clinical trials (Tables 2 and 3). In the real world, patients present a wide range of diag-

Table 3
Main Areas of Inquiry Addressed in Postmarketing Studies[33]

Area of Inquiry	Examples
Long-term effects	
that manifest after long periods of use	use of exogenous estrogen during menopause and endometrial cancer
that manifest after long latency periods	adenocarcinoma of the vagina due to diethylstilbestrol
Low-frequency effects	
that can be detected only in large populations	aplastic anemia: phenylbutazone; colitis: clindamycin; jaundice: halothane
Relative effectiveness in customary practice	
patients	children, pregnant or elderly women
therapeutic situations	concurrent pathologies and several simultaneous treatments, flexible dosages, tolerance, noncompliance, nonresponse
healthcare settings	emergencies, ambulatory care accord-
healthcare professionals	ing to training, specialty, information sources
Efficacy in new indications	
discovered after marketing	propranolol as an antihypertensive medication, captopril in rheumatoid arthritis, amantadine in Parkinson's disease, antihistamines in motion sickness
including secondary effects	antihypertensive medications for prevention of cardiovascular disease, hypoglycemic agents to prevent complications of diabetes
Modifiers of efficacy	
concurrent drugs	a decrease of sodium intake can improve the efficacy of some diuretics in hypertension
disease severity	patients with severe asthma do not respond to metaproterenol without supplementary therapy
lifestyle	risk of myocardial infarction in women who use oral contraceptives may be increased by smoking cigarettes

noses, lifestyles, and exposures to other drugs and environmental agents. In brief, drug epidemiology deals with what Lasagna[34,35] calls the most important question for therapeutics: How does a drug actually perform in clinical practice?

The performance of a drug in clinical practice or under general medical practice conditions is referred to as the effectiveness of the drug. Variability in the patient population, comorbidities, or noncompliance may make the drug less effective than its efficacy or effect achieved in the strictly controlled conditions of the clinical trial. Experimental designs and the randomized, blind clinical trial are excellent to establish the efficacy of the drug, while the observational methods of pharmacoepidemiology are particularly suited to evaluate the effectiveness of the drug under general medical practice conditions.

Both *experimental* (i.e., random allocation of treatments) and *observational* (i.e., nonexperimental) epidemiologic methods are used by drug epidemiologists. As further explained in Chapter 4, randomized clinical trials (the paradigm of experimental studies) tend to be more common before a drug is marketed; observational studies (e.g., cross-sectional surveys, follow-up studies, case–control studies) usually are conducted after marketing. The rationale for postmarketing epidemiologic studies becomes apparent when the strengths and limitations of premarketing clinical trials are considered. We first address these premarketing limitations, then introduce the reader to the rationale for postmarketing studies, and subsequently explain the major strengths of experimental studies.

LIMITATIONS OF PREMARKETING CLINICAL TRIALS

Clinical evaluation of a drug in the premarketing phase seeks to validate scientific premises by the drug's extensive use in common therapeutic practice.[36] Although the randomized, controlled clinical trial is the most powerful tool available to clinical scientists and epidemiologists, its limitations—mostly due to ethical, practical, and economic reasons—should be recognized.

As we just mentioned, much of the rationale for PMS arises from the limits of clinical trials in Phases I–III (Tables 2 and 3). Premarketing trials study the efficacy and risks of a drug for selected clinical indications before the drug is marketed. Clinical trials in Phase III include a small number of nonrepresentative patients—nonrepresentative of the population and indications for which the drug eventually will be used. In such trials, patients are followed for short periods of time and under very strictly defined conditions (e.g., double-blindness, random allocation of treatments, frequent and thorough examinations, placebo treatments, fixed-dose regimens, tertiary care hospitals)[33,36-43] (see also Chapters 2 and 3).

Furthermore, it is important to understand the "nature" of the question posed in any particular study: premarketing studies usually choose an *explanatory* or knowledge-oriented question (focusing, as we just saw, on the efficacy of the drug under strict experimental conditions); in turn, postmarketing studies often take a more *pragmatic* or decision-oriented approach (focusing on the effectiveness of the drug under usual clinical circumstances). The explanatory/pragmatic distinction, which actually constitutes a rich conceptual framework, was first proposed by Schwartz and Lellouch[44] in 1967 and by Schwartz et al.[45] for randomized clinical trials; yet it is relevant also for observational studies.[46]

It should also be noted that patients admitted to randomized clinical trials must be able to receive any of the study therapies, according to the result of randomization. A major consequence of this ethical and methodologic requirement is that patients with a definitive indication for one of the therapies will be excluded from the trial, since it would not be ethical to withhold a drug they clearly need. Consequently, therapeutic agents are often not tested in those most likely to receive it.[47] These patients will have to be observed in PMS.

BEYOND PHASE III

In recent years, the US Food and Drug Administration (FDA) and other regulatory agencies in several countries have attempted to remedy some pitfalls in Phase III studies. Consequently, Phase III clinical trials are often multicentric and attempt to include a spectrum of patients more representative of the population that would eventually receive the drug under study. Furthermore, study size is largely determined by the potential population of patients; for example, for an antihypertensive drug, a study population between 1000 and 3000 could be required; for an orphan drug, 50–100 patients might be sufficient.

Phase IV clinical trials are defined as those conducted after a drug has been marketed (Table 2). These are not always mandated by regulatory agencies, such as the FDA, but are often negotiated between the manufacturer and the agencies such as the FDA as a condition for new drug approval (see Chapters 2 and 19).[48-50] In addition, Phase IV clinical trials can be initiated on signals originating from pharmacovigilance or adverse-event spontaneous reporting systems (see Chapter 5) or as pharmacoeconomic studies to establish the cost–effectiveness of one treatment over another. The objectives, design, and sample size are at times similar to those of Phase III clinical trials. In Phase IV clinical trials, however, larger and more heterogeneous populations usually are available, and a stronger emphasis is placed on reproducing the usual clinical care conditions[51-53] (Table 3).

In part because of their larger sample size, Phase IV studies provide additional information on the benefits and risks of drugs. Sample size is a direct determinant of the probability of detecting drug effects that occur with a low frequency (Table 4). The "rule of three" states that to detect an unintended drug effect (UDE) that occurs at a particular frequency, the number of subjects that one needs to follow up is three times that of the estimated frequency of the event.[54] For example, if a UDE is suspected to occur in 1 of 10 000 drug users, we will need to observe 30 000 users in order to be 95% likely to detect it. Smaller numbers of patients will be needed if a lower statistical power is chosen. More complex, specific calculations will be required by different study designs.[51,55-71] The larger sample sizes used in Phase IV clinical studies allow for the assessment of drug effects with a low incidence. As shown in Table 2, during PMS, both experimental and observational methods[72-74] have a role. PMS studies will sometimes be clearly epidemiologic and sometimes typically clinical (e.g., case series, case reports). Beyond the purely methodologic dimension, in the real world, particularly for companies and governments, a major challenge is to establish efficient surveillance schemes, to select appropriate research strategies, and to synthesize and interpret the evidence available from a variety of sources (see Chapter 17).

While the routine monitoring of drug uses and effects is always necessary and in many ways possible, conducting specific epidemiologic studies is often not necessary or feasible. Therefore, in recent years, growing attention has been given to the following question: *When is it warranted to undertake a postmarketing study? Should it be undertaken as soon as marketing approval is granted?* Table 5 displays some guidelines suggested by a

Table 4
Number of People Exposed to a Drug Necessary to Detect True Frequencies of Unintended Drug Effects[54]

Frequency	Statistical Power[a]			
	95%	90%	80%	63%
1/100	300	231	161	100
1/500	1500	1152	805	500
1/1000	3000	2303	1610	1000
1/5000	15 000	11 513	8048	5000
1/10 000	30 000	23 026	16 095	10 000
1/50 000	150 000	115 130	80 472	50 000

[a]Statistical power: the probability of detecting an unintended drug effect if it really occurs in the population under study (e.g., studying 8048 users of the drug will allow 8 of 10 times the detection of an unintended drug effect's occurring in 1 of 5000 exposed people). Most epidemiologists try to achieve sample sizes yielding a statistical power of 80% or 90%.

Prevalence of the disease	**Table 5**
Severity of the medical condition	Factors That May
Expected duration of therapy	Warrant the Conduct of
New chemical entity status	Postmarketing
Chemical class with demonstrated acceptable safety	Epidemiologic
Safety profile of the drug in premarketing trials	Studies[75]
Formulation of the agent	
Availability of safe and efficacious alternatives	

group of experts.[75] In summary, the need for postmarketing (Phase IV) studies increases if the prevalence of the disease under treatment is high, if its severity is low, if it predominantly affects children or other special population groups, if the drug is indicated for use in relatively healthy individuals, if the projected market share of the new drug is high, if the drug is likely to be used in combination with other agents, if there are safe and cost-effective alternative therapies available, if the expected duration of drug exposure is long, if one is dealing with a chemical entity whose mechanism of action is new or with a new compound belonging to a chemical class with known problems of safety, if the safety profile of the drug in premarketing trials raised relevant questions, if such trials were poorly designed or conducted, if the drug was not approved for marketing in other countries, and if the agent will be marketed for outpatient use.[75] Surely, a detailed analysis of these factors will, in every circumstance, raise a myriad of issues. Such a set of factors is important to decide not only whether and when to undertake a formal epidemiologic study, but also, if the decision is to proceed, to design, conduct, analyze, and interpret the study.

To put PMS—and, more generally, the role of pharmacoepidemiology—into a proper perspective, it is critical to realize that:

1. answers to questions on the safety and efficacy of drugs sometimes cannot be provided even by the most valid, complex, and lengthy Phase III studies;
2. it is often more reasonable to expect that such an answer be obtained by Phase IV epidemiologic studies; and
3. it may be ethically correct, scientifically sound, and politically wise to allow a drug to be marketed if well-designed epidemiologic studies are initiated at the very moment of marketing approval.

When all these assumptions hold, pharmacoepidemiology can help to hasten the drug approval process and to protect citizens, companies, and governments against unsubstantiated claims of risk.[76] No doubt, beyond the criteria mentioned in Table 5, the decision of why, when, and how to conduct a formal postmarketing study also has wide economic, commercial, and policy implications[77-79] (see Chapters 18 and 24). Phase IV studies can make significant contributions to drug development (e.g., in terms of labeling changes, length of the administrative process, pricing negotiations, marketing).

STRENGTHS OF RANDOMIZED, CLINICAL TRIALS

Randomized, controlled clinical trials are generally regarded as "the most scientifically rigorous method of hypothesis testing available in epidemiology."[80] Clinical trials are an excellent tool to assess the efficacy and safety of pharmaceuticals and to assess health technology in general.[51,60] Whereas they are part of the pharmacoepidemiologic armamentarium, there is no question that they are also used by other epidemiologic and nonepidemiologic disciplines, notably clinical medicine and clinical pharmacology. Strictly speaking, not all clinical trials can be viewed as falling within the domain of drug epidemiology (Table 2).

In any case, specialty limits are rarely decisive in actual practice; what really matters is the innovative nature of hypotheses, the feasibility of study designs, the validity of findings, and, most importantly, the clinical and population relevance of any knowledge gained through research. To achieve these ambitious aims, both experimental and observational methods deserve attention. Furthermore, the methodologic strengths and weaknesses of any given study will generally have to be appraised within the context of the available substantive knowledge on the specific issue that the study addressed. If little is known, the study may have a more exploratory nature, and a lesser level of methodologic sophistication may be required; conversely, if basic answers already exist, application of highly complex methods may not be justified.

Random allocation of treatments (randomization) is the most essential feature of clinical trials and makes this design so powerful. Randomization is almost always the only way to control for a specific confounder: the *indication* for the drug. Broadly speaking, confounding is a situation in which the effects of two or more processes are fused or mixed. A confounding variable or confounder is a variable that (1) can cause or prevent the outcome of interest and (2) is associated or "linked" with the exposure of interest (traditionally, it has also been said that a confounder could not be an intermediate variable in the causal pathway between exposure and outcome[80]). Confounding by indication generally occurs when patients who are prescribed a given drug have a poorer prognosis than those who are not receiving the drug.[25,33,36,81-88] Naturally, this is precisely why a health professional often decides that a certain drug is indicated and, hence, it is fully logical from a clinical perspective. Nevertheless, it does pose a problem from a scientific point of view, as Sir Austin Bradford Hill noted long ago[72] (Table 6). In other words, a set of clinical signs, symptoms, or an *indication* for treatment whatsoever (e.g., lack of response to a "standard" bronchodilator, centrilobular emphysema, and persistent, severe airways obstruction in a patient with bronchial asthma), assessed by a health professional, is associated with both the prescription of a *drug* (e.g., a new, apparently more effective bronchodilator) and a higher probability of a particular *outcome* (asthma attack). In fact, even if the new bronchodilator reduces the risk of an asthma death, an observational study may find mortality to be apparently higher among patients treated with the new drug than among patients treated with the older drug. The higher rate of attacks among the former may be due to their poorer prognosis before the drug was prescribed (see Chapter 20). Similarly, high levels of anxiety and emotional distress during and shortly after a myocardial infarction, to an extent that sedatives are required, may simply identify a subset of high-risk patients (e.g., patients with a more severe infarct, experiencing intense

"The treatment of patients with a particular disease is unplanned but naturally varies according to the decision of the physician in charge. To some patients a specific drug is given, to others it is not."	**Table 6** An Early Vision of *Confounding by the Indication* by Sir Austin Bradford Hill[a]

"The progress and prognosis of these patients are then compared. But in making this comparison in relation to the treatment the fundamental assumption is made — and it must be made — that the two groups are equivalent in all respects relevant to their progress, except for the difference in treatment. It is, however, almost invariably impossible to believe that this is so. *Drugs are not ordered by doctors at random, but in relation to a patient's condition* when he first comes under observation and also to the subsequent progress of his disease. The two groups are therefore not remotely comparable and more often than not *the group given the specific drug is heavily weighted by the more severely ill.* No conclusion as to its efficacy can possibly be drawn."

In the late 1970s and early 1980s, during the "prelude" or "overture" of modern epidemiology, explicit and formal analyses of confounding by indication were published by Miettinen, Slone, and Shapiro.[33,36,81,82] The most comprehensive attempt at characterizing the confounding web and, in particular, an exhaustive search for alternatives to randomization is due to Strom, Miettinen, and Melmon.[25,83,84]

[a]The clinical trial (1951)[72] [italics added].

pain, or with a more anxious personality). While just *associated* or *linked* to it, sedatives may erroneously appear to cause an increase in the risk of reinfarction and death.[89]

Thus, confounding by indication stems from an initial lack of similarity in the prognostic expectations of treated and nontreated subjects.[87] The consequence is that, although the observed "results" may be true (in the example, patients treated with the new bronchodilator die more often), any *inferences* based on them may not be true (i.e., conclusions will not be valid). For an in-depth discussion of this problem and suggestions to overcome it, see Chapter 20.

Of course, assessing the degree of *validity* of a given study—the extent to which biases are absent—is a central question in research; as such, it must always take precedence over statistical issues (e.g., precision of estimates). Bias can occur through a large number of mechanisms. Because of this, the assessment of bias should not be done in an abstract or general fashion. It is too easy to *imagine* a bias! Rather, judgments must be based on reasonable evidence on the specific underlying mechanisms that are likely to have caused bias in the study. In pharmacoepidemiology, as elsewhere, the design, conduct, analysis, and interpretation of studies must be based on the following[90]:

1. a *causal model hypothesis*, which includes knowledge of the basic and clinical pharmacology of the drug and of the molecular biology, pathophysiology, and clinical course of the disease; and
2. a *healthcare pathway hypothesis*, which in turn includes knowledge of patient behavior, referral patterns, actual diagnostic and therapeutic strategies, as well as other aspects of the functioning of the health system relevant to the assessment of potential selection and information biases.

Confounding by indication shares many features with what is called "susceptibility bias"[91] and "procedure selection bias."[92] Methods other than randomization that may sometimes help control for this confounding effect have been proposed, and the issue continues to constitute one of the most challenging issues in the field.[25,33,36,81-88] Once again, no statistical or methodologic recipe will be of help without an in-depth knowledge of the two models just mentioned, as relevant to the issue at stake.

DRUGS POSE UNIQUE RESEARCH PROBLEMS

Drugs present problems to researchers that are uncommon in other branches of epidemiology (e.g., environmental, nutritional, occupational epidemiology). The main reason lies in the complex *mechanisms of reasoning and decision-making* that usually involve exposure to drugs. Health professionals and patients (as well as relatives and social acquaintances in general) all play important roles. For example, seldom will someone change from one NSAID to another at random[93,94]; thus, the reasons for changing drugs will have to be considered as potential confounders. In addition, it is not uncommon to find that the use of psychotropic drugs and analgesics is *associated* with problems, such as interpersonal problems at work or at home.[95] In contrast, many environmental exposures (e.g., air pollution, electromagnetic fields, or even the type of drinking water) are influenced to a lesser extent by self-perception of health than is the intake of drugs. Certainly, different types of selection bias may operate in occupational settings, the "healthy worker effect" being the best-known case.[96]

All factors and processes leading to drug exposure (e.g., prescription, self-medication, compliance) must be considered in the study design, its implementation, analysis, and interpretation. Assumptions that often are true in other epidemiologic and clinical studies are rarely valid when studying drugs. For example, the possibility that concomitant illnesses, subclinical disease, or early and mild symptoms influence drug exposure, the assessment of drug exposure, the diagnostic pathway, or the labeling of the entity must always be kept in mind, so that drugs are not wrongly held responsible for clinical events whose origin actually preceded drug intake. Hence, one sees the importance of carefully choosing the "exposure time-window" in case-control and cohort studies; again, such choice must be grounded as much as possible on hypotheses based on the *causal model* and on the *healthcare pathway model* previously mentioned. The variety of potential mechanisms through which NSAIDs may act in such radically heterogeneous scenarios as the causation of gastrointestinal hemorrhage and the prevention of colorectal cancer and selected cardiovascular diseases underscores that decisions which might seem "purely methodologic" (e.g., the choice of the exposure time-window) are actually not; thus, they must not be made in a methodologic "vacuum"; that is, they must not rely solely on the advice of methodologic experts. Rather, during the design, analysis, and interpretation of a study, absolute precedence should be given to knowledge of the pharmacology of the drug, the pathophysiology and clinical features of the disease, and patient and physician behaviors.

Measurement errors[97-100] (particularly in assessing drug exposure) and their main consequence, misclassification biases, are also of great importance in drug epidemiology[101-104] (see Chapter 11). In general, independence of exposure classification and disease classification[105-110] cannot be taken for granted if a physician, pharmacist, or nurse intervenes in the data collection. In clinical practice, the diagnostic pathway is often influenced by patient characteristics (e.g., age, severity of symptoms); such characteristics may in turn be associated with specific exposures, so that diagnostic certainty may actually be related to the appraisal of risk factors. For example, histologic confirmation of a suspected cancer may be less likely in very old patients and in patients whose past exposure to drugs and other agents may differ from that of younger patients undergoing biopsies or full staging of their disease.[111-114] Often, knowledge that a particular drug has been taken guides the search for specific effects, the assessment of these effects, and their labeling. Sometimes, a particular diagnosis (e.g., Stevens–Johnson syndrome) may more likely be made if it is known that the patient took a particular drug (e.g., a sulfonamide). Sackett[92] has called "diagnostic suspicion bias" the distortions that occur when knowledge of the subject's prior exposures influences both the intensity and the outcome of the diagnostic process (again, a process that is fully logical from a clinical perspective but one that can distort scientific inferences). As Inman[115] points out, UDEs are often clinically and pathologically indistinguishable from events that can occur spontaneously in untreated patients; for example, thrombosis in a woman taking oral contraceptives cannot be distinguished from thrombosis in a nonuser. Although the diagnosis can be verified by a professional blinded to the patient's drug history, a hospital-based study may still suffer from selection bias.[81]

In survival analysis, it is sometimes assumed that the reasons for censoring (e.g., loss to follow-up) are independent of treatment. However, it is particularly important to ensure that the follow-up of patients who have been lost to or withdrawn from treatment is as intense as for patients who continue treatment.[116] Withdrawing from treatment cannot be assumed to be unrelated to the risk of a poor outcome. Thus, failure to follow up a group experiencing more adverse events may underestimate the risk.

Let us briefly look at another interesting illustration of the specific mechanisms through which bias can happen in pharmacoepidemiology, a finding made during a follow-up study of cimetidine users.[117-119] It was observed that a greater number of patients on cimetidine were admitted to a hospital than age- and gender-matched controls from the community. The increased frequency of hospital admission among cimetidine users was largest for patients with diseases of the digestive tract, but it also was higher for those with diseases of the musculoskeletal system, cancers, respiratory diseases, and diseases of other major systems. Because the study was nonrandomized (observational), the most plausible explanation seemed to lie in contributory causes to the conditions for which cimetidine is actually prescribed. Thus, smoking is a risk factor for peptic ulcer and respiratory diseases (including lung cancer); NSAIDs used in musculoskeletal diseases can also produce dyspepsia; a peptic ulcer that bleeds may lead to iron-deficiency anemia; and so on. Again, subjects exposed to cimetidine appeared to have more risk factors for a variety of ailments than do subjects not exposed to the drug.[117-119] This explanation is logically and clinically appealing. As the sayings go: "health and disease are not randomly distributed,"[120] and "usually people who take drugs are sick." Nevertheless, great caution is needed if valid causal inferences are to be made. Simple advice would be that, when judging a difference between two treatment outcomes, ask two questions: (1) Why was each treatment prescribed?; and (2) Could those reasons help explain the observed difference in outcome? Pharmacoepidemiology is, hence, a rather peculiar branch of epidemiology because of the many subtle factors that affect drug exposure and the assessment of drug effects.

Broadly speaking, observational epidemiologic studies are those in which the investigator does not have "control" over the exposures of interest (e.g., there is no random allocation of treatments). Observational epidemiologic methods were applied to the study of drug effects and uses well before the terms pharmacoepidemiology or drug epidemiology ever appeared in print.[1-3] Observational methods include vital and morbidity statistics,[121-123] case-control studies,[124,125] cohort studies,[126-127] descriptive studies of drug utilization,[19,94,128-134] and other approaches.[3,24,135-145] The strengths and weaknesses of these methods are discussed in detail elsewhere in this book, particularly in Chapter 4.

One of the most promising developments facilitating the use of observational methods is automated databases. They usually cover large, well-defined populations, they can provide follow-up data on drug effects, and they allow for relatively fast and cost-effective studies of delayed as well as short-term effects[146-170] (see Chapter 14). However, the validity and completeness of data are not an uncommon limitation; in particular, it is not rare that databases lack accurate information on potential confounding factors such as smoking, drinking alcohol, diet, or occupational exposures. This is why access to clinical records and to patient interviewing is often crucial. Descriptive studies on drug utilization may also occasionally provide information on confounders.[133] Studies using computerized databases should not replace traditional ad hoc epidemiologic designs when the latter are ethically and logistically feasible.[52,53,171-173]

Further Issues, Further Opportunities

One of the health services issues that is relevant to pharmacoepidemiology is the role of drugs within the healthcare system, that is, the system in which diseases are perceived, detected, and diagnosed; decisions are made for treatment (or no treatment); and diseases are modified during their "natural" course.[174-187]

To study the metabolic processes of a particular organism, *markers* (e.g., radioactive substances) are sometimes administered. Markers allow observation of the interactions of the physical and chemical components in the human body. Metaphorically speaking, drugs may be considered markers for the study of the healthcare system's "metabolism." To quote from Kunin,[188]

> *The therapeutic or prophylactic decisions made by providers or consumers represent the final common pathway of virtually all of the critical factors related to the appropriateness and efficacy of medical care. These decisions represent the synthesis of the mixed ingredients of behavioral, social, cultural, economic, and educational concepts and beliefs about health and disease in populations.*

Hence, drugs reflect not only the prevalence of some health problems,[189-193] but also how humans experience health and cope with suffering.[176] Drug prescribing is one of the most visible indicators of physician practice patterns, because it is observable, can be documented, and is rather frequent.[194] Patient compliance with drugs has been found to be an outcome variable for the quality of patient–physician interaction, for the patient's belief in the efficacy of the treatment, and for the effectiveness of patient education.[195] Drugs allow health services researchers to follow the way the medical and lay communities interact in selecting solutions through pharmacologic intervention. Thus, if we study how drugs are developed, promoted, and used, they become excellent markers of the functional processes of the healthcare system.[176,196-198] The expression "pharmacokinetics in the community" also signifies the tasks of professionals interested in the interaction of drugs, the healthcare system, and society at large.[199]

After emerging from basic molecular and cell biology research, many new techniques (e.g., polymerase chain reaction, recombinant DNA, and the production of monoclonal antibodies via cell fusion) have now come of age. Often based on these and other techniques, as well as on a body of knowledge dramatically increasing, new products have entered the marketplace. Although substantially different from traditional pharmacologic agents, products based on biotechnology should be evaluated in the pharmaceutical context rather than upon the production techniques used. The products of biotechnology are essentially a new class of human therapeutic agents and, as such, are going through the conventional regulatory approval process and marketing channels. However, because of the unique production techniques used and their different mode of action, it is likely that new pharmacoepidemiologic methodologies will need to be developed.

Summary

Drugs and vaccines present challenges to researchers that are uncommon in epidemiologic studies of other types of exposures, such as environmental pollutants, occupational carcinogens, or food nutrients. Attention must be paid to the complex mechanisms of reasoning and decision-making that usually involve the use of drugs.

Although pharmacoepidemiology was not widely recognized as a distinct discipline until the early 1980s, its practice is not new. Epidemiologic, clinical, and laboratory studies of drugs and vaccines captured epidemiologists' interest at least since the beginning of this century.[1] What is different today is the technologic, scientific, societal, and regulatory context within which drugs are developed and used (see Chapter 24). As with other branches of epidemiology and pharmacology, a formal scientific evaluation of the actual contributions and accomplishments of pharmacoepidemiology has been undertaken only partially.[2,11-14,42,139-143,200-206] However, in recent years, drug epidemiology has experienced many developments in substantive, methodologic, and operational issues. Important questions are addressed, meaningful answers to these questions are generated, and, increasingly, policy-makers implement a reasonable proportion of recommendations.[77-79] Clinical pharmacologists and other health professionals often use epidemiologic methods and evidence in their research, practice, and teaching. This has naturally resulted in an expansion of journals and courses devoted to pharmacoepidemiology.[3]

One could contend that pharmacoepidemiology constitutes classic quantitative epidemiology techniques applied to a specific content area, namely, drugs. The specificity of the techniques, evidence, and reasoning used in drug epidemiology and the unique problems that drugs present to practitioners and researchers provide a unique identity to the discipline of pharmacoepidemiology. Conversely, drugs can contribute to the study of the frequency and origins of human illness, as well as to the functioning of the healthcare system. Development of new therapeutic agents based on biotechnology will stimulate the design of innovative, feasible, and valid pharmacoepidemiologic techniques. The uniting, common aim is to foster the optimal use of therapeutic agents by contributing to evidence-based clinical decision-making.

The authors thank the students of "Methods and Issues in Pharmacoepidemiology" (University of North Carolina [UNC] School of Public Health, 1985) for their comments on a previous version of this chapter. The manuscript stemmed from a Working Paper submitted in 1984 by M.S. Porta to Barbara S. Hulka, MD, MPH, then Chair of the Department of Epidemiology of UNC. Further work was made possible by a grant from The Wellcome Fund to the UNC School of Public Health (M.S. Porta). Additional comments and suggestions provided by Linda Wastella, Xavier Carné, Magí Farré, and Ferran Sanz are also gratefully acknowledged. Originally published in *Drug Intelligence and Clinical Pharmacy* (1987;21:741-7), the manuscript was later extensively revised for the successive editions of this book.

References

1. Porta M, Ruiz X, Hartzema AG. Pharmacoepidemiology: the name is new; what else is new? Drug News Perspect 1988;1:243-5.

2. Alvarez-Requejo A, Porta M. Pharmacoepidemiology in practice: current status and future trends. Drug Saf 1995;13:1-7.
3. Porta M, Carné C. Pharmacoepidemiology. In: Olsen J, Trichopoulos D, eds. Teaching epidemiology—what you should know and what you could do. Oxford: Oxford University Press, 1992:285-304.
4. Vineis P, Porta M. Causal thinking, biomarkers and mechanisms of carcinogenesis. J Clin Epidemiol 1996;49:951-6.
5. Fletcher RH. Clinical medicine meets modern epidemiology—and both profit. Ann Epidemiol 1992;2:325-33.
6. Wynder EL. Studies in mechanisms and prevention: striking a proper balance. Am J Epidemiol 1994;139:547-9.
7. Sackett DL. Basic research, clinical research, clinical epidemiology, and general internal medicine (Zlinkoff Honor Lecture). J Gen Intern Med 1987;2:40-7.
8. Sackett DL. Inference and decision at the bedside. J Clin Epidemiol 1989;42:309-16.
9. Sackett DL, Rosenberg WM. On the need for evidence-based medicine. J Public Health Med 1995;17:330-4.
10. Sackett DL, Rosenberg WM. The need for evidence-based medicine. J R Soc Med 1995;88:620-4.
11. Vandenbroucke JP. Epidemiology in transition: a historical hypothesis. Epidemiology 1990;1:164-7.
12. Vandenbroucke JP. How trustworthy is epidemiologic research? Epidemiology 1990;1:83-4.
13. Susser M. Epidemiology today: "a thought-tormented world." Int J Epidemiol 1989;18:481-8.
14. Cole P. The hypothesis generating machine. Epidemiology 1993;4:271-3.
15. Porta M. La epidemiología clínica: ¿un puente entre el individuo y la comunidad? Rev Med Fam Comunity 1994;4:156-7.
16. Porta M, Malats N, Alguacil J, Soler M, Rifà J. La búsqueda de factores de riesgo para el cáncer de páncreas: práctica, paciencia y paradigmas. Gastroenterol Hepatol 1997;20:259-73.
17. Hemminki E, Paakulainen A. The effect of antibiotics on mortality from infectious diseases in Sweden and Finland. Am J Public Health 1976;66:1180-4.
18. Rose G. Prophylaxis with β-blockers and the community. Br J Clin Pharmacol 1982;14:45S-8S.
19. Westerholm B, Agenäs I, Dahlström M, Nordenstam I. Relation between drug utilization and morbidity pattern. Acta Med Scand Suppl 1984;683:95-9.
20. Mackenbach JP, Looman CWN. Secular trends of infectious disease mortality in the Netherlands, 1911–1978: quantitative estimates of changes coinciding with the introduction of antibiotics. Int J Epidemiol 1988;17:618-24.
21. Casper M, Wing S, Strogatz D, Davis CE, Tyroler HA. Antihypertensive treatment and U.S. trends in stroke mortality, 1962 to 1980. Am J Public Health 1992;82:1600-6.
22. McKeown T. The role of medicine: dream, mirage or nemesis? London: The Nuffield Provincial Hospitals Trust, 1976.
23. Rose G. The strategy of preventive medicine. Oxford: Oxford University Press, 1992.
24. Strom BL, ed. Pharmacoepidemiology: the science of postmarketing drug surveillance. New York: Churchill Livingstone, 1989.
25. Strom BL, Miettinen OS, Melmon KL. Postmarketing studies of drug efficacy: why? Am J Med 1985;78:475-80.

26. Paganini-Hill A. Aspirin and colorectal cancer (editorial). BMJ 1993;307:278-9.
27. Heath CW. Rheumatoid arthritis, aspirin, and gastrointestinal cancer (editorial). J Natl Cancer Inst 1993;85:258-9.
28. Baron JA, Greenberg ER. Could aspirin really prevent colon cancer (editorial)? N Engl J Med 1991;325:1644-6.
29. Silagy CA, McNeil JJ, Donnan GA, Tonkin AM, Worsam B, Campion K. Adverse effects of low-dose aspirin in a healthy elderly population. Clin Pharmacol Ther 1993;54:84-9.
30. Fuster V, Dyken ML, Vokonas PS, Hennekens C. Aspirin as a therapeutic agent in cardiovascular disease. Special Writing Group. Circulation 1993;87:659-75.
31. Canadian Task Force on the Periodic Health Examination. Periodic health examination, 1991 update. 6. Acetylsalicylic acid and the primary prevention of cardiovascular disease. Can Med Assoc J 1991;145:1091-5.
32. Fuster V, Cohen M, Halperin J. Aspirin in the prevention of coronary disease (editorial). N Engl J Med 1989;321:183-5.
33. Slone D, Shapiro S, Miettinen OS, Finkle WD, Stolley PD. Drug evaluation after marketing. Ann Intern Med 1979;90:257-61.
34. Lasagna LL. A plea for the "naturalistic" study of medicines. Eur J Clin Pharmacol 1974;7:153-4.
35. Lasagna LL. Randomized clinical trials (letter). N Engl J Med 1976;295:1086-7.
36. Miettinen OS. Efficacy of therapeutic practice: will epidemiology provide the answers? In: Melmon KL, ed. Drug therapeutics. Edinburgh: Churchill Livingstone, 1980:201-8.
37. Jick H, Miettinen OS, Shapiro S, Lewis GP, Siskind V, Slone D. Comprehensive drug surveillance (letter). JAMA 1979;213:1455.
38. Wardell WM, Tsianco MC, Anavekar SN, Davis HT. Postmarketing surveillance of new drugs: I. review of objectives and methodology. J Clin Pharmacol 1979; 19: 85-94, and II. case studies. J Clin Pharmacol 1979;19:169-84.
39. Strom BL, Melmon KL. Can postmarketing surveillance help to effect optimal drug therapy? JAMA 1979;242:2420-3.
40. Castle WM, Nicholls JT, Downie CC. Problems of postmarketing surveillance. Br J Clin Pharmacol 1983;16:581-5.
41. Bell RL, Smith EO. Clinical trials in post-marketing surveillance of drugs. Control Clin Trials 1982;3:61-8.
42. Rossi AC, Knapp DE, Anello C, et al. Discovery of adverse drug reactions: a comparison of selected Phase IV studies with spontaneous reporting methods. JAMA 1983;249:2226-8.
43. Borden EK, Gardner JS, Westland MM, Gardner SD. Postmarketing drug surveillance (letter). JAMA 1984;251:729.
44. Schwartz D, Lellouch J. Explanatory and pragmatic attitudes in therapeutic trials. J Chronic Dis 1967;20:637-48.
45. Schwartz D, Flamant L, Lellouch J. Clinical trials. (English translation of the 1970 first French edition). London: Academic Press, 1980.
46. Porta M. The relevance of the explanatory/pragmatic distinction for experimental and observational studies (abstract). Clin Res 1986;34:831A.
47. Charlson ME, Horwitz RI. Applying results of randomized trials to clinical practice: impact of losses before randomization. Br Med J 1984;259:1281-4.
48. Mattison N, Richard BW. Postapproval research requested by the FDA at the time of NCE approval, 1970–1984. Drug Inf J 1987;21:309-29.

49. Richard BW, Melville A, Lasagna L. Postapproval research as a condition of approval: an update, 1985–1986. J Clin Res Drug Dev 1989;3:247-57.
50. Bailly GB, Pierredon M, Rondel R, Steru L, Szapiro E. Phase IV and Europe. Drug Inf J 1989;23:105-15.
51. Meinert CL. Clinical trials: design, conduct, and analysis. New York: Oxford University Press, 1986.
52. Tognoni G, Franzosi MG, Garattini S, Maggioni A, Lotto A, Mauri F, et al. The case of GISSI in changing the attitudes and practice of Italian cardiologists. Stat Med 1990;9:17-27.
53. Tognoni G, Alli C, Avanzini F, Bettelli G, Colombo F, Corso R, et al. Randomised clinical trials in general practice: lessons from a failure. BMJ 1991;303:969-71.
54. Sackett DL, Haynes RB, Gent M, Taylor DW. Compliance. In: Inman WHW, ed. Monitoring for drug safety. 2nd ed. Lancaster, England: MTP Press, 1986:471-83.
55. Hulley SB, Cummings SR, eds. Designing clinical research. An epidemiologic approach. Baltimore: Williams & Wilkins, 1987:139-50,215-20.
56. Freiman JA, Chalmers TC, Smith H, Kuebler RR. The importance of beta, the type II error, and sample size in the design and interpretation of the randomized controlled trial. Survey of 71 "negative" trials. In: Bailar JC, Mosteller F, eds. Medical uses of statistics. 2nd ed. Waltham, MA: New England Journal of Medicine Books, 1992:357-73.
57. Strom BL, ed. Pharmacoepidemiology: the science of postmarketing drug surveillance. New York: Churchill Livingstone, 1989:27-37.
58. Fleiss JL. Statistical methods for rates and proportions. New York: John Wiley, 1981: 33-49.
59. Fleiss JL. The design and analysis of clinical experiments. New York: John Wiley, 1986:369-76.
60. Pocock SJ. Clinical trials. A practical approach. Chichester, UK: John Wiley, 1983: 123-41.
61. Schlesselman JJ, Stolley PD. Case-control studies. Design, conduct, analysis. New York: Oxford University Press, 1982:144-70.
62. Detsky AS, Sackett DL. When was a "negative" clinical trial big enough? Arch Intern Med 1985;145:709-12.
63. Blackwelder WC. "Proving the null hypothesis" in clinical trials. Control Clin Trials 1982;3:345-53.
64. Blackwelder WC, Chang MA. Sample size graphs for "proving the null hypothesis." Control Clin Trials 1984;5:97-105.
65. Lwanga SK, Lemeshow S. Estimating sample size in health studies. A practical manual. Geneva: World Health Organization, 1991.
66. Kraemer HC, Thiemann S. How many subjects? Statistical power analysis in research. Newbury Park, CA: Sage, 1987.
67. Florey C. Sample size for beginners. BMJ 1993;306:1181-4.
68. Ederer F, Church TR, Mandel JS. Sample sizes for prevention trials have been too small. Am J Epidemiol 1993;137:787-96.
69. Church TR, Ederer F, Mandel JS, Watt GD, Geisser MS. Estimating the duration of ongoing prevention trials. Am J Epidemiol 1993;137:797-810.
70. Carné X, Moreno V, Porta M, Velilla E. El cálculo del número de pacientes necesarios en la planificación de un estudio clínico. Med Clin (Barc) 1989;92:72-7.
71. Porta M, Moreno V, Sanz F, Carné X, Velilla E. Una cuestión de poder. Med Clin (Barc) 1989;92:223-8.

72. Hill AB. The clinical trial. Br Med Bull 1951;7:278-82.
73. Hill AB. The clinical trial. N Engl J Med 1952;247:113-9.
74. Hill AB. Observation and experiment. N Engl J Med 1952;248:995-1001.
75. Rogers AS, Porta M, Tilson HH. Guidelines for decision-making in postmarketing surveillance of drugs. J Clin Res Pharmacoepidemiol 1990;4:241-51.
76. Porta M. Los ensayos clínicos de fase IV: porqué, cuándo y ¿cómo? In: García Alonso F, Bakke OM, eds. Metodología del Ensayo Clínico. Barcelona: Fundación Dr. Antonio Esteve/ediciones Doyma, 1991:31-9.
77. Anderson GM, Spitzer WO, Weinstein MC, Wang E, Blackburn JL, Bergman U. Benefits, risks, and costs of prescription drugs: a scientific basis for evaluating policy options. Clin Pharmacol Ther 1990;48:111-9.
78. Spitzer WO. Drugs as determinants of health and disease in the population. J Clin Epidemiol 1991;44:823-30.
79. Ray WA, Griffin MR, Avorn J. Evaluating drugs after their approval for clinical use. N Engl J Med 1993;329:2029-32.
80. Last JM, ed. A dictionary of epidemiology. 3rd ed. New York: Oxford University Press, 1995.
81. Miettinen O, Slone D, Shapiro S. Current problems in drug-related epidemiologic research. In: Colombo F, Shapiro S, Slone D, Tognoni G, eds. Epidemiological evaluation of drugs. Littleton, MA: PSG Publishing, 1977:295-303.
82. Miettinen OS. The need for randomization in the study of intended effects. Stat Med 1983;2:267-71.
83. Strom BL, Miettinen OS, Melmon KL. Postmarketing studies of drug efficacy: when must they be randomized? J Clin Pharmacol 1983;34:1-7.
84. Strom BL, Miettinen OS, Melmon KL. Postmarketing studies of drug efficacy: how? Am J Med 1984;77:703-8.
85. Walker AM. Confounding by indication (editorial). Epidemiology 1996;7:335-6.
86. Horwitz RI, McFarlane MJ, Brennan TA, Feinstein AR. The role of susceptibility bias in epidemiologic research. Arch Intern Med 1985;145:909-12.
87. Porta MS, Hartzema AG. The contribution of epidemiology to the study of drug effects. Drug Intell Clin Pharm 1987;21:741-7.
88. Porta M. Confounding by indication and past clinical trials (letter). Epidemiology 1997;8:219-20.
89. Wiklund I, Oden A, Sanne H, Ulvenstam G, Wilhelmsson C, Wilhelmesen L. Prognostic importance of somatic and psychosocial variables after a first myocardial infarction. Am J Epidemiol 1988;128:786-95.
90. Porta M. Métodos de investigación clínica: errores, falacias y desafíos. Med Clin (Barc) 1990;94:107-15.
91. Feinstein AR. Clinical epidemiology. The architecture of clinical research. Philadelphia: WB Saunders, 1985:461-7,44-5,285-6,303-5.
92. Sackett DL. Bias in analytic research. J Chronic Dis 1979;32:51-63.
93. Walker AM, Chan KW, Yood RA. Patterns of interchange in the dispensing of nonsteroidal anti-inflammatory drugs. J Clin Epidemiol 1992;45:187-95.
94. Chan KW, Walker AM, Yood RA. An equilibrium model of drug utilization. J Clin Epidemiol 1993;46:113-21.
95. Appelberg K, Romanov K, Honkasalo ML, Koskenvuo M. The use of tranquilizers, hypnotics and analgesics among 18,592 Finnish adults: associations with recent interpersonal conflicts at work or with a spouse. J Clin Epidemiol 1993;46:1315-22.

96. Choi BC. Definition, sources, magnitude, effect modifiers, and strategies of reduction of the healthy worker effect. J Occup Med 1992;34:979-88.
97. Hulley SB, Cummings SR, eds. Designing clinical research. An epidemiologic approach. Baltimore: Williams & Wilkins, 1987:31-52.
98. Kleinbaum DG, Kupper LL, Morgenstern H. Epidemiologic research. Principles and quantitative methods. Belmont, CA: Lifetime Learning Publications, 1982:221-41.
99. Rothman KJ. Modern epidemiology. Boston: Little, Brown, 1986:77-97.
100. Sudman S, Bradburn NM. Asking questions. A practical guide to questionnaire design. San Francisco: Jossey-Bass, 1987.
101. Harlow SD, Linet MS. Agreement between questionnaire data and medical records: the evidence for accuracy of recall. Am J Epidemiol 1989;129:233-48.
102. Kelly JP, Rosenberg L, Kaufman DW, Shapiro S. Reliability of personal interview data in a hospital-based case-control study. Am J Epidemiol 1990;131:79-90.
103. Graham DJ, Smith CR. Misclassification in epidemiologic studies of adverse drug reactions using large managerial data bases. Am J Prev Med 1988;4(suppl 2):15-24.
104. de Jong PCM, Huijsmans AA, Nienhuis HE, Nijdam WS, Zielhuis GA, Eskes TKAB. Validation of a questionnaire on medical drug use during pregnancy. Am J Epidemiol 1991;134:998-1002.
105. Brenner H, Savitz DA, Gefeller O. The effects of joint misclassification of exposure and disease on epidemiologic measures of association. J Clin Epidemiol 1993;46: 1195-202.
106. Walker AM, Blettner M. Comparing imperfect measures of exposure. Am J Epidemiol 1985;121:783-90.
107. Walker AM, Lanes SF. Misclassification of covariates. Stat Med 1991;10:1181-96.
108. Kristensen P. Bias from nondifferential but dependent misclassification of exposure and outcome. Epidemiology 1992;3:210-5.
109. Wacholder S, Dosemeci M, Lubin JH. Blind assignment of exposure does not always prevent differential misclassification. Am J Epidemiol 1991;134:433-7.
110. Mertens TE. Estimating the effects of misclassification. Lancet 1993;342:418-21.
111. Porta M, Malats N, Piñol JL, Rifà J, Andreu A, Real FX, for the PANKRAS I Project Investigators. Diagnostic certainty and potential for misclassification in exocrine pancreatic cancer. J Clin Epidemiol 1994;47:1069-79.
112. Porta M, Malats N, Piñol JL, Real FX, Rifà J. Relevance of misclassification of disease status in epidemiologic studies of exocrine pancreatic cancer. J Clin Epidemiol 1996;49:601-3.
113. Modan B, Wagener DK, Feldman JJ, Rosenberg HM, Feinleib M. Increased mortality from brain tumors: a combined outcome of diagnostic technology and change of attitude toward the elderly. Am J Epidemiol 1992;135:1349-57.
114. Greenberg ER, Baron JA, Dain BJ, Freeman DH Jr, Yates JW, Korson R. Cancer staging may have different meanings in academic and community hospitals. J Clin Epidemiol 1991;44:505-12.
115. Inman WHW. Prescription-event monitoring. Acta Med Scand Suppl 1984;683:119-26.
116. Mosteller F, Gilbert JP, McPeek B. Controversies in the design and analysis of clinical trials. In: Shapiro SH, Louis TA, eds. Clinical trials. Issues and approaches. New York: Marcel Dekker, 1983:13-64.
117. Colin-Jones DG, Langman MJS, Lawson DH, Vessey MP. Post-marketing surveillance of the safety of cimetidine: twelve-month morbidity report. Q J Med N Ser 1985;54:253-68.

118. Colin-Jones DG, Langman MJS, Lawson DH, Vessey MP. Postmarketing surveillance of the safety of cimetidine: 12 month mortality report. Br Med J 1983;286: 1713-6.
119. Colin-Jones DG, Langman MJS, Lawson DH, Vessey MP. Postmarketing surveillance of the safety of cimetidine: mortality during second, third, and fourth years of follow-up. Br Med J 1985;291:1084-8.
120. Stallones RA. To advance epidemiology. Annu Rev Public Health 1980;1:69-82.
121. Stolley PD. The use of vital and morbidity statistics for the detection of adverse drug reactions and for monitoring of drug safety. J Clin Pharmacol 1982;22:499-504.
122. Stolley PD. Asthma mortality: why the United States was spared an epidemic of deaths due to asthma. Am Rev Respir Dis 1972;105:883-90.
123. Edlavitch SA, Feinleib M, Anello C. A potential use of the National Death Index for postmarketing drug surveillance. JAMA 1985;253:1292-5.
124. Jick H, Vessey MP. Case-control studies in the evaluation of drug-induced illness. Am J Epidemiol 1978;107:1-7.
125. Ibrahim MA, Spitzer WO, eds. The case-control study: consensus and controversy. New York: Pergamon Press, 1979.
126. Royal College of General Practitioners. Oral contraceptives and health. London: Pitman, 1974.
127. Vessey M, Doll R, Peto R, Johnson B, Wiggins P. A long-term follow-up study of women using different methods of contraception—an interim report. J Biosoc Sci 1976;8:373-427.
128. WHO Collaborating Centre for Drug Statistics Methodology. Drug utilization bibliography. Copenhagen: World Health Organization Regional Office for Europe, 1989.
129. WHO Collaborating Centre for Drug Statistics Methodology. Drug utilization bibliography. Publications and reprints from January 1989 to January 1993. Copenhagen: World Health Organization Regional Office for Europe, 1993.
130. Dukes MNG, ed. Drug utilization studies. Methods and uses. WHO regional publications. European Series No. 45. Copenhagen: World Health Organization Regional Office for Europe, 1993.
131. Bergman U, Grimsson A, Wahba AHW, Westerholm B, eds. Studies in drug utilization. Methods and applications. Copenhagen: World Health Organization Regional Office for Europe, 1979.
132. Sjoqvist F, Agenas I, eds. Drug utilization studies: implications for medical care. Proceedings from ANIS Symposium, Sanga-Saby, Sweden, June 8–9, 1982. Acta Med Scand Suppl 1984;683:127-34.
133. Porta M. Some comments. In: Kunin CM, ed. Meeting report. International Clinical Epidemiology Network (INCLEN) meeting on pharmacoepidemiology. Tarrytown, NY: The Rockefeller Foundation, 1988:79-80.
134. Laporte JR, Porta M, Capella D. Drug utilization studies: a tool for determining the effectiveness of drug use. Br J Clin Pharmacol 1983;16:301-4.
135. Colombo F, Shapiro S, Slone D, Tognoni G, eds. Epidemiological evaluation of drugs. Amsterdam: Elsevier/North Holland, 1977.
136. Tognoni G, Bellantuono C, Lader M, eds. Epidemiological impact of psychotropic drugs. Amsterdam: Elsevier/North Holland, 1981.
137. Inman WHW, ed. Monitoring for drug safety. Lancaster, UK: MTP Press, 1980.
138. Walker SR, Goldberg A, eds. Monitoring for adverse drug reactions. Lancaster, UK: MTP Press, 1984.
139. Venning GR. Identification of adverse reactions to new drugs. I. What have been the important adverse reactions since thalidomide? Br Med J 1983;286:199-202.

140. Venning GR. Identification of adverse reactions to new drugs. II. How were 18 important adverse reactions discovered and with what delays? Br Med J 1983;286: 289-92.

141. Venning GR. Identification of adverse reactions to new drugs. II (continued). Br Med J 1983;286:365-8.

142. Venning GR. Identification of adverse reactions to new drugs. III. Alerting processes and early warning systems. Br Med J 1983;286:458-60.

143. Venning GR. Identification of adverse reactions to new drugs. IV. Verification of suspected adverse reactions. Br Med J 1983;286:544-7.

144. Porta M, Bolúmar F, Hernández I, Vioque J. N of 1 trials, crossover clinical trials and the case-crossover design (letter). BMJ 1996;313:427.

145. Matoren GM, ed. The clinical research process in the pharmaceutical industry. New York: Marcel Dekker, 1983.

146. Roos LL, Roos NP, Cageorge SM, Nicol JP. How good are the data? Reliability of one health care data bank. Med Care 1982;20:266-76.

147. Roos LL, Nicol JP. Building individual histories with registries. A case study. Med Care 1983;21:955-69.

148. Feinleib M. Data bases, data banks and data dredging: the agony and the ecstasy. J Chronic Dis 1984;37:783-90.

149. Jick H, Madsen S, Nudelman PM, Perera DR, Stergachis A. Postmarketing follow-up at Group Health Cooperative of Puget Sound. Pharmacotherapy 1984;4:99-100.

150. Tilson HH. Getting down to bases—record linkage in Saskatchewan (editorial). Can J Public Health 1985;76:222-3.

151. Strand LM. Drug epidemiology resources and studies: the Saskatchewan data base. Drug Inf J 1985;19:253-6.

152. Morse ML. The COMPASS data base. Drug Inf J 1985;19:249-52.

153. Strom B, Carson JL, Morse L, LeRoy AA. The computerized on-line Medicaid pharmaceutical analysis and surveillance system: a new resource for postmarketing drug surveillance. Clin Pharmacol Ther 1985;38:359-64.

154. Jick H. Use of automated data bases to study drug effects after marketing. Pharmacotherapy 1985;5:278-9.

155. Connell FA, Diehr P, Hart LG. The use of large data bases in health care studies. Annu Rev Public Health 1987;8:51-74.

156. Avorn J. Medicaid-based pharmacoepidemiology: claims and counterclaims. Epidemiology 1990;1:98-100.

157. Roos LL, Sharp SM, Cohen MM. Comparing clinical information with claims data: some similarities and differences. J Clin Epidemiol 1991;44:881-8.

158. Von Korff M, Wagner EH, Saunders K. A chronic disease score from automated pharmacy data. J Clin Epidemiol 1992;45:197-203.

159. Charlson ME, Pompei P, Ales KL, MacKenzie CR. A new method of classifying prognostic comorbidity in longitudinal studies: development and validation. J Chronic Dis 1987;40:373-83.

160. Lurie N. Administrative data and outcomes research (editorial). Med Care 1990;28: 867-9.

161. Quaak MJ, Westerman RF, Van Bemmel JH. Comparisons between written and computerised patient histories. Br Med J 1987;295:184-90.

162. Tennis P, Andrews E, Bombardier C, Wang Y, Strand L, West R, et al. Record linkage to conduct an epidemiologic study on the association of rheumatoid arthritis and lymphoma in the province of Saskatchewan, Canada. J Clin Epidemiol 1993; 46:685-95.

163. Tennis P, Bombardier C, Malcolm E, Downey W. Validity of rheumatoid arthritis diagnoses listed in the Saskatchewan hospital separations database. J Clin Epidemiol 1993;46:675-83.
164. Shapiro S. Reasons for the successes and failures of specific models in drug epidemiology. In: Kewitz H, Roots I, Voigt K, eds. Epidemiological concepts in clinical pharmacology. Berlin: Springer-Verlag, 1987:11-22.
165. Shapiro S. The role of automated record linkage in the postmarketing surveillance of drug safety: a critique. Clin Pharmacol Ther 1989;46:371-86.
166. Faich GA, Stadel BV. The future of automated record linkage for postmarketing surveillance: a response to Shapiro. Clin Pharmacol Ther 1989;46:387-9.
167. Strom BL, Carson JL. Automated data bases used for pharmacoepidemiology research. Clin Pharmacol Ther 1989;46:390-4.
168. Shapiro S. Automated record linkage: a response to the commentary and letters to the editor. Clin Pharmacol Ther 1989;46:395-8.
169. Jick H, Walker AM. Uninformed criticism of automated record linkage. Clin Pharmacol Ther 1989;46:478-9.
170. Tilson HH. Pharmacoepidemiology: the lessons learned; the challenges ahead (letter). Clin Pharmacol Ther 1989;46:480.
171. Yusuf S, Collins R, Peto R. Why do we need some large, simple randomized trials? Stat Med 1984;3:409-20.
172. Green SB, Byar DP. Using observational data from registries to compare treatments: the fallacy of omnimetrics. Stat Med 1984;3:361-73.
173. Byar DP. Why data bases should not replace randomized clinical trials. Biometrics 1980;36:337-42.
174. Hulka BS. Epidemiological applications to health services research. J Community Health 1978;4:140-9.
175. Hulka BS, Wheat J. Utilization patterns. Med Care 1985;23:438-60.
176. Tognoni G, Liberati A, Pello L, Sasanelli F, Spagnoli A. Drug utilization studies and epidemiology. Rev Epidemiol Sante Publique 1983;31:59-71.
177. Tognoni G. Drug use and monitoring. In: Holland WW, ed. Evaluation of health care. Oxford: Oxford University Press, 1983:207-25.
178. Janes CR, Stall R, Gifford SM, eds. Anthropology and epidemiology. Interdisciplinary approaches to the study of health and disease. Dordrecht: Reidel, 1986.
179. Zola IK. Culture and symptoms—an analysis of patients' presenting complaints. Am Sociol Rev 1966;31:615-30.
180. Twaddle AC. Sickness and the sickness career: some implications. In: Eisenberg L, Kleinman A, eds. The relevance of social science for medicine. Dordrecht: Reidel, 1981:111-33.
181. Mechanic D. Social psychologic factors affecting the presentation of bodily complaints. N Engl J Med 1972;286:1132-9.
182. Eisenberg L. Psychiatry and society. A sociobiologic synthesis. N Engl J Med 1977;296:903-10.
183. Eisenberg L. What makes persons "patients" and patients "well"? Am J Med 1980;69:277-86.
184. Eisenberg L. The subjective in medicine. Perspect Biol Med 1983;1:40-8.
185. Kleinman A, Eisenberg L, Good B. Culture, illness, and care. Clinical lessons from anthropologic and cross-cultural research. Ann Intern Med 1978;88:251-8.
186. Eisenberg L. Treating depression and anxiety in primary care. Closing the gap between knowledge and practice. N Engl J Med 1992;326:1080-4.

187. Rothenberg LS. Molecular medicine in the U.S.: can three paradigms shift simultaneously (editorial)? Lancet 1993;341:1379-80.

188. Kunin CM, ed. Meeting report. International Clinical Epidemiology Network (INCLEN) meeting on pharmacoepidemiology. Tarrytown, NY: The Rockefeller Foundation, 1988.

189. Aquilonius SM, Granat M, Hartvig P. Utilization of antiparkinson drugs in Norway, Sweden, Denmark and Finland in 1975–1979. Acta Neurol Scand 1981;64: 47-53.

190. Anderson DW. A survey approach for finding cases of epilepsy. Public Health Rep 1985;100:386-93.

191. Maggini M, Salmaso S, Alegiani SS, Caffari B, Raschetti R. Epidemiological use of drug prescriptions as markers of disease frequency: an Italian experience. J Clin Epidemiol 1991;44:1299-307.

192. Papoz L, EURODIAB Subarea C Study Group. Utilization of drugs sales data for the epidemiology of chronic diseases: the example of diabetes. Epidemiology 1993;4:421-7.

193. Sartor F, Walckiers D. Estimate of disease prevalence using drug consumption data. Am J Epidemiol 1995;141:782-7.

194. Parish PA. Sociology of prescribing. Br Med Bull 1974;30:214-7.

195. Haynes RB, Taylor DW, Sackett DL, eds. Compliance in health care. Baltimore: Johns Hopkins University Press, 1981.

196. Cirera L, Porta M, Monteis J, Camí C. Trends in acute drug poisoning in the Hospital del Mar (Barcelona), and the relative impact of "Prosereme," Spain's drug review program. J Pharmacoepidemiol 1995;4:3-19.

197. Fernàndez E, Porta M, Alonso J, Antó JM. Epidemiology of prostatic disorders in the city of Barcelona. Int J Epidemiol 1992;21:959-65.

198. Juncosa S, Porta M. Effects of primary health care reform on the prescription of antibiotics: a longitudinal study in a Spanish county. Eur J Public Health 1997;7:54-60.

199. Baksaas I, Lunde PKM. Drug utilization: pharmacokinetics in the community. Trends Pharmacol Sci 1981;2(2):V-VII.

200. Susser M. Epidemiology in the United States after World War II: the evolution of technique. Epidemiol Rev 1985;7:147-77.

201. Rossi AC, Knapp DE. Discovery of adverse drug reactions: a review of the Food and Drug Administration's spontaneous reporting system. JAMA 1984;252:1030-3.

202. Sheps MC. The clinical value of drugs: sources of evidence. Am J Public Health 1961;51:647-54.

203. Weinshilboum RM. The therapeutic revolution. Clin Pharmacol Ther 1987;42:481-4.

204. Porta M. Prólogo: ¿para qué necesitamos la farmacoepidemiología? In: Matos L, ed. Farmacoepidemiología. Santiago de Compostela: Xunta de Galicia, 1995:9-12.

205. Stolley PD, Lasky T. Investigating disease patterns. The science of epidemiology. New York: Scientific American Library/HPHLP, 1995.

206. Stolley PD. A public health perspective from academia. In: Strom BL, ed. Pharmacoepidemiology. New York: Churchill Livingstone, 1989:51-5.

2

The FDA Drug Approval Process

Ann M Myers
James R Hunter
Steven R Moore

Abstract

Critical to the understanding of pharmacoepidemiology is an insight into the process by which new drugs are reviewed and approved for marketing in the US. Information gathered during the drug development and review process can potentially lay the foundation for pharmacoepidemiologic studies after the application is approved and the drug is marketed. This chapter presents an overview of the drug review process in the US. A brief description is provided of the review process in the US, in terms of the responsibilities of the sponsor in submitting a marketing application for review to the Food and Drug Administration (FDA) and the FDA's organizational procedures for reviewing and then approving those applications with the requisite scientific data. A brief history of the legislation regarding the FDA's responsibility in the drug review area is discussed along with recent regulations, legislation, and FDA initiatives aimed at improving and expediting the drug development and review process. The discussion is limited to the regulation of drugs; somewhat different regulations govern the review and regulation of biologic products, abbreviated new drug applications (generic drugs), and medical devices. The discussion is based on the process in the US; although the details differ, the logic is similar around the world where drug applications are reviewed and approved.

Outline

1. Brief history of drug regulations and current initiatives
2. The Center for Drug Evaluation and Research and the review process
3. The traditional drug development process
   Postmarketing surveillance
4. Initiatives to expedite the availability of certain drugs for severe illnesses

Subpart E regulations
Treatment investigational new drugs
Parallel track proposal
Accelerated drug approval proposal
5. Summary
6. References

B y law, the Food and Drug Administration (FDA) is responsible for determining whether a new drug is safe and effective before it is approved for marketing in the US and for monitoring its use after approval. The FDA's authority over drug review and approval began with the Food and Drug Act of 1906. This Act (often referred to as the Wiley Act or Heyburn Act) made it unlawful to manufacture adulterated or misbranded foods or drugs within any state or territory of the US and the District of Columbia, and banned adulterated or misbranded foods or drugs from interstate commerce. However, the law was limited in that the burden of proof was on the FDA to show that the labeling was false or fraudulent before the product could be taken off the market and that the manufacturer intended that the labeling was false or fraudulent.

The limitations of the 1906 act prompted further legislation, and in 1938 Congress passed the federal Food, Drug, and Cosmetic Act, which prohibited marketing new drugs unless they had been tested adequately to show they were safe for use under the conditions prescribed on their labels. This legislation was passed the year following the elixir of sulfanilamide tragedy, in which more than 100 people died as a result of ingesting ethylene glycol that was used as a solvent in an untested new drug formulation. This act put the burden on manufacturers to prove that a product was safe prior to marketing.

In 1962 Congress passed the Kefauver–Harris amendments to the Food, Drug, and Cosmetic Act, which included an additional burden on manufacturers to prove efficacy as well as safety before a drug could be marketed. This requirement was applied retroactively to 1938, when the Food, Drug, and Cosmetic Act was passed. Pre-1938 drugs were, to some extent, "grandfathered," provided no evidence of problems with safety or efficacy developed and no changes were made in the way the drug was marketed. The amendment also stated that the FDA must be notified when drugs are being tested on humans.

More recent changes to the Act include congressional actions that provide initiatives to manufacturers to develop drugs for limited populations. For example, Congress enacted the Orphan Drug Act in 1983, which allows the manufacturers that are developing drugs and other products for rare diseases the benefits of tax deductions for much of the cost of clinical development. Firms that are the first on the market with a designated orphan product are also granted exclusive marketing rights for 7 years when the orphan products are approved. In addition, the FDA can grant special funding for such research on orphan products.

More recent regulatory changes provide mechanisms for expediting the evaluation and early availability of new drugs for people with serious or life-threatening diseases for which no comparable or satisfactory alternative drug or other therapy exists. The treatment investigational new drug (IND) regulations, issued in 1987, increase widespread early access of promising investigational drugs to patients prior to product approval. In 1988, Subpart E regulations provided a program that commits the FDA to early and ongoing consultation with sponsors in the design of drug trials, provides for more expansive early trials to permit earlier risk/benefit assessment, and provides for FDA-sponsored regulatory research.

In 1990, the FDA published a proposed policy known as parallel track that makes promising investigational drugs more widely available to people with AIDS and HIV-related diseases through studies conducted in parallel with the controlled clinical trials.

Proposed regulations for an accelerated approval process for new drugs to treat serious and life-threatening illnesses were published in the *Federal Register* on April 15, 1992. These regulations contain several new provisions that allow for an approval based upon trials using surrogate clinical end points but require completion of studies using definitive clinical end points to confirm the surrogate-based evidence of safety and effectiveness. It is important to recognize that this "accelerated" approval does not, per se, accelerate the review process for these products but, rather, accelerates the development process by allowing the use of surrogate end points as primary evidence of efficacy.

In 1992, the enactment of the Prescription Drug User Fee Act paved the way for additional resources to be allocated to the review of new drug applications (NDAs). Although "user fees" have been charged for many years in insulin certification, in 1992, the Prescription Drug User Fee Act expanded the collection of fees to include specific drug and biologic products. In particular for the drug review area, fees are collected for original NDAs, some supplements that require clinical studies (i.e., efficacy), and manufacturing establishments covered under the Prescription Drug User Fee Act.

Under the provisions of this Act, additional revenues generated by the fees paid by sponsors are dedicated for use in improving the new drug review process in accordance with the prescribed performance goals developed by the FDA and the drug industry. For example, from October 1994 to 1996, the FDA reviewed and acted on a prescribed percentage of original NDAs and efficacy supplements within 12 months. Manufacturing supplements were reviewed and acted on within 6 months of receipt.

To achieve the challenging performance goals set forth by the Prescription Drug User Fee Act agreements, the FDA is involved in information technology initiatives aimed at improving and increasing the efficiency of the review of drug applications. As part of this effort, the FDA is promoting the electronic submission of data from the drug industry to the Agency. Sections of the application, such as the clinical portion with detailed clinical trial information or, in some cases, all parts of the NDA can be submitted to the FDA in a format that can be reviewed and analyzed by reviewers electronically. Internal initiatives include developing electronic review and document management tools geared to support electronic archiving, searching, and routing capabilities. More information regarding these recent drug approval initiatives is included later in this chapter.

The Center for Drug Evaluation and Research and the Review Process

The Center for Drug Evaluation and Research is the FDA component responsible for regulating the review and approval of new drug products intended for human use. The Center's director and senior staff provide the highest level of policy-making and program management. Within the Center, the main offices responsible for drug review oversight are the Office of Review Management and the Office of Pharmaceutical Science. Support for the review process is also provided by the Office of Compliance, the Office of Management, and the Office of Training and Communications that are also organizationally located within the Center (Figure 1).

Within the Office of Review Management, there are five Offices of Drug Evaluation that provide direct oversight over the actual drug review divisions. At this time, there are 13 drug review divisions organized by medical specialty that are responsible for the actual evaluation and review of specific types of new drugs (Figure 2).

The management and review structures of each review division are organizationally similar (Figure 3). Each has a division director and some, but not all, have a deputy director. The division review team is composed of a scientific team leader who is usually a medical officer, the medical reviewer, the pharmacologist, and the project manager who is in charge of the regulatory and administrative management of each application. A microbiology review is also required for some applications, such as for antimicrobial and large-volume parenterals.

Although located organizationally outside the drug review divisions, other components of the Center provide direct input to the review. Within the Office of Review Management, primary statistical reviews are conducted by the Office of Epidemiology and Biostatistics. Within the Office of Pharmaceutical Science, the chemistry review and a biopharmaceutics review are also conducted (Figure 4).

Each member of the review team performs a review of submitted information based on regulatory guidelines and precedents. Periodically, reviewers meet to discuss issues, progress, and problems, and meetings are arranged frequently with the applicant (sponsor) to discuss certain issues or to summarize the status of the application. To ensure consistency of the

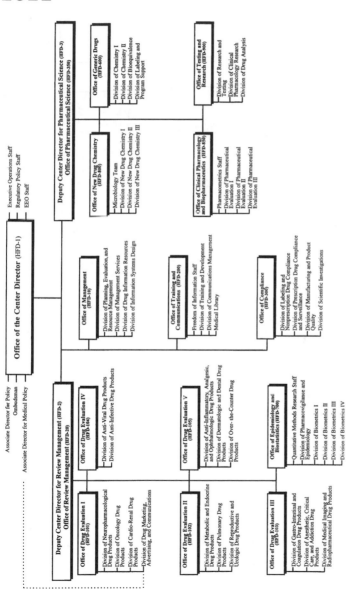

Figure 1
Center for Drug Evaluation and Research

Figure 2
Center for Drug Evaluation and Research: Office of Review Management

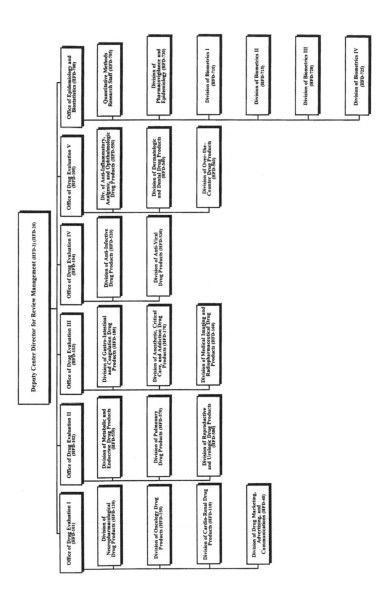

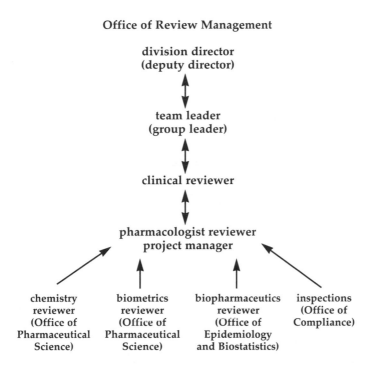

Office of Review Management

Figure 3
Functional
Organization
Chart of the
Reviewing Team

division director
(deputy director)

team leader
(group leader)

clinical reviewer

pharmacologist reviewer
project manager

| chemistry reviewer (Office of Pharmaceutical Science) | biometrics reviewer (Office of Pharmaceutical Science) | biopharmaceutics reviewer (Office of Epidemiology and Biostatistics) | inspections (Office of Compliance) |

drug review process across review divisions, the Center has developed a Manual of Policies and Procedures (called MaPPs) in which procedures and policies are outlined.

In addition, the Office of Compliance oversees the clinical investigators involved in preclinical and clinical trials and the inspection of manufacturing facilities. These inspections take place before and after approval of the drug.

Once all reviews have been completed (including the chemistry, statistical, and any necessary biopharmaceutical reviews), an "action package" consisting of a draft action letter, the reviews, and other pertinent information is prepared by the project manager. This package is circulated to the review staff, including team leaders, supervisors, and the division director, for concurrence and signatures. Final signature authority resides at different levels of the organization, based on the chemical classification of the product. For example, applications such as new molecular entities, new combinations, significant new indications, and novel routes of administration must then be forwarded to the appropriate director's office of the Office of Drug Evaluation for upper-level final clearance and final action (either approval, not approval, or approvable).

Figure 4
Center for Drug Evaluation and Research: Office of Pharmaceutical Science

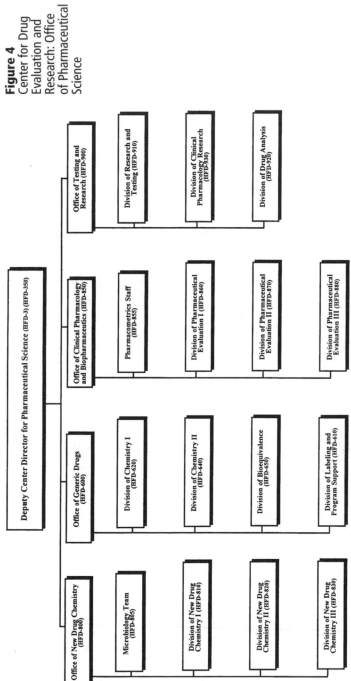

The Traditional Drug Development Process

From the perspective of the FDA, new drug development can be broadly divided into four phases (Figure 5): (1) preclinical research and development, (2) clinical research and development (also called the IND phase), (3) NDA review, and (4) postmarketing surveillance (PMS).

The preclinical research and development of a new drug include the discovery and initial identification of the drug, its synthesis and purification, and initial chemical work-up. This first phase also includes the generation of laboratory data showing that the experimental drug may be therapeutically useful. Animal testing focuses on both acute and chronic toxicity. In addition, the initial bioavailability and pharmacokinetics studies in animals help to predict a reasonable starting dose in humans. The goal at this stage of preclinical testing is to gather adequate in vitro and animal data to define a drug's initial pharmaceutical and toxicologic profile to support human testing and to gather data to assist the design of the initial clinical protocols.

While preclinical testing is going on and when the risk/benefit ratio appears to be acceptable, a commercial drug sponsor or sponsor-investigator develops a clinical protocol (plan) for the initial studies in humans. To study the new drug in humans in the US, a sponsor must file an IND with the FDA.[1] This mechanism in the Food, Drug, and Cosmetic Act provides exemptions for interstate shipment of INDs from the requirement of having an approved NDA. Regulations permit the interstate shipment of new drugs if they are intended solely for investigational use by experts whose scientific training and experience qualify them to investigate the safety and effectiveness of a drug.

The sponsor must submit the IND application with a signed Form 1571 and must ensure that a Form 1572 was submitted by the investigator (Figures 6 and 7). The sponsor must submit results of all animal studies that were conducted prior to submitting the IND application to document that the drug will not impose an unreasonable risk to human subjects. The following information also needs to be submitted:

- descriptive name of the drug and the route of administration;
- complete list of components, quantitative composition, source of the new drug, and chemical and manufacturing information;
- preclinical test results (any clinical studies or experience);
- clinical protocol;
- scientific training and experience of investigators;
- statements to the effect that the sponsor will notify the FDA when and why studies have been discontinued; and

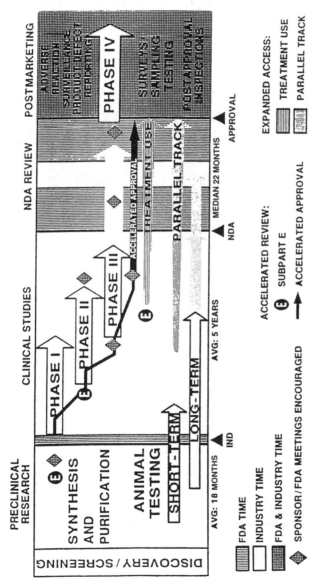

Figure 5
New Drug
Development
AVG = average;
FDA = Food and
Drug
Administration;
IND = investiga-
tional new drug;
NDA = new drug
application.

DEPARTMENT OF HEALTH AND HUMAN SERVICES PUBLIC HEALTH SERVICE FOOD AND DRUG ADMINISTRATION **INVESTIGATIONAL NEW DRUG APPLICATION (IND)** *(TITLE 21, CODE OF FEDERAL REGULATIONS (CFR) PART 312)*	Form Approved: OMB No. 0910-0014. Expiration Date: February 29, 1996. See OMB Statement on Reverse. NOTE: No drug may be shipped or clinical investigation begun until an IND for that investigation is in effect (21 CFR 312.40).

Figure 6
Investigational New Drug Application

1. NAME OF SPONSOR	2. DATE OF SUBMISSION
3. ADDRESS *(Number, Street, City, State and Zip Code)*	4. TELEPHONE NUMBER *(Include Area Code)*

5. NAME(S) OF DRUG *(Include all available names: Trade, Generic, Chemical, Code)*	6. IND NUMBER *(If previously assigned)*

7. INDICATION(S) *(Covered by this submission)*

8. PHASE(S) OF CLINICAL INVESTIGATION TO BE CONDUCTED: ☐ PHASE 1 ☐ PHASE 2 ☐ PHASE 3 ☐ OTHER _____
(Specify)

9. LIST NUMBERS OF ALL INVESTIGATIONAL NEW DRUG APPLICATIONS (21 CFR Part 312), NEW DRUG OR ANTIBIOTIC APPLICATIONS *(21 CFR Part 314)*, DRUG MASTER FILES *(21 CFR Part 314.420)*, AND PRODUCT LICENSE APPLICATIONS (21 CFR Part 601) REFERRED TO IN THIS APPLICATION.

10. *IND submission should be consecutively numbered. The initial IND should be numbered "Serial number: 000." The next submission (e.g., amendment, report, or correspondence) should be numbered "Serial Number: 001." Subsequent submissions should be numbered consecutively in the order in which they are submitted.*	SERIAL NUMBER _ _ _

11. THIS SUBMISSION CONTAINS THE FOLLOWING: *(Check all that apply)*
☐ INITIAL INVESTIGATIONAL NEW DRUG APPLICATION (IND)   ☐ RESPONSE TO CLINICAL HOLD

PROTOCOL AMENDMENT(S):	INFORMATION AMENDMENT(S):	IND SAFETY REPORT(S):
☐ NEW PROTOCOL	☐ CHEMISTRY/MICROBIOLOGY	☐ INITIAL WRITTEN REPORT
☐ CHANGE IN PROTOCOL	☐ PHARMACOLOGY/TOXICOLOGY	☐ FOLLOW-UP TO A WRITTEN REPORT
☐ NEW INVESTIGATOR	☐ CLINICAL	

☐ RESPONSE TO FDA REQUEST FOR INFORMATION   ☐ ANNUAL REPORT   ☐ GENERAL CORRESPONDENCE
☐ REQUEST FOR REINSTATEMENT OF IND THAT IS WITHDRAWN,   ☐ OTHER _____
INACTIVATED, TERMINATED OR DISCONTINUED   *(Specify)*

CHECK ONLY IF APPLICABLE

JUSTIFICATION STATEMENT MUST BE SUBMITTED WITH APPLICATION FOR ANY CHECKED BELOW. REFER TO THE CITED CFR SECTION FOR FURTHER INFORMATION.

☐ TREATMENT IND 21 CFR 312.85(b)   ☐ TREATMENT PROTOCOL 21 CFR 312.35(a)   ☐ CHARGE REQUEST/NOTIFICATION 21 CFR312.7(d)

FOR FDA USE ONLY

CDR/DBIND/DGD RECEIPT STAMP	DDR RECEIPT STAMP	IND NUMBER ASSIGNED:
		DIVISION ASSIGNMENT:

FORM FDA 1571 (1/96)   PREVIOUS EDITION IS OBSOLETE.

- notice that an institutional review board will be responsible for continuing review of the proposed study and that informed consent will be obtained.

The sponsor must wait 30 calendar days after submitting the IND application before beginning the initial test in humans. This period allows the FDA to determine whether there are any safety problems that would not permit the drug's use in humans. If there are concerns, the FDA places the application on clinical hold, and the investigator may not begin testing in humans until changes are made to eliminate the safety problems.[2] In the absence of a clinical hold, the investigator may begin testing in humans. Following the initial submission of an IND application, further clinical trial protocols require only notification to the FDA (i.e., no further 30-d wait).

Figure 7
Statement of Investigator

DEPARTMENT OF HEALTH AND HUMAN SERVICES PUBLIC HEALTH SERVICE FOOD AND DRUG ADMINISTRATION **STATEMENT OF INVESTIGATOR** ***(TITLE 21, CODE OF FEDERAL REGULATIONS (CFR) PART 312)*** (See instructions on reverse side.)	Form Approved: OMB No. 0910-0014. Expiration Date: February 29, 1996. *See OMB Statement on Reverse.* NOTE: No investigator may participate in an investigation until he/she provides the sponsor with a completed, signed Statement of Investigator, Form FDA 1572 (21 CFR 312.53(c)).

1. NAME AND ADDRESS OF INVESTIGATOR

2. EDUCATION, TRAINING, AND EXPERIENCE THAT QUALIFIES THE INVESTIGATOR AS AN EXPERT IN THE CLINICAL INVESTIGATION OF THE DRUG FOR THE USE UNDER INVESTIGATION. ONE OF THE FOLLOWING IS ATTACHED.

☐ CURRICULUM VITAE ☐ OTHER STATEMENT OF QUALIFICATIONS

3. NAME AND ADDRESS OF ANY MEDICAL SCHOOL, HOSPITAL OR OTHER RESEARCH FACILITY WHERE THE CLINICAL INVESTIGATION(S) WILL BE CONDUCTED.

4. NAME AND ADDRESS OF ANY CLINICAL LABORATORY FACILITIES TO BE USED IN THE STUDY.

5. NAME AND ADDRESS OF THE INSTITUTIONAL REVIEW BOARD (IRB) THAT IS RESPONSIBLE FOR REVIEW AND APPROVAL OF THE STUDY(IES).

6. NAMES OF THE SUBINVESTIGATORS *(e.g., research fellows, residents, associates)* WHO WILL BE ASSISTING THE INVESTIGATOR IN THE CONDUCT OF THE INVESTIGATION(S).

7. NAME AND CODE NUMBER, IF ANY, OF THE PROTOCOL(S) IN THE IND FOR THE STUDY(IES) TO BE CONDUCTED BY THE INVESTIGATOR.

FORM FDA 1572 (1/96) PREVIOUS EDITION IS OBSOLETE.

The number of active INDs (both commercial and research) submitted to the FDA is displayed in Figure 8.

Clinical testing is typically divided into three consecutive regulatory phases.

Phase I. The first phase of human testing is directed at determining the safety of the drug, its pharmacokinetics, and its acute dose-limiting toxicities and possible levels of toxicity. These studies are usually conducted on 20–80 healthy volunteers. About 70% of drugs successfully complete this phase and go on to Phase II.

Phase II. The second phase of human testing is performed on closely monitored patients to learn more about the drug's safety and effectiveness. The number of patients monitored in this phase depends on the nature of the drug, but usually there are about 200. Most Phase II testing is directed at the treatment or prevention of a specific disease.

Additional animal testing is usually undertaken concurrently to gain further safety information on more chronic toxicities. If the tests show that the drug may be useful in treating a disease, and if long-term animal testing indicates no unwarranted harm, the sponsor then proceeds to Phase III testing. Approximately 33% of drugs successfully complete Phase II and go on to Phase III.

Phase III. This phase involves the most extensive testing. Phase III studies are designed to further assess the safety, effectiveness, and most desirable dosage of the drug in treating a specific disease in a large group of patients (usually several hundred to several thousand, depending on the drug).[3] During Phase III, the drug is used the way it is intended to be administered when marketed. Additional testing intended to define more specifically any drug-related adverse effects is also done in Phase III. The Food, Drug, and Cosmetic Act requires evidence of safety and effectiveness from adequate and well-controlled clinical trials for a drug to be approved for marketing in the US. Approximately 25–30% of drugs will clear Phase III.

As the investigational studies progress, the IND application must be amended to include new protocols, progress reports, and stability data. Once Phase III is completed and the sponsor believes the drug is safe and effective under specific conditions, the sponsor can submit an NDA to the FDA for approval to market the drug. Approximately 20% of the drugs that enter Phase I testing are eventually approved (Figure 9).[4] A study[5] con-

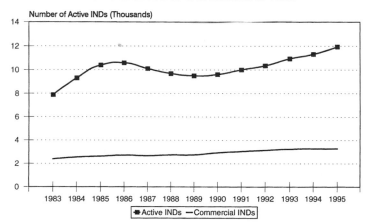

**NUMBER OF ACTIVE INDs
AT THE CLOSE OF THE CALENDAR YEAR**

Number of Active INDs (Thousands)

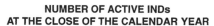

Figure 8
Number of Active
Investigational
New Drugs (INDs)
at the Close of
the Calendar Year

ducted of INDs filed from 1980 to 1984 analyzed the reasons for terminating the IND trial. The study indicated that 43% of those terminations that occurred at least 4 years after filing were for economic reasons, 31% were for efficacy reasons, and only 21% were for safety issues. Thus, economic consideration was the primary reason underlying late-stage termination of clinical research.

By the time an NDA is submitted, a drug has usually been studied in several hundred to several thousand patients, and sufficient data exist to determine whether the product is safe and effective (i.e., the benefits outweigh the risk for the condition to be treated), utilizing current regulatory standards. The applicant must submit a signed Form 356h (Figure 10) and two copies of the NDA (an archival and a review copy). The archival copy is a complete copy of the application that serves as a permanent reference source for the FDA, and it includes some of the case report forms and tabulations on the clinical studies.

The NDA is the formal application requesting approval to market a new drug for human use. Within 60 days after receiving an NDA, the FDA determines whether the application is suitably complete or "fileable."[6] The decision to file an NDA does not address the safety or effectiveness that the data suggest; therefore, it is neither a decision to approve the drug nor an implication that approval is imminent or likely. After the application has been filed, the FDA multidisciplinary review team continues to review the data in the application in depth to determine whether the product has met the requirements for commercial marketing.

Early in the review process, all NDAs and commercially sponsored INDs are classified by chemical type and therapeutic potential, as described in Figure 11. The chemical classification of a particular application is determined by comparing the active ingredient(s) with other prod-

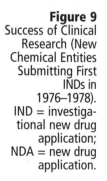

Figure 9 Success of Clinical Research (New Chemical Entities Submitting First INDs in 1976–1978). IND = investigational new drug application; NDA = new drug application.

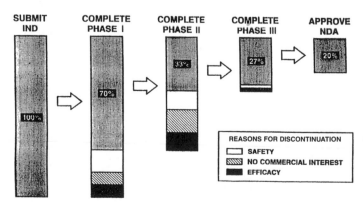

DEPARTMENT OF HEALTH AND HUMAN SERVICES
PUBLIC HEALTH SERVICE
FOOD AND DRUG ADMINISTRATION

APPLICATION TO MARKET A NEW DRUG FOR HUMAN USE OR AN ANTIBIOTIC DRUG FOR HUMAN USE

(Title 21, Code of Federal Regulations, 314)

Form Approved: OMB No. 0910-0001. Expiration Date: December 31, 1995. See OMB Statement on Page 3.

FOR FDA USE ONLY

DATE RECEIVED	DATE FILED
DIVISION ASSIGNED	NDA/ANDA NO. ASS.

NOTE: No application may be filed unless a completed application form has been received *(21 CFR Part 314)*.

NAME OF APPLICANT — DATE OF SUBMISSION

TELEPHONE NO. *(Include Area Code)*

ADDRESS *(Number, Street, City, State and ZIP Code)* — NEW DRUG OR ANTIBIOTIC APPLICATION NUMBER *(if previously issued)*

DRUG PRODUCT

ESTABLISHED NAME *(e.g., USP/USAN)* — PROPRIETARY NAME *(if any)*

CODE NAME *(if any)* — CHEMICAL NAME

DOSAGE FORM — ROUTE OF ADMINISTRATION — STRENGTHS (S)

PROPOSED INDICATIONS FOR USE

LIST NUMBERS OF ALL INVESTIGATIONAL NEW DRUG APPLICATIONS *(21 CFR Part 312)*, NEW DRUG OR ANTIBIOTIC APPLICATIONS *(21 CFR Part 314)*, AND DRUG MASTER FILES *(21 CFR 314.420)* REFERRED TO IN THIS APPLICATION:

INFORMATION ON APPLICATION

TYPE OF APPLICATION *(Check one)*

☐ THIS SUBMISSION IS A FULL APPLICATION *(21 CFR 314.50)* ☐ THIS SUBMISSION IS AN ABBREVIATED APPLICATION (ANDA) *(21 CFR 314.55)*

IF AN ANDA, IDENTIFY THE APPROVED DRUG PRODUCT THAT IS THE BASIS FOR THE SUBMISSION

NAME OF DRUG — HOLDER OF APPROVED APPLICATION

TYPE SUBMISSION *(Check one)*

☐ PRESUBMISSION ☐ AN AMENDMENT TO A PENDING APPLICATION ☐ SUPPLEMENTAL APPLICATION

☐ ORIGINAL APPLICATION ☐ RESUBMISSION

SPECIFIC REGULATION(S) TO SUPPORT CHANGE OF APPLICATION *(e.g., Part 314.70(b)(2)(iv))* ______

PROPOSED MARKETING STATUS *(Check one)*

☐ APPLICATION FOR A PRESCRIPTION DRUG PRODUCT *(Rx)* ☐ APPLICATION FOR AN OVER - THE - COUNTER PRODUCT *(OTC)*

FORM FDA 356h (5/95) PREVIOUS EDITION IS OBSOLETE. Page 1

Figure 10a
Form 356h.

ucts previously approved or marketed. Therapeutic classification is the FDA's subjective estimate of the drug's therapeutic benefit over what is currently marketed. In general, a priority application represents a drug with the potential to provide a significant improvement in the safety or effectiveness of the treatment, diagnosis, or prevention of a disease when compared with existing alternatives.

If the FDA determines that it would be useful, an advisory committee composed of non-FDA expert consultants convenes in either a public (open) meeting or, if warranted, a closed meeting. A closed meeting occurs only when it is necessary to discuss proprietary (i.e., confidential, commercial) information. Committee members make specific recommendations to

Figure 10b
Form 356h.

CONTENTS OF APPLICATION
This application contains the following items: *(Check all that apply)*
1. Index
2. Summary (21 CFR 314.50) (c))
3. Chemistry, manufacturing, and control section (21 CFR 314.50 (d) (1))
4. a. Samples (21 CFR 314.50 (e) (1)) (Submit only upon FDA's request)
b. Methods Validation Package (21 CFR 314.50 (e) (2) (i))
c. Labeling (21 CFR 314.50 (e) (2) (ii))
i. draft labeling *(4 copies)*
ii. final printed labeling (12 copies)
5. Nonclinical pharmacology and toxicology section (21 CFR 314.50 (d) (2))
6. Human pharmacokinetics and bioavailability section (21 CFR 314.50 (d) (3))
7. Microbiology section (21 CFR 314.50 (d) (4))
8. Clinical data section (21 CFR 314.50 (d) (5))
9. Safety update report (21 CFR 314.50 (d) (5) (vi) (b))
10. Statistical section (21 CFR 314.50 (d) (6))
11. Case report tabulations (21 CFR 314.50 (f) (1))
12. Case reports forms (21 CFR 314.50 (f) (1))
13. Patent information on any patent which claims the drug (21 U.S.C. 355 (b) or (c))
14. A patent certification with respect to any patent which claims the drug (21 U.S.C 355 (b) (2) or (j) (2) (A))
15. OTHER *(Specify)*

I agree to update this application with new safety information about the drug that may reasonably affect the statement of contraindications, warnings, precautions, or adverse reactions in the draft labeling. I agree to submit these safety update reports as follows: (1) 4 months after the initial submission, (2) following receipt of an approvable letter and (3) at other times as requested by FDA. If this application is approved, I agree to comply with all laws and regulations that apply to approved applications, including the following:
1. Good manufacturing practice regulations in 21 CFR 210 and 211.
2. Labeling regulations in 21 CFR 201.
3. In the case of a prescription drug product, prescription drug advertising regulations in 21 CFR 202.
4. Regulations on making changes in application in 21 CFR 314.70, 314.71, and 314.72.
5. Regulations on reports in 21 CFR 314.80 and 314.81.
6. Local, state and Federal environmental impact laws.
If this application applies to a drug product that FDA has proposed for scheduling under the Controlled Substances Act I agree not to market the product until the Drug Enforcement Administration makes a final scheduling decision.

NAME OF RESPONSIBLE OFFICIAL OR AGENT	SIGNATURE OF RESPONSIBLE OFFICIAL OR AGENT	DATE
ADDRESS *(Street, City, State, ZIP Code)*	TELEPHONE NO. *(Include Area Code)*	

(WARNING: A willfully false statement is a criminal offense. U.S.C. Title 18, Sec. 1001.)

FORM FDA 356h (8/95)   PREVIOUS EDITION IS OBSOLETE.   Page 2

Figure 10c

Public reporting burden for this collection of information is estimated to average 20 minutes per response, including the time for reviewing instructions, searching existing data sources, gathering and maintaining the data needed, and completing and reviewing the collection of information. Send comments regarding this burden estimate or any other aspect of this collection of information, including suggestions for reducing this burden to:

PHS, Reports Clearance Officer
Paperwork Reduction Project (0910-0001)
Hubert H. Humphrey Building, Room 737-F
200 Independence Avenue, S.W.
Washington, DC 20201

Chemical Types[a]

Type 1. New molecular entity: A drug for which the active moiety (either as the unmodified base [parent] compound or an ester, salt, clathrate, or other noncovalent derivative of the base [parent] compound) has not been previously approved or marketed in the US for use in a drug product, either as a single ingredient or as part of a combination product, or as part of a mixture of stereoisomers. The term "new molecular entity" is used interchangeably with "new chemical entity."

Type 2. New ester, new salt, or other noncovalent derivative: A drug for which the active moiety has been previously approved or marketed in the US, but for which the particular ester, salt, clathrate, or other noncovalent derivative or the unmodified base (parent) compound, is not yet approved or marketed in the US, either as a single ingredient, part of a combination product, or part of a mixture of stereoisomers.

Type 3. New formulation: A new dosage form or formulation, including a new strength, when the drug has already been approved or marketed in the US by the same or another manufacturer. The indication may be the same as that of the already-marketed drug product or may be new.

Type 4. New combination: A drug product containing two or more active moieties that have not been previously approved or marketed together in a drug product by any manufacturer in the US. The new product may be a physical or a chemical (ester or noncovalent) combination of two or more active moieties.

Type 5. New manufacturer: The product duplicates a drug product (same active moiety, same salt, same formulation, or same combination) already approved or marketed in the US by another firm.

Type 6. New indication: The product duplicates a drug product (same active moiety, same salt, same formulation, or same combination) already approved or marketed in the US by the same or another firm, except that it provides for a new indication.

Type 7. Drug already marketed, but without an approved new drug application (NDA): The application is the first NDA for a drug product containing one or more drugs marketed at the time of application or in the past without an approved NDA. Includes (1) first post-1962 application for products marketed prior to 1938, and (2) first application for DESI-related products first marketed between 1938 and 1962 without an NDA. The indication may be the same as, or different from, the already-marketed drug product.

Figure 11
Classification of Chemical Type and Therapeutic Potential of INDs.

[a]Chemical types are mutually exclusive except in the case of new combinations. That is, a new combination (Type 4) may also contain a new molecular entity (Type 1), a new salt (Type 2), or a new formulation (Type 3). In such cases, both numbers are included in the overall classification number for the drug. For example, a new molecular entity representing an important therapeutic gain would be classified Type 1A. However, if the entity were in a new combination, it would be classified Type 1, 4A. DESI = Drug Efficacy Study Implementation (Project); INDs = investigational new drugs.

Figure 11
(continued)

Therapeutic Potential

Type P. Priority review, therapeutic gain: The drug, if approved, would be a significant improvement, compared with marketed products, in the treatment, diagnosis, or prevention of a disease. Improvement can be demonstrated by, for example: (1) evidence of increased effectiveness in treatment, prevention, or diagnosis of disease; (2) documented enhancement of patient compliance; (3) elimination or substantial reduction of a treatment-limiting drug reaction; or (4) evidence of safety and effectiveness in a new subpopulation of patients with the disease.

Type S. Standard review, substantially equivalent: The drug appears to have therapeutic qualities similar to those of one or more already-marketed drugs. All nonpriority applications will be considered "standard" applications.

Auxiliary Codes

Type AA: The drug is indicated for the **treatment of AIDS or HIV-related disease.**

Type V: Designated orphan drug: The sponsor of the drug has officially requested and received orphan designation pursuant to section 526 of the Orphan Drug Act (Public Law 97-414 as amended).

Type E: The drug was developed and/or evaluated under the special procedures for drugs intended to **treat life-threatening and severely debilitating illnesses.**

---

the FDA on complex and/or difficult issues that have arisen during the drug review process and on the approvability of the drug. However, the recommendations of the committee are advisory, and the FDA makes the final decision to approve or not to approve an NDA, not the advisory committee.

The FDA advisory committees may also consider pharmacoepidemiologic evidence of adverse reactions to an already-marketed drug. For example, the FDA received reports of serious reactions, including deaths, to Omniflox (temafloxacin) in the first 3 months of marketing, resulting in the manufacturer's voluntarily withdrawing the drug from the market. However, because this drug was one of a newer class of antiinfective drugs (the fluoroquinolones), the FDA asked its Anti-Infective Drugs Advisory Committee to discuss the problem and consider implications for other quinolones under development[7] and those already marketed.

The number of NDAs and new molecular entities approved by year is shown in Figure 12. There is tremendous interest in the amount of time it takes the FDA to review and approve drugs. Table 1 displays total times to approval for NDAs, including the new molecular entities. The total time to approval is defined as the time from initial receipt of the application to the time it is actually approved. It also includes the time the sponsor takes to respond to questions or deficiencies.

There has been notable progress made in recent years since the inception of the Prescription Drug User Fee Act in 1992 to decrease the total time to approval. NDA median approval time in 1992 was 26.7 months compared with 16.5 months for NDAs approved in 1995. Approval times for

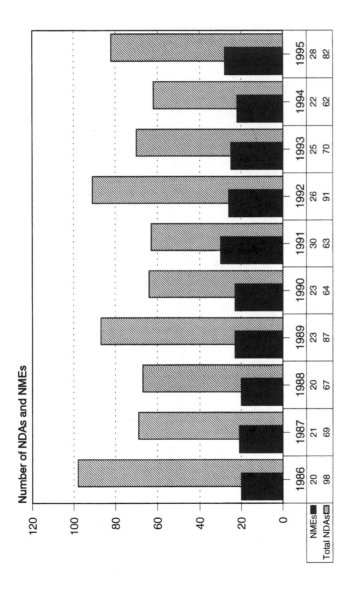

Figure 12
Number of New Drug Applications (NDAs) and New Molecular Entities (NMEs) Approved by Year.

new molecular entities dropped from the median approval time of 22.6 months in 1992 to 15.9 months in 1995.

It is believed that this reduction in the total time to approval is due to an increased emphasis on quality and complete submissions by the pharmaceutical industry in addition to the additional resources allocated to the Center because of the Prescription Drug User Fee Act. Some evidence of this increased quality of submissions is the fact that a greater percentage of applications are "fileable" at the current time compared with pre-Prescription Drug User Fee Act years. In any case, the FDA is far exceeding the performance goals of the Prescription Drug User Fee Act set to date.

POSTMARKETING SURVEILLANCE

The PMS phase (Phase IV) follows NDA approval. This phase, which is continuous while the drug remains on the market, includes collection,

Table 1 Comparison of FDA Total Approval Times for NDAs and NMEs, 1988–1995.		Median (mo)	Mean (mo)	No. Approved
	1988			
	NDAs	17.9	24.5	67
	NMEs	27.2	29.2	20
	1989			
	NDAs	19.2	24.1	87
	NMEs	23.6	25.4	23
	1990			
	NDAs	22.6	25.0	64
	NMEs	23.8	25.1	23
	1991			
	NDAs	21.4	25.7	63
	NMEs	22.2	27.8	30
	1992			
	NDAs	20.0	26.3	91
	NMEs	22.6	28.5	26
	1993			
	NDAs	20.8	24.1	70
	NMEs	21.0	25.7	25
	1994			
	NDAs	19.0	25.5	62
	NMEs	17.5	19.7	22
	1995			
	NDAs	16.5	22.7	82
	NMEs	15.0	19.6	28

FDA = Food and Drug Administration; NDAs = new drug applications; NMEs = new molecular entities.

reporting, and evaluation of adverse drug events (ADEs), and periodic inspections of drug manufacturing facilities and products.[8] The FDA is responsible for monitoring the use of the drug after its approval to ensure that changes and reports of ADEs are reflected accurately in the drug labeling, so that the benefits of the drug are still considered to outweigh any newly learned risks of the product. The FDA's PMS regulations require that drug manufacturers report ADEs on a regular basis, but reporting by other health professionals and consumers is voluntary. These reports are used to identify signals of potentially serious ADEs.

Sometimes the FDA requests that the NDA sponsor conduct formal studies during Phase IV. These postmarketing studies may be requested prior to marketing approval. In an analysis of new molecular entities approved between 1987 and 1993, approximately 53% have included some form of postmarketing research as part of their initial approval. During these years, each of the Phase IV drugs has, on average, involved a commitment to conduct four studies.[9]

The design of these studies spans the spectrum between epidemiologic studies and controlled clinical trials. These studies are sometimes designed to answer important, but not critical, questions that arise during the review of clinical data in the NDA. They usually further characterize the proper use of the drug. For example, Phase IV studies may be used to identify other patient populations in which the drug may be useful, refine dosing recommendations, or explore potential drug interactions.

To make a change in a product following its approval, sponsors are required to submit and obtain approval of a supplement to their NDA or, in some cases, to report changes in their annual report. Changes include, for example, adding a new indication, revising an approved indication, relaxing or increasing limits of specification for drug substances, establishing new regulatory analytical methods, changing the synthesis of the drug substances, changing manufacturing facilities, changing ingredients in drug products, changing packaging, extending expiration date, and changing labeling.

Initiatives to Expedite the Availability of Certain Drugs for Severe Illnesses

Demonstrating the safety and efficacy of a new drug is a complex and often time-consuming process. The time from initial discovery of an active compound to marketing approval is about 8 years on average.[3] To make promising new drugs available sooner in the development process to people with severe life-threatening illnesses, the FDA has initiated several modifications to the traditional development and review process. These modifications streamline certain steps in both the development and the FDA evaluation process for new drugs and have impacted access times significantly. They also provide new mechanisms for making certain drugs available to well-defined patient populations prior to full marketing approval. These modifications reflect a recognition that caregivers and patients are generally willing to accept greater risks from drugs intended to treat life-threatening illnesses than from drugs intended to treat less serious illnesses.[10] Therefore, these modifications generally apply only to significantly promising new drugs to treat people with life-threatening and severely debilitating diseases, such as AIDS or cancer, who are without satisfactory alternative therapy.

SUBPART E REGULATIONS

In October 1988, the FDA published regulations committing the Agency to more extensive and intensive participation in the development of new drugs to treat people with life-threatening and severely debilitating illnesses. Early and frequent consultation with the FDA by drug sponsors is one of the key components of these regulations. Traditionally, the FDA is not directly involved in the drug development process, except for the formulation of guidelines, until an IND application is submitted by a sponsor. However, under Subpart E, the FDA works closely with sponsors to design efficient animal and human studies before an official IND submission is made.

The intent of this early consultation is to minimize wasted efforts and time on studies that are flawed or less than optimal in design. Properly designing and conducting early basic research to establish the safety of a new drug allow studies to proceed in patients more quickly.[11] This more consultative approach between the FDA and the drug sponsor continues throughout all phases of the drug's development. An analysis of recent approvals from 1994 to mid-1996 showed the median total time to approval for NDAs classified as Subpart E to be 7.8 months, compared with 18.7 months for other NDA approvals.

Subpart E procedures provide for periodic meetings between the FDA and drug sponsors to review and discuss early study results and to plan for the design of the Phase II trials. As mentioned earlier, Phase II studies are usually the first controlled trials of a new drug. One goal in the design of Phase II studies for Subpart E drugs is to provide sufficient data on the drug's safety and efficacy to support a decision for marketing approval. This contrasts with traditional drug development, where results from Phase III trials are usually used to support approval. Phase II studies for Subpart E drugs are typically more extensive than Phase II studies for non-Subpart E drugs so as to be sufficiently robust to allow extrapolation to the affected population at large.

The FDA usually requires that results from well-controlled studies sufficiently demonstrate drug safety and efficacy for approval. Under Subpart E, one multicenter study of a drug to treat a life-threatening illness may be adequate to support approval if the evidence is unusually dramatic and convincing. These multicenter studies should have more than one independent investigator, each with an adequate number of available patients to generate independently robust results. The approval of zidovudine in 1987 for the treatment of people with AIDS is one example of this process. To increase the likelihood that a worthwhile therapy can be shown to be safe and effective in the shortest possible time, the FDA generally advises that sponsors of Subpart E drugs conduct two concurrent pivotal trials so that the results of both studies will be available for analysis and review at approximately the same time. If the results of the expanded Phase II trials do not satisfy scientific criteria for approval, additional Phase II or Phase III testing will be necessary.

A traditional role of the FDA has been to review information provided by others, usually the drug's sponsor. Subpart E rules establish a role for the FDA to undertake focused regulatory research when a sponsor lacks the resources or expertise to generate information deemed critical to the continued development of an important drug.

PMS studies play a potentially large role in the development of a drug under Subpart E. If a drug is approved primarily on the basis of information from expanded Phase II trials, the total number and diversity of the patient population receiving this drug will usually be more limited than if the drug had completed Phase III testing. This poses some unique problems and concerns: (1) adverse effects occurring with low incidence are less likely to be detected, (2) important drug interactions may not be well characterized, (3) dosing schedules may need to be better defined and optimized, and (4) other patient populations in whom the drug may be safe and effective may not have been studied. To address some of these limitations, the FDA and the NDA sponsor may work together to design post-marketing (Phase IV) studies at the time the drug is approved for marketing. For example, following the approval of zidovudine, the drug's sponsor (Glaxo Wellcome) initiated several Phase IV studies. These studies focused on answering questions regarding the use of the drug in children with AIDS, the safety and efficacy of alternative dosing regimens in adults, and the safety and efficacy in patients with less advanced disease.

TREATMENT INVESTIGATIONAL NEW DRUGS

On May 22, 1987, the FDA issued treatment-use IND regulations to increase widespread early access to promising investigational drugs to desperately ill patients. A treatment IND authorizes the use of an investigational drug in a defined group of patients with a serious or life-threatening disease before it is formally approved for marketing. To be considered for a treatment-use application, the following conditions must be met[12]:

- the drug must be intended to treat a serious or life-threatening disease;
- there is no comparable or satisfactory alternative therapy available;
- the drug is actively under investigation in a controlled clinical trial under an IND application, or all the clinical trials required for approval have been completed; and
- the sponsor of the controlled trial is actively pursuing marketing approval.

If these criteria are met, patients who were shown to benefit from the drug during the controlled trials may receive the drug while the NDA is being prepared and final marketing approval considered. To date, 39 treatment INDs have been allowed to proceed: 11 for AIDS-related therapies, 11 for cancer treatments, and the remainder for a variety of serious conditions including Alzheimer disease, amyotrophic lateral sclerosis, multiple sclerosis, and respiratory distress syndrome in premature infants. This mechanism was used to make ganciclovir, aerosolized pentamidine, didanosine, and zidovudine available to some HIV-infected patients prior to the drugs' being approved for marketing. Manufacturers may be allowed to recover the cost for a drug under an easier mechanism when it is in treatment IND status.

PARALLEL TRACK PROPOSAL

Another mechanism to make promising investigational drugs for HIV-related diseases more widely available to patients at an early stage of development is the parallel track mechanism. This mechanism was proposed by the FDA in the *Federal Register* on May 21, 1990. Under this mechanism, trials to monitor safety are conducted in parallel with the principal controlled trials. Enrollment into parallel track protocols is limited to people with AIDS and HIV-related diseases who cannot participate in the ongoing clinical trials. Existing IND regulations allow such open, nonconcurrently controlled studies (i.e., studies in which all patients receive the investigational drug, and there is no appropriate comparison group).

The parallel track policy provides unique safeguards, such as having a national human subjects' protection panel that serves as a national institutional review board, careful product selection criteria, and a program for patient and physician education. Studies conducted under the parallel track proposal are usually open-label, nonconcurrently controlled studies similar to those conducted under a treatment IND. Because they are uncontrolled in design, these studies are typically unsuitable for demonstrating drug effectiveness but may yield valuable safety information that would appear in the drug's approved labeling (i.e., a pharmacoepidemiologic surveillance function). The evidence of efficacy supporting such use spans the spectrum from the minimal evidence suggesting possible efficacy to that just short of what is required for FDA approval. The only drug to date to use the parallel track mechanism was the antiviral drug stavudine, which was approved in June 1994.[13]

ACCELERATED DRUG APPROVAL PROPOSAL

The FDA published proposed procedures for an accelerated drug approval program in the *Federal Register* on April 15, 1992.[14] To be eligible for this program, products must be intended for use in serious or life-threatening illnesses and potentially must provide meaningful therapeutic benefits to patients beyond existing treatments. This proposal provides for several new mechanisms that allow a significant new therapy to be approved for marketing at the earliest possible point at which safety and effectiveness are reasonably established under existing law. Under this program, the FDA has approved 13 NDAs since 1992. The median approval time for these applications has been 5.9 months, compared with 20.6 months for all NDAs approved during the same time frame. It is important to recognize that this "accelerated" approval does not, per se, accelerate the review process for these products but rather accelerates the development process by allowing use of surrogate end points as primary evidence of efficacy.

One principal element of this program is that approval of a drug could be accelerated by demonstrating a favorable effect on a well-documented clinical surrogate end point in humans to predict clinical benefit instead of requiring the completion of longer studies that demonstrate actual clinical benefit. Surrogate end points include laboratory tests or physical signs that are not in themselves evidence of a significant clinical benefit but are likely to be predictive of benefits, such as survival or relief of disease symptoms.

If an approval is granted using surrogate markers, the sponsor is required to complete ongoing studies to validate the surrogate to confirm the product's effectiveness as measured by traditional clinical benefit end points. In certain circumstances, the sponsor must agree to restricted distribution of the product. In addition, if the further trials to demonstrate actual clinical benefit do not bear out the product's effectiveness or if restricted distribution is inadequate to ensure safe use, approval of the product would be withdrawn through a streamlined process.

The first drug product to be approved under an accelerated drug approval program was didanosine (Videx) on October 9, 1991. Didanosine was approved primarily on the basis of data derived from early clinical trials that demonstrated the drug's positive effect on an immunologic or surrogate marker (CD4 cells) in patients with advanced stages of HIV disease. This use of surrogate end points allowed the approval of didanosine earlier in its development than if traditional clinical benefit end points were required, such as survival or incidence of opportunistic infections. Demonstration of actual clinical benefit of didanosine therapy was confirmed from the results of a large clinical trial that were submitted to the FDA and published in the *New England Journal of Medicine* on August 27, 1992.[14]

Under this initiative, the FDA has also expanded the use of the accelerated approval process for cancer treatment, based on verified and recognized demonstration of objective tumor shrinkage, for example.

Summary

The FDA as a federal regulatory agency upholds high scientific standards to ensure that products whose established benefits outweigh their known risks are available to the American public. Through changes in its procedures and regulations in recent years, the FDA has demonstrated its commitment to ensure that important drugs become available to patients with serious and life-threatening illness as soon as possible.

The policies, practices, and procedures of the FDA remain a dynamic force in the medical marketplace. More than ever, rapidly evolving changes in technology and scientific innovation challenge the FDA to balance issues of safety, efficacy, and drug availability in coherent public policies. In addition, with the advent of user fees, the FDA is committed to reducing review times for all new drugs. With the additional resources used to hire and train new review staff and increase process efficiency through electronic information technology, mechanisms for speeding the review process and providing early and complete feedback to sponsors regarding deficiencies in their applications are being identified, implemented, and refined. Providing early access to appropriate drugs and drug approval remains a dynamic process undergoing continual improvement by the FDA as permitted in the interest of public safety.

References

1. 21 CFR 312.
2. 21 CFR 312.42.
3. Food and Drug Administration. From test tube to patient: new drug development in the United States. An FDA consumer special report. Rockville, MD: US Food and Drug Administration, 1995:6.
4. The outcome of research on new molecular entities commencing clinical research in the years 1976–1978. An Office of Planning and Evaluation Study, May 1988. Washington, DC: US Government Printing Office, 1988.

5. Di Masi J. Success rates for new drugs entering clinical testing in the United States. Clin Pharmacol Ther 1995;58:1-14.

6. 21 CFR 314.101.

7. Food and Drug Administration. From test tube to patient: new drug development in the United States. An FDA consumer special report. Rockville, MD: US Food and Drug Administration, 1995:30.

8. 21 CFR 314.80.

9. DHHS Office of the Inspector General. Postmarketing studies of prescription drugs. OEI-03-94-00760. Washington, DC: US Department of Health and Human Services, 1996.

10. 53 Federal Register 41518.

11. Cooper EC. The Food and Drug Administration's interim rule for expedited development and approval of drugs for life threatening illnesses: pro-active approach to the regulation of therapeutic agents for patients with human immunodeficiency virus infection, clinical considerations. Regul Aff 1989;1:191-200.

12. Investigational new drug, antibiotic, and biological drug product regulations; treatment use and sale; final rule, May 22, 1987. 52 Federal Register 19466-77.

13. FDA highlights: speeding approval/expanding access. In: FDA backgrounder. Rockville, MD: US Food and Drug Administration, 1995.

14. HHS news. P91-26. Washington, DC: US Department of Health and Human Services, 1991:2.

3 Safety Profiles of New Drugs at the Time of Initial Marketing
Bert Spilker

Abstract

A critical element in pharmacoepidemiology is the determination of the amount of safety data required when a new drug is marketed. The perspective is primarily that of a pharmaceutical company developing a new drug, but perspectives of a regulatory agency and a practicing physician are mentioned also. Limitations of safety data usually present at the time a drug is initially marketed are discussed. The greater the benefit/risk ratio of a new drug over existing treatments, the smaller the safety package may be at the time of the drug's initial approval. The two most important influences on the size of the safety package usually are the sponsor and the regulatory agency. A third major influence is the nature of the disease being treated. Acceptable safety packages are discussed for the following types of drugs: breakthrough drugs, "me-too" drugs, average new drugs with substantial medical value for some patients, lifesaving drugs, and orphan drugs that are not lifesaving. Delaying some safety studies from Phase III to Phase IV affects major breakthrough drugs and does not represent a trend that will affect the development of most new drugs.

Outline

R esearch- and development-based pharmaceutical companies frequently address the question of the amount of clinical safety data, efficacy
data, and other types of data (e.g., pharmacokinetic, quality of life)
necessary for inclusion in the initial regulatory submission (e.g.,
product license application [PLA] or new drug application [NDA]) for each
new drug under development. This chapter discusses how a company may
identify the amount of safety data required when a new drug is marketed.
Both general and specific factors that influence this decision are discussed.
The perspective used is primarily that of a pharmaceutical company developing a drug, but perspectives of a regulatory agency and a practicing
physician are mentioned also.

Limitations of Safety Data at the Time of Initial Marketing

Before a description of the factors that influence the decision of the
quantity of data to collect, it is important to understand the limitations of
safety data that usually are present when a drug is initially marketed. The
reasons for those limitations should also be understood. It would be ideal
if the full profile of the unintended drug effects (UDEs), as well as the incidence of each of these, were known at the time of marketing. This is impossible for several reasons.

First, only several hundred to a few thousand patients usually are evaluated at the time a new drug is marketed. This number is insufficient to
identify the nature and clinical importance of rare UDEs, although most
common and unusual ones will be known. It was estimated that zomepirac
sodium was administered to 15 million patients before it was withdrawn
as a result of a rare, severe anaphylactic reaction. An incidence of 0.007%
resulted in five deaths (0.00003% of all users).[1] The number of patients that
must be studied to be reasonably sure of having observed any specific
adverse reaction usually is three times the UDE incidence. Thus, to identify a UDE with an incidence of 1 in 5000 patients, 15 000 patients must be
studied. Algorithms, global introspection, and other techniques are used to
identify whether any specific adverse event is drug related. See Chapters 5
and 11 for a more detailed discussion of these issues.

The problem of having safety data on too few patients to understand
which uncommon adverse reactions are drug related at the time of initial
marketing is even more severe when a drug is developed to treat a rare disease. Data on fewer than 100 patients may be all that can be included in a
regulatory application; therefore, relatively few safety data will be available at the time of marketing. In the 1980s, pimozide was approved for
Tourette's syndrome, using data from approximately 60 patients, although
it did not have an orphan drug designation (personal communication,
Abbey Meyers, National Organization for Rare Disorders, September 1989).
Since the Orphan Drug Act in 1983, several drugs have been approved for
marketing with data on fewer than 100 patients (e.g., hemin, L-carnitine,

sodium benzoate, sodium phenylacetate; personal communication, Aleta Sindelar, RN, Office of Orphan Products Development, Food and Drug Administration, October 1989). Risk/benefit considerations often suggest that orphan drugs should be made available rapidly to patients, despite what may be obvious shortcomings in their safety profile.

The second reason limited safety information usually is available when a new drug is first marketed is that some severe UDEs may not be recognized until many years after the drug is marketed. Diethylstilbestrol is an example of this situation.[2] The potential for precancerous and cancerous genital lesions that sometimes occur with this agent many years after maternal exposure are difficult, if not impossible, to recognize in the early years of a drug's development and marketing. Major improvements in toxicologic methods and standards that are used to evaluate drugs since diethylstilbestrol was first marketed should minimize and perhaps prevent future occurrences of this type of problem. These changes include the necessity of conducting teratology studies and more elaborate reproduction studies in animals to evaluate fertility, reproductive function, and perinatal and postnatal aspects.

Third, it is impossible to study fully or even to predict all areas in which safety problems may arise. There is an almost infinite combination of concurrent diseases, potential drug interactions, patient ages, genetic predispositions, and other factors that may affect the safety of a new drug. Few of these possible factors can or should be specifically studied during Phase III, unless there are particular reasons to do so.

Fourth, drugs often are used for nonapproved indications in patients who differ significantly from those participating in clinical trials. These patients may have quite different UDE profiles.

Fifth, there are increasing pressures in society from consumer groups, politicians, and others to make important new efficacious drugs (i.e., breakthrough drugs) available for medical treatment at an earlier time than ever before. This means that some of the human safety studies traditionally conducted during Phases II and III are now delayed until Phase IV. This is appropriate when the risk/benefit ratio favors the new treatment over existing therapy. Examples of the types of drugs targeted for abbreviated Phase III development and for rapid regulatory review include important anti-AIDS and anticancer drugs.

Sixth, certain patient populations are either excluded from all clinical trials or so few patients are studied that their UDE profile is virtually unknown. This includes both children and pregnant women.

Seventh, the optimal method of treating patient overdose often is not established when the drug is marketed initially. The profile of clinical effects observed after an accidental or purposeful overdose may be incomplete or even unknown, because few cases of overdose may have occurred. As a result, determining the optimal method to treat those patients would be mere speculation.

Total Safety Package Required for New Drugs

There is no simple formula to define an acceptable size of a safety package for new drugs. The algebraic sum of interactions, pressures, and opinions of groups shown in Figure 1 will determine the appropriate size. Not all groups shown in Figure 1 are always involved, and other groups may express opinions on this issue, particularly for controversial drugs. *Although a single, precise formula cannot be established, an important principle is that the greater the risk/benefit ratio of a new drug over existing treatments, the smaller the safety package may be at the time of the drug's initial approval.* In situations in which the risk/benefit ratio of a new drug represents a clinically significant improvement over current therapy, there should be a shifting of some (or all) of the Phase III trials to Phase IV. This last point has not been generally accepted by the regulatory agencies, except for a number of clinically important breakthrough drugs.

The most important groups that influence the size of the safety package are usually the sponsor and the regulatory agency. Other groups generally play little, if any, role. For novel and newsworthy drugs such as

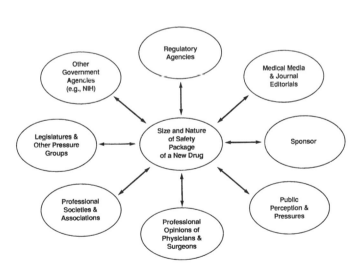

Figure 1
Groups That Influence the Relative Size of a New Drug's Safety Package

The arrows are double headed to illustrate that there may be influences moving back and forth between each group and those people responsible for establishing the size and nature of the safety package of a new drug. NIH = National Institutes of Health.

anistreplase (tissue plasminogen activator), most of the groups shown in Figure 1 became heavily involved in attempting to influence the size and nature of the efficacy package required.

Three types of safety studies are conducted on new drugs: (1) the basic package of safety studies, which is generally similar in nature, and often size, for most new drugs; (2) specialized safety studies that depend on the particular drug in terms of its use or its similarity to other drugs or compounds (e.g., dermatologic, ophthalmologic, gonadal, electroencephalographic, or sleep studies); and (3) additional safety studies that explore abnormalities observed or possible safety issues raised in clinical trial or in toxicologic studies.

BASIC PACKAGE OF SAFETY STUDIES

The basic package of safety studies required on all new drugs includes evaluations of laboratory parameters (e.g., electrolytes, basic chemistry analytes, basic hematology analytes), complete physical examinations with vitals signs and body weights, electrocardiograms, ophthalmologic examinations, and assessment of any observed UDEs. The number of patients who should have a complete battery of assessments generally is at least 100 for almost any new drug. Virtually all patients exposed to a drug during the investigational period should have at least a minimal safety profile obtained. This number usually varies from 1000 to 3000 patients, but numerous exceptions occur that may make the safety package required for marketing either greater or lesser than this range. There must be some balance in the number of patients studied in each of the tests of the basic safety package. This means that it makes little sense to have data on only 25 patients with complete hematologic profiles to demonstrate a lack of drug effect, and totally negative data on 500 patients with multiple 12-lead electrocardiograms on a new drug to treat a noncardiac disease. Any abnormal safety findings or unexpected signals of potential safety issues require a sufficient number of additional studies and patients to convince the sponsor, regulatory agencies, and physicians that there is either no problem or the problem has been adequately explored and described.

NUMBER OF PATIENTS EXPOSED TO A DRUG

Clinical safety evaluations must be determined at therapeutic dose concentrations of a drug. If a drug studied for several years at a dosage of 50 mg/d is found to be ineffective, and if a dosage of 250 mg/d is necessary to provide clinical benefits, then the basic safety package must be reassembled and possibly redone at the higher dose.

The number of patients required to be evaluated with a new drug does not refer to the total number of patients entered in a study but to those exposed to therapeutic concentrations. The total number of patients treated with a therapeutic dose for the full treatment period usually is far fewer than the number who receive the drug under various other conditions. Numerous reports state, for example, that the safety profile of drug X is based on data from 3000 patients. However, closer examination of the data often reveals that this number includes the following: (1) patients given placebo, (2) subtherapeutic doses, (3) therapeutic doses for inadequate treatment periods, (4) doses for patients with other indications in pilot studies, or (5) patients receiving active drugs who were used as controls.

SPECIALIZED PACKAGE OF SAFETY STUDIES

A number of specialized safety studies are almost always conducted prior to a drug's approval, based on data from the basic package of safety and efficacy studies, as well as on knowledge of the chemical class of a drug. These studies may focus on a particular target organ (e.g., eyes, heart, liver, lungs), on a particular physiologic function (e.g., digestion, metabolism, absorption), or on certain interactions (e.g., with other drugs, with food). The exact nature of these specialized studies varies from drug to drug, but the following is the most important principle in determining how many data are required: Enough data must be gathered so that a physician prescribing the drug can understand the relative risks of the drug from the package insert and can assess the risk/benefit ratio for the particular patient being treated.

The specialized package of safety studies overlaps the third category of safety studies, which explore any abnormal results observed. The principles for guiding both types of studies are similar, so a separate discussion of this type of study is not presented.

Three major factors affect the decision of the amount of clinical safety data to include in the initial submission of a new drug for marketing approval: the regulatory strategy adopted, the type of drug being developed, and the nature of the disease being treated. Each of these is discussed below.

Regulatory Strategies

Regulatory agencies vary widely in the type and amount of clinical safety data they require before they are willing to approve a new drug for marketing.[3] A company that first attempts to attain regulatory approval in a less-demanding country may take either of two views. It may decide to seek more rapid approval by submitting a minimal safety data package, or it may wait until a relatively complete safety package of data has been assembled. The strategy of submitting a minimal amount of safety data may easily backfire if the regulatory agency requests more data, and this delays the drug's approval. If a company wants to minimize the total amount of work required for rewriting reports, assembling and reassembling documents, and submitting regulatory applications, it makes sense to obtain a relatively complete amount of data before submitting the initial application.

The actual quantity of safety data included in regulatory applications on a single drug submitted to different national agencies often varies widely. This depends on the year of submission, rather than on an attempt to withhold data. Figure 2 illustrates two models of how clinical safety packages are assembled for multiple regulatory submissions. The simultaneous model minimizes the difference in time between regulatory submissions compared with potential differences that arise if a company follows the sequential model. In this model, it is possible that safety reports in regulatory applications sent to agencies A, D, and F not only contain different quantities of safety data, but may also contain conflicting information, interpretations, and conclusions. This could readily lead to multiple regulatory problems for a company if different safety results or interpretations were present, although the company would not be guilty of any wrongdoing. In fact, pending PLA and NDA regulatory submissions in multiple countries may (and in some sense should) be updated periodically to minimize any substantial differences between them. The practice of frequent updating, however, is frowned upon by regulatory agencies, although they generally are interested in a final updating of safety data shortly before the drug's approval.

Companies may be unable to utilize the simultaneous model for a variety of practical reasons. In situations in which the sequential model is used,

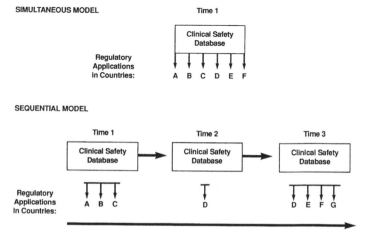

Figure 2
Models of Clinical Safety Package Assembly for Multiple Regulatory Submissions

the duration of time between submissions to major agencies should be kept to a minimum. The longer this time becomes, the greater the number of new personnel at both the company and the regulatory agencies. The new people will have to familiarize themselves with the data and are more likely to challenge the conclusions reached than are the individuals who previously worked with the data.

The components of regulatory applications in the simultaneous model vary in the amount of data presented, but the database from which the information is drawn does not. Expert reports are critical evaluations of up to 25 pages that summarize one type of study (e.g., clinical, preclinical safety). These reports are required for PLA regulatory submissions in many countries and usually are prepared by experts either in academia or within the pharmaceutical company. It becomes more problematic to prepare multiple versions of these reports when they are based on a changing database. The question that must be addressed concerns the types of changes in the database that require a new expert report to be written.

A company may initially submit an application to a less-demanding regulatory agency but intend to follow up rapidly with applications to more demanding authorities. The simultaneous model still makes the most sense in that situation. One of the difficulties in using the simultaneous model is that it requires more time and effort to acquire necessary data than if a company wanted to market its drug as rapidly as possible. The counterargument is that acquiring postmarketing data in one or more countries often helps speed regulatory approval elsewhere. A corollary of this view is that a drug should be marketed first in a major area where postmarketing data may be obtained and not in a minor market with little scientific or commercial significance.

The preceding discussion demonstrates that the regulatory strategy established for a particular drug depends on more than just the nature of the drug and its therapeutic usefulness. Other critical factors that influence regulatory strategies are the nature and transactions of the company, its leaders' personalities, and the degree of risk they are comfortable taking.

The clinical development plan indicates which studies will be conducted for a regulatory submission. At some stage during a drug's development, each of the studies that will be conducted is identified. The number of studies and number of patients targeted for enrollment in each study for any specific drug vary with different companies. At one extreme, these clinical development plans are designed to be lean or skimpy; the company decides to accumulate the least amount of safety and efficacy data possible to achieve marketing authorization. At the other extreme, the company adopts a "fat" plan and accumulates many more data than necessary for market approval. Of course, it is possible to propose a development plan in which a fat plan is chosen for efficacy data and a lean plan for safety data (or vice versa). Clinical and regulatory strategies are discussed elsewhere in much greater detail.[4,5]

Type of Drug Being Developed

A company that uses the simultaneous model for regulatory submissions must determine the standards to be used in acquiring clinical data. These standards depend to a large degree on the type of drug being developed. An acceptable safety package is discussed for the following types of drugs. This classification is a convenient one proposed for this discussion.
- Breakthrough drugs
- "Me-too" drugs
- Average new drugs with substantial medical value for some patients
- Lifesaving drugs
- Orphan drugs that are not lifesaving

A single drug may fit two of these categories. In the description of these categories, the primary focus is what safety questions should be addressed, if not answered, at the time of initial marketing. A related question is: What safety information may be reasonably delayed to Phase IV?

BREAKTHROUGH DRUGS

The amount of safety data necessary at the time of initial marketing for a breakthrough drug traditionally has been viewed as approximately the same as that for an average new drug with substantial medical value. One of the arguments for requiring a smaller safety package for marketing this category of drugs would be the desire of companies, physicians, and the public to reach the market more rapidly with an acknowledged medically superior drug. Whether regulatory agencies agree with this premise and would approve a drug for earlier marketing under these circumstances is uncertain. However, they do not always agree whether a drug represents a true medical breakthrough.

Most regulatory agencies accept the logic of deferring some safety assurances for breakthrough drugs to the postmarketing period. Nonetheless, two successive drugs of this type could be treated entirely differently by a single regulatory agency. Discussions with regulatory authorities to achieve an agreement and commitment to defer some safety studies to Phase IV would be an ideal solution to reach at the end of Phase II. The Food and Drug Administration welcomes these discussions. Unfortunately, those types of discussions and commitments are the exception worldwide rather than the rule, and companies must use their own judgment about whether or not to submit a PLA without Phase III data. Propranolol and cimetidine are examples of breakthrough drugs that were not lifesaving treatments of previously untreatable diseases. The sponsors of these drugs had to conduct substantial Phase III trials prior to their approval for marketing in the US and other countries.

ME-TOO DRUGS (FAST FOLLOWERS)

Me-too drugs represent agents that are relatively equivalent to one or more drugs already on the market. The exact number is arbitrary and depends on the type of drug, the differences between them, and the views of the persons referring to them as me-too drugs. These drugs often are developed because some or many patients are not receiving adequate treatment with their current therapy or have developed tolerance or UDEs. The rationale for developing and marketing me-too drugs is that some of the patients who are being inadequately treated might be helped with a related but different drug. This occurred with nonsteroidal antiinflammatory drugs (NSAIDs). Another reason for the development of NSAIDs is that some of these drugs were major breakthroughs at the time of their discovery and early development, but were beaten to the market by a number of competitors. Yesterday's breakthrough drugs may become today's me-too drugs.

A commercial reason for developing me-too drugs is that attaining even a small share of a very large market often justifies the development effort. Market research may suggest that there is a chance the total market will expand, that the drug will become widely used, or that other drugs will lose market share and development should continue.

Two points of view are often expressed about safety packages for me-too drugs. The first is that, since there are several (or many) similar drugs on the market (e.g., beta-blockers, thiazide diuretics, calcium-channel blockers), their safety has been firmly established and potential problems are well understood. The proponents of this view state that companies and regulatory agencies should not require as substantial a total safety package as for a new drug that is chemically and medically unique.

The opposite perspective is also widely heard and states that, because there are other similar drugs available, it is mandatory to acquire as many, if not more, safety data on a me-too drug to get its application approved. Companies that develop me-too drugs with the philosophy of acquiring a limited safety package prior to regulatory submission risk the chance that their drug will be expeditiously approved in a major market. They also risk the possibility that regulatory agencies will raise safety questions that brand the drug with a negative stigma. Usually most stigmas are difficult to erase. The company also may be branded with a negative stigma within the regulatory agency. Therefore, a lean safety package for me-too drugs is inadvisable.

Little, if any, pressure is ever placed on a regulatory agency to approve me-too drugs, and in numerous cases, these applications sit for many years on regulators' desks. When these applications eventually are picked up and reviewed, the safety data may be found lacking by new, higher standards used at that time. The regulators then can easily justify their denial of marketing approval for the drug, or they may request additional safety data. The latter response places companies in a difficult position because of the possibility that this cycle will continue. Similar problems also may occur for efficacy data on me-too drugs.

This negative approach to me-too drugs usually is practiced at important regulatory agencies and must be considered if a decision is made to develop a me-too drug. Nonetheless, there often are sound medical and commercial reasons (described above) for developing me-too drugs, and no company should eschew this practice. Additional points about me-too drugs are presented by Spilker.[4]

AVERAGE NEW DRUGS WITH SUBSTANTIAL MEDICAL VALUE FOR SOME PATIENTS

This category represents drugs that do not have special labels such as breakthrough, lifesaving, orphan, or me-too. They may be second-generation drugs that offer important medical benefits for some patients who are unable to tolerate UDEs of other drugs of the same class (e.g., NSAIDs). The appropriate safety package of drugs in this group is judged on an individual basis as described in other sections.

LIFESAVING DRUGS

There is universal agreement that the safety package of a new lifesaving drug may be smaller than that for most other new drugs. Despite this agreement, there is no consensus on the definition of lifesaving drugs and exactly how much smaller the safety package may be. The difficulty of identifying which drugs are lifesaving arises because most clinical situations and responses to drugs cannot be described simply. Some of the issues that complicate this definition are the following:

- If alternative therapies currently used to treat the disease are adequate or almost adequate, when could the new drug be considered as lifesaving?
- Must a new drug be more effective than existing therapy to be considered lifesaving (e.g., if current therapy is lifesaving)?
- If a drug is agreed to be lifesaving, but the quality of a patient's life is severely compromised by UDEs, should the size of the safety package be smaller than that for other drugs at the time of initial approval?

- What percentage of patients with a disease must find the drug to be lifesaving before that label is appropriate?

After these and other issues are determined, the issue of how much smaller the safety package may be for the new drug remains to be determined. This should be addressed in the same manner as for breakthrough drugs.

ORPHAN DRUGS THAT ARE NOT LIFESAVING

The safety package for orphan drugs that are not lifesaving must be determined case by case. Each of the factors influencing the safety package must be considered. Regardless of which definition of orphan drugs is accepted, there are many types or categories of orphan drugs, representing a heterogeneous group of investigational and marketed drugs. The vast majority do not represent breakthrough or lifesaving treatments. In fact, many are developed for diseases that already have treatments, albeit inadequate ones. A well-known example is Wilson's disease, which is treated with penicillamine, Dimaval (2,3-dimercaptopropane 1-sulfonate), trientine, or zinc sulfate. The need for new therapies varies widely among orphan diseases, and the appropriate safety package for a new orphan drug depends on the need for the drug in terms of its medical value and safety.

Nature of the Disease Being Treated

The third major element in determining the amount of safety data to obtain on a new drug relates to the disease being treated. If the disease is one with high morbidity or mortality and is not adequately treated (e.g., primary pulmonary hypertension, adult respiratory distress syndrome), then a smaller safety package may be acceptable at the time of initial marketing. The less the morbidity and mortality of a disease (e.g., allergic rhinitis, nausea, hiatal hernia), the greater must be the safety package of a drug used to treat it. The exact size of the safety package required depends, however, on an overall assessment by various regulatory agencies of the medical importance of the drug being developed, as well as on other factors described in this chapter. Drugs given on a continuing basis to prevent a disease (e.g., by decreasing a risk factor such as hypertension) must have a relatively extensive safety package at the time of marketing.

Summary

There has been a change in recent years to delay some safety studies on new drugs from Phase III to Phase IV, but this primarily affects major breakthrough drugs that are also lifesaving and does not represent a trend that will affect the development of most new drugs. The optimal relationship between Phase III and Phase IV requirements for safety is a relative one, depending on the perspective of the person or group addressing the question, the medical importance of the drug, its relative safety as demonstrated in investigational trials, and the time when this relationship is being defined. The factors to consider when designing a safety package are described.

References

1. Reines SA, Fong D. Clinical evaluation of drug candidates. In: Williams M, Malick JB, eds. Drug discovery and development. Clifton, NJ: Humana Press, 1987:327-52.
2. Chalmers TC. The impact of controlled trials on the practice of medicine. Mt Sinai J Med 1974;41:753-9.
3. Walker SR, Griffin JP. International medicines regulations: a forward look to 1992. Dordrecht: Kluwer, 1989.
4. Spilker B. Guide to clinical trials. New York: Raven Press, 1991.
5. Spilker B. Multinational pharmaceutical companies: principles and practices. New York: Raven Press, 1994.

4

Pharmacoepidemiology Study Methodologies

Stanley A Edlavitch

Abstract

This chapter describes and discusses the strengths and limitations of the major pharmacoepidemiologic study methodologies used in postmarketing drug surveillance. Special attention is given to study design considerations that permit causal inferences. The main methodologies used in pharmacoepidemiology include controlled clinical trials, observational epidemiologic studies (cohort, case–control, cross-sectional), ecologic studies, drug use surveys, and spontaneous reports of unintended drug effects. Examples of pharmacoepidemiologic studies using each of these methodologies are presented. When a question arises about the efficacy, effectiveness, safety, or value of a marketed drug, typically a mixture of these methodologies is used. Finally, critical factors are suggested for the growth of pharmacoepidemiology as a scientific discipline, including the value that society places on the questions addressed by this discipline, the availability and use of high-quality data to understand drug efficacy and safety and to provide outcomes data for economic evaluations, the development of training programs to prepare pharmacoepidemiologic scientists, and the expansion of currently existing forums for exchanging knowledge.

Outline

A s discussed in other chapters, an increased awareness of the potential effectiveness of drugs for preventing and treating disease, coupled with an awareness of the potential for some drugs to cause unwanted adverse effects, has led to the emergence of the challenging scientific discipline, pharmacoepidemiology. This chapter discusses the major pharmacoepidemiologic study methodologies used in postmarketing drug surveillance.

In Chapter 1, Porta et al. list the main questions that should be addressed by postmarketing drug studies. These include discovery of chronic or latent drug effects, discovery of rare effects, determination of efficacy in customary practice as well as in new indications, and identification of modifiers of a drug's efficacy and the comparative value of alternative therapies.

Because there are more than 35 000 prescription drugs (more than 2000 molecular entities) and 300 000 over-the-counter products on the market in the US, for example, it is impossible to conduct individual, continuous, formal studies for each marketed drug. To further complicate the scientific challenge, our knowledge and questions are not static. We continuously develop questions about a drug's efficacy and safety for current and new indications and either formally or informally evaluate the drug's efficacy, toxicity, and effectiveness in comparison with alternative therapies. Furthermore, the manufacturer may change the drug's formulation and, once the patent for the innovator drug expires, a number of generic versions with similar, but not exact, bioavailability normally appear on the market.

Issues surrounding postmarketing surveillance (PMS) have generated vigorous, healthy, and sometimes heated scientific debate.[1-6] Somewhat esoteric discussions of study design, statistical significance, and comparison of diagnostic algorithms have dominated these debates, but almost all parties agree on a few principles.

Areas of agreement include the following.

1. Premarketing clinical evaluations of a new drug may leave unanswered important questions about its optimal use. The limitations of premarketing studies include relatively small numbers of patients, short duration of therapy, highly screened volunteers, and exclusion of children, pregnant women, and the elderly. These limitations are addressed in Chapters 4 and 7.
2. The number of "unsafe" drugs that have reached the market is relatively small compared with the total number of marketed drugs. The manufacturers' caution during pharmaceutical development, Food and Drug Administration (FDA) enforcement of US federal drug regulations and similar diligence by regulatory agencies in other countries, and the vigilance of physicians, nurses, pharmacists, other

health practitioners, and the public have all contributed to the presence of relatively few medical disasters in the marketing of drugs.

3. In most countries, standards and/or expectations for medical care are very high. With few exceptions, we exhibit very low tolerance when pharmaceutical manufacturers or regulatory agencies permit the marketing of unsafe or ineffective drugs.

4. In most cultures, physicians and patients have different perspectives on drug effectiveness and safety. As a generality, physicians and pharmacists are advised to consider the efficacy, cost–effectiveness, and risk/benefit ratio of one drug versus another or of various regimens; the patient is concerned primarily with whether the drug is effective and affordable (or covered by insurance) and whether the unintended drug effects (UDEs) that the patient associates with the drug are tolerable.

5. There is no simple, single approach to postmarketing drug surveillance. Some postmarketing discoveries of UDEs and new indications have been serendipitous, but drug surveillance cannot rely on chance alone.[7-10] The complexity of monitoring the effectiveness and safety of all drugs and the desire to identify rare events require the use of modern population methods, in particular, the use of epidemiology and biostatistics.[11-15]

6. A PMS system must involve pharmaceutical manufacturers, the drug regulatory agency, physicians, nurses, pharmacists, third-party payers, the academic community, the general public, legislators, and the legal community.

7. A PMS system should provide quantitative data to aid in making therapeutic and regulatory decisions. These data must be adequate to measure the beneficial effects and the risks associated with drugs as they are used in actual practice and should provide information that can be used to determine the value of the drugs.

8. Epidemiologic study techniques and reasoning are essential to evaluate the safety, effectiveness, and value of drugs.

UNINTENDED DRUG EFFECTS

A UDE can be defined as a noxious and unintended response to a drug in humans that occurs at usually recommended doses.[16] In Chapter 5, Rogers discusses the distinction between the pharmacologic categories of UDEs and the importance of the reaction on patient morbidity and mortality. The effects on patients' physical, mental, and social functioning and on quality of life are difficult to measure and evaluate, but they are important considerations. UDEs affect the health professional as they relate to patients and their families.

Rawlins and Thompson[17] proposed a useful dichotomy of UDEs (adverse drug reactions [ADRs]) into two broad classes, type A reactions and type B reactions. Type A reactions result from exaggerated pharmacologic effects, and type B reactions are rare, unpredictable, and often more serious. Improvement in premarketing pharmacokinetic and pharmacodynamic studies, physician prescribing, and patient compliance could reduce the incidence of type A reactions. However, type B reactions can be discovered only through PMS.

The foundation to any PMS system is the quality of information available for decision-making. Therefore, the most important roles played in PMS are those of the healthcare professionals who are relied on to correctly identify and report unusual or unwanted life events as well as therapeutic successes to their colleagues, the manufacturer, and regulatory agencies and to cooperate with epidemiologic investigations.

A critical role belongs to patients who best know how they are feeling but who have not traditionally been encouraged to recognize and report adverse events to their physician, the manufacturer, or drug regulatory authorities. Patient input may also be lost when the physician or pharmacist chooses not to report patients' complaints about drugs to the drug regulatory authority.

In the US, the FDA (for practical reasons) traditionally has returned patient-initiated reports with a request to the patient to ask his/her physician to resubmit the report. This system reinforces the message that only health professionals can objectively identify when a drug is not working as well as expected. Although in the past the pharmacist's potential pivotal role was not adequately acknowledged, today there is a changing perception that the pharmacist can play a critical role in identifying UDEs and in educating patients on the proper administration of medications and about potential UDEs and drug interactions.

Because of the public health importance of ensuring that the risk/benefit of a marketed drug is acceptable to individual patients and to society, the application of epidemiologic methodologies has traditionally been oriented toward identifying UDEs. Cost containment and healthcare reform are important considerations worldwide. As a result, epidemiologic techniques are used to collect data so that decision-makers can make better-informed decisions about the value of various medical services. This applies particularly to pharmaceuticals, which continue to account for a small proportion of total healthcare expenditures in developed countries (higher in developing countries) but account for a substantial proportion of out-of-pocket and discretionary healthcare expenses in these systems.

In describing the various methodologic designs used by pharmacoepidemiologists, this chapter includes a definition of the basic design, information on popular modifications to the design, data requirements for the design, comments on methodologic flaws/considerations, and an indication of the information provided by the study design for clinical practice and public health/epidemiology decisions, as a basis for pharmacoeconomic analysis. In addition, comments are included on limitations in interpreting data from each approach and a few examples of applications of the approach. The purpose of this chapter is to provide an overview and/or review of important principles. Books have been written on each of these designs, and readers unfamiliar with the conduct of epidemiologic research are encouraged to refer to one of these references prior to embarking on a specific study.[18]

Pharmacoepidemiologic studies may be conducted to describe drug use; to generate hypotheses about drug use and health-related outcomes; to provide evidence to support a hypothesis generated from descriptive studies, theory, or other sources; to test hypothesized relationships; and to provide economic data on the cost of diseases and therapeutic interventions. Pharmacoepidemiologic studies use standard epidemiologic study design techniques. Pharmacoepidemiologic studies draw on the knowledge and techniques of a number of related disciplines, particularly epidemiology, biostatistics, pharmacology, clinical medicine, psychology, sociology, and economics.

Epidemiologic study designs are typically presented in two broad categories, descriptive and analytic. Because analytic studies always contain a descriptive component and descriptive studies usually contain analyses, the division is helpful mostly for understanding the purpose of the studies. Descriptive studies generally are conducted *to generate hypotheses* on the cause of a disease or a UDE in various patient groups or regions or for purposes of public health administration and economic planning. Analytic studies focus on the determinants of a disease or a UDE by *testing the hypotheses* that are generated by the descriptive studies. The ultimate goal of analytic studies is to provide evidence on the causality of a relationship of a particular exposure to the occurrence of a disease or a UDE [17] or other health outcome.

The data that are derived from pharmacoepidemiologic studies contribute to determining the risk/benefit of various drug therapies. In the conceptualization that value = expenditures/outcomes, epidemiologic studies have typically been conducted to provide many of the data on outcomes. Recently, epidemiologic studies have been conducted with the primary purpose of collecting both outcomes data and data on direct costs, indirect costs, and intangible costs.

RATES

Epidemiology is generally considered to be the study of the distributions and determinants of diseases and health in human populations. In

Last's book, *A Dictionary of Epidemiology*,[19] a broadened definition of epidemiology was suggested: "The study of the distribution and determinants of health-related states or events in specified populations, and the applications of this study to the control of health problems."

Epidemiologic study designs are scientific approaches that permit the collection of meaningful valid data to describe the distribution and determinants of disease and health. Comparisons of the occurrence of disease or other measures of health between groups of individuals with certain characteristics or drug exposures are normally expressed in comparisons of rates. Each of the study designs presented in this chapter has as an ideal goal to provide information on rates of various measures of health in individuals with different histories, characteristics, or drug exposures and to compare these rates to reach conclusions about disease etiology or the costs and/or effectiveness of various interventions.

A rate used for comparison purposes is calculated as:

$$\text{rate} = \frac{\text{no. of events, cases, or deaths (may be adjusted) in defined time period}}{\text{population at risk to exhibit the event in defined time period}}$$

CAUSATION

One of the prime purposes of a pharmacoepidemiologic study is to determine whether drug exposure causes an improvement in health or a UDE. The pharmacoepidemiologist tries to determine whether the drug is unrelated to the outcome, a sufficient cause of the outcome, a necessary cause of the outcome, a necessary and sufficient cause, or in the causal chain but neither sufficient nor necessary. A drug is a sufficient cause if, whenever the drug is present, the outcome occurs. It is a necessary cause if the outcome does not occur unless the drug exposure is present.

The issue of establishing causation from epidemiologic studies and whether it is critical to understand causation to develop public health policy has led to fascinating and somewhat heated debates among epidemiologists and philosophers. Chapter 5 discusses causation in pharmacoepidemiology in more detail. The reader is further referred to *Causal Inference,* edited by Rothman,[20] for a sophisticated collection of essays on these issues.

Many epidemiologists keep in mind a proposal from Hill[21] as a model for evaluating evidence from a study (or studies) to support a causal relationship between a drug exposure and an outcome. In biologic systems, hard and fast rules do not necessarily apply, because biologic systems do not always behave logically, at least based on our current state of knowledge. The Hill proposal is a guideline, not a hard and fast rule. Hennekens et al.[18] have enhanced Hill's model and proposed a useful framework for interpreting epidemiologic evidence from a study:

Hill's Model of Supporting a Causal Relationship à la Hennekens.
A. Is there a valid statistical association? How well was the study designed?
   Is the association likely due to chance? That is, was there power to reach a conclusion?
   Is the association likely to be due to bias?
   Is the association likely to be due to confounding?
B. If valid statistically, is the evidence consistent with a causal relationship?
   Is the association strong?
   Is the causal theory biologically plausible?
   Do other studies give consistent findings?
   Is the time sequence compatible with causation?
   Is there a dose–response relationship?
   Is the relationship specific?

Another approach attributed to Popper,[20] that causal inference in epidemiology should be based on predictability and testability, has a great deal of appeal, and the merits of each are discussed in Rothman's book.

DISEASE—PRESENT OR ABSENT?

For many conditions, coronary artery disease being a good example, it can be misleading to think in terms of studying the presence or absence of the disease. A more accurate formulation of the research question is disease: how much is present or how little is present (absent)? The purpose in raising this topic is as a reminder that most medical conditions do not present in dichotomies. In research, as well as in clinical practice, we use shorthand to describe a disease as present or absent. In actuality, we naturally and immediately grade the disease on the basis of severity. Moreover, we recognize that the pathologic processes that lead to clinically detectable levels of disease have usually been occurring for years prior to our recognizing their clinical emergence.

These considerations are extremely important in every epidemiologic study. First, the study investigator needs to determine the level of consistency and the degree of thoroughness that will be used in making diagnoses and screening for disease. Valid comparisons of associations in different groups of patients will depend on our understanding of how alike the patients are and how similar their likelihood is of developing the study outcome. For example, patients who are diagnosed early or preclinically (women with a few changes in the morphology of cells from a breast biopsy) will have a survival history from date of "early" diagnosis. However, it is not always clear that their total life expectancies will differ when compared with women diagnosed at a slightly later stage (an interesting discussion of the controversy over the value of routine mammography in women aged 40–49 years is found in the January 1994 issue of the *American Journal of Public Health*).[22-24]

Study Design Strategies

The major epidemiologic design strategies are presented in Table 1. The specific study approaches will be described in succeeding sections. Each of these contributes to our goal to describe and understand causal relationship.

Sequence of Discovery of a Causal Association — General.

Before looking specifically at these designs and UDEs, we find it helpful to look more specifically at the sequence for discovery of a causal association using epidemiologic approaches (Table 1). Typically, there are five steps[22]:

1. *clinical observation of a possible causal association between a factor and a disease*
2. *descriptive epidemiologic analysis establishing the association on a population level*
3. *analytic epidemiologic studies establishing the association on an individual level*

Table 1
Overview of
Epidemiologic Design
Strategies Used in
Pharmacoepidemiology

Descriptive observational studies
  Individual based
    Case reports
    Case series
  Population based (correlational studies)
    Secular trend analyses (ecologic studies)
    Cross-sectional studies
    Drug utilization studies
Analytic studies
  Observational studies
    Cohort studies
    Case–control studies
    Hybrid studies
      Nested case–control studies
      Case–crossover studies
      Case–cohort studies
  Interventional studies (trials)
    Controlled clinical trials
    Randomized, controlled clinical trials (blinded or unblinded)
    N of 1 trials
    Simplified clinical trials

4. *experimental reproduction of the disease by the risk factor and/or elucidation of the pathologic mechanism of the factor in the disease*
5. *observation that removal of the risk factor (or modification of the host response to it) decreases the incidence of the disease*

These steps may be repeated several times as new information is learned at each stage.

Sequence of Discovery of a Causal Association — UDEs.

Applying the same five steps to issues around UDEs (the same applies to other health outcomes):

1. observation of a possible causal association between a drug and a UDE(s) (descriptive epidemiologic approaches, e.g., spontaneous reports, MedWatch Program of the FDA; vaccines, Vaccine Adverse Events Reporting System [VAERS] of the Centers for Disease Control and Prevention [CDC]; permanent epidemiologic surveillance systems)
2. descriptive epidemiologic analysis establishing the association on a population level (descriptions of case series, drug use analyses, cross-sectional studies, vital statistics, secular analysis)
3. analytic epidemiologic studies establishing the association on an individual level (cohort, case–control studies)
4. experimental reproduction of the UDEs by the drug and/or elucidation of the biologic mechanism causing the UDEs (randomized clinical trials)
5. observation that removal of the drug (or modification of the host response to it) decreases the incidence of the UDE (descriptive epidemiologic approaches, secular trend analysis, vital statistics)

OBSERVATIONAL STUDIES

Observational studies are those in which the investigator has no control over who receives what kind of drug.

Case Reports. The most basic descriptive study is a detailed report by a physician, other healthcare provider, or a patient of the profile of single individuals.

Case reports are published frequently in the medical literature. They tend to document unusual occurrences and may provide early clues about the development of a disease or the occurrence of rare UDEs. According to Hennekens et al.,[18] a single case report of pulmonary embolism in a 40-year-old woman exposed to oral contraceptives led to formulation of the hypothesis that oral contraceptive exposure can lead to venous thromboembolism.[25]

The fundamental limitation of observations from single case reports is that each is based on the experience of only one patient. In general, it is not possible to determine whether an observed relationship is causal or coincidental. Several articles have warned against publication bias and the temptation to overinterpret case reports in the literature.[26]

On the other hand, while also warning about bias and against overinterpretation, the book by Fletcher et al.[25] includes a brief interesting discussion on the value and previous contribution of case reports (pages 189–191). Although it is usually very difficult, if not impossible, to generalize from single patients to entire populations without the rigor of study criteria, case reports have sometimes been instrumental in elucidating causal relationships, particularly when the outcome is rare and not related to underlying disease or clearly drug related. Examples in which case reports have been instrumental include the identification of vaginal adenocarcinoma in young women exposed in utero to diethylstilbestrol[27] and the confirmation of hepatitis caused by halothane.

Case Series. A case series is a description of a number of patients who exhibit the same exposure, disease, or UDEs. Spontaneous ADR reports are the classic example of a case series that is used in pharmacoepidemiology. A single case report may indicate an individual reaction and/or an extremely rare phenomenon. A case series provides evidence that a finding, even though still rare, is repeated. The major advantage of case series is that they often serve as an early warning system. See Chapter 9 on spontaneous reporting and the MedWatch Program for a discussion of how spontaneous drug event reporting is conducted in the US. In the US, vaccine-related events are reported to the US CDC in Atlanta (VAERS). See Chapter 17 for information about how UDEs are reported outside the US and for examples of the value of spontaneous reports for generating hypotheses about specific UDEs.

In a definable population, a case series may be useful for quantifying the incidence or prevalence of a UDE or for characterizing patients who exhibit a UDE. Since information is not collected in a similar manner on controls, case series analyses normally lead to the development of causal hypotheses, but they are not on their own adequate to substantiate causation.

In 1993, Bégaud et al. in Bordeaux published an interesting treatise on their work of the past several years to apply statistical approaches to interpreting spontaneous reports received through the French Pharmacovigilance System.[28] They provide insights into the nature of spontaneous reporting and suggest that, in certain instances in which good data on drug use are available and information on underreporting can be substantiated, incidence rates of UDEs for some drugs in a class may be calculated and compared. The authors correctly point out the potential limitations of this approach and the conditions in which it may be applicable. On the other hand, they also correctly point out that, with certain UDEs, it may be possible to estimate underreporting rates reliably and, in those instances, case series (spontaneous reports) become valuable as an analytic as well as a descriptive tool.

The approach of Bégaud et al. is appealing because we accumulate a tremendous quantity of drug use data and information on UDEs each year. This approach is a useful attempt to quantify the numerator and denominator more accurately so that we can calculate and appropriately compare UDE rates.

Case series collected over a long time period may be affected by the availability of newer diagnostic tools. For example, between 1970 and 1980 and between 1980 and 1990, there were significant advances in the development and availability of reasonably priced cardiac enzyme tests in most hospitals in the US. As a result, the number of non-Q-wave infarcts was shown to increase. Likewise, computed tomography (CT) scans and magnetic resonance imaging (MRI) are now widely available to the medical diagnostician. Thus, the potential exists to identify other previously subclinical disease and label it as a UDE. Such changes in the sensitivity and specificity of our diagnostic tools need to be considered when case series are collected over many years.

Another consideration in interpreting case series is that diagnostic accuracy may sometimes be very poor. One example of this problem was reported by Funch et al.,[29] who found that only 26% (25/98) of the reports of liver disease in rheumatoid patients who received methotrexate could be verified as cases.

One additional consideration that affects the interest in reporting a UDE is the time since the drug was launched on the market or proximity to publicity or regulatory action. This is discussed in Chapter 11. From a methodologic perspective, we must always consider whether new diagnostic tools, changes in standard practice, or other factors affect the identification of UDEs.

Secular Trend Analyses (Ecologic Studies). In a secular trend, time series analysis, or ecologic study, the effect of a particular drug or risk factor on the occurrence of a particular end point is measured at least twice, before and after the drug is introduced or before and after the drug is withdrawn from a marketplace. In a multiple time series analysis, the introduction or withdrawal of the drug is measured at varying times in varying populations and locations. Secular trend analyses are useful for providing additional data to investigate a hypothesis. Normally, the data are readily available, so the analysis can be conducted efficiently.

In all pharmacoepidemiologic studies, the data appear to support the hypothesis better when a positive high correlation between a rate of exposure and a level of outcome can be demonstrated. The concept is similar to dose–response curves familiar to all clinicians and pharmacologists. This also applies to time series analyses. When multiple points in time are measured and exposure can be measured (sales, patients, defined daily doses [DDD]) and when the rate or severity of disease or number of UDEs is correlated to the exposure level, the data strengthen the hypothesized relationship. Most frequently, the evidence does not meet the criteria to support a causal relationship in the Hill causality model presented earlier and can only contribute to the hypothesis, not prove its correctness.

When multiple exposure trends coincide with that of the disease, it may not be possible to differentiate which exposure is causally related. This has been a problem in developed countries since the Industrial Revolution. Frequently, we have observed deteriorating environments (e.g., worsening air quality), increased individual high-risk behavior (e.g., cigarette smoking, sedentary behavior), and changes in health outcomes (e.g., cardiovascular disease, lung cancer, bronchitis). Since we are aware that genetic factors, the environment, and our behavior contribute to health, in a changing environment ecologic data can generally only be suggestive or supportive of a biologic hypothesis.

A particular type of secular trend analysis relates to the monitoring of data available from demographic studies and vital statistics. The health of a population can be studied by evaluating its vital statistics. Vital statistics data collected from ongoing recording or registration of vital events include births, adoptions, deaths, fetal deaths, marriages, divorces, legal separations, and annulments.[30]

The CDC keeps records of abortions, congenital malformations, rubella, nosocomial infections, tuberculosis, and other conditions that may have a preventable component. All states have a common list of more than 45 reportable diseases that physicians are supposed to report to their state health departments, which in turn forward the information to the CDC.

In the US, the National Center for Health Statistics (NCHS) manages the National Death Index (NDI), a central computerized registry of death certificates from all states.[31] For approved research, it is possible to trace individuals lost to follow-up in epidemiologic studies for mortality status and often to obtain death certificates from the individual states. This system is particularly useful for longitudinal studies in which participants lost to follow-up could be an important factor in interpreting the results.

Studies of vital statistics have prompted many investigations and helped formulate a number of important questions about disease incidence and mortality. For example, why have stomach cancer rates decreased so dramatically in this century? Why has there been a linear decrease in stroke rates since the mid-1900s (which is prior to the introduction of antihypertensive medications)? Why was there an increase in coronary heart disease mortality rates until 1968, but a steady decrease since then?

Secular trend analyses of vital statistics have also influenced drug safety monitoring by exposing links between drugs and disease. For example, secular trend analyses provided evidence that the introduction of oral contraceptives may be related to thromboembolism and pulmonary embolism, and that large doses of a halogenated hydroxyquinoline may be related to subacute myelo-optic neuropathy in Japan. In the US, vital statistics also provided evidence that methyldopa was strongly implicated as a cause of cancer of the biliary ducts and that saccharin use is not closely related to bladder cancer.[15] Pearce et al.[32-34] in New Zealand found that the mortality rates due to asthma increased significantly with the introduction of fenoterol in the 1970s and decreased suddenly and markedly with the withdrawal of fenoterol from the marketplace in the early 1990s. This is discussed in detail in Chapter 20. Burgess et al.[33] and Woodman et al.[34] used this analysis to generate and support a hypothesis that they then carefully investigated through use of a number of epidemiologic approaches. Another example relates to bendectin. McKeigue et al.[35] provided a convincing argument that bendectin alone was not the cause of the suspected birth defects in bendectin-exposed mothers by showing that there has been virtually no change in the incidence of suspected congenital abnormalities with the withdrawal of bendectin from the market.

An interesting secular trend analysis was reported by the Western Australian Monitor Trends in Cardiovascular Disease Program (MONICA) of the World Health Organization (WHO).[36] The investigators noted a striking change in the use of aspirin prehospitalization and beta-blockers in the hospital from their population-based register of acute coronary events. They correlate these data with the decreasing coronary mortality observed in Australia and hypothesize that drugs may be playing a role in this decline.

Cross-sectional Studies. Another name for a cross-sectional study is a prevalence study. In this study design, exposure and disease status or drug effect are determined simultaneously among members of a well-defined population. The data may be collected at the same point in time or over a short period of time for all study subjects. Cross-sectional studies are often based on a probability sample of the general population. A cross-sectional survey may be launched to gather only a few pieces of information, or a more elaborate survey might include quite extensive interviews and well-developed procedures and instruments for data collection. The US census is probably the best-known cross-sectional survey.

The interpretation of cross-sectional data differs, depending on the acuteness of the onset of the disease or outcomes studied, the acuteness of the exposure, and the length of time the individual experiences the disease or outcome. Some measures clearly are not related to drug exposure. For example, gender and race are determined at birth and are permanent characteristics of an individual that are not related to exposures after birth. The relationship of other characteristics to disease status or exposure may not be certain. For example, job status changes periodically and may or may not precede and be related to the development of a disease or UDEs.

Cross-sectional studies are more typically useful for suggesting the etiology of diseases of slow onset and long duration for which medical care may not be sought until at a very advanced stage. Examples of conditions might include elevated cholesterol, hypertension, and osteoarthritis. An example of a cross-sectional study conducted for these purposes was reported by Barrett-Connor and Palinkas.[37] They conducted a cross-sectional population-based study in a California adult care community to determine whether an association exists between low blood pressure and depressive symptoms in older men. Kelsey et al.[26] point out that case–control studies (see next section) that usually identify incident cases at the point medical care is first sought and cohort studies that would require long follow-up are more difficult to perform than cross-sectional studies. Cross-sectional studies are not advised for diseases or reactions of short duration, because few people would demonstrate the disease or UDEs at any point in time.

These studies may contribute to evidence of a causal relationship between a drug exposure and an outcome. However, they are most useful for describing current practice and hypothesis generation. There are two major disadvantages of conducting cross-sectional studies to study causal associations. The first, mentioned above, is that the exposure and outcome data are collected at the same point in time, and it is often impossible to tell which came first. A second disadvantage of these studies is that persons who die quickly or recover quickly from the disease or UDEs are less likely to be included as having the characteristic studied. Every cohort study that identifies participants after birth is affected by the prior selective survivorship of the birth cohort. This is particularly important when interpreting the results of cross-sectional studies. The bias introduced by missing fatal and short episodes of disease or UDEs is known as the prevalence-incidence bias or Neyman bias.[38]

Cross-sectional studies are used particularly by pharmacoepidemiologists to establish disease prevalence, drug prescribing patterns, current health status, and changes in medical practice. They sometimes serve as the first step and basis for conducting a case–control study (see Chapter 10).

The most extensive cross-sectional health study undertaken in this country is the National Health Survey, which has been conducted for more than 20 years by the NCHS. The National Health Survey collects data periodically through a number of programs, including the Health Interview Surveys of 40 000 households, Health Examination Surveys of people aged 1–74 years, the National Discharge Survey, the National Nursing Home Survey, and the National Family Growth Survey. Of particular interest to pharmacoepidemiology is the ongoing National Ambulatory Care Survey, which asks physicians to report on medical conditions and drugs prescribed (restricted almost exclusively to prescription drugs) during 1 week of practice. Aside from providing valuable information on health and health practices, NCHS has made major contributions to survey and biostatistics methodologies. In addition to numerous publications, another source of NCHS survey data is "public use" tapes[39] that can be purchased at nominal charges through the Scientific and Technical Information Branch, NCHS. The Center is also putting many of the raw survey data on floppy disks formatted for personal computers.

On a much smaller scale than NCHS surveys, surveillance data are collected in large research programs. One such example is the community survey data from the Minnesota Heart Survey,[40] which collects information on prescription and over-the-counter medications and on health histories and measures cardiovascular risk factors for a sample of 5000 Minneapolis–St. Paul residents. The Florida Geriatric Research Program has conducted three 1-year cross-sectional surveys over the 13-year period from 1978 to 1990 to determine the frequency and pattern of hypolipidemic drug use in an ambulatory elderly population.[41]

The Health of the Population Study conducted in Stockholm, Sweden, in 1984 and 1985 has provided some interesting insights into the use of sedatives and hypnotics in Stockholm.[42] The WHO-initiated multicountry MONICA surveillance effort begun in the early 1980s has resulted in more than 160 publications and provides valuable information on cardiovascular risk factors and drug use (selected centers only) on an international basis.[43,44]

Drug Use Studies. Drug use methods are reviewed in some detail in Chapter 6. A few of the concepts from Chapter 6 are repeated here because of their methodologic importance.

One of the major sources of drug use data in the US is IMS America, Inc. IMS America conducts several ongoing surveys of drug use. Although IMS has numerous surveys, two that have been used frequently by the FDA and by pharmacoepidemiologists are the National Prescription Audit (NPA) and the National Disease and Therapeutic Index (NDTI). The National Drug Audit, initiated in 1964, is a prescription-based audit, collected at the point of sale. Data are now collected from a panel of 20 000+ computerized retail pharmacies, mass merchandisers, and food stores.[45,46] The NDTI, initiated in 1956, is a physician-office-based audit of a quarterly sample of 29 specialties and 2790 office-based physicians who report on all patients treated in a 48-hour time window. Data on dispensed prescriptions for most developed and several developing countries are available from IMS International.[47]

An additional source of drug use data for the US is available from Walsh PDS. Walsh PDS collects point-of-sale information from 31 000+ pharmacies and patient-based data on several million beneficiaries.

Although the data from IMS and PDS encompass information on millions of covered lives, the data sometimes have limited usefulness for pharmacoepidemiologic studies. In the managed care arena, there are several sources of drug use data. One of these sources is Diversified Pharmaceutical Services (DPS), a pharmacy management company formerly owned by United Health Care (DPS now owned by SmithKline Beecham), which has dispensing data on approximately 10 million covered individuals.

Typically, dispensing data have been shown to be highly accurate. Pharmacists are paid on the basis of the drug dispensed, and large insurers audit claims to ensure that dispensing charges are accurate. On the other hand, the pharmacist and physician are paid for information directly related to claims processing. They are not necessarily paid for accurately capturing patient age, recording diagnoses, or entering prescribing instructions. Moreover, since both the New Drug Application data and the PDS Alpha database are based on prescriptions, not patients, it is not always possible to calculate how many individuals are prescribed drugs that could potentially interact. This lack of completeness is compounded when patients go to multiple medical care providers and fill their prescriptions at multiple pharmacies that do not share common databases. A patient-based database solves this problem to a limited extent.

The user of pharmacy prescription data must be careful to inquire whether all medications under study are captured in the database. For example, generic erythromycin and generic digoxin may be available at a cost below the patient copay under a particular insurance plan. In these instances, the insurance plan or health maintenance organization (HMO) data may include only dispensed and paid-for prescriptions. The less expensive erythromycin or digoxin would never appear. The same applies to more expensive medications that are not covered and to medical services that are covered, but are restricted. This problem is encountered with all computerized record-linked databases. In some pharmacy databases, all prescriptions are entered into the database, regardless of payment source. In other pharmacy databases, only covered prescriptions are captured.

An example of a drug use study that combines many of the elements of an ecologic study was reported by Schor et al.,[48] who studied changes in the use of antipsychotic drug and other psychotropic drug use in Tennessee Medicaid enrollees from April 1, 1989, to September 30, 1991. The study was conducted to determine whether there was a decrease in antipsychotic drug use with the Nursing Home Reform Amendments included in the 1987 Omnibus Budget Reconciliation Act.

Several investigators have suggested using drug use data as an indicator for disease prevalence. This approach is most reliable when good-to-excellent drug use data, diagnostic data, and census data are available and when the drugs being studied are used almost exclusively for the condition being considered. For example, beta-blockers that are used for a number of indications including hypertension, cardiac arrhythmia, and anxiety do not meet these criteria. On the positive side, a thoughtful investigation of this approach applied to diabetes was reported by Papoz.[49]

The reader is encouraged to refer to Chapter 6, which more fully addresses the approaches used to measure drug use, the problems associated with classifying drugs, and the epidemiologic uses of drug utilization review data.

ANALYTIC STUDIES

Cohort Studies. A cohort refers to a group of people who have something in common at a defined (index) point in time. A cohort study is a study of a cohort of people who have not exhibited the study outcome (disease, UDEs) when the cohort is formed and who are followed for an adequate period of time to develop the outcome of interest. Normally, the cohort is stratified by individuals who have certain characteristics or into subsets of individuals who have been exposed to alternative drugs.

The analytic (observational) study design that most closely resembles the controlled clinical trial is the *controlled cohort study.* In this type of study, cohorts are characterized by exposure to the drug being evaluated, with a second cohort being untreated or exposed to an alternative drug. Controlled cohort studies are scientifically preferable to uncontrolled cohort studies in which there is no control group.

One way to characterize cohort studies is on a time axis. If the cohort is created in the present and followed into the future, then the study is a prospective cohort design (also referred to in the literature as a prolective cohort design). If the cohort existed in the past, can be defined according to exposure in the past, and is followed forward in time from the time of exposure, the study is a historical cohort design (also referred to in the literature as a nonconcurrent, historical, or retrolective cohort design).[30] The two designs are illustrated in Figure 1.

The design of a completely prospective cohort study becomes clear from Figure 1. What sometimes is confusing is the fact that a historical cohort study can be conducted completely from existing data (retrospective historical cohort study) or with outcomes that occur in the present or future (prospective historical cohort study). To confuse matters further, some studies are ambidirectional; that is, they capture data on exposures and outcomes that have occurred in the past and on outcomes that will occur in the future).

One additional study design variation frequently used in evaluating preventive and therapeutic agents comprises a prospectively followed cohort of treated individuals compared with a cohort of historical controls.[50]

Figure 1
Basic Cohort
Study Designs

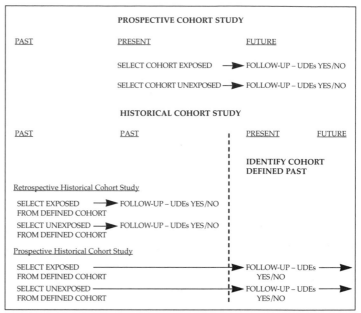

UDE = unintended drug effect.

This design applies when there is a great deal of confidence that past experience with the disease and/or drug used to select the control group has not changed over the time that the control group was followed. If secular changes in morbidity or mortality occurred, the results of such a study may be impossible to interpret.

If a drug was hypothesized to be a teratogen and also possibly to affect childhood development, it would be possible to identify a population of women who have taken the suspected teratogen during pregnancy in an HMO database (see Chapter 14) and to examine pregnancy outcome. For live births, data on birth defects could be captured from existing medical records. These children also may be followed prospectively annually from ages 1 to 7 years to determine developmental abnormalities. The Mayo Clinic provides an ideal environment in which to conduct historical cohort studies. Since 1907, it has kept complete records, including prescriptions written for outpatient visits and hospitalization for Olmsted County patients.[51]

Selection of Cohorts for Study. Cohorts may be selected for reasons of convenience (e.g., medical records are available, volunteers) or because the cohort is known to have experienced an exposure of interest (e.g., the first 10 000 people to receive a prescription for a newly marketed drug).

Historical cohort studies are possible only when existing clinical records permit correct classification of the individual's past exposures. The longitudinal information characteristic of these studies covers time intervals from the past to the present or to the future. The integrity of this study design depends on the completeness of the record-keeping system that is being relied upon to provide data from the past.[51]

Sample Size Considerations. Prior to conducting any cohort study, it is important that proper attention be paid to the statement of a clear hypothesis, to collecting existing data on possible outcomes, and to using existing data and hypothesized results to determine a correct sample size to test for statistical significance.

The advantages and disadvantages of cohort studies follow.

Advantages of Cohort Studies.
- Temporal relationships can be established; for example, exposure precedes the diagnosis of clinical disease or UDE.
- More efficient for studying rare exposures.
- Multiple outcomes, diseases, and UDEs can be studied.
- No selection bias based on disease outcome.
- May be used when randomized assignment of treatments is ethically prohibited.
- Retrospective cohort studies are usually less expensive than prospective cohort studies or clinical trials.
- Prospective data collection usually can be determined by the investigator with respect to quality, quantity, and frequency of collected information.
- Special cohorts with high expectation of developing a rare outcome may be studied versus cohorts representing the general population. For example, it would be reasonable to study the development of seizures in epilepsy patients exposed to one drug versus a second. The question would not be pertinent or practical in general population cohorts.
- Cohorts may be heterogeneous or homogeneous with respect to a previous exposure.

Disadvantages of Cohort Studies.
- Often require large numbers of participants.
- May be impractical to study rare outcomes, diseases, and UDEs.
- May require years of follow-up for sufficient disease or UDEs to develop.
- Therapeutic biases are possible, since participants are often seen more frequently than in normal practice, and consistent diagnostic information is gathered for each participant.
- Dropouts may be considerable.
- Often very costly.
- Data for various cohorts may not be comparable. Historical cohort

studies (retrospective and prospective) rely on data that exist in current records for exposure and other pertinent characteristics. The accuracy of prior data collection, the completion of all pertinent items uniformly, and the number of data points may differ among exposure cohorts. For example, individuals who are beginning to exhibit early symptoms of an illness may seek medical care more frequently. More frequent visits may lead to an increased number of tests and diagnoses not related to the exposure being studied.

Criteria for Evaluating Cohort Studies. DESIGN CONSIDERATIONS IN COHORT STUDIES. Table 2 lists criteria for evaluating cohort study designs (modified from Hartzema et al.[52] and Greenberg.[53] These criteria apply to both ran-

Table 2 Design Criteria for Cohort Studies	1. Is the study hypothesis stated clearly in terms that are meaningful and answerable from this design and sample size? 2. Randomization in exposure; this will ensure that exposed and nonexposed subjects have equal susceptibility for developing the UDEs relative to factors other than drug exposure. 3. The exposed and nonexposed cohort should be comparable with respect to demographics and other background characteristics that may affect the likelihood of developing the UDEs. (This is ensured by randomization when it is feasible.) 4. The exposed and nonexposed cohort should be comparable with respect to clinical characteristics (pharmacogenetics), which may affect the likelihood of developing the UDEs. 5. Drug exposure including compliance should be ascertained equally in both groups and should be thorough and accurate. Duration and amount of exposure should be captured. 6. Exposed individuals are classified correctly with respect to exposure and amount of exposure, and that both exposed and nonexposed individuals are representative of all patients with respect to risk of disease or UDEs. 7. Medical surveillance for the UDEs should be equal in the exposed and nonexposed cohorts. 8. The same diagnostic criteria and examinations should be used in the exposed and nonexposed cohorts. 9. Dropout rates and characteristics of dropouts in the exposed and nonexposed cohorts should be similar. 10. The cohort should be representative of the population that normally uses the drug. 11. The cohort should have the characteristics of an inception cohort; that is, the subjects are followed from the beginning of the drug exposure. 12. Is possible bias considered in interpreting the results?

UDE = unintended drug effect.

domized studies and observational cohort studies. They suggest that randomization is preferable scientifically whenever possible to ensure that exposed and nonexposed subjects are alike. With or without randomization, these criteria suggest that the cohorts should be treated the same and be representative of the population of patients who normally would be expected to use the drug.

As listed in Table 2, one of the important aspects of cohort studies is assurance that the participants who drop out are similar to individuals who remain in the study or, when this is not the case, that the reasons for dropout are not related to drug exposure. Some of the important factors to consider when evaluating dropouts are listed below.

Dropouts in Cohort Studies. Incomplete data on patients who cannot be fully followed (dropouts) can prove to be a major problem in a cohort study. The following guidelines may prove useful.

1. STUDY DURATION. The longer the follow-up period, the more individuals will be lost.
2. INTENSITY OF DETECTION OF THE UDEs. The more intense the follow-up is or when more effort is expected from the individuals (e.g., participation in extensive medical examinations or filling out lengthy questionnaires), the more individuals will be lost for follow-up.
3. MATURATION OF THE COHORT POPULATION. In elderly populations (most drugs are used by the elderly), individuals may be lost through death by natural or other causes.
4. CONVENIENCE OF ALTERNATE TREATMENTS OVER THE STUDY TREATMENT. The difference in treatment intensity or efficacy between the drug under examination and other drugs on the market may adversely affect the dropout rate. The perception of the severity of the UDEs may also affect the dropout rate.

Examples of Cohort Studies. Fourteen years ago, large prospective postmarketing cohort studies (7607–22 653 patients) were reviewed by Rossi et al.[54] for cimetidine hydrochloride, cyclobenzaprine hydrochloride, and prazosin hydrochloride. The authors expressed specific concerns about the designs of these studies, each of which was very expensive and failed to discover adverse reactions that were not already known from premarketing trials. They also found that reporting of adverse reactions occurred at substantially lower rates in postmarketing versus premarketing studies. The frequency of reporting decreased with the length of the study, and despite the fact that the practitioners were very willing to agree to participate in these studies, compliance with the protocol was found to be poor.[55]

There are also numerous reports of successful prospective cohort studies, both uncontrolled and controlled.[13,56,57] A large, successfully conducted multicenter prospective cohort study was the Collaborative Perinatal Project, sponsored by the National Institute of Neurological and Communicative Disorders of the National Institutes of Health. Between 1959 and 1965, it enrolled 50 282 mother–child pairs in 12 medical centers. Although this study did not identify any "new thalidomides," new methods to analyze the enormous amount of information that is collected in large prospective cohort studies were developed. In addition, reference data on the expected incidence of various types of malformations helped in the design of future studies.[58]

Two current European initiatives using a cohort study approach are prescription-event monitoring (PEM) in the UK and prescription-sequence analysis in the Netherlands.

Prescription-Event Monitoring. In the early 1980s, Professor Bill Inman, formerly director of England's spontaneous reporting system (the Yellow Card System) initiated a new event monitoring approach in the UK called PEM.[59-61] The basis of the approach is to create a cohort of newly prescribed individuals for all newly marketed drugs. The study ideally is initiated soon after drug approval. Information on who prescribes the drug is obtained from the UK Prescription Pricing Authority. The physician is queried periodically during the year following the prescription to report any life event experienced by the patient. In this way, prospective information is available on potential UDEs.

Information and associations derived from PEM are clearly useful for hypothesis generation. They are less useful for hypothesis confirmation and testing for two reasons. First, the response rates of prescribing physicians have been somewhat low for most studies (<70%). Second, the best comparison group is a PEM of another drug used to treat patients with the same condition and of equal severity. Comparisons are useful if issues of confounding and information bias can be eliminated or controlled. This may not be possible, since PEM data reflect decisions made in normal medical practice. Early in 1994, Professor Inman retired, and Professor Ron Mann (formerly of the Medicines Control Agency and the Royal College of Physicians) succeeded him.

Prescription-Sequence Analysis. Petri et al.[62] and Petri and Urquhart[63] in the Netherlands have proposed an interesting drug cohort study technique that can sometimes be very useful when a second drug is used to treat (iatrogenic) disease caused by another drug. They suggest that, if a UDE is caused by the first drug, an increased frequency (above that expected) of use of the second drug will be observed. They have applied prescription-sequence analysis to studying an alleged link between use of the antivertigo drug flunarizine and mental depression. In this instance, there was no clustering of use in antidepressants in flunarizine users, and the authors concluded that prescription-sequence analysis did not support the hypothesis of a causal link with depression.[64]

Case–Control Studies (Case–Referent Studies). Probably the least expensive, the simplest, and often the most controversial design to implement and interpret is the case–control study.[5,10,11,30,65-70] The case–control design can be very elegant and useful in pharmacoepidemiology. It is a cost-effective method for studies in which the UDEs have a low incidence or a long latency time. Case–control studies are also cost-effective alternatives to cohort studies.

General Design Case–Control Study. In a case–control study, patients are selected according to carefully defined criteria and compared with controls who do not have the disease being studied. Existing medical records and/or interviews and surveys are used to determine past exposure in both case and control groups to some characteristic of interest (e.g., past use of a drug). Case–control studies are sometimes called case–referent studies, case–comparison studies, and retrospective studies.

Nested Case–Control Study. There are a number of hybrid designs that combine aspects of cohort designs and case–control designs. These are discussed in Chapter 5 of the thorough textbook on epidemiologic research by Kleinbaum et al.[71] One specific hybrid design is very important and often used. This is the ambidirectional or nested case–control study. In this study, a defined population is followed for a period of time until a number of incident cases of a disease or UDE are identified. At a specified point in time, all cases and a sample of noncases (controls) are compared with regard to prior exposure to a risk factor. It is also particularly useful when the hypothesis being tested is generated after the prospective cohort study has been initiated. This design is particularly attractive when stored biologic specimens are available and has been encouraged for consideration in those instances by the National Institutes of Health.[72] When this approach is used, some data may be prospectively available on all participants. Other data must be collected retrospectively on the cases and controls included in the nested study.

A few recent examples of the application of this study design include a study of fatal and nonfatal venous thromboembolism in women using oral contraceptives with differing oral progestagen components,[73] a study of risk factors for HIV type 1 seroconversion among injection drug users,[74] and a study conducted by the Mayo Clinic[75] of trends of hospitalizations for gastrointestinal bleeding among patients with rheumatoid arthritis in Rochester, Minnesota.

The general case–control study and nested case–control study are depicted in Figure 2.

Rare Versus Frequent Outcomes: Rare Versus Frequent Exposures. Case–control studies are usually considered first when the outcome being studied occurs rarely and/or is suspected to be a latent effect of the exposure. This is because, with rare outcomes and/or latent effects, a cohort study may be impractical. For example, it is more feasible to assemble 100 cases of a rare cancer to study than it is to assemble and follow an adequately large healthy exposed population until 100 cases develop. Ideally, the amount of exposure in the control population is equal to the expected level of exposure in the general population represented by both cases and controls. There is an assumption that controls are as likely to develop the disease or UDEs as cases to be exposed to the drug if there is no relationship between the drug and the disease. When the expected exposure is rare, this design is not practical. Our understanding of the best choice of design, given how rare the study outcome and the drug exposure are expected to be, is listed in Table 3. When both the expected exposure and outcome are rare occurrences, there is no efficient study design. Epidemiologists normally are called upon to address issues that affect large numbers of persons. However, this is not always the case.

Considerations in Case–Control Studies. To ensure that differences in the experiences of cases and controls can be attributed to the drug or risk factor being studied, the study design must incorporate the following considerations.

1. *Diagnoses should be accurate and equivalent* for cases and controls.
2. *Confounding* the progression of the illness under study *with exposure* to the drug of interest must be considered and, where identified, accounted for through matching of controls and/or analytic techniques.

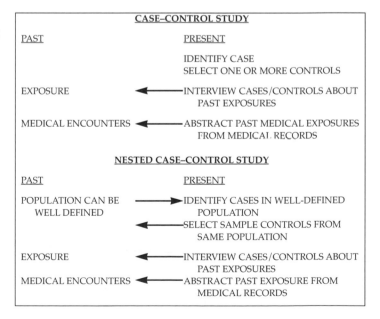

Figure 2
Basic
Case–Control
Designs

3. Patients included for study should have a *reasonable probability* of having been *exposed* to the drug of interest (e.g., men with breast cancer have almost no chance of being previously exposed to oral contraceptives).
4. *Very rare drug exposures* can often *not be studied.*
5. *Exposure levels* should be *adequate,* so that if an excess risk of a UDE exists, there is a reasonable expectation of identifying the relationship.
6. *Sample sizes* should be determined for *desired power.*
7. It is important to guard against *selection biases* in cases and controls. Preferably, only newly diagnosed patients will be included, so that patients who died immediately from the disease or were cured quickly are not excluded.
8. The *same eligibility criteria* should apply to both cases and controls.
9. Control subjects should be *comparable with* patients in all relevant ways *except they should not have the disease or other UDE under study,* nor should they be more or less likely than those with the disease or UDE to take the drug under question (protopathic bias). Patients with conditions that are indications for drug use or contraindications for the drug must be excluded, as must patients with conditions known to be caused by or prevented by the drug. For example, in a study of the relationship of salicylates to Reye's syndrome, you would want to exclude hospitalized children with rheumatoid arthritis or other rheumatic diseases because hospitalized children are likely to use aspirin for rheumatoid conditions.[76]

Likelihood of Exposure — Cases/Controls. One of the most important assumptions underlying the validity of case–control studies is that controls are just as likely as cases to be exposed to the drug under study. Miettinen[67] suggests that the appropriate strategy for case–control studies is to identify the study base represented by cases and controls or the referent series.

	Prevalence or Incidence of Outcome		
		Not Rare	Rare
Drug Exposure	Not Rare	either cohort or case–control	case–control
	Rare	cohort	no efficient design; cohort only possibility

Table 3
Frequency of Disease Outcome and Drug Exposure

For example, hospitalized patients in a single hospital do not necessarily represent all hospitalized patients in that community or all persons in the community. Patient and physician preferences, hospital capabilities and reputation, and risk of out-of-hospital mortality are just a few of a number of factors that are easily recognized in differentiating hospitalized patients.

If the study base is defined a priori, it will be easier to ensure that the controls are representative of that referent base and to control for covariants that could act as confounders. It is preferable to include all cases of disease or UDE in the defined population. If the referent populations differ significantly in drug exposure, then comparison of UDE risk may be misleading. For example, a chronic user of a nonsteroidal antiinflammatory drug (NSAID) has a different exposure and risk of a UDE than does the user who takes a single dose a few times a year for pain relief.

Measuring Exposure (Case–Control Studies). The goal is to collect information thoroughly in the same way in both cases and controls. Biases listed on page 100, such as information bias, recall bias, and measurement bias, should be recognized and avoided. Data collection should be standardized, monitored, and performed by trained personnel.

Exposure information is frequently not recorded completely in medical records. For example, in HMOs, drug-dispensing information may be accurate, but patient consumption and compliance may be unavailable, incomplete, or inaccurate in existing records. When the patient is asked to recall past behavior, it is extremely important to use corroborating data to ensure that cases and controls provide comparable data.

Selecting Cases (Case–Control Studies). Where possible, a study based on incident or new cases of disease or UDEs is preferred. The problem with using only new cases is that it may be necessary to wait a period of time until enough new cases are diagnosed (particularly for rare outcomes). As discussed previously, prevalent cases of disease or UDEs underestimate cases of short duration or cases who die prior to being eligible for inclusion in the study.

The diagnostic/inclusion criteria for cases should be both sensitive (captures true cases) and specific (does not include noncases). It is important that cases represent a homogeneous disease entity. The only way to ensure that this occurs is that the criteria for selecting cases (incident or prevalent) are clearly specified and strictly adhered to.

Selecting Controls (Case–Control Studies). CASES/CONTROLS FROM SAME POPULATION. Occasionally, it is possible to estimate the relative risk in case–control studies by accurately defining the population from which the cases derive. An accurate definition of this population allows one to select the controls from the same population. This is possible when: (1) we know all cases or have a sample of cases included in the study and are able to define precisely the population from which these cases are derived, and (2) the matching control group is representative of the same population. Under these conditions, estimates of the probabilities of the UDEs in exposed and nonexposed individuals can be established and used to calculate estimates of the relative risk. Both the nested case–control and the case–cohort study (hybrid design) approaches meet these criteria and permit relative risk calculations.

GENERAL POPULATION CONTROLS. When cases come from a defined general population and a census of eligible individuals or households exists, controls can be randomly selected. If no census exists, a partial census must be created. However, it can be expensive to identify an appropriate sample from the general population by using this approach.

A popular solution for identifying eligible controls is to use random-digit dialing. This method provides a random sample of households with telephones. Biases introduced by excluding individuals who do not have telephones or who refuse to consider telephone solicitations need to be considered.

MATCHED CONTROLS. Matching controls to cases may make it possible to control the impact of confounding factors that are difficult to measure directly and therefore cannot be controlled by analyses. For example, occupational exposures may be controlled for by selecting controls who work at the same job.

Types of Matching. TWINS. The most compatible matching among human beings occurs with the case and the control being identical twins. Identical twins who have the same genes often are raised together and thus have been exposed to the same environment. Consequently, in an observational study, a strong scientific inference can be made if appropriate pairs of twins are found. If one had identical twins raised in the same environment and one of the twins smoked and the other did not, then prospective follow-up for the incidence of lung cancer, general health, and survival experience could provide quite strong scientific inferences as to the health effects of smoking.

The difficulty with twin studies is that sufficient numbers of identical twins cannot be located such that one of the twins is exposed to the drug while the other is not. There are limited numbers of identical twins, and it is most likely that both are exposed or not exposed. Thus, the number of epidemiologic studies using twins is small, and no pharmacoepidemiologic studies using this design have been reported in the literature. Although this approach is logistically not feasible, other methodologic approaches can be taken.

MATCHED PAIRS. A control or multiple controls are identified for each case on the basis of similarity (or identity) with regard to all variables pertinent to the study except for the UDE outcome. Thus, in many studies, individuals are matched with regard to age, gender, race, and some indicator of social or economic status. Still, the possibility exists that the case and control are not truly comparable because of some unrecognized variable.

MATCHED CONTROL GROUP. An entire control group is selected. Through careful consideration of the study question and insight, it is assumed that the control group will in some sense mirror the case group with regard to the distribution of the pertinent variables.

Normally, the first step is to identify key characteristics of the cases that the investigator determines should be the same for the control group. When these characteristics are determined for the cases, a control group is selected to meet the criterion that the distribution of the characteristics is the same in both the case and control populations. For example, if 30% of the cases are married and 80% are older than 65 years, controls might be selected randomly from married individuals and from older and younger individuals so that the control group has a similar marital status and age distribution.

PROXIMITY MATCHING. Cases and controls are not matched on specific variables but somewhat intuitively on the basis of proximity in the process of case selection. The procedures often used are to select the next person after a case with the same gender and in the same age range with an appointment in the clinic or admitted to the hospital, or one might have a case designate a friend of the same age and gender. The rationale behind this approach is that, by being a friend, the control will tend to have the same social and economic environment and often will have similar ethnic characteristics. Hospital controls or other patient groups may not be representative of the general population.

STATISTICAL ADJUSTMENT TO MATCHING. Two groups are selected according to a protocol, and pertinent variables are measured, such as the variables that one considers for matching. An analytic model then is used to make statistical adjustments to estimate what the comparisons would have been had the two groups been comparable. Two approaches can be taken: stratified analysis and analytic matching.

Stratified analysis is a more straightforward way to adjust for matching variables. In stratified analysis, one separates the data into a set of two or more 2×2 tables. For example, if we expect an age effect (± 55 y) and the age distribution in the cases and controls to be different, the data are further partitioned in strata for those younger than 55 years old and those older than 55 years. Analysis is performed on the two resulting 2×2 tables. In particular, the Mantel–Haenszel statistic is used for testing the overall association between drug exposure and UDE for the combined strata in a manner that controls for potential confounding from the stratification factor. Methods that control for confounding through analytic modeling include analysis of covariance and logistic regression. When the dependent variable is dichotomous, the logistic model is commonly used; when the dependent variable is continuous, analysis of covariance is used.

The selection of the controls in a case–control study is based to a large extent on the skills and expertise of the researcher. Critical considerations are to identify cases and controls that are comparable for all variables that may confound the study outcome and to ensure that cases and controls are derived from the same defined population, even though the nature of the population may not be clearly known.

Criteria for evaluating case–control studies are shown in Table 4.

Advantages of Case–Control Studies.

- Can be used to study rare outcomes.
- Can often be used with study populations of relatively smaller size than prospective cohort studies or clinical trials.
- Often less expensive than cohort or clinical trial studies.
- Efficiency of size and cost is advantageous for studying rare conditions or conditions that appear after long latency periods.
- Do not require waiting until disease or UDE develops.

Disadvantages of Case–Control Studies

- Often difficult to determine and select cases and appropriate controls.
- Controls from the general population can be expensive to identify and enroll.

Table 4
Evaluation Criteria for Case–Control Studies

1. Selection method for cases and controls should be defined before the study starts.
2. Level of drug exposure should be established before data analysis.
3. Data collection should be unbiased by the use of blinded interviewers relative to case–control status of subjects and the use of structured data-collection instruments.
4. Patients' drug exposure recall should be equivalent in cases and controls.
5. Exclusion criteria should be unbiased for cases or controls.
6. Equal diagnostic examination based on explicit criteria should be implemented for cases and controls.
7. Similar intensity of medical surveillance for cases and controls before enrollment in the study should be observed.
8. Equal demographic susceptibility for the use of the drug by cases and controls should be ensured.
9. Equal clinical susceptibility, or pharmacogenetic attributes, by cases and controls should be ensured.
10. Berkson's bias should be avoided: Cases and controls should arrive from a common defined population rather than selected from patients admitted to a hospital, because patients who are both exposed and diseased are often more likely to be hospitalized than those who are unexposed and diseased or exposed and nondiseased.

- May be hard to collect valid/consistent retrospective data from records.
- Retrospective exposure data may not be detailed.
- Possibility of biased results (e.g., recall bias).
- Problem of interpreting the results to remove the effects of confounding factors (factors associated with exposure to the drug and with the disease or UDEs under study).
- Normally not possible to calculate a direct estimate of UDE incidence rates, except in nested case–control studies (see Chapter 10 for discussion and exceptions).
- Sizes of the underlying exposed and unexposed populations usually unknown.[77]

Examples of Case–Control Studies. There are numerous examples of important case–control studies. As mentioned earlier, the classic, small definitive case–control study consisted of only 8 cases and 32 controls and was responsible for definitively establishing the link between maternal diethylstilbestrol therapy and adenocarcinoma of the vagina in daughters.[23]

Examples that illustrate the difficulties in designing and interpreting case–control studies are the controversies generated by the studies linking endometrial cancer with estrogen use, Reye's syndrome with aspirin, and breast cancer with reserpine.

Hundreds of investigations of drug–disease relationships were conducted using case–control methodologies by the Boston Collaborative Drug Surveillance Program (BCDSP) and the Slone Epidemiology Unit (SEU), formerly the Drug Epidemiology Unit. The BCDSP and SEU have maintained in-hospital monitoring studies that identify patients hospitalized with diseases that are potentially drug induced and sufficiently serious to warrant ongoing drug surveillance efforts. General cautions concerning confounding, patient deficiencies in drug recall, and difficulties with assessing the validity of medical records apply to these databases.[4,78,79] The BCDSP research program is now oriented toward automated databases. However, limited hospital surveillance continues under their auspices.

Ongoing in-hospital monitoring studies are conducted by the SEU. Histories of drug use and current medical status are collected for patients hospitalized with targeted conditions. These include myocardial infarction, agranulocytosis, peptic ulcer, various cancers, and hepatic diseases. More than 40 000 hospitalized patients have been interviewed by nurse abstractors in hospitals in Boston, Baltimore, New York, Tucson, Philadelphia, Kansas City, and London, Ontario.

An example of an important case–control study is the multinational study of the risk of NSAIDs and aplastic anemia, called the International Agranulocytosis and Aplastic Anemia Study (IAAAS),[80] which demonstrated both the possibility of applying this approach to UDEs of extremely low incidence and the difficulties in practically conducting a multinational investigation.

Case–Crossover Designs.

Maclure[81] suggests that, when a *brief exposure* causes a *transient change* in the *risk of a rare acute outcome,* periods of time in the past when the patient was not exposed could provide control data. He suggests that, in some instances when the briefness of exposure, the transient change, and acute outcome criteria are satisfied, using the patient as his/her own control may eliminate the impact of confounding on the study outcomes. The approach is best suited to answer the question of whether the patient was doing anything unusual prior to the acute event under study. Rate ratios are calculated for the exposed and unexposed time periods.

Maclure suggests using Mantel–Haenszel statistics to analyze these rate ratios. An article by Marshall and Jackson[82] provides a general maximum likelihood method to approaching the risk estimation problem. The latter article examines the sensitivity of the assumption of brief and acute exposure (lasts ≤ 24 h) by analyzing data on the risk of recent alcohol exposure on acute myocardial infarction from Auckland Heart Study data.

Although this approach eliminates some potential confounding, there are several design issues that need to be considered for the approach to provide useful data. These include the following: the assumption about the duration of the change in risk must be valid; results will be affected if subjects modified their behavior on the basis of prior experience with similar outcomes or related symptoms; information bias is very possible; selection bias based on disease severity is often an issue; and information may not be available for individuals who refused to participate or were eliminated (e.g., patients who died prior to interview).

Case–Cohort Studies.

Another hybrid design suggested by Prentice[83] is a case–cohort design. This design is similar to that of the nested case–control study, but the non-cases (controls) are selected randomly from the original cohort. This study design has been suggested as being an economic alternative to a standard cohort design.[84,85] The design permits direct estimation of risk ratios without the assumption that the disease under study is rare, a normal assumption when odds ratios are calculated in traditional case–control studies.

An example of this approach was published by van der Klauw et al.[86] who conducted a case–cohort study of drug-induced anaphylaxis in the Netherlands. Cases consisted of all admissions in 1987 and 1988 to all Dutch hospitals with anaphylaxis as the principal diagnosis and a sample of all other admissions. The referent population comprised all persons in the catchment areas of a sample of pharmacies during the same period. The study generated high relative risks associated with NSAIDs, glafenine, amoxicillin, and diclofenac exposure.

Design Issues Common to All Observational Analytic Studies. BIAS. Bias is defined as systematic error (vs. random error) in design, data collection, patient selection, or follow-up that is likely to lead to a distortion in study conclusions.

SELECTION BIAS. Noncomparable criteria are used to select exposed and unexposed participants. This is a concern whenever comparison groups are selected. An example of selection bias is Berkson's bias. Since hospitalized patients often have more than one disease, selection of hospital controls may lead to a false conclusion about the relationship of a drug exposure and disease outcome.

INFORMATION BIAS. This bias is a systematic difference in collecting information from various exposure or outcome groups. It may be related to measurements and to patient or physician behavior/recall. Examples are recall bias and measurement bias.

Recall bias. Individuals with different health histories, diseases, or UDEs may be motivated to recall past exposures with varying thoroughness. For example, mothers of children with birth defects are more likely to recall/report exposures during pregnancy than are mothers of healthy children.

Measurement bias. The presence of a UDE affects the measurement of the exposure or recording of the exposure.

Confounding. Confounding is defined as the mixing of effects among the drug exposure, the outcome (disease, UDEs), and a third factor that independently affects the risk of developing the disease or UDEs. For a factor to be a confounder, it must be associated with the outcome of interest and be associated with the drug exposure. For example, in a study of the relationship between NSAID use and gastrointestinal bleeding, preexisting abdominal problems (e.g., ulcers) are probably related to the reason for NSAID use and the possibility of gastrointestinal bleeding independent of NSAID use and, if not recorded, would potentially be a confounder.

CONFOUNDING BY INDICATION. Whenever an observational noninterventional study of medical care is conducted, the question is raised whether patients treated with alternative therapies had the same severity of illness, were followed similarly, and were diagnosed and treated similarly. Frequently, the choice of therapy is affected by the severity of the illness at baseline and the preconceived notions of the physician that one therapy will be more effective than an alternative. In those instances, confounding by indication occurs and may affect our ability to correctly interpret the observational data that have been collected.

In an effort to encourage a systematic approach to determining the effect of confounding by indication, Neutel[87] has suggested that three types of confounding by indication be considered: confounding by prescriber expectancy, confounding by severity, and confounding by disease history.

The Neutel article also provides an interesting table of terms used for confounding by indication. In the example above concerning NSAID use, if one NSAID was selected by patients with the worst pain in preference to other NSAIDs, confounding by severity could occur. If physicians expected increased gastrointestinal problems with certain NSAIDs, confounding by provider expectancy would be an issue; if certain NSAIDs were prescribed for or selected by patients with a history of ulcers versus other NSAIDs, confounding by disease history would be an issue.

Effect Modification (Interaction). When the association between the drug exposure under study and a disease outcome or UDE varies by the level of a third factor, the third factor is considered an effect modifier. For the example of NSAIDs above, if an NSAID were related to gastrointestinal bleeding differently according to the patient's ethnic background, then ethnic background would be an effect modifier. (Since ethnic background may be related to a number of factors including genetic composition, diet, and lifestyle, measured differences among various ethnic groups could remain confounders, however.)

INTERVENTIONAL STUDIES

Clinical Trials.

A controlled clinical trial is a specific type of experimental prospective cohort study that involves assigning participants to various treatment and control cohorts in a manner in which the cohorts, independent of the intervention, are at equal risk of developing the study outcome(s). Cohort members may be treated with an active drug, a placebo, or both.

The treatment, follow-up, end points, and data collection for each cohort are specified in advance. The purpose of conducting a controlled clinical drug trial may be to assess the efficacy of drug therapy in either preventing disease (prophylactic trials) or treating established disease (therapeutic trials), to provide data on the costs of various outcomes (economic clinical trials), or to compare the safety of alternative therapies. Clinical trials may also alert us to potential safety issues that will best be studied through a combination of postmarketing epidemiologic strategies.

Randomized, Controlled Clinical Trials.

A randomized, controlled clinical trial is a controlled clinical trial in which participants are assigned to treatment or control groups in a random unbiased fashion, based on probability. The main reasons for randomization are (1) to avoid selection biases that could be introduced by patients' or medical care providers' preferences, and (2) to try to ensure that the alternative study cohorts are the same with respect to known and unknown prognostic factors.

Many scientists believe randomized, controlled clinical trials are the "gold standard" for establishing the efficacy of various therapeutic regimens.[11,12,18,30] This is particularly true when the trial is a randomized, double-blind, or triple-blind design.

Warning: Randomization is not a guarantee that the alternative study cohorts are the same with either known or unknown prognostic factors. When the investigator observes that the groups are different for known prognostic factors, often analytic techniques can be used to adjust for these differences.

Blinding. Blinding means that the treatment assignment is not known to certain persons involved with the study. Blinding is introduced into clinical trials to avoid potential biases that might be introduced by having the participant's treatment known.

> *Single blinded.*   Treatment assignment is unknown to the patients.
> *Double blinded.* Treatment assignment is unknown to either the patient or the provider.
> *Triple blinded.*   Treatment assignment is unknown to the patient, the provider, and the epidemiologist/statistician or other investigators.

Sample Size. The number of subjects required to conduct a clinical trial is determined by a clear statement of the hypothesis to be tested and by the level of difference and statistical confidence in the findings that would be considered statistically, clinically, and practically important. See Chapter 10 for considerations on sample size and type I and type II errors.

Sampling. Ideally, the participants in a clinical trial are a representative and unbiased sample of the cohort or population at risk to an exposure and outcome that you want to study. Even when potential participants are selected in a completely unbiased fashion, for practical and design reasons, study participants may not be an unbiased representative sample of the general population. The major reasons are the following.

1. Inclusion/exclusion criteria tend to select patients who are more alike than is the general patient population that is at risk. For example, many trials exclude persons with multiple diseases, the elderly, pregnant women, and illiterate patients.
2. Compliance is a factor if patients are excluded if their likelihood of compliance is considered too low. Most trials include numerous reinforcements to the patients, not found in actual therapy settings, so that they will comply with therapy.
3. The trial includes persons willing to volunteer. This may exclude individuals who are mentally or physically unable or unwilling to make the effort to adhere to the study regimentation.[88]

Efficacy Versus Effectiveness. One critical difference between most clinical trials and population-based epidemiologic studies conducted to find out how well a drug works is whether the study was designed to demonstrate efficacy or effectiveness.

- Efficacy relates to whether an intervention *can* accomplish a particular outcome. A clinical trial answers this question in a protocol environment.
- Effectiveness deals with whether the intervention *does* accomplish a particular outcome as it is used in real-world situations.

Neither efficacy nor effectiveness is an inherent characteristic of the intervention. Additional information is needed for either term to have meaning.

A clinical trial provides data on how well an intervention accomplishes its goal in a protocol environment when certain kinds of patients, diagnosed according to specific criteria, are treated with certain doses and are monitored for certain outcomes. In other words, can the drug work at a specified dose in certain kinds of patients?

The same detail is needed to discuss effectiveness rationally. The difference is that the question now becomes, does the drug work at a specified dose in certain kinds of patients in real-world practice?

The reader is encouraged to use these terms carefully and accurately when describing studies and presenting results. This is particularly important when the results of multiple studies are being compared.

Ethical Issues. In any investigation in which the study changes or determines a patient's care, it is extremely important that the investigator adheres to the highest ethical conduct. Entire books have been published on the subject of ethics, and courses on ethics in medical research and randomized clinical trials are conducted regularly. In the US and in most countries, studies (particularly experimental studies) must be reviewed and approved by an independent committee of scientists and nonscientists before the study can be conducted.

Following are five ethical guidelines for medical professionals conducting clinical trials.[88]

1. None of the treatment options should be known to be inferior. If a standard regimen exists, it should be used as the control treatment.
2. The question should be clinically important.
3. There must be informed patient consent.
4. It should be reasonably feasible to complete the trial, based on design, number of patients required, and so on, or the trial should not be initiated.
5. If in the course of the trial it becomes scientifically clear from external or internal evidence that one treatment option being tested is

clearly superior to the other or that one is clearly inferior, then the trial must be halted in the first instance or modified in the second (stopping rules).

The importance of an independent committee that represents and balances general ethical issues and local risk/benefit considerations cannot be overemphasized. When the underlying incidence and prevalence of diseases with very high mortality and morbidity affect a community, the community may be willing to accept higher-risk experimental interventions. These issues are currently being faced in the development of malaria and AIDS vaccines for regions with high disease incidence and high mortality.

Advantages of Randomized Clinical Trials.

- Randomization protects against patient selection for a particular therapy based on subjective factors or judgmental factors related to the outcome of interest.
- Randomization helps to ensure that the comparison groups are the same on unknown prognostic factors.
- The level of detail of the information collected can be specified.
- Prospective data collection leads to ensuring that pertinent information is collected consistently and accurately.
- Blinding protects against bias.
- Randomization provides direct estimates of efficacy and the risk of developing an adverse event.
- When the trial fails to demonstrate a difference between therapies, it is possible to evaluate the probability that this lack of difference is an error and may be due to variation alone (power of the trial).
- Findings of well-designed clinical trials are generally widely accepted.[89-91]

Disadvantages of Randomized Clinical Trials.

- Randomization requires extensive planning.
- Randomization cannot be initiated quickly.
- Randomization often requires long follow-up.
- Randomization is generally limited in measuring the effects of prolonged drug use and in determining latency.
- Patient compliance/dropouts may affect results.
- Participants may cross over to alternative therapies.
- Randomization is not exploratory. The cost and complexity of most clinical trials dictate that information is usually collected to answer questions specified in advance and that "superfluous" data are often not recorded.
- Randomization is expensive.

- Randomization is not efficient for studying rare outcomes; it requires large numbers.
- Randomization is limited in generalizing to the total population that may be treated with the study drug.[18,30,49,69]

Other advantages and limitations of postmarketing clinical trials are discussed later in this book. Excellent references on clinical trial design, conduct, and interpretation are available.[72]

Examples of Randomized Clinical Trials. Major postmarketing clinical trials have been conducted to study the effectiveness of drug therapy in reducing the consequences of disease, such as the Aspirin Myocardial Infarction Study (AMIS)[92] and the Veterans Administration[93] and US Public Health Service trials of the treatment of mild hypertension[94,95]: the Hypertension Detection and Follow-up Program (HDFP),[96,97] the Multiple Risk Factor Intervention Trial (MRFIT),[98] the Lipid Research Clinics (LRC), and the Systolic Hypertension in the Elderly Program (SHEP).[99]

Other Experimental Approaches.

Smaller and Smaller Trials. N OF 1 CLINICAL TRIALS. Another interesting approach for optimizing therapy for an individual patient is the N of 1 randomized clinical trial proposed by Guyatt et al.[100,101] and Sackett et al.[102] In these studies, the patient serves as his own control in a drug crossover design. This type of study can be conducted in individual patients when the condition being studied is chronic and relatively stable and when the drugs being compared manifest an effect on an outcome in a relatively short period of time and the effect is reversed in a similarly short period of time. Those authors make an excellent suggestion that an N of 1 trial might be conducted to help determine eligibility criteria for larger randomized clinical trials. Jaeschke et al.[103] have also considered N of 1 trials for quality-of-life measurement.

SIMPLIFIED CLINICAL TRIALS. Senior researchers have debated whether placebo-controlled or randomized clinical trials are ethical and necessary.[14,104,105] To avoid assigning patients to placebo therapies, researchers should consider alternative study designs (e.g., historical controls) that may be appropriate in special situations.

Strom et al.[12,13] have published very provocative articles on the necessity of conducting experimental studies (e.g., randomized clinical trials) to study a marketed drug's efficacy. The essential idea is that we conduct randomized studies to protect against selection bias when the efficacy of a drug on a particular outcome can be confounded by the health status of the patient when the drug was prescribed. For example, confounding occurs if patients with more severe diseases receive the drug and patients with better prognoses do not receive the drug, so the drug appears less effective than it actually is. Randomization is helpful in solving the problem, because it helps to produce two groups with comparable baseline status. When the indication for treatment can be fully characterized, randomization may not be essential. When Strom et al. applied these criteria to 100 of the approved drugs (since 1978), representing 131 potential drug uses, they found that the efficacy of 68% of the drugs could be evaluated from clinical observations, 10.7% could be evaluated by experimental or nonexperimental studies, 4.6% only by experimental studies, 8% only by nonexperimental studies, and 22.1% "could not be studied by either technique."[12,13,106]

Faich[107] has for several years suggested conducting simpler targeted clinical trials, the principle being that the costs of conducting the clinical trial are often compounded by the complexity of the data collected, the number of visits, and the overall trial management. When a specific question or a few questions can be posed, such as whether a drug is responsible for a specific UDE, it may be possible to simplify the clinical trial and thus eliminate some of the overhead. When the population entering the trial is representative of the community or patient population that may be exposed to the drug and when the follow-up does not affect normal care, randomization permits the calculation of accurate rates of drug effectiveness for alternative therapies.

Larger and Larger Clinical Trials. During the past 10 years, we have witnessed a trend toward the conduct of larger and larger clinical trials. In certain instances, the scientific community has concluded that the only way a protective effect of a public health intervention can be proven or safety issue resolved is to conduct a clinical trial that is large enough to measure and confirm what once were considered differences too small to detect by using clinical trial approaches. Several examples of this are worth mentioning. There are three primary prevention antioxidant trials in cancer research. The Alpha-Tocopherol, Beta-Carotene (ATBC) lung cancer trial was completed in Finland in 1993.[108] The Global Utilization of Streptokinase and Tissue Plasminogen Activator for Occluded Arteries (GUSTO) study randomized more than 40 000 patients with myocardial infarctions into one of four thrombolytic protocols.[109,110] The randomized 29 246 male smokers (5+/d) aged 50–69 years demonstrated a 25% reduction in lung cancer. The Physicians' Health Study is studying beta carotene in 22 071 healthy men, and the Women's Health Study will report on beta carotene and vitamin E in 40 000 healthy women. The SEU recently completed a randomized trial of ibuprofen versus acetaminophen in 84 000 children to demonstrate the safety and effectiveness of the two drugs in children.

A potential problem that may apply to any study is of particular concern when these newer mega trials are conducted. With larger studies, it is possible to achieve statistical significance without biologic importance. Investigators and readers need to require both statistical and biologic significance for evidence to be important in elucidating causal relationships. As trials become larger and larger, very small differences between group means for a variable may become statistically significant. This is because the statistical tests used in most instances are themselves a function of the true size of the difference and the variability of the estimate of the difference that is inversely related to sample size.

Observations

GENETIC CONSIDERATIONS — PHARMACOGENETICS

There has been significant progress in characterizing individuals who either metabolize certain drugs quickly or, conversely, metabolize other drugs slowly. As pharmacokineticists and pharmacogeneticists learn more about classes of fast and slow acetylators, we should be able to understand iatrogenic disease better, and we may be able to explain the inconsistencies among the findings from various epidemiologic studies. Currently, differences in individual drug metabolism serve as a confounder in most epidemiologic studies.

FUTURE TRENDS

The frustration at wanting solid, irrefutable evidence before initiating drug interventions that could affect millions of patients has led to the recent trend for larger and larger clinical trials. An example of the discomfort with observational epidemiologic evidence is typified by the article by a leading epidemiologist, Dr. Lynn Rosenberg,[111] who questions the weight of evidence that leads to exposing millions of women to hormone replacement therapy. Rosenberg thoughtfully urges caution and is most comfortable with the evidence that will be available a decade from now from three large clinical trials in women that are now being undertaken in the US (the Postmenopausal Estrogen/Progestin Trial, a secondary trial of postmyocardial women, and the Women's Health Initiative). I expect that as a society we will not heed her advice and wait for the results. On the other hand, hopefully her caution and the fact that these large trials are under way are good signs that we will not permit large segments of the population to be exposed to any intervention without epidemiologic studies in place to ensure long-term safety. Unfortunately, as pointed out above, clinical trials are not infallible, and size alone will not guarantee multiple conclusions about the meaning of the data once they are completed. Better science, not necessarily larger numbers, is required.

Our colleagues in pharmacogenetics have made amazing advances in the past few years in understanding how individuals metabolize certain drugs. In the next 5–10 years, hopefully these advances will reach the clinic at low cost and apply to the majority of frequently used drugs, and we will see a reversal of the necessity to conduct these mega trials. While I am discouraged by the trend for larger and larger clinical trials, I am encouraged by the work of the McMaster group and others[100,101] to conduct smaller studies and to improve our analysis of current data.

An interesting approach to conducting multiple mega clinical trials has recently been implemented by Spitzer[112] and others.[113-115] To address the question of whether gestadone containing oral contraceptives causes cardiovascular disease, they initiated three concurrent observational epidemiologic studies. One is a case–control study in Germany, the second is a historical cohort study in the Saskatchewan Health database, and the third is a concurrent cohort study in the Venous Arterial Management Protection system. This important program should permit one study to confirm and complement the results of the other. I hope that we see further comprehensive efforts of this nature in which independent complementary studies are initiated in a coordinated manner to answer important public health questions.

For the immediate future, pharmacoepidemiologists will be challenged to provide data on outcomes for pharmacoeconomic analyses. This is appropriate. The demands for economic evaluations are immediate and acute. The epidemiologist will play an important role to ensure that the science that contributes to the outcomes and cost measurements will be sound and generalizable. There is a tendency to concentrate on the economic aspects of the risk/benefit considerations. These efforts should not replace, but supplement, our diligence in ensuring that safety issues are addressed for marketed drugs.

COMMENT

Regardless of which methodology is elected in pharmacoepidemiology, good scientific technique is required to ensure valid results. As in all biologic sciences, this includes reviewing the scientific literature, clearly specifying study objectives, selecting study methodology, pretesting and validating data collection procedures, and conducting careful data analyses and interpretation of the results from statistical and biologic vantage points.

While pharmaceutical scientists have concentrated on the risk/benefit of drugs in a comprehensive sense, a number of our colleagues now concentrate on the value of alternative drugs expressed in economic terms. Pharmacoepidemiologists play an important role providing data to answer these questions. The growth of pharmacoepidemiology as a scientific discipline depends on the value that society places on the questions this discipline examines (i.e., with respect to the safety and value of drugs). The availability of scientific techniques and high-quality data to pursue the answers, the continued development of high-quality training programs, the useful organization of the growing body of knowledge, and the support of forums for exchanging knowledge are critical factors for the health of the discipline. Finally, increased recognition that pharmacoepidemiology has contributed with successful applications of this new knowledge to important problems is essential.

References

1. Blackwell B, Stolley PD, Buncher R, Klimt CR, Temple R, Venn D, et al. Panel 4: Phase IV investigations. Clin Pharmacol Ther 1975;18:653-6.
2. Borden EK, Gardner JS, Westland MM, Gardner SD. Postmarketing drug surveillance (letter). JAMA 1984;251:729-30.
3. Gross FH, Inman WHW. Drug monitoring. New York: Academic Press, 1977.
4. Slone D, Shapiro S, Miettinen OS, Finkle WD, Stolley PD. Drug evaluation after marketing. Ann Intern Med 1979;90:257-61.
5. Wardell WM, Tsianco MC, Anavekar SN, Davis HT. Postmarketing surveillance of new drugs. I. Review of objectives and methodology. J Clin Pharmacol 1979;19:85-94.
6. Feinstein AR, Sosin DM, Wells CK. The Will Rogers phenomenon: state migration and new diagnostic techniques as a source of misleading statistics for survival in cancer. N Engl J Med 1985;312:1604-8.
7. Venning GR. Identification of adverse reactions to new drugs. I. What have been the important adverse reactions since thalidomide? Br Med J 1983;286:199-202.
8. Venning GR. Identification of adverse reactions to new drugs. II. How were 18 important adverse reactions discovered and with what delays? Br Med J 1983;286: 289-92.
9. Venning GR. Identification of adverse reactions to new drugs. II (continued). How were 18 important adverse reactions discovered and with what delays? Br Med J 1983;286:365-8.
10. Venning GR. Identification of adverse reactions to new drugs. III. Alerting processes and early warning systems. Br Med J 1983;286:458-60.
11. Remington RD. Post-marketing drug surveillance: a comparison of methods. Am J Pharm 1978;150:72-80.
12. Strom BL, Miettinen OS, Melmon KL. Postmarketing studies of drug efficacy: when must they be randomized? J Clin Pharmacol 1983;34:1-7.
13. Strom BL, Miettinen OS, Melmon KL. Postmarketing studies of drug efficacy: how? Am J Med 1984;77:703-8.
14. Gehan EA, Freireich EJ. Non-randomized controls in cancer clinical trials. N Engl J Med 1974;290:198-203.
15. Strom BL, ed. Pharmacoepidemiology. 2nd ed. West Sussex, England: John Wiley & Sons, 1994.
16. Stolley PD. Prevention of adverse effects related to drug therapy. In: Clark DW, MacMahon B, eds. Preventive and community medicine. 2nd ed. Boston: Little, Brown, 1981:141-8.
17. Rawlins MD, Thompson JW. Pathogenesis of adverse drug reaction. In: Davis DM, ed. Textbook of adverse drug reactions. Oxford: Oxford University Press, 1977:44.

18. Hennekens CH, Buring JE, Mayrent SL, eds. Epidemiology in medicine. Boston: Little, Brown, 1987.
19. Last JM, ed. A dictionary of epidemiology. Toronto: Oxford University Press, 1995:55.
20. Rothman KJ, ed. Causal inference. Chestnut Hill, MA: Epidemiology Resources, Inc., 1988.
21. Hill AB. The environment and disease: causation or association? Proc R Soc Med 1965;58:295-300.
22. Cole P, Amoateng-Adjepong Y. Cancer prevention: accomplishments and prospects (editorial). Am J Public Health 1994;84:8-9.
23. Skinner CS, Strecher VJ, Hospers H. Recommendations for mammography: do tailored messages make a difference? Am J Public Health 1994;84:43-9.
24. Andrews HF, Kerner JF, Zaauber AG, Mandelblatt J, Pittman J, Struuering E. Using census and mortality data to target small areas for breast, colorectal, and cervical cancer screening. Am J Public Health 1994;84:56-61.
25. Fletcher RW, Fletcher SW, Wagner EH. Clinical epidemiology: the essentials. 2nd ed. Baltimore: Williams & Wilkins, 1988.
26. Kelsey JL, Thompson WD, Evans A. Methods in observational epidemiology. New York: Oxford University Press, 1986.
27. Herbst AL, Ulfelder H, Poskanzer DC. Adenocarcinoma of the vagina: association of maternal stilbestrol therapy with appearance in young women. N Engl J Med 1971;284:878-81.
28. ARME-P, ed. Methodological approaches in pharmacoepidemiology: applications to spontaneous reporting. Amsterdam: Elsevier, 1993.
29. Funch D, Dryer NA, Bassin LG, Crawley JA, Brickley MG, Walker AM. The validity of case reports in a pharmacoepidemiologic study of adverse. Postmarketing Surveillance 1993;7:283-9.
30. Mausner JS, Kramer S. Epidemiology: an introductory text. Philadelphia: WB Saunders, 1985.
31. National Center for Health Statistics. DHHS Publication No. (PHS) 83-1200. Hyattsville, MD: US Department of Health and Human Services, 1983.
32. Beasly R, Pearce N, Crane J, Burgess C. The withdrawal of fenoterol and the end of the New Zealand asthma mortality epidemic. Int Arch Allergy Immunol 1995;107:325-7.
33. Burgess C, Pearce N, Thiruchelvan R, Wilkinson R, Linaker C, Woodman K, et al. Prescribed drug therapy and near-fatal asthma attacks. Eur Respir J 1994;7:498-503.
34. Woodman K, Pearce N, Beasly R, Burgess C. Albuterol and deaths from asthma in New Zealand from 1969 to 1976: a case–control study. Clin Pharmacol Ther 1992;51:566-71.
35. McKeigue PM, Lamm SH, Linn S, Kutcher JSF. Bendectin and birth defects: I. A meta-analysis of the epidemiologic studies. Teratology 1994;50:27-37.
36. Thompson PL, Parsons RW, Jamrozik K, Hockey RL, Hobbs MS, Broadhurst RJ. Changing patterns of medical treatment in acute myocardial infarction. Observations from the Perth MONICA Project 1984–1990. Med J Aust 1992;157:87-92.
37. Barrett-Connor E, Palinkas LA. Low blood pressure and depression in older men: a population based study. BMJ 1994;308:446-8.
38. Neyman J. Science 1955;122:401.
39. Catalog of public use data tapes from the National Center for Health Statistics. DHHS Publication No. (PHS) 81-1213. Hyattsville, MD: US Department of Health and Human Services, 1980.

40. Gillum RF, Hannan PJ, Prineas RJ, Jacobs DR Jr, Gomez-Marin O, Luepker RV, et al. Coronary heart disease mortality trends in Minnesota, 1960–80: the Minnesota Heart Survey. Am J Public Health 1984;74:360-2.
41. Stewart RB, Marks RG, May FE, Hale WE. Hypolipidemic drug use in an ambulatory elderly population. Postmarketing Surveillance 1993;7:299-308.
42. Bostrom G, Hallqvist J, Hagland BJ, Romelsjo A, Svanstrom L, Diderichsen F. Socioeconomic differences in smoking in an urban Swedish population. The bias introduced by non-participation in a mailed questionnaire. Scand J Soc Med 1993;21:77-82.
43. Ginter E. Cardiovascular risk factors in the former communist countries. Analysis of 40 European MONICA populations. Eur J Epidemiol 1995;11:199-205.
44. Ecological analysis of the association between mortality and major risk factors of cardiovascular disease. The World Health Organization MONICA Project. Int J Epidemiol 1994;23:503-16.
45. Baum C, Kennedy D, Forbes M, Jones J. Drug use in the United States in 1981. JAMA 1984;25:1293-7.
46. Draft of guidelines for postmarketing reporting of adverse drug reactions. Rockville, MD: Division of Drug and Biological Products Experience, Center for Drugs and Biologics, 1985 (docket no. 85D-0249).
47. IMS America, Ltd.
48. Schor RI, Fought RI, Ray WA. Changes in antipsychotic drug use in nursing homes during implementation of the OBRA-87 regulations. JAMA 1994;271:358-62.
49. Papoz, L. EURODIAB Subarea C Study Group. Utilization of drug sales data for the epidemiology of chronic disease: the example of diabetes. Epidemiology 1993;4:421-7.
50. Lilienfeld D, Stolley P. Foundations of epidemiology. 3rd ed. New York: Oxford University Press, 1994.
51. Kurland LT, Molgaard CA. The patient's record in epidemiology. Sci Am 1981;245:54-63.
52. Hartzema AG, Porta MS, Tilson HH, eds. Pharmacoepidemiology: an introduction. 2nd ed. Cincinnati: Harvey Whitney Books Company, 1991.
53. Greenberg RS. Medical epidemiology. Norwalk, CT: Appleton & Lange, 1993.
54. Rossi AC, Knapp DE, Anello C, O'Neill RT, Graham CF, Mendelis PS, et al. Discovery of adverse drug reactions. A comparison of selected Phase IV studies with spontaneous reporting methods. JAMA 1983;249:2226-8.
55. Edlavitch SA. Practical perspectives on postmarketing surveillance—phase IV. In: Nwangwu PU, ed. Concepts and strategies in new drug development. New York: Praeger, 1983:223-42.
56. Jabbari B, Bryan GE, Marsh EE, Gunderson CH. Incidence of seizures with tricyclic and tetracyclic antidepressants. Arch Neurol 1985;42:480-1.
57. Vessey MP, Lawless M, Yeates D. Oral contraceptives and stroke: findings in a large prospective study. Br Med J 1984;289:530-1.
58. Heinonen OP, Slone D, Shapiro S. Birth defects and drugs in pregnancy. Littleton, MA: PSG, 1977.
59. Inman WHW. Postmarketing surveillance of adverse drug reactions in general practice. II. Prescription-event monitoring at the University of Southampton. Br Med J 1981;282:1216.
60. Rawson NSB, Inman WHW. Prescription-event monitoring. Recent experience with 5 NSAIDs. Med Toxicol 1986;1(suppl 1):79.
61. Inman WHW, ed. Monitoring for drug safety. 2nd ed. Lancaster, PA: MTP Press, 1986:673.

62. Petri H, Leufkens H, Naus J, Silkens R, Hessens P, van Urquhart J. Rapid method for estimating the risk of acutely controversial side effects of prescription drugs. J Clin Epidemiol 1990;43:433-9.
63. Petri H, Urquhart J. Channeling bias in the interpretation of drug effects. Stat Med 1991;10:577-81.
64. Petri H, de-Vet HC, Naus J, Urquhart J. Prescription sequence analysis: a new and fast method for assessing adverse reactions of prescription drugs in large populations. Stat Med 1988;11:1171-5.
65. Sartwell PE. Retrospective studies: a review for the clinician. Ann Intern Med 1974;81:381-6.
66. Spitzer WO. Ideas and words: two dimensions for debates on case controlling (editorial). J Chronic Dis 1985;38:541-2.
67. Miettinen OS. The "case–control" study: valid selection of subjects. J Chronic Dis 1985; 38:543-8.
68. Schlesselman JJ. Valid selection of subjects in case–control studies. J Chronic Dis 1985; 38:549-50.
69. Axelson O. The case–referent study: some comments on its structure, merits, and limitations. Scand J Work Environ Health 1985;11(suppl 3):207-13.
70. Miettinen OS. Author's response. J Chronic Dis 1985;38:557-8.
71. Kleinbaum DG, Kupper LL, Morgenstern H. Epidemiologic research: principles and quantitative methods. New York: Van Nostrand Reinhold, 1982.
72. Ernster VL. Nested case–control studies. Prev Med 1994;23:587-90.
73. Jick H, Jick SS, Gurewich V, Myers MW, Vasilakis C. Risk of idiopathic cardiovascular death and nonfatal venous thromboembolism in women using oral contraceptives with differing progestagen components. Lancet 1995;346:1589-93.
74. Chitwood DD, Griffin DK, Comerford M, Page JB, Trapido EJ, Lai S, et al. Risk factors for HIV-1 seroconversion among injection drug users: a case–control study. Am J Public Health 1985;85:1538-42.
75. Matteson EL, Yachyshyn V, Yachyshyn J, O'Fallon WM. Trends in hospitalizations for gastrointestinal bleeding among patients with rheumatoid arthritis in Rochester, Minnesota, 1950–1991. J Rheumatol 1995;22:1471-7.
76. Hurwitz ES, Barrett MJ, Bregman D, Gunn WJ, Schonberger LB, Fairweather WR, et al. Public Health Service study on Reye's syndrome and medications. Report of the pilot phase. N Engl J Med 1985;313:849-57.
77. Feinstein AR. The case–control study: valid selection of subjects. J Chronic Dis 1985; 38:551-2.
78. Lawson DH, Jick H. Comparative drug utilization in hospitalized patients. In: Hollman M, Weber E, eds. Drug utilization studies in hospitals. Stuttgart, Germany: FK Schattauer Verlag, 1980:39-41.
79. Strom BL, ed. Pharmacoepidemiology. 2nd ed. Sussex: Wiley, 1994.
80. Risks of agranulocytosis and aplastic anemia. A first report of their relation to drug use with special reference to analgesics. The International Agranulocytosis and Aplastic Anemia Study. JAMA 1986;256:1749-57.
81. Maclure M. The case–crossover design: a method for studying transient effects on the risk of acute events. Am J Epidemiol 1991;133:144-53.
82. Marshall RJ, Jackson JT. Analysis of case–crossover designs. Stat Med 1993;12:2333-41.
83. Prentice RL. A case–cohort design for epidemiologic cohort studies and disease prevention trials. 1986;73:1-11.

84. Wacholder S. Practical considerations in choosing between the case–control and the nested case–control designs. Epidemiology 1991;2:155-8.
85. Sato T. Risk ratio estimation in case–cohort studies. Environ Health Perspect 1994; 102(suppl 8):53-6.
86. van der Klauw MM, Stricker BH, Herrings RM, Cost WS, Valkenberg HA, Wilson JH. A population based case–cohort study of drug induced anaphylaxis. Br J Clin Pharmacol 1993;35:400-8.
87. Neutel CI. A new, "user-friendly" terminology for confounding by indication in the study of adverse drug reactions. Postmarketing Surveillance 1993;7:363-9.
88. Miettinen OS, Cook EF. Confounding: essence and detection. Am J Epidemiol 1981;114:593-603.
89. Meinert C. Clinical trials: design, conduct, analysis. Oxford: Oxford University Press, 1986.
90. Friedman LM, Furberg CD, Demets DL. Fundamentals of clinical trials. Boston: John Wright, PSG, Inc., 1984.
91. Louis TA, Shapiro SH. Critical issues in the conduct and interpretation of clinical trials. Annu Rev Public Health 1983;4:25-46.
92. Aspirin Myocardial Infarction Study Research Group. A randomized, controlled trial of aspirin in persons recovered from myocardial infarction. JAMA 1980;243: 661-9.
93. Veterans Administration Cooperative Study on Antihypertensive Agents. Effects of treatment on morbidity in hypertension. I. Results of patients with diastolic blood pressure averaging 90 through 114 mm Hg. JAMA 1970;213:1143-51.
94. Smith WM, the US Public Health Service Hospitals Cooperative Study Group. Treatment of mild hypertension: results of a ten-year intervention trial. Circ Res 1977;40(suppl):I-98-105.
95. Smith WM, Edlavitch SA, Krushat WM. Public Health Service hospitals intervention trial in mild hypertension. In: Onesti G, Klimt C, eds. Hypertension determinants, complications and intervention. New York: Grune & Stratton, 1977:381-99.
96. Hypertension Detection and Follow-up Program Cooperative Group. The hypertension detection and follow-up program. Prev Med 1976;5:207-15.
97. Hypertension Detection and Follow-up Program Cooperative Group. Five-year findings of the hypertension detection and follow-up program. I. Reduction in mortality of persons with high blood pressure, including mild hypertension. JAMA 1979;242:2562-71.
98. Multiple Risk Factor Intervention Trial Research Group. Multiple Risk Factor Intervention Trial: risk factor changes and mortality results. JAMA 1982;248:1465-77.
99. Hulley SB, Furberg CD, Gurland B, McDonald R, Perry HM, Schnaper HW, et al. Systolic Hypertension in the Elderly Program (SHEP): antihypertensive efficacy of chlorthalidone. Am J Cardiol 1985;56:913-20.
100. Guyatt G, Sackett D, Taylor DW, Chong J, Roberts R, Pugsley S. Determining optimal therapy — randomized trials in individual patients. N Engl J Med 1986;314: 889-92.
101. Guyatt GH, Heyting A, Jaeschke R, Keller J, Adachi JD, Roberts RS. N of 1 randomized trials for investigating new drugs. Control Clin Trials 1990;11:88-100.
102. Sackett DL, Haynes RB, Guyatt GH, Tugwell P. Clinical epidemiology: a basic science for clinical medicine. Boston: Little, Brown, 1991.
103. Jaeschke R, Guyatt GH, Keller J, Singer J. Interpreting changes in quality-of-life in N of 1 randomized trials. Control Clin Trials 1991;12(4 suppl):226s-33s.

104. Byar DP, Simon RM, Friedewald WT, Schlesselman JJ, DeMets DL, Ellenberg JH, et al. Randomized clinical trials. Perspectives on some recent ideas. N Engl J Med 1976;295:74-80.
105. Feinstein AR. Should placebo-controlled trials be abolished (editorial)? Eur J Clin Pharmacol 1980;17:1-4.
106. Strom BL, Miettinen OS, Melmon KL. Postmarketing studies of drug efficacy. Why? Am J Med 1985;78:475-80.
107. Faich GA. Pharmacoepidemiology and clinical research (editorial). J Clin Epidemiol 1991;44:821-2.
108. The ATBC Cancer Prevention Study Group. The Alpha-Tocopherol, Beta-Carotene Lung Cancer Prevention Study: design, methods, participant characteristics, and compliance. Ann Epidemiol 1994;4:1-10.
109. Gore JM, Granger CB, Simoons ML, Sloan MA, Weaver WD, White HD, et al. Stroke after thrombosis. Mortality and function outcomes in the GUSTO-I trial. Global use of strategies in open occluded coronary arteries. Circulation 1995;92:2811-8.
110. Agnelli G. Thrombolytic and antithrombotic treatment in myocardial infarction: main achievements and future perspectives. Int J Cardiol 1995;49(suppl):S77-87.
111. Rosenberg L. Hormone replacement therapy: the need for reconsideration. Am J Public Health 1993;83:1670-3.
112. Spitzer WO. Three epidemiological studies in the low-dose oral contraceptive research programme: a coherent strategy. Pharmacoepidemiol Drug Saf 1993;2:17-20.
113. Suissa S, Hemmelgarn B, Spitzer WO, Brophy JP, Collet R, Côte R, et al. Pharmacoepidemiol Drug Saf 1993;2:33-50.
114. Spitzer WO, Thorogood M, Heinemann LAJ. Trinational study of oral contraceptives and health. Pharmacoepidemiol Drug Saf 1993;2:21-32.
115. Lis Y, Spitzer WO, Mann RD, Cockburn I, Chukwujindu J, Thorogood M, et al. A concurrent cohort study of oral contraceptive users from the VAMP Research Bank. Pharmacoepidemiol Drug Saf 1993;2:51-64.

5

The Detection and Identification of Unintended Drug Effects

Audrey Smith Rogers

Abstract

Pharmacoepidemiology requires an insight into the complex relationship among the many methods of defining unintended drug effects (UDEs), the duration of clinical experience with a specific drug, and the strategies for detection of UDEs. The development of a precise and generally accepted definition of a UDE has been complicated by not only the number of factors that can be considered, but also the very purpose of defining the event. The assessment of patient experience for individual clinical management represents a different situation than measurement within a research protocol.

A fundamental axiom of pharmacoepidemiology is that all therapeutic interventions will produce unintended drug effects (UDEs). While there will never be an absolute guarantee of drug safety, it is important that a drug's safety profile be defined. The rapidity with which this is done and the strategies used to do it have prompted debate that focuses on questions of how much safety information is necessary, when it should be required in the process of drug development, and how much this knowledge will cost.

Defining Unintended Drug Effects

Simple definitions ("any undesirable effect produced by a drug"[1]) include experiences such as overdose, drug abuse, and expected adverse effects. Although appropriate for purposes such as cost–benefit analysis related to societal impact, this approach complicates the estimate or determination of risk associated with both drug evaluation and therapeutic drug use.

RESEARCH APPLICATION

Premarketing Research. Every use of an experimental drug in humans must be viewed as a unique clinical experiment. The evaluation of an individual's response can be guided by available toxicologic and animal data, but it cannot be restricted by it. Consequently, subject assessment must be comprehensive and, while an item-specific checklist is an efficient strategy, the evaluation must also accommodate a global and open-ended approach.

The comprehensiveness of the premarketing evaluation must extend to the determination of efficacy or safety differences between men and women if the agent is expected to be used therapeutically in both genders. Focusing on homogeneity among research subjects to reduce unexplained variance in clinical studies and to promote more efficient assessments of efficacy has precluded studying the heterogeneous populations in which important toxicity trends might emerge. Consequently, new attention has been directed at increasing participation by women in clinical trials.[2]

If the drug will be used in the very sick, very elderly[3,4] persons, or very young pediatric populations,[5] adequate safety data should be collected from them to define specific pharmacokinetic and pharmacodynamic parameters for the drug's use; data from healthy volunteers do not suffice. If the judgment is made to establish safety data for special populations, toxicity end points need to be redefined to conform to the clinical reality of the underlying disease or condition.

Commonly, clinicians are asked to judge whether a UDE should be attributed to the experimental drug. Many have come to believe that this clinical judgment about attribution may be of little value. At this very early stage of drug development, clearly too little experience has accumulated upon which to base such a judgment. This can be illustrated with a simplistic example. Fever due to a gastroenteritis can be easily dismissed as not attributable to a drug for depression or hypertension; however, if the drug in fact caused an unpredictable immunologic alteration that made individuals more susceptible to infection, this whole association would be missed if analysis were restricted based on attribution status.

The collection of safety data should focus on the population likely to receive the drug and should consist of a comprehensive assessment of adverse events grouped by physiologically related body systems. The safety profile will emerge from an analysis of the frequencies of expected adverse effects based on the drug's pharmacology, as well as any clustering of events in particular body systems.

Postmarketing Research. Formal research projects conducted after a drug is marketed will examine population-based UDE experience with the drug. Causation judgments based on epidemiologic evidence accumulated in well-designed case–control or cohort studies rely on these accepted criteria[6]:

1. Strength of association: What is the relative risk estimate derived from the study, and what values are bounded by the associated confidence intervals?
2. Specificity of the association: Does this medical event occur frequently, and has it been linked to other, perhaps multiple, causes? Alternatively, the association is more likely to be real when the outcome event is a specific form of medical condition; for example, a site- and histologic-specific cancer is a more credible candidate than a drug association with cancer in general.
3. Consistency of the association: Does the association between drug and event remain the same when different subgroups of the population are examined? It may be true that a particular subset is at greater risk or the only group at risk, but this conclusion can be reached only if it can be determined that the increased risk in that particular subset is not due to an extraneous factor operating only in that subset.
4. Dose–response: When controlled for all other factors, if the dose is increased, does the intensity and/or frequency of the UDE increase in the population?
5. Biologic plausibility: Are there experimental or animal data that support the cause-and-effect link?

6. Concordance among studies: Do investigations generally concur on the presence, direction, and strength of the drug–event relationship?

CLINICAL APPLICATION

For the clinician managing an individual patient, the broadest definition of a UDE might apply in immediate management decisions. Any event, occurring during therapy, that is unacceptable to either the patient or the physician can be viewed as an adverse experience. Examples include a patient's proclivity to abuse a particular agent, intolerance of fully expected adverse effects, and even therapeutic failure. Termination of a specific therapy solves the immediate clinical dilemma, but long-term clinical management will require a thoughtful and systematic consideration of the patient's experience. The corresponding clinical judgment about attribution can be no better than the data supporting it. UDE assessment should contain information specific to the event, the drug, and the patient (Table 1). Information on demographics, concurrent disease, and concomitant drug therapy permits the examination of risk in particular subsets. Information on dose, duration, and route gives an indication of any dose–response relationship. An examination of the event itself may elucidate the pharmacologic mechanism of action for the adverse experience and demonstrate any necessary induction time. This kind of information is valuable to the clinician in analyzing the experience of a particular patient.

Determining the exact role a drug plays in an untoward patient experience can become a difficult process of sorting out the effects of the disease being treated, other therapies, and the influence of lifestyle (e.g., smoking, obesity, alcoholism). Numerous standardized assessment methods[7-9] have been devised to aid in this determination, and they propose that certain common criteria be applied to clinical situations to assess causation.

In routine clinical practice, causality can be assumed when these criteria are met:

1. Nature: The character of the UDE is consistent or predictable, based on the pharmacology of the drug; that is, the event is a known or predictable response to the drug.
2. Timing: If the event was compatible with the pharmacologic action of the drug, it occurred after an appropriate interval consistent with the pharmacokinetic parameters of the drug.
3. Dose: The intensity of the event was related to the dose or serum concentration of the drug. Serum concentrations were higher than predicted based on dose.
4. Experience: Events of this nature have been reported previously in the literature.

Table 1
Probable Timing of Unintended Drug Effect Detection

If an unintended drug effect exists:

Increasing probability of detection ——————————————→

Premarketing evaluation			Approval	Postmarketing evaluation		
Phase I	**Phase II**	**Phase III**	marketing	**Phase IV-A**	**Phase IV-B**	**Phase IV-C**
3 years	3 years	4 years		2 years	8 years	>10 years
healthy volunteers	selected patients	multicenter patients		preliminary experience in limited populations	routine use in general population	chronic effects and dose accumulation

expected adverse effects ----→

limited dose-related toxicity from dose-finding studies → toxicity/overdose experience[a] ----→

excessive pharmacologic effects in some patients[a] ----→

unexpected, unintended effects in some patients[a] ----→

allergic or hypersensitivity events in a few patients[a]

idiosyncratic events in a few patients

cancer, other chronic diseases

[a]Detection will always be a function of the size of the population exposed and the true rate of the unintended drug effect of interest.

5. Dechallenge/rechallenge: The event abated when the drug was withdrawn. It recurred when the drug was restarted.
6. Alternative etiologies: The effects of the disease being treated, other therapies being used, or the influence of lifestyle are not likely to be responsible for the event.

Although these criteria appear clear and direct, their application in the clinical situation is not always possible. Rawlins[10] has categorized events as type A or type B reactions. Type A reactions are those that are consistent with the agent's pharmacology, are commonly occurring, usually dose dependent, and fairly predictable. Type B reactions represent allergic and idiosyncratic reactions to the drug and are independent of its pharmacologic effect. These occurrences are rare, are not dose related, and cannot be predicted. The criteria for assessing causality outlined above do not address type B reactions. Furthermore, the criterion for corroborating published reports is not practical during early clinical use, nor is it frequently feasible to attempt drug rechallenge. Data on the influence of such other factors as interactions with concurrent drugs or lifestyle characteristics are often unavailable. Despite these limitations, this set of criteria provides a useful framework for systematic clinical evaluation of the event. Ultimately, the clinician is left in uncertainty to decide pragmatically the best course for the individual patient by weighing the risks of continuing treatment against those of discontinuing it.

PUBLIC HEALTH APPLICATION

Regarding drug safety, prescribing clinicians have a particular responsibility to the public's health beyond their obligation to the individual patient. This responsibility entails the reporting of adverse clinical experiences associated with drug use. The acceptance of UDE reporting as a professional responsibility requiring no reimbursement has been documented.[11] UDEs should be reported to those authorities charged with monitoring drug safety, specifically the spontaneous reporting system MedWatch of the US Food and Drug Administration (FDA)[12] (see Chapter 9). If the event is well documented, simultaneous reporting in the medical literature should be considered for wider distribution of toxicity information to colleagues (although editorial and publication delays do not necessarily make distribution more timely).

For any spontaneous reporting system to be an effective sentinel system, it must be selective in data collection.[13] It should focus on serious UDEs that cause new hospitalizations, prolong current hospitalizations, are associated with congenital anomaly, cause cancer, or lead to death. Events that are serious clinical conditions (e.g., drug-associated liver disease or renal impairment) not meriting hospitalization (because new reimbursement practices may make such hospitalizations unlikely) should also be reported. Of all types of targeted events, the two that the system may have the most difficulty tracking would be congenital anomalies and cancers, since considerable time must elapse between drug exposure and clinical outcome; often the earlier drug prescriber is not the later clinician evaluating a medical condition of unknown etiology.

Another point to remember about sentinel surveillance systems is that their very purpose is to generate signals whose investigations are pursued through more formal study. Therefore, it is not important for the physician to be convinced that the suspected drug was responsible for the UDE (although certain circumstances to be reviewed later should hold), nor should reports be filtered through stringent hospital committee criteria that may confuse and frustrate reporting clinicians.[14] If the system is operating effectively, it is the frequency and pattern of drug-associated clinical events that signal the need for closer examination. Thus, every serious UDE should be reported, whether it is documented in the literature or not, because no physician would be in the position to detect trends in the frequency or nature of rare events.

For clinicians who plan to submit the UDE for publication as a case report, Soffer[15] lists the following additional necessary information: the individual's prior adverse experiences with drugs of a similar class, ancillary information from pharmaceutical manufacturers and regulatory agencies, and data on previous publications relating to the same or similar events.

Duration of Experience with a Specific Drug

The probable timing of UDE detection is a function of the nature of the event and the frequency with which it occurs. This is discussed in the following sections and graphically presented in Table 2.

PROBABLE DETECTION IN PREMARKETING PERIOD

Premarketing clinical research (Phases I–III) should define all common unfavorable dose-related effects, regardless of whether they are predictable on the basis of the drug's pharmacology. These effects are likely to be exhibited with varying intensity in many patients. Information on the drug's full safety profile is limited as a consequence of the five "too's" of premarketing drug evaluation: too few, too simple, too median-aged, too narrow, and too brief.

Too Few: The number of people exposed to a drug prior to its approval in the US is usually less than 2000. However, to have a 95% probability of detecting even a single instance of an adverse medical event that an investigational drug is suspected of producing once in every 10 000 exposed persons, the drug experience of 30 000 individuals would have to be studied. Even reducing the probability of detecting this same 1 in 10 000 occurrence from 95% to 80% still requires the evaluation of 16 000 drug exposures (see Chapter 3). In fact, with the 2000 or so exposed persons commonly studied, the risk of UDE associated with the drug exposure would have to be substantial for it to be detected prior to marketing (e.g., the investigational drug would have to increase about 13 times the risk of a medical event that would normally occur in the population once per 1000 individuals to be detected with 95% probability). Thus, establishing drug safety to this extent prior to marketing would entail prohibitive expense and usually is not feasible.

Too Simple: Because an ineffective drug, however safe, is useless, the primary objective of premarketing studies is the determination of efficacy. Patients with complicated medical conditions or receiving concurrent drug therapies usually are excluded from premarketing studies to simplify the evaluation of drug efficacy.

Too Median-Aged: The very young and the very old are rarely represented in clinical trials. Once marketed, the agent will be prescribed to both groups if there is a perceived need.

Too Narrow: The indications for which an investigational drug is used are specified and well defined in all study protocols. Once a drug is marketed, however, it may be used for other related conditions for which the risk/benefit ratio may be radically different.

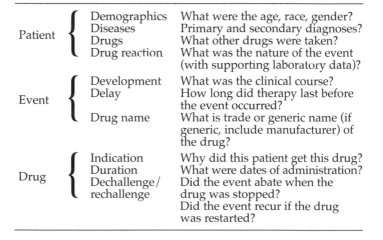

Table 2 Information Required in a Comprehensive Unintended Drug Effect Report			
Patient		Demographics	What were the age, race, gender?
		Diseases	Primary and secondary diagnoses?
		Drugs	What other drugs were taken?
		Drug reaction	What was the nature of the event (with supporting laboratory data)?
Event		Development	What was the clinical course?
		Delay	How long did therapy last before the event occurred?
		Drug name	What is trade or generic name (if generic, include manufacturer) of the drug?
Drug		Indication	Why did this patient get this drug?
		Duration	What were dates of administration?
		Dechallenge/ rechallenge	Did the event abate when the drug was stopped? Did the event recur if the drug was restarted?

Too Brief: UDEs that occur after years of chronic therapy with an agent or that require an extended incubation period after single exposure (e.g., vaginal carcinoma after intrauterine exposure to diethylstilbestrol) cannot be known when a drug is approved for marketing.

In summary, the only safety information that is definitively available at the time a drug is approved for marketing consists of a frequency description of expected adverse effects; dose-related toxicity information from dosing studies (Phase I); and the toxicologic, teratogenic, and carcinogenic evaluations in animals. (The extent, duration, and number of animal studies performed depend on the expected length of therapy with the drug, its proposed indication, and characteristics of the target population. Positive findings in animal studies can indict the drug or identify concerns requiring closer scrutiny in subsequent human studies, but negative studies can never fully guarantee the drug's safety.) If serious UDEs exist, the ones with any reasonable probability of detection by this stage of limited drug use are those that occur commonly. For a drug frequently exhibiting serious UDEs to reach this stage of approval, a special case must exist. Such situations include treatment of uniformly fatal diseases for which there are no therapeutic alternatives or serious diseases for which the new drug represents a demonstrated improvement in the balance between risk and benefit.

There are two cases in which these data limitations should be addressed before the drug is brought to market: (1) when the drug is indicated for use in treating a highly prevalent disease and large numbers of people (increasing the probability of those with unusual genetic and physical characteristics) may be treated, and (2) when the drug is indicated for use in medically complicated populations. It is essential that the occurrence of occasional serious events (1/100–1/500) be clinically proven unlikely to occur in the target populations or, if demonstrated, be worth the risk, given the expected benefit. Therefore, if either of these cases holds, Phase III trials should widen the detection net by increasing the numbers and/or medical complexity of enrollees.

It is unlikely that other, more frequent UDEs, if they exist, will be observed at this stage of limited exposure. The detection of these events will occur after the drug is marketed and used for extended periods of time in larger numbers of patients of all ages with more complicated disease states.

POSSIBLE DETECTION IN POSTMARKETING PERIOD

Allergic or idiosyncratic reactions, because they occur so infrequently, have little likelihood of detection during the premarketing phase, as discussed in Chapter 3. Other UDEs unlikely to emerge prior to marketing include those that (1) occur rarely (1/10 000–1/100 000), (2) require a long induction period, or (3) result from a specific interaction with personal characteristics, concurrent disease, or concomitant drug therapies. These UDEs are noted to be only "possibly detected" during the postmarketing period, since their identification will be a function of the integrity and efficiency of existing surveillance systems.

Strategies for Detection of Unintended Drug Effects

After drug marketing, safety data are collected from sentinel surveillance systems and population-based epidemiologic studies.

SENTINEL SURVEILLANCE SYSTEMS

Sentinel surveillance systems are mechanisms for detecting signals of possible drug toxicity. Their strengths include an unparalleled timeliness, the potential to draw on the universe of drug experience, and open participation to all prescribers. However, their contribution must be kept in perspective by their limitations, for the reports these systems generate are, in Avorn's words,[16] "only numerators in search of their denominators." The nature of these reports is frequently confounded by comorbidity, concurrent drugs, and lifestyle factors that can be evaluated only in the context of population experience. In fact, because these reports depend on voluntary reporting behavior and the complexity of factors that can produce either underreporting or a flurry of cases,[17] the ultimate issue of actual risk can never be answered by surveillance data.

The national-level sentinel surveillance system for the US—the spontaneous reporting system (MedWatch)—is maintained by the FDA. The system is described extensively elsewhere in this book (see Chapter 9). Case reports of UDEs are received directly from health professionals or through the efforts of pharmaceutical manufacturers. MedWatch may serve as an early warning system for serious UDEs, but it depends on voluntary professional reporting. The rate of physician reporting of UDEs in the US has lagged far behind the rates in other Western countries.[18] For the system to be an effective sentinel, practicing clinicians must be aware of it, have the means of reporting (this includes ease of access and convenience), and be willing to participate. The degree of underreporting in the US showed that these conditions were not being met, and generated FDA support of innovative local programs to stimulate physicians' reporting of UDEs.[19,20] These projects, wider dissemination of the reporting forms, and enhanced guidelines for manufacturers' reporting contributed to a major increase in UDE reporting from all sources between 1984 and 1989 compared with the prior 5-year period.[21] In addition, the FDA has issued new rules recently to strengthen reporting of safety problems. The rules will promote international cooperation and sharing of safety information on marketed agents by using definitions, reporting periods, and formats that correspond with the recommendations of international organizations, such as the International Conference on Harmonization and the World Health Organization's Council for International Organizations of Medical Sciences.[22]

Direct, professional, UDE reporting has been demonstrated to be the most efficient and productive source of serious drug reactions that resulted in labeling changes for the drug.[23] Milstien et al.[24] have demonstrated that pharmacists play an important role in encouraging direct physician reporting to the FDA. Over the last decade, the emerging capacity of drug information units in industry has enhanced the effectiveness of the system.

If reports are received in a timely manner, both the investigation and appropriate action can occur more quickly. In those circumstances in which the evidence is clear and a specific drug is judged unequivocally responsible for producing serious reactions that are judged disproportionate to clinical benefit, regulatory action restricting its use can ensue.[25] (See example in Chapter 17.)

More commonly, however, spontaneous reports alone present inconclusive evidence for drug causality. It remains crucial, therefore, that the anecdotal reports generated by this surveillance system never assume more importance than they merit, because many require verification and some may be no more than false positive reports.[26] Venning[27] assessed the validity of all suspected UDEs reported in four major medical journals in 1963 to determine what proportion was ultimately verified 18 years later. Ten percent of the 52 articles on UDEs were planned scientific studies; the remaining 47 articles consisted of anecdotal reports. Of these, 28 articles demonstrated satisfactory evidence of validity at publication, and 7 others were subsequently satisfactorily verified, leaving 12 articles with an unclear status. Eight of these 12 articles reported rare clinical events (7 hematologic) that may have represented conditions with such extremely low incidences that similar cases had not yet occurred or been reported. The other 4 articles involved the association between frequently used drugs and common clinical syndromes, and they would have required epidemiologic evaluation. With varying probabilities corresponding to the evidence in each case, there also exists the possibility that all 12 articles on UDEs may represent false positive reports. No reason exists to assume that the nature of reports in the FDA system is any different from that of these published reports. Indeed, without the editorial filter that journals provide and adequate governmental staffing to pursue missing data, the quality of the reports is probably worse. Spontaneous reports can fulfill their potential only when they are evaluated in systematic, population-based surveillance and in epidemiologically and clinically sound studies to determine whether they represent coincidence, artifact, or a genuine problem in toxicity.[16] However, despite limitations, spontaneous reporting systems may be the only affordable means of detecting rare and serious UDEs, and attempts to improve function are necessary. The contribution of the pharmacist in monitoring, collecting, and reporting the UDE of drug therapy is an important component of the spontaneous reporting systems.

POPULATION-BASED EPIDEMIOLOGIC STUDIES

Epidemiologic studies undertaken after a drug is marketed can be hypothesis generating or hypothesis testing. Either has the capacity to generate a rate of adverse event occurrence that makes these studies more informative and clinically relevant than the numerator reports from sentinel systems. Hypothesis-testing studies confer the additional advantage of producing estimates of the relative risk associated with particular drug use. The choice of study design is usually a function of the time period in which such studies are initiated.

Postmarketing Surveillance Projects. The purpose of projects that begin within the first 3 years after marketing is to collect information on the nature, severity, and incidence of UDEs in the general population and, in effect, to compensate for the premarketing deficiencies discussed above (the 5 "too's"). Such projects have included efforts called Phase IV studies, as they can be viewed as a continuation of safety data collection from the premarketing Phases I–III.[28] Although these studies have defined populations and specified exposures, the outcomes of interest are not limited to any one medical condition; rather, they use the "event-monitoring" approach of Inman.[29] An outcome is defined as "any new diagnosis, unexpected deterioration, or improvement in a pre-existing condition (whether or not related to the condition for which the drug was prescribed), and any accident or complaint of symptoms that were not present before the treatment was started."[29] These projects are deemed hypothesis generating because, in general, they lack specific a priori hypotheses. Consequently, it is only serendipitous when these studies have adequate statistical power to evaluate the full significance of the UDE rates that may emerge. However, these projects can be useful in understanding the limits of a drug's toxicity, because they usually have sufficient statistical power to detect major toxicity events if they were to be present in large numbers. Postmarketing surveillance (PMS) projects using an event-monitoring outcome definition were conducted in the evaluation of cimetidine in Great Britain[30,31] and in the US.[32] Obviously, a project that follows many patients and records all events over a long period is expensive, and the technical and statistical problems encountered in analysis of such data can be formidable.

Every drug brought to market merits a systematic, thorough, and scientific review of unanswered safety questions. However, large-scale evaluation of every marketed drug would be neither cost effective nor possible. Public health and clinical considerations may necessitate supplemental epidemiologic information on drug safety.[33] The decision to perform an event-monitoring postmarketing study should result from a careful examination of these factors: (1) known safety information for the drug including animal data, premarketing clinical data, and evidence from population use in countries where the drug may have already been marketed; (2) prevalence and severity of the disease for which the drug is indicated; (3) the probability of exposure to the drug; and (4) the efficacy and safety profile of currently available treatment.

Studies Examining Specific Research Hypotheses. The other type of population-based epidemiologic study occurring after the drug is marketed and has been in general use for 4 or more years is designed to answer a specific research hypothesis. These drug safety questions are usually generated from case reports of UDEs associated with drug use and require validation by accepted epidemiologic methods. Such projects have a defined population, stated exposure criteria, and specific medical conditions of interest. Data from these studies produce incidence and risk estimates of specific UDEs with a given drug exposure. The safety information gathered is limited to the research questions posed, but if the study design and analysis are valid and the study has adequate statistical power, that information may often be considered definitive as it relates to the specific question studied if the effect of evolving clinical practice has been evaluated.[34]

In summary, the probable timing of the detection of any event depends on the size of the susceptible, exposed population and the rate of exposure, as well as the true rate of the UDE itself. A drug's safety profile is dynamic rather than static; it unfolds over time, and it may be modified as the drug is used to treat different conditions or is used in combination with new or unusual therapies. The natural history of its original indication may change and thereby alter the risk/benefit ratio for the drug's use. As the US population ages with accompanying changes in pharmacokinetics and pharmacodynamics,[3] UDEs may become more frequent at commonly used dosages. Furthermore, when established drugs are used in combination with newer agents, unexpected drug interactions may be encountered.

Regulatory Action

Often, the event does not emerge from a controlled observational study, but is reported as a single occurrence or a small cluster of reports demanding a regulatory response. In this situation, it is imperative to obtain as detailed and comprehensive a report as possible on the individual case and to evaluate the type of evidence provided. In the absence of valid epidemiologic data from controlled trials, Venning[27] proposes use of the following criteria to develop operating guidelines for regulatory agencies deciding on the drug–event link: (1) rechallenge data, (2) experimental data demonstrating mechanisms of pathogenesis, (3) immediate and acute UDEs, (4) local reactions at the site of administration, (5) a first report of reaction with a new route previously recognized with another method of administration, and (6) repeated occurrence of rare events. Given these types of evidence, regulators must weigh the nature of the event: Is it reversible, and at what cost? Does it result in permanent disability or death? They must estimate the incidence of the event and the proportion of the population that might be exposed. How many individuals could experience this event? They must evaluate the contribution this agent makes to the overall treatment of the disorder for which it is indicated. Is this the only drug available, or one of many? All these factors must be carefully considered in deciding on regulatory action.

Summary

Attempts to strengthen spontaneous reporting systems, such as MedWatch, and new methods for examining drug safety after marketing may be useful in preventing unnecessary delay in the public availability of new and efficacious agents while fulfilling safety requirements. At the same time, examination of past drug safety issues has clarified the type of evidence required to link the event with a drug. Certainly no one believes a drug could and therefore should be certified as safe before human use. Given the new appreciation of the limits of our knowledge about a drug's safety at any point of its temporal evolution, the current task is to make wise decisions about drug safety evaluation that safeguard the public health, provide physicians with therapeutic options, and secure industry investment in necessary research.

References

1. Karch FE, Lasagna L. Adverse drug reactions: a critical review. JAMA 1975;234:1236-41.
2. Committee on the Ethical and Legal Issues Relating to the Inclusion of Women in Clinical Studies, Division of Health Sciences Policy, Institute of Medicine. Scientific considerations. In: Mastroianni AC, Faden R, Federman D, eds. Women and health research: ethical and legal issues of including women in clinical trials. Washington, DC: National Academy Press, 1994.
3. Ray WA, Griffin MR, Shorr RI. Adverse drug reactions and the elderly. Health Aff (Millwood) 1990;9:114-22.
4. International working group standardizes drug testing requirements in elderly. Am J Hosp Pharm 1994;51:2776,2779.

5. Jensen P, Vitiello B, Leonard H, Laughren T. Design and methodologic issues for clinical drug trials in children and adolescents. Psychopharmacol Bull 1994;30:3-8.
6. Lilienfeld AM, Lilienfeld DE. Foundations of epidemiology. Oxford: Oxford University Press, 1980:289-321.
7. Karch FE, Lasagna L. Toward the operational identification of adverse drug reactions. Clin Pharmacol Ther 1977;21:247-54.
8. Kramer MS, Leventhal JM, Hutchinson TA, Feinstein AR. An algorithm for the operational assessment of adverse drug reactions. I. Background, description, and instructions for use. JAMA 1979;242:623-32.
9. Naranjo CA, Busto U, Sellers EM, Sandor P, Ruiz I, Roberts E, et al. A method for estimating the probability of adverse drug reactions. Clin Pharmacol Ther 1981;30: 239-45.
10. Rawlins MD. Clinical pharmacology: adverse reactions to drugs. Br Med J 1981;282: 974-6.
11. Rogers AS, Israel E, Smith CR, Levine D, McBean AM, Valente C, et al. Physician knowledge, attitudes, and behavior related to reporting adverse drug events. Arch Intern Med 1988;148:1596-600.
12. Kessler DA. Introducing MedWatch: a new approach to reporting medication and device adverse effects and product problems. J Adolesc Health 1994;15:281-5.
13. Faich GA, Castle W, Bankowski Z, the CIOMS ADR Working Group. International reporting on adverse drug reactions: the CIOMS project. Int J Clin Pharmacol Ther Toxicol 1990;28:133-8.
14. Jeurgens JP. Controversies in adverse drug reaction reporting (letter). Am J Hosp Pharm 1990;47:76-7.
15. Soffer A. The practitioner's role in the detection of adverse drug reactions (editorial). Arch Intern Med 1985;145:232-3.
16. Avorn J. Reporting drug side effects: signals and noise (editorial). JAMA 1990;263: 1823.
17. Roeser HP, Rohan AP. Post-marketing surveillance of drugs. The spontaneous reporting scheme: role of the Adverse Drug Reactions Advisory Committee. Med J Aust 1990;153:720-6.
18. Griffin JP, Weber JCP. Voluntary systems of adverse reaction reporting. Adverse Drug React Acute Poisoning Rev 1986;1:23-55.
19. Rogers AS. FDA-sponsored project to promote physician reporting of adverse drug events in Maryland, 1985–1988. Clin Res Pract Drug Regul Aff 1990;8:29-43.
20. Scott HD, Thacher-Renshaw A, Rosenbaum S, Waters WJ Jr, Andrews LG, Faich GA. Physician reporting of adverse drug reactions: results of the Rhode Island Adverse Drug Reaction Reporting Project. JAMA 1990;263:1785-8.
21. Faich GA. National adverse drug reaction reporting. Arch Intern Med 1991;151: 1645-7.
22. Nightingale S. New rules to strengthen reporting of safety problems. JAMA 1994; 272:1814.
23. Rossi AC, Knapp DE. Discovery of new adverse drug reactions: a review of the Food and Drug Administration's spontaneous reporting system. JAMA 1984;252: 1030-3.
24. Milstien JB, Faich GA, Hsu JP, Knapp DE, Baum C, Dreis MW. Factors affecting physician reporting of adverse drug reactions. Drug Inf J 1986;20:157-64.
25. Dukes MNG. The importance of adverse reactions in drug regulation. Drug Saf 1990;5:3-6.

26. Fletcher AP. An appraisal of spontaneous adverse event monitoring. Adverse Drug React Toxicol Rev 1992;11:213-27.
27. Venning GR. Validity of anecdotal reports of suspected adverse drug reactions: the problem of false alarms. Br Med J 1982;284:249-52.
28. Fletcher AP. Spontaneous adverse drug reaction reporting vs event monitoring: a comparison. J R Soc Med 1991;84:341-4.
29. Inman WHW. Postmarketing surveillance of adverse drug reactions in general practice. II. Prescription–event monitoring at the University of Southampton. Br Med J 1981;282:1216-7.
30. Colin-Jones DG, Langman MJS, Lawson DH, Vessey MP. Postmarketing surveillance of the safety of cimetidine: 12 month mortality report. Br Med J 1983;286:1713-6.
31. Colin-Jones DG, Langman MJS, Lawson DH, Vessey MP. Postmarketing surveillance of cimetidine: mortality during second, third, and fourth years of follow-up. Br Med J 1985;291:1084-8.
32. Gifford LM, Aeugle ME, Myerson RM, Tannenbaum PJ. Cimetidine postmarketing outpatient surveillance program: interim report on Phase I. JAMA 1980;243:1532-5.
33. Rogers AS, Porta M, Tilson HH. Guidelines for decision-making in postmarketing surveillance of drugs. J Clin Res Pharmacoepidemiol 1990;4:241-51.
34. Joseph KS. The evolution of clinical practice and time trends in drug effects. J Clin Epidemiol 1994;47:593-8.

6

Drug Utilization — Measurement, Classification, and Methods

Darrel C Bjornson
Joaquima Serradell
Abraham G Hartzema

Abstract

This chapter describes the history, development, and current status of drug utilization and focuses mainly on population-based drug utilization methodologies. The requirement for a standardized unit of measurement to quantify drug use in populations is discussed. The defined daily dose (DDD) is a unit of measurement that estimates the proportion of patients within a community who receive a particular drug. Clearly, it has limitations, and other measurements have been proposed. However, the DDD remains the most widely used measure, and the drug utilization literature is replete with studies using this methodology. Various drug classification systems are discussed and include the American Hospital Formulary Service and the Anatomical-Therapeutic Chemical Classification systems. Major sources of drug utilization data are discussed. These sources include market surveys, third-party payers or health maintenance organizations (HMOs), institutional or ambulatory settings, and pharmacoepidemiologic studies designed for monitoring and evaluating exposure-related outcomes. The chapter concludes with examples of drug utilization studies that have focused on several areas of research to include (1) use in specific populations; (2) patterns of use, both over time and cross-sectional; (3) use in specific disease states; (4) detection of adverse outcomes; (5) use as a surrogate for disease states; (6) use as a public policy tool; (7) use across countries; and (8) the effects of demographic variables. When used appropriately in conjunction with analytic studies on drug effects and other epidemiologic methods, drug utilization studies become a powerful scientific tool for ensuring the rational use of drugs in our society.

Outline

T his chapter discusses the units of measurement used in drug use or utilization studies, describes the major sources of drug use data, reviews prescribing patterns based on national and international comparative drug use data analysis, and defines the contribution of drug utilization studies to pharmacoepidemiology.

Drug utilization has been defined as "the prescribing, dispensing, administering, and ingesting of drugs."[1] This definition recognizes that several steps and factors are involved in drug utilization and that, consequently, in each of these steps problems in drug use can arise. Factors that can contribute to these problems may have historical, social, cultural, organizational, political, economic, technologic, and physiologic or pharmacologic origins.

The World Health Organization (WHO) expands on this definition by including outcome variables in the definition. Drug utilization is defined by the WHO as "the marketing, distribution, prescription, and use of drugs in society, with special emphasis on the resulting medical, social, and economic consequences."[2] Tognoni[3] stresses the importance of these outcomes when he notes that the point of observation in drug utilization studies is the act of prescribing the drug, and that quantitative data need to be obtained on the extent and variability in use and costs of drug therapy, from which medical and social qualitative consequences can be extrapolated. In drug-monitoring studies, the focus is on the observable effects of the drug that, depending on the specific aims of the method selected, are limited to the type and extent of drug exposure. The general goals of drug utilization studies include the following: (1) description of patterns of drug use in specific populations; (2) identification and definition of likely problems; (3) general analysis of the problem with regard to its importance, cause, and consequence; (4) establishment of a weighted basis for decisions on problem-solving; and (5) assessment of the effects of the action taken.[4]

The users of drug utilization studies may include healthcare policymakers, the pharmaceutical industry, the academic and clinical health professions, social scientists, economists, and consumers. The complexity of the drug utilization process often calls for an interdisciplinary approach to methodology development and consequently fosters improved communication among the health science disciplines. In fact, important linkages are now being made between pharmacoepidemiology and pharmacoeconomics.[5]

This chapter focuses mainly on population-based drug utilization research. As such, drug utilization has a strong descriptive character. Drug utilization review (DUR) and drug use evaluation (DUE) are important components evaluating drug use. Typically, DUR is a retrospective study that summarizes who prescribed the drug, which drug was prescribed, and when the drug was prescribed. DUE is a prospective study of the same prescribing parameters but also includes the reasons for the prescription and the outcome. Although labor intensive, DUE is a unique tool that can help to define criteria for the use of certain drugs, determine who fits these criteria, and find out whether the criteria need to be changed. DUR programs that monitor drug selection and use in hospitals (DUE) and in long-term care facilities (drug regimen review [DRR]) are discussed briefly. They are not, however, the focus of this chapter.

The Unit of Measurement

Population-based drug utilization studies were pioneered in Europe during the late 1960s and early 1970s. The primary focus of these studies was determined by the needs of program administrators. Drug use statistics published in these studies were not linked to population data. However, in later studies, a shift toward a more epidemiologic approach occurred, with the population denominator becoming increasingly important. In addition, more adequate measures for drug utilization data or numerator data were developed. Although drug utilization studies have used different methodologic approaches for quantifying drug use, three units for quantification of drug use are used predominantly: cost data, prescription volume, and the defined daily dose (DDD).

In the early studies, gross sales data were the most commonly used indicator. This information is widely available and can be obtained from manufacturers or wholesalers. However, using data based on drug cost can introduce measurement errors, because differential pricing occurs according to the distribution channels used, quantity purchased, import duties and currency exchange rate differences among countries, and regulatory policies that affect pricing. These problems with the interpretation of drug cost data are compounded by the different classification systems used for drugs in different countries. Studies based on cost data may make it difficult to perform cross-national comparisons, comparisons between different programs within one nation, or longitudinal studies.[6] Consequently, cost data introduce considerable limitations in the interpretation of drug utilization studies, although such analyses may have a role if data are weighted by the gross national product (GNP), per capita income, and other important economic factors.

The number of prescriptions written or dispensed for a particular drug product is used as a measure of drug use in DUR studies. Databases such as the National Prescription Audit of the International Marketing Services (IMS) America, Ltd., and the Source Prescription Audit (SPA) from Scott-Levin, a division of PMSI Scott-Levin, Inc., contain information compiled from prescription records. However, the quantity of the prescription items varies from prescription to prescription, and the supply per prescription can be for any time period, with no adequate assessment provided of the amounts of drugs prescribed or dispensed. Drug use data based on prescription records are difficult to obtain without the aid of computer systems. The main sources for these data are computerized pharmacies, health maintenance organizations (HMOs), or third-party databases (e.g., Medicaid in the US and Sickness Funds in Europe).

THE DEFINED DAILY DOSE

Although drug utilization based on prescription data is more accurate for epidemiologic purposes than cost data in estimating true drug utilization, the need to develop a more adequate index for drug utilization was deemed necessary. To overcome the inherent shortcomings of drug utilization studies based on cost data or prescription volume, a new unit of analysis was developed in the early 1980s, called the DDD. The DDD was developed based on an assumed average dose per day for a drug product used for its major indication in everyday practice. The dosing levels have been defined according to recommendations in the medical literature and are thought to be the average maintenance dose when used for the major indication of a particular drug. The DDD is a purely technical unit of measurement and comparison and, as such, provides a rough estimate of the proportion of patients within a community who would receive that particular drug. It also enables comparisons across time and geographic areas. Two basic assumptions underlie the use of DDD: first, that patients take the medication (in other words, the patients are compliant) and, second, the doses used for the major indication are the average maintenance doses. An example of DDD calculation is provided in Figure 1.

Naturally, there are limitations to the use of the DDD. Serradell and Patwell[7] showed that a large percentage (about 30%) of drugs are used for

Figure 1
Number of Defined Daily Doses Consumed, Calculated According to the Formula

$$\text{DDDs}/1000 \text{ people}/\text{day} = \frac{\text{amount of drug (mg) sold in 1 year}}{\text{DDD (mg)} \times 365 \text{ days} \times \text{no. of people}} \times 1000$$

An example follows. The DDD of diazepam is 10 mg. Assume that 400 million doses of the 5-mg tablet are sold in a country with a population of 50 million during a 1-year period. The consumption, expressed in DDDs/1000 people/day, would be:

$$\frac{5\text{-mg tablet} \times 400\,000\,000 \text{ doses}}{10 \text{ mg} \times 365 \text{ days} \times 50\,000\,000 \text{ people}} \times 1000 = 10.96 \text{ DDD}/1000 \text{ people}/\text{day}$$

This means that about 11 people of 1000 in this population will be taking diazepam 10 mg each day.

DDD = defined daily doses.

off-label indications and hence may be used at different dosages than the average maintenance dose for the major indication. Wessling and Boethius[8] evaluated the accuracy of the DDD/1000 inhabitants/unit time by comparing DDD figures with data from the actual prescriptions dispensed. They found a large variance, depending on the drug. The DDD for digoxin was 40% below actual use, 17% below for bendroflumethiazide, 80% below for naproxen, and 4% below to 28% above for antibiotics. The authors concluded that the DDD methodology was a valuable first step in overall drug measurement, but for more precise estimates of drug use it must be supplemented by other techniques.

To overcome limitations of the DDD, which, as mentioned, is based on the standard doses for the major indication for the drug and does not reflect actual prescribing patterns, US researchers and many others have been using the prescribed daily dose (PDD). These researchers argue that the PDD reflects drug exposure more accurately in the US population than the DDD, because the PDD is based on actual doses ordered by physicians for new prescriptions. PDDs can, for example, be derived from the IMS National Prescription Audit.

Ried and Johnson[9] have proposed a new standard of drug use intensity, the minimum marketed dose (MMD), using anxiolytic drugs as models. The MMD is based on the assumption that the minimum dosage strength marketed by the manufacturer is the minimum dose that will produce a desired therapeutic concentration. A study to assess the reliability and validity of the MMD showed that the magnitude of the average correlation for the MMD measure of drug use intensity was greater than the total number of prescriptions and the total number of dosage units. Discriminant validity was demonstrated because the MMD was not correlated with measures in unrelated therapeutic categories. Summed MMD units were shown to significantly predict physical impairment (criterion validity). The authors concluded that the MMD is a valid and reliable measure of drug use intensity for anxiolytic drugs. However, the DDD remains the most widely used measure of drug exposure.

Studies on the application of the DDD are confined mostly to the European literature. By applying such a measure to a defined population, it is feasible to (1) examine changes in drug consumption over time, (2) make international comparisons, (3) evaluate the effect of educational programs directed at either the prescriber or the patient, (4) document the "relative therapy intensity" with various groups of drugs, (5) follow changes in the use of a class of drugs, and (6) evaluate effects on prescription patterns caused by regulatory changes.[10] A review of DDDs, with possible applications in the institutional setting and pharmacy and therapeutics committees, is provided by Wertheimer.[11]

In addition, literature suggests that there are other uses for the DDD. Drug use comparisons using the DDD can assess use differences in subpopulations, for example, between different social classes,[12] urban versus rural,[13] and in pregnancy.[14] The DDD can also be used in drug utilization studies in which drugs are used as surrogates for estimating disease prevalence[15,16] and disease-related hospitalizations.[17] Drug utilization studies using the DDD have also been used to measure drug use in clinical research studies.[18,19] In the US, drug utilization with the DDD has been used as a trend analysis tool in resource management.[20] Differences in drug use between countries using the DDD methodology are described,[21-24] and studies have used the DDD for within-country comparisons as well.[25-28]

The following is a classic study illustrating the application of DDD methodology in a drug utilization study that led to a program that changed prescribing behavior.[29] In 1979, Malmöhus County of Sweden led the list of counties in the sales of hypnotics, sedatives, and minor tranquilizers, with sales of 82.9 DDDs/1000 inhabitants/day. In comparison, the national mean was 64.4 DDDs/1000 inhabitants/day. This observed difference led to an investigation in which prescriptions for hypnotics, sedatives, and minor tranquilizers dispensed at pharmacies in the city of Malmö were further analyzed. The results showed that 10–15 physicians accounted for a very high prescription volume in psychotropics; the remaining physicians were responsible for only a moderate number of prescriptions. These findings led to a consensus conference at which guidelines for the prescribing of hypnotics, sedatives, and minor tranquilizers were established. An information letter containing these guidelines was sent by the local medical association to all physicians in the area, including the indications for and the precautions to be taken in the prescribing of these drugs. In a follow-up study done in 1981, the consumption in DDD units for Malmöhus County had decreased to 76.8 DDDs/1000 inhabitants/day. The provision of prescribing information proved to be effective, even though the consumption of these drugs was still above the national mean. Demographic and morbidity information would be needed to further assess these differences. A study by Ekedahl et al.[30] showed that the mean 1981–1990 benzodiazepine sales were 62.0 DDDs/1000 inhabitants/day in Malmöhus County, still higher than in other geographic areas of Sweden, but showing a continuing downward trend from the data in 1979 and 1981. The authors state that much of the high use of benzodiazepines is in Helsingborg, a large city in Malmöhus County. This county is close to Denmark, which has consistently had the highest sales expressed in DDDs of any of the four Nordic countries. The authors conclude that the higher usage of benzodiazepines may be partly related to higher psychiatric morbidity and more psychosocial problems, but deviant prescribing habits among a minority of physicians are important also.

Drug Classification Systems

There is clearly a need for a standardized classification system for drugs that can be used in DUR and other pharmacoepidemiologic studies. Such a system would allow for drug use comparisons within or between countries and across periods of time. The classification systems can be by therapeutic or pharmacologic category, by indication, or by chemical structure. Unfortunately, there has been no standardized, international system that has been universally accepted by researchers.

There have been systems that have categorized drugs therapeutically. In the US, the American Hospital Formulary Service System (AHFS), published by the American Society of Health-System Pharmacists in Bethesda, Maryland, is frequently used. This system broadly defines drugs and is of some use in DUR studies. The classification of drugs in this system is by the pharmacologic-therapeutic category, with the 30 major therapeutic categories and index numbers provided in Table 1.[31] This arrangement permits easy review of information on a group of drugs with similar activities and uses, and it allows the reader to determine quickly the similarities and differences among drugs within a group. The names of the drugs are the United States Adopted Names (USAN). There may be multiple subcategories under the major category (Figure 2). The system allows for classes and subclasses of drugs to be coded numerically for drug utilization studies. The AHFS has more than 30 years of continuous service and therefore is a well-known system in the US. It has been part of a widely used complete drug information source (*AHFS Drug Information*) for use by healthcare professionals, and it often has been placed in patient-care areas for ready access by healthcare professionals in hospitals, extended care facilities, nursing homes, and HMOs. Unfortunately, the classification system does not categorize individual drugs nor fixed combinations, and therefore cannot be used in certain drug utilization studies that require extensive detail.

A second system, the Anatomical-Therapeutic Classification System, is used by the European Pharmaceutical Market Research Association (EPhMRA) and by the International Pharmaceutical Market Research Group (IPMRG).[32] It has been adopted by various European countries and the US, and it is also used by IMS, which conducts surveys for the pharmaceutical industry. Drugs are divided into 14 main categories according to organs or body systems, with subsequent categorization into a second level (main therapeutic group) and a third level (therapeutic subgroup). The system, like the AHFS, does not allow the identification of a particular drug nor does it classify fixed-dose combinations.

There is another system chosen by the Nordic Council on Medicines as a common classification system for all medicines in Nordic countries.[33]

Essentially it was developed by the Norwegian Medical Depot and allows for the complete chemical and therapeutic classification of each compound. This system, the Anatomical-Therapeutic Chemical classification system (ATC), is also recommended by the WHO to be used in DUR studies. The ATC classification system is based on the same main principles as the Anatomical Classification developed by the EPhMRA and the IPMRG. Again, the basic system divides drugs into 14 main groups (first level) with two subdivisions, a second and a third level, which are therapeutic subgroups. The ATC classification system comprises two additional levels, a fourth level being a chemical/therapeutic subgroup and a fifth level for the single chemical substance (Figure 3). The ATC system has proved suitable for DUR studies at all levels and contributes to a further standardization of individual drugs for national and international drug utilization statistics.

Table 1
American Hospital Formulary Service Pharmacologic-Therapeutic Categories[31]

Major Category	Index No.
Antihistamine drugs	4:00
Antiinfective agents	8:00
Antineoplastic agents	10:00
Autonomic drugs	12:00
Blood derivatives	16:00
Blood formation and coagulation	20:00
Cardiovascular drugs	24:00
Central nervous system agents	28:00
Contraceptives	32:00
Dental agents	34:00
Diagnostic agents	36:00
Disinfectants	38:00
Electrolyte, caloric, and water balance	40:00
Enzymes	44:00
Antitussives, expectorants, and mucolytic agents	48:00
Eye, ear, nose, and throat preparations	52:00
Gastrointestinal drugs	56:00
Gold compounds	60:00
Heavy metal antagonists	64:00
Hormones and synthetic substitutes	68:00
Local anesthetics	72:00
Oxytocics	76:00
Radioactive agents	78:00
Serums, toxoids, and vaccines	80:00
Skin and mucous membrane agents	84:00
Smooth muscle relaxants	86:00
Vitamins	88:00
Unclassified therapeutic agents	92:00
Devices	94:00
Pharmaceutical aids	96:00

The advantages of the ATC system can clearly be seen because it is able to identify drugs at their chemical level.

Standardized drug classification systems can provide a useful tool that would allow researchers to perform DUR studies within or between countries and across time intervals.

Drug Utilization Data—Sources and Variables

Pharmacoepidemiologic databases, including DUR databases, can be organized by using the following taxonomy: (1) population databases including both drug and diagnostic data, (2) population databases including diagnostic data only, and (3) population databases with drug data only. Population databases with both drug and diagnostic data can be divided into outpatient databases (e.g., Medicaid Management Information System [MMIS], the Computerized Online Medicaid Pharmaceutical Analysis and Surveillance System [COMPASS] databases), and inpatient databases (e.g., the Boston Collaborative Drug Study Program). Furthermore, in population databases with diagnosis and drug data, diagnosis-specific population databases (e.g., the American Rheumatism Association), drug-specific population databases (e.g., SmithKline Beecham Cimetidine Cohort Database),

28:00 Central nervous system agents	
28:12 Anticonvulsants	
28:12.04 Barbiturates	
28:12.08 Benzodiazepines	
28:12.12 Hydantoins	
28:12.16 Oxazolidinediones	
28:12.20 Succinimides	
28:12.92 Miscellaneous anticonvulsants	

Figure 2
Example of Major Therapeutic Categories (Central Nervous System Agents) Along with Appropriate Subcategories and Index Numbers

1st level	N — central nervous system	(anatomical group)
2nd level	N05 — psycholeptics	(therapeutic main group)
3rd level	N05B — tranquilizers	(therapeutic subgroup)
4th level	N05BA — benzodiazepines	(chemical/therapeutic subgroup)
5th level	N05BA01 — diazepam	(chemical substance group)

Figure 3
Example of Central Nervous System Agents, Using the Anatomical-Therapeutic Chemical Classification System with Appropriate Indices and Groupings

and spontaneous drug event reporting systems (e.g., the Food and Drug Administration [FDA] Spontaneous Drug Event Reporting System, the National Registry of Drug-Induced Ocular Side Effects) are included. In some European countries, data are available via retail pharmacy computer systems. For example, the Danish retail pharmacies' drug subsidy system is completely computerized. The data are person-identifiable, making it possible to chart the population's drug use from the perspective of the individual user.[34]

Examples of the other two main categories of databases are the Population Database Diagnosis Data Only, an example being the Framingham Study; and Population Databases Drug Data Only, examples including IMS databases. A thorough discussion of databases is provided in Chapter 14.

A commercially available compendium containing descriptive information on drug and diagnosis databases is the *International Drug Benefit/Risk Assessment Data Resource Handbook*,[35] prepared under the auspices of Ciba-Geigy. Separate volumes of the compendium have been prepared for data sources in North America, the UK, Japan, Germany, the Netherlands, and Switzerland.

Four major sources of DUR data that are the major vehicles for drug utilization studies are discussed below in more detail. The sources are (1) market surveys based primarily on sales data or prescription volume data, (2) third-party payers or HMOs, (3) institutional and ambulatory settings, and (4) pharmacoepidemiologic studies designed for monitoring and evaluating exposure-related outcomes.

MARKET SURVEYS

These data often are collected by commercial database vendors who resell the aggregate data to pharmaceutical firms for marketing studies. One such commercial vendor includes IMS America, which surveys physician–patient contacts for diagnoses and therapies, monitors prescriptions dispensed in pharmacies, and collects sales data from hospitals and drugstores.

IMS provides the following information[36]:

National Prescription Audit. Based on a panel of about 1400 computerized pharmacies and 600 noncomputerized pharmacies, the National Prescription Audit (NPA) measures the prescription volume that moves out of pharmacies into the hands of consumers. These data are derived only from retail pharmacies; however, it is estimated that retail pharmacies account for nearly 90% of the prescriptions dispensed in the US. Other outlets, such as supermarkets and mail-order pharmacies, are not included. The unit of measurement is the prescription; thus, the data obtained do not reflect an exact dollar amount or units of medication, because prescription size fluctuates.

National Disease and Therapeutic Index. This index provides descriptive information on disease patterns and treatments in private, office-based medical practices in the US. The NDTI physician panel now represents up to 92 primary specialties grouped into 27 specialty groups. A 6-year history is available on compact disc. Physicians salaried by hospital or government agencies are not eligible to participate. Physicians are randomly selected for recruitment to the National Disease and Therapeutic Index (NDTI) panel from the American Medical Association and American Osteopathic Association. Each participating physician reports on his or her medical practice for all patient contacts for two consecutive working days for each calendar quarter. The NDTI uses the term "mentions" for drug reports. Mentions are not directly equivalent to prescriptions or patients, since only about 65% of drugs recorded during a physician–patient contact involve issuance of a formal outpatient prescription. However, mentions reflect use, since the remainder are drugs administered directly, given as samples, recommended, or discussed but not issued. The data include mentions of hospital drug use, but do not include refill prescriptions that do not involve patient contact.

IMS also provides several other databases. Mail Order Prescription Audit measures the level of prescriptions that are dispensed from non-government mail-order pharmacy services to patients via the US Postal Service, United Parcel Service, and other home delivery services. A database called Xponent monitors prescription activity at retail and mail-order outlets, and custom projects prescriptions generated by more than 650 000 individual prescribers every month. A similar database called Xponent Hospital monitors prescriptions that are written in the hospital yet filled at retail pharmacies. Long-term Care Audit is a database that measures the dispensing of prescription by nursing homes with in-house pharmacies and by nursing home provider pharmacies in the US.[37]

Other sources of data are available to researchers and policy-makers. These sources often are required to assemble and integrate data from different databases. For example, the US Department of Health and Human Services conducts a continuing National Health Care Expenditure Survey that has data on drug use as well as the utilization of other health and social services. The National Ambulatory Care Survey by the National Center for Health Statistics is another information source available on drug use. A summary of the results of prescription drug use in office practice has been published.[38] McCaig and Hughes[39] used the National Ambulatory Medical Care Survey to assess changes in oral antimicrobial drug prescribing by office-based physicians from 1980 to 1992, with emphasis on the treatment of otitis media and sinusitis. Results showed that increased prescribing was found for the more expensive, broad-spectrum antimicrobial drugs (e.g., cephalosporins), and that decreasing rates were observed for less expensive antimicrobials with a narrower spectrum (e.g., penicillins).

Furthermore, the Retired Persons Services organization, which operates approximately 12 pharmacies throughout the US on behalf of the American Association of Retired Persons, has an extensive drug utilization database. Other important sources are special registries established for groups of patients thought to be at higher risk, including the National Registry of Drug-Induced Ocular Side Effects, Registry of Tissue Reactions to Drugs, Dermatological Adverse Reaction Reporting System, Hepatic Events Registry, and the International Registry of Lithium Babies. These registries are also particularly important as spontaneous drug–event reporting systems. In the four major Nordic countries (Denmark, Finland, Norway, Sweden), sales data are available from the Nordic Council on Medicines. These data are available by the ATC system as discussed in the section on drug classification systems, and researchers have used these data along with the DDD to describe prescribing patterns in the Nordic countries.[29,30]

THIRD-PARTY PAYERS/HMO/MEDICAID

Noncommercial national and international drug utilization sources include the FDA's postmarketing surveillance (PMS) system and the Swedish Diagnosis and Therapy Survey. Drug utilization information originating from the FDA includes drug utilization trends over time, by age and gender distribution, and by drug category. The primary focus of the FDA's PMS system has been capturing information on unintended drug effects (UDEs) to assess risks. Many of these data come from various group health organizations in which the continuity of care of an enrolled population allows for the linkage of pharmacy records with medical charts. Clinical databases that allow for record linkage are discussed in greater detail in Chapter 14.

The Medicaid health insurance system in the US is a computerized medical and pharmaceutical care billing system of which selected data items from the computerized files have been used for DUR studies. For example, one combined database of such data from several states is COMPASS.[40] State Medicaid programs make data available without patient identification to researchers at a nominal cost. Although Medicaid data reflect consumption of a changing and nonrandom patient population skewed to lower income groups, it can have value, especially for identifying trends of utilization. The Congress of the US passed the Omnibus Budget Reconciliation Act of 1990 (OBRA '90), which mandated both prospective and retrospective DUR programs. OBRA '90 required that each state establish a DUR program for covered outpatient drugs in its Medicaid programs by January

1, 1993. The objective of the DUR program is to identify patterns of fraud, abuse, gross overuse, or inappropriate or medically unnecessary care.[41]

Medicaid databases have been used for drug utilization studies to examine the effects of formulary restrictions on drug expenditures and drug use, to provide cost analysis of specific disease states, and to assess the influence of demographic variables on prescription drug use.[42-45] A recent report reviewed and summarized state DUR initiatives described in the first annual reports submitted by 48 states and the District of Columbia under a mandate of OBRA '90. Although the review points out problems in the reporting by states, it summarizes that the state reports do have the potential to describe the difficulties of implementing broad-based programs to monitor the quality of healthcare service and to provide constructive lessons about creative approaches to quality improvement in diverse settings.[46]

In Sweden, the prescribing of medicines to ambulatory care patients has been collected in the Diagnosis and Therapy Survey since 1978. Copies of prescription, containing not only drugs, but also diagnosis and/or symptoms, are collected from a stratified, randomized sample of physicians. This survey connects the diagnosis/symptoms for which the drugs are prescribed and allows for the important diagnosis–therapy link.[30] In New Zealand, a patient database has been developed by the Ministry of Health. This database, although modest in size, may prove to be a valuable resource in performing Phase IV studies.

INSTITUTIONAL/AMBULATORY SETTINGS

It is important for administrators and health professionals to know patterns of drug use, along with population changes and disease prevalence. As mentioned earlier, descriptive data are readily available on the extent of drug use, where drugs are used, local differences in the choice of drugs, use in various groups, and changes over time. However, there is a need for information on the outcomes of treatments, drug intake, and prescribing patterns for different indications. These factors require in-depth studies using individualized data on a longitudinal basis correlated with healthcare use data.[47] Patterns of drug use data provide information on how the effects of drugs, as predicted from clinical trials and from known prescribing practice, are related to recommended treatment regimens.[48] As mentioned in the introduction, DUR studies are the major source of this information in institutional settings. In the hospital, they are referred to as DUE and, in long-term-care facilities, as DRR. Regardless, DUR is the common nomenclature for all quality assurance studies examining the relationship between diagnosis and drug therapy.

In the US, DUR activities generally are mandated by Professional Review Organizations (PROs) and by institutional accrediting bodies, such as the

Joint Commission on the Accreditation of Healthcare Organizations.[49] PROs were initiated to help the federal government curb its expenditures for Medicaid recipients while ensuring quality of care. The PROs include peer review in the use of services, quality assurance activities, and credentialing, with their emphasis focused primarily on hospital-oriented activities. An extensive amount of literature on DUR studies in institutional care has been published, providing the researcher access to data on the use of drugs in the clinical practice setting. Readers are referred to the several articles on the published results of a workshop on DUR for definitive information.[50] Most DUR data are collected retrospectively. Concurrent DUR, at the point of service, is now a requirement under OBRA '90. OBRA '90 also included a requirement that each Medicaid agency implement retrospective DURs in January 1993. Prescription drug claims are to be analyzed for intrapatient therapeutic conflicts such as drug–patient, drug–drug, and drug–condition, as well as for aberrant interpatient prescribing, dispensing, or consumption patterns. When formulating this requirement, legislators presumably acted on the experience of practitioners who administer retrospective DUR programs for various state Medicaid agencies and private companies.

Medical Audit. DUR data provide information about drug patterns, prescriber's performance, and patient contacts with the healthcare system. Therefore, drug utilization data can be used as an indicator to evaluate, at the macro level, the functions of the healthcare system. The medical audit concept serves to evaluate differences in prescribing between individual prescribers or between groups. Medical audits examine differences between institutional and community prescribers at the local or national level or among countries.

The objective of the medical audit is to identify problems associated with prescribing and to be able to provide recommendations leading to a solution for the problems identified. This then facilitates appropriate prescribing to maintain high standards of care.[51] Although the self-audit has value, such data must be questioned with regard to validity and reliability because the data are self-reported.

Another approach to medical audits is to study the prescribing patterns of care given at community, state, or national levels. This is often called peer audits. Thus, studies can be conducted not only in institutions, but also in the community where most of the drugs are used.

The advantages of medical audits over other types of available drug use data are that they provide the diagnosis on which the prescribing has taken place, thus providing documentation for the diagnosis–therapy relationship. Some studies have suggested that the medical audit may threaten the physician's ability to change prescribing behavior.[46,52] Therefore, it is important to perform medical audits objectively and with physicians' input. In this way, the important link between diagnosis and drug therapy can be affected and rational drug prescribing can be enhanced.

MONITORING AND EVALUATING EXPOSURE-RELATED OUTCOMES

Another source of information on drug use and performance is specific studies designed to address pharmacoepidemiologic questions. This type of drug utilization research involves epidemiologic methodologies, such as case–control and cohort studies.[53,54] Herbst et al.,[55] for example, demonstrated that, with only eight cases and four controls per case, a significant association between diethylstilbestrol therapy and vaginal and cervical adenocarcinoma in young women could be established. Case–control studies usually are not designed as DUR studies, but instead they are designed to test hypotheses. In fact, they generally are used to confirm or refute reported UDEs associated with a defined pharmacologic agent in PMS.

Another epidemiologic design, the cohort study, follows a cohort of individuals over time who have been exposed to a drug thought to be a potential risk factor for an adverse outcome. An example of a cohort study is one performed by Jick et al.,[56] which showed an association between replacement estrogens and endometrial cancer. Case–control and cohort designs, which are appropriate for PMS, are not ideally suited for DUR studies. Pharmacoepidemiologic methodologies used in postmarketing studies with a strong analytic and etiologic orientation are discussed in Chapter 4.

Drug utilization data obtained by the methodologies discussed under the four major data sources above are used for a wide variety of inquiries and studies that are detailed in the next section. Pharmacoepidemiologic inquiries include the use rate for a class of drugs, estimates of the population at risk for the use of a defined causal agent, prescribing rates as an indicator of the prevalence for a nonreportable disease,[57] quantification of the incidence of a UDE, evaluation of shifts in prescribing patterns to document secondary indications for labeling purposes, and the establishment of causality between a reported event and a pharmacologic agent. The nature of the inquiry determines the appropriate drug utilization data course and the pharmacoepidemiologic method. An understanding of the validity of drug use data and the methodology by which these data are obtained is essential in examining any of these inquiries.

Drug Utilization Studies—A Focus on Descriptive Pharmacoepidemiology

Drug utilization studies explore what drugs are used, in what quantity, by whom, how they are used, and the context in which they are used.

These studies have focused on several areas of research to include (1) use in specific populations; (2) patterns of use, both over time and cross-sectional; (3) use in specific disease states; (4) detection of adverse outcomes; (5) use as a surrogate for disease states; (6) use as a public policy tool; (7) use across countries; and (8) the effects of demographics.

SPECIFIC POPULATIONS

Drug utilization studies have reviewed drug use in specific populations. For example, Olubadewo and Ikponmwamba[58] surveyed outpatient drug use in a pediatric population and found that three pharmacotherapeutic categories (antiinfectives/chemotherapeutics, central nervous system agents, respiratory agents) make up more than three-fourths of all prescribed medications. A study in the ambulatory elderly population showed that health-status indicators are better predictors of the use of prescription medications than over-the-counter (OTC) medications and that antihypertensive and cardiac medications make up more than one-half of prescribed medications.[59] Analgesic medications and laxatives represent more than half of all OTC drugs used by the elderly. Drug utilization studies in the elderly are important because people are living longer and consume a disproportionate percentage of medications in the population.[60,61] Jörgensen et al.,[62] in a study of drug use among the elderly in a Swedish municipality, found extensive drug use among those 85 years and older, an age group that is increasing in numbers. The most commonly prescribed drug categories were cardiovascular, psychotropic, and analgesic agents. Kotzan et al.[44] used the Medicaid database in Georgia to show that the patient's age and race significantly influenced the number of prescription drugs used. Patients who were white, female, and 65 years or older had the greatest mean number of prescriptions per patient. Melnick et al.[63] assessed racial differences in the use of antibiotics in an urban population of the Minneapolis–St. Paul, Minnesota, area. They found that significant independent predictors of antibiotic use were younger age, white race, and female gender. Potential explanations for these differences include differences in patient access, physician-prescribing behaviors, and cultural and other factors. Fillenbaum et al.[64] showed that about one-third of the variance in a multivariate health services model for prescription drug use was explained by race. These data compared the characteristics of African-American and white elderly who represented all socioeconomic levels and who live in both urban and rural settings in a defined geographic area.

PATTERNS OF USE

Studies on patterns of drug use have been done at various times for specific drugs or drug categories and also over time to show trends. A cross-sectional study of psychotropic medication by Hohmann et al.[65] using the data from the National Ambulatory Medical Care Survey showed excessive use of minor tranquilizers, the continuing use of first-generation psychotropic medications, and the lack of concordance between diagnoses and prescribed psychotropic medications. Another cross-sectional study, by Hume et al.,[66] used point prevalence estimates and showed that the prevalence of antidepressant use had increased in population-based samples between 1981 and 1993. Bjornson and Wertheimer[67] used the Prescription Card System (PCS), which provides secondary data on third-party prescriptions, to look at patterns of use of oral and topical acyclovir in nearly 3000 patient records. Results suggested that topical acyclovir was being used for indications other than initial genital herpes infections and that oral acyclovir was being used extensively for recurrent infections and suppressive therapy. Use patterns may be beyond currently recommended FDA indications, and further pharmacoepidemiologic studies were recommended. Another study examining the extent and patterns of use of acyclovir in an HMO (northwest region of Kaiser Permanente) showed that women used two-thirds of the prescriptions and that people 15–45 years of age received 80% of the prescriptions. Most oral acyclovir prescriptions were for the treatment of genital herpes, with more than 60% used for first treatment, more than 30% for repeat treatment, and about 6% for continuing (suppressive) therapy.[68] Grasela and Green[69] used the Drug Surveillance Network, a nationwide network of clinical pharmacists in nearly 400 hospitals who are organized to collect drug experience data prospectively from targeted patient populations. One nationwide survey of prescribing patterns for thrombolytic drugs showed that use of these agents varied markedly across institutions and that clinical pharmacists may play a major role in implementing appropriate prescribing changes. Another surveillance study looked at use patterns and infusion-related adverse events of amphotericin B from 397 hospitalized patients. The data showed that nearly three-fourths of the patients experience at least one episode of an infusion-related adverse event and that test doses may not provide much benefit.[70]

Drug utilization studies have also been conducted to look at drug use patterns over time. Data published in the FDA's 1985 review summarized the following trends in overall drug use. From 1971 to 1985, both the number of prescriptions dispensed and the population size increased by 16%, while the prescription size (the average number of capsules, tablets, or other units in a prescription) increased by 29%. In major therapeutic classes, cardiovascular drugs held 15% of the 1985 prescription drug market and were the most frequently dispensed, followed by antiinfectives (13%) and psychotherapeutics (9%).[71,72] Wysowski and Baum[73] used the data from the NPA and the NDTI to study the trends in the use of prescription sedative-hypnotic drugs in the US from 1979 through 1989. Data show trends indicating shifts from longer to shorter acting, and from higher to lower dose, benzodiazepine prescriptions; increasing use of antidepressant drugs for insomnia; female predominance of use; and increasing use with age. Another study that examined the long-term use of benzodiazepines was done by Isacson et al.[74] A cohort of all benzodiazepine users in 1976, aged 15–84 years, was identified and followed for 8 years. Nearly one-third of the cohort continued using benzodiazepines during all 8 years of follow-up. Heavy use, previous use of benzodiazepines, and age were of great importance for predicting long-term use, while gender and type of benzodiazepine were of minor importance. In the MONICA Augsburg project (MONItor trends in CArdiovascular diseases), a cohort of 3324 men and women randomly selected from the population was surveyed in 1984–1985 and again in 1987–1988 regarding antihypertensive medications.[75] The prevalence of antihypertensive drug use increased from 7.8% to 11.2%, with nearly one-half of the persons having their therapy changed during the 3-year follow-up period. Drug class changes showed a marked decrease in diuretic combinations and an increase in calcium-channel blockers. About one-fourth of the patients were taking triple therapy. Prospective analysis showed an underlying discontinuation rate of 49%.

Psaty et al.[76] described the changing patterns of antihypertensive medication use before and after the publication of the results of three major clinical trials of the treatment of hypertension in older adults between 1989 and 1992. Results showed that, among starters of antihypertensive therapy, persons using diuretics increased over time. Among continuous users, the numbers of persons taking diuretics, beta-blockers, and vasodilators generally decreased during the 3-year period, while those taking angiotensin-converting enzyme inhibitors and calcium-channel blockers increased. The temporal trends in antihypertensive therapy coincided in time with and may have reflected, in part, the influence of the major clinical trials on the pattern of clinical practice. Gabriel and Fehring[77] used the NPA and NDTI from IMS America to study the trends in the utilization of nonsteroidal antiinflammatory drugs (NSAIDs) over time. These data illustrate that, in contrast to the rapid rise in NSAID prescriptions from 1973 (27.5 million) to 1983 (66.7 million), NSAID prescriptions between 1986 (66.5 million) and 1990 (66.2 million) have been remarkably stable. However, between 1986 and 1990, NSAIDs have been increasingly prescribed concomitantly with antiulcer and gastroprotective agents from 21 000 "mentions" in 1986 to more than 1 million "mentions" in 1990.

DISEASE STATES

Drug utilization studies have also been conducted to document patterns of use in specific disease states. Thompson et al.[78] reported on a descriptive study that documented drug therapy trends compiled for the years 1984–1990 in acute myocardial infarction. Results showed striking changes in the use of aspirin before admission to the hospital (4–18%). During the stay in the hospital, the use of beta-blockers increased steadily from 52% to 76%, while the use of aspirin increased 3.5-fold from 25% to 88% and the use of streptokinase increased 13.5-fold from 2.4% to 32.4%. The proportion of patients prescribed beta-blockers on discharge from the hospital increased from 46% to 65%, and that for aspirin rose from 16% to 83%. A study by Bjornson et al.[79] used a hospital pharmacy computer database to document prescription drug use patterns of patients infected with HIV and being treated with zidovudine. About one-third of the patients were unable to take the full dose, presumably because of hematologic toxicity. Nearly one-half of the patients were taking systemic antifungals, about one-third were on antivirals or topical fungicides, and about one-fourth were on NSAIDs. The study documented that the HIV-infected patient is being treated concomitantly with many pharmacologic agents prescribed by various medical specialists. The potential for significant drug interactions is evident, and the possibility for long-term toxicities is high. Venturini et al.[80] reported a prospective DUR survey that reviewed thrombolytic therapy for the management of acute myocardial infarction in 58 general hospitals in Italy. After reviewing data on 676 patients, they found that thrombolytic therapy varied significantly according to different demographic and clinical parameters such as age, gender, and delay from the onset of symptoms to admission.

DETECTION OF ADVERSE OUTCOMES

DUR studies have also been used to detect adverse outcomes or risks of therapy. In a study by Oster et al.,[81] pharmacy claims submitted to a health insurance plan operated by Blue Cross/Blue Shield were used to identify nearly 5000 persons who had been prescribed benzodiazepines along with a matched control group. By linking these records with medical claims records that provided diagnosis, they were able to determine that accident-related care was more likely among persons who had been prescribed benzodiazepines. Among those persons, the probability of an accident-related medical encounter was higher during the months in which a prescription for a benzodiazepine had recently been filled compared with other months. Persons who had filled three or more prescriptions for these agents in the 6 months following initiation of therapy had a significantly higher risk of an accident-related medical event than those who had filled only one such prescription. Approximately twofold risks of accident-related care were found, after controlling for age, gender, and prior use. Using a continuous prescription recording system in Jämtland County in Sweden,

Isacsson et al.[82] traced the prescription patterns of 80 individuals who committed suicide from 1970 to 1984 and found that suicide patients obtained 1.5 times more prescription drugs than did matched controls. While the use of psychotropics was high in the suicide group, only about 10% of the patients received antidepressants, often in low doses. The authors conclude that the low rate of antidepressant prescriptions in patients committing suicide may reflect insufficient diagnosis and treatment of depressive disorders. McLeod et al.[83] conducted a retrospective medical record review of concurrently treated patients with streptokinase or r-alteplase for acute myocardial infarction. The objective of the study was to compare the incidence and type of bleeding complications after the use of these agents. The study, performed in 32 participating hospitals in the US, showed that no thrombolytic-related differences were found in the incidence or severity of bleeding following the use of the two thrombolytics. Zito et al.[84] conducted a field trial for hospitalized patients to determine the long-term effectiveness of clozapine in patients with schizophrenia. The authors conclude that the response rate at 12 weeks was similar to that found in the major, double-blind, 6-week, controlled, clinical trial of clozapine. The authors state that, despite the methodologic problems of the naturalistic study design, the data provide a reasonably accurate description of the use of clozapine in a large, systematized program for allocation of scarce resources.

SURROGATE FOR DISEASE STATES

Drug utilization studies can be used as surrogate markers to study the prevalence of a disease or other factor. In Italy, all citizens are covered by the National Health Service, and medical records of individual prescription drugs are computerized through a procedure titled EPIFAR. EPIFAR makes it possible to link simultaneous as well as subsequent prescriptions for each person. Maggini et al.[85] used EPIFAR to provide estimates of tuberculosis prevalence and compared their data with routine surveillance data. The EPIFAR procedure identified a total number of tuberculosis patients seven times higher than that from official notifications. In a preventive health use of drug use information, Grabenstein and Hayton[86] used a hospital pharmacy computer database in a small US Army hospital to search for drugs used to treat patients with diagnoses that warranted vaccination against influenza or pneumococcal pneumonia. Screening by pulmonary, cardiovascular, and hypoglycemic drug use identified the largest numbers of patients in need of vaccination, as did age over 64 years. Of the records screened, nearly three-fourths had valid indications for immunizations.

PUBLIC POLICY

Public policy issues can be addressed with drug utilization studies. Weintraub et al.[87] compared psychotropic medication prescribing and Med-

icaid expenditures before and after institution of the New York State triplicate benzodiazepine regulations. The data sources used were from the
NPA, Medicaid, and Blue Cross/Blue Shield. Results showed that the triplicate regulations have decreased benzodiazepine prescribing; however,
there was an undesirable increase in the prescribing of less-acceptable medications. The effects of removing a propoxyphene napsylate product from a
state Medicaid drug program were examined by Kreling et al.[88] Using the
MMIS in a before–after study, researchers showed that program expenditures increased because of prescribing changes to more expensive products. However, the authors state that other qualitative outcomes should be
considered, such as any therapeutic advantages of replacement products.
Walker et al.[89] found that about one-half of NSAID prescriptions were followed by another NSAID prescription within 2 months and that about 15%
of those patients received a different NSAID. NSAIDs that were frequently
changed for lack of efficacy or for prior toxicity of other NSAIDs were not,
as a whole, associated with more frequent changes for the same reasons.
This study is an example of how a drug utilization study provides information that is essential to increase validity for etiologic studies (e.g., on the
differential distribution of confounding factors and susceptibilities among
those exposed to different NSAIDs). Sclar et al.[90] evaluated the use of the
sulfonylureas using the Medicaid database to see whether the use of second-generation sulfonylureas resulted in a reduction of healthcare expenditures and an enhanced quality of life relative to those of first-generation
drugs. Results showed that there were increases in prescription drug, outpatient hospital, and eye care expenditures with the second-generation
drugs. However, there were decreases in hospital, laboratory, physician,
home health, and clinic expenditures.

ACROSS COUNTRIES

Patterns of drug use in different countries can be found in the drug utilization literature; these consumption patterns often provide clues to the
cause of the observed differences. Baksaas,[22] studying the use of drugs to
control hypertension in the Nordic countries, found that 10% of the population received these drugs on a chronic basis. In Sweden, only about three-
fourths of the beta-blockers and thiazide diuretics were used in the treatment of hypertension, showing that these drugs that are traditionally thought
to be markers for hypertension are used for other indications. The drug of
choice to treat hypertension varies from country to country, but diuretics
are the most widely used, with Danish physicians being especially high
prescribers of thiazide diuretics. Another study comparing drug use for
hypertension in Spain with that in Nordic countries showed that the consumption of antihypertensive drugs measured in DDDs was much lower
in Spain than in the Nordic countries. The use of beta-blocking agents, syn-

thetic hypotensives, and diuretics was also lower in Spain than in the Nordic countries. Only *Rauwolfia* preparations, including combinations with other antihypertensives, were more commonly prescribed. However, thiazides and other diuretics were the most commonly prescribed drugs for hypertension.[91] A study by Kiivet et al.,[24] comparing drugs used in Estonia with those used in Nordic countries, found that many drugs were used in large quantities in Estonia, although they are no longer considered to be first-line medications in the Nordic countries because of their high risk/benefit ratio. Among the factors influencing drug use, it appears that economic status, the ordering and invoicing routines of the pharmaceutical services, and therapeutic traditions were the main reasons for the differences found. A classic international study by Kohn and White[92] used household interview surveys to compare medication use by 48 000 respondents representing 15 million persons in 12 study areas. Six areas were in North America, two in Yugoslavia, and one each in Buenos Aires, Poland, Liverpool, and Helsinki. They found that women are generally more likely than men to use medicines for every age group in all the study areas. One exception was found for men aged 65 years and older residing in Yugoslavia. They also found that drug use rates increase with age, except for women in the six North American study areas, where women of reproductive age (15–44 y) showed a slightly higher usage rate than did those aged 45–64 years. This phenomenon can be explained by oral contraceptive use. Analyzed by therapeutic class, systemic antiinfectives were the most frequently mentioned products, followed by cardiovascular drugs.

DEMOGRAPHICS

Drug utilization studies have also examined the effect of demographic variables on drug use. A study by Moore et al.[93] used a cohort design to determine whether sociodemographic characteristics of patients influence drug therapy in practice. They found that, among patients infected with HIV, African-Americans were significantly less likely than whites to have received antiretroviral therapy or *Pneumocystis carinii* pneumonia prophylaxis. Melnick et al.[63] assessed racial differences in the use of antibiotics in a population-based survey as part of the Minnesota Heart Survey. They found that significant independent predictors of antibiotic use were younger age, white race, and female gender.

Other approaches to comparative analysis of drug utilization patterns are possible. This chapter provides some examples of comparative analytic strategies that are published in the medical and pharmaceutical literature. A more comprehensive bibliography of drug utilization studies can be obtained from the WHO Collaborating Centre for Drug Statistics Methodology, P.O. Box 100, Veitvet, 0518 Oslo 5, Norway.[94]

While the numerous methods reviewed here are important approaches to comparative analysis, traditional pharmacoepidemiologic studies will, by necessity, have to address other issues. Drug utilization studies assess the population using a particular drug to qualify individuals who meet the inclusion and exclusion criteria for clinical trials. Pharmacoeconomic analysis, in the form of cost–effectiveness or cost–benefit studies, will use decision analysis modeling to make rational decisions on therapeutic choices.[95] Safety and efficacy of products now will be looked at in light of overall costs to the healthcare system. Australia and Canada have required cost–benefit data to accompany new drug applications. These data may eventually be required in the European Community Drug Registration Office and by the FDA. Healthcare outcome measures, to include quality-of-life and quality-adjusted life years, will have to be taken into account. Outcome measures can help regulatory agencies, manufacturers, and managed care organizations to obtain relative efficacy data and to enable them to compare adverse effects and other adverse drug reaction profiles of alternative products. In addition, drug utilization studies may help to define off-label drug use to assist in therapeutic outcomes research. Although quality of life has been difficult to measure because of its subjective nature, valid instruments are being developed as the healthcare industry realizes the importance of measuring this variable.[96]

Drug use patterns are influenced by patient characteristics, such as diagnosis, disease severity, related physical conditions, culture, and age. Health system characteristics also have an impact on drug use patterns. Prescribing and consumption are affected and protected by national and regional prescribing norms, traditions, economics, payment systems, number of physicians, the role of advertising, and patient education levels. Moreover, it appears that these patterns evolve regularly and continuously. Therefore, drug use data cannot be used without consideration of these and other confounding variables.

Drug Utilization—The Future

There are increasingly more effective drugs on the market today than ever before. Variations in the utilization of drugs and in the prediction of that utilization, together with the generation of hypotheses exploring those variations, are the objective of pharmacoepidemiology. Drug utilization has captured the attention of researchers internationally, and proper methods needed to conduct DUR studies along with appropriate use of the results of these studies have become the focus of at least one book.[97] Patients are better educated, have greater expectations from health care, and frequently use multiple sources of care. A high correlation between the use of healthcare services, particularly physician contacts, and the use of prescribed drugs can be observed. However, not all prescribing is based on patient needs, and not all patient needs are met with drug therapy. Consequently, there is as much concern about inappropriate and expensive prescribing as there is about underprescribing.

The assessment of the rationality of drug therapy through drug utilization studies is of particular interest in some of the developed countries.[98] For instance, in Sweden, there are several reasons for this interest: (1) the population in general believes there is an imbalance between the beneficial effects and the UDEs of drug therapy and between the importance of pharmacologic and nonpharmacologic treatment; (2) primary care physicians are mandated to have better knowledge of the sociomedical status of patients in their practice areas, including prescription drug use patterns; and (3) limited resources available in the healthcare system necessitate the review of drug therapy outcomes. In the US, DUR studies have been used widely in state Medicaid programs to control inappropriate prescribing. However, there have been few rigorous studies of their impact.[99,100] Lipton and Bird[101] recommend an expanded DUR policy research agenda, strongly suggesting that priority be given to studies in (1) DUR criteria development and validation; (2) prevalence of prescribing problems and their association with patient outcomes; (3) efficacy, toxicity, and costs of therapeutic alternatives; and (4) DUR program evaluation.

The assessment of the rationality of drug use in less-developed countries continues to be problematic.[102] Issues are related to three major areas: (1) national drug policies have been established without referring to the need for assessing drug utilization; (2) healthcare practices and services suffer from communication problems, lack of guidelines, and poor control over the introduction of new medications on the market; and (3) education and training programs for healthcare professionals have generally lacked emphasis in newer pharmacologic concepts.

In addition, major changes are under way in the US that will impact prescribing practice and, consequently, drug utilization in the near future, as is discussed in Chapter 24. The prepaid care practice format referred to as "managed care" is making a profound impact on patterns of drug use in US managed care organizations, since health insurers play an aggressive role in directing and controlling the use of services. Examples include directing patients to specific hospitals, clinics, or practitioners and implementing drug formularies with a focus on multisource products. All of this will clearly influence established drug utilization trends. Moreover, buying arrangements with selective manufacturers will direct demand for products made by those manufacturers, which may be different from local prescribing patterns. Managed care organizations, through the use of payment sanctions to prescribers and dual copayment levels to patients, will succeed in modifying previous drug use patterns. In addition, state-of-the-art electronic data management systems, integrated healthcare data interchange, and strong customer communication between managed care organizations and their clients will potentially revolutionize the DUR process.[103]

The interpretation of drug utilization data is essential for clinical researchers, regulatory agencies, and manufacturers to evaluate marketed drugs for both therapeutic efficacy (primary and secondary effects) and unexpected reactions not identified during Phase I, II, and III premarketing studies. These data are needed in an effort to endorse the selection of efficacious and comparatively less toxic drugs based on the incidence of UDEs in larger populations.

The population at risk for a given medical condition must be known to justify the level of drug use for the specific diagnosis in the defined population. Descriptive data on drug use are easy to obtain and provide the most common information originating from drug utilization studies. These data have important applications in pharmacoepidemiology, with each of these applications placing different demands on the methodologic rigor with which the data are collected. Drug utilization frequencies provide information on the use of classes of drugs or the use of drugs over time. Usage frequencies also define the sample frame of the population at risk for a UDE. Expressed in rates, drug utilization data can provide the numerator data to assess drug use per population unit or patient population with a defined diagnosis. Used as denominator data with the incidence of UDEs defining the numerator, drug use data can be used to calculate the incidence rate and the relative risk of a UDE for the drug under investigation. Each of these applications of drug use data requires the correct unit of measurement, which can be sales data, prescription volume, or DDD.

Care is needed in interpreting drug utilization data as a health indicator. Discrepancies between geographic patterns of morbidity and drug sales can be attributed to factors such as diagnostic criteria, differences in the age distribution of the population, access to health care, and the prevalence of disease.[104,105] Moreover, drug sales do not necessarily reflect drug intake. Medication compliance needs to be addressed; it often is assumed in drug utilization studies that all drugs are being taken as directed by the physician. Drug utilization studies provide the necessary denominator data to be used in more pharmacoepidemiologic research. Drug utilization methods, in conjunction with in-depth observational studies (cohort, case–control) and other surveillance methods, can ensure that future drug use will become more rational, safe, and efficacious.

References

1. Brodie DC. Drug utilization and drug utilization review and control. NCHS-RD-70-8. Rockville, MD: Department of Health, Education, and Welfare, 1970.

2. World Health Organization. The selection of essential drugs. Report of a WHO expert committee. Technical report. Series no. 615. Geneva: World Health Organization, 1977.
3. Tognoni G. Drug use and monitoring. In: Holand WW, ed. Evaluation of health care. Oxford: Oxford University Press, 1983:207-25.
4. Lunde PKM, Baksaas I. Epidemiology of drug utilization—basic concepts and methodology. Acta Med Scand 1988;721(suppl):7-11.
5. Garattini S, Tognoni G. Drug utilization review and pharmacoeconomics. Interaction after parallel development? PharmacoEconomics 1993;4:162-72.
6. Scruba TJ. International comparison of drug consumption: impact of prices. Soc Sci Med 1986;22:1019-25.
7. Serradell J, Patwell JT. Unlabeled drug use patterns in a contemporary outpatient setting. J Pharmacoepidemiol 1991;2:19-43.
8. Wessling A, Boethius G. Measurement of drug use in a defined population. Evaluation of the defined daily dose methodology. Eur J Clin Pharmacol 1990;39:207-10.
9. Ried LD, Johnson RE. Evaluation of the reliability and validity of a measure of anxiolytic drug-use intensity for pharmacoepidemiologic studies. Ann Pharmacother 1992;26:1441-6.
10. Lunde PKM. Drug statistics and drug utilization. In: Columbo F, Shapiro S, Slone D, Tognoni G, eds. Epidemiologic evaluation of drugs. Littleton, MA: PSG Publishing, 1977.
11. Wertheimer AI. The defined daily dose system (DDD) for drug utilization review. Hosp Pharm 1986;21:233-41,258.
12. Benitez J, Puerto AM, Diaz JA. Differences in antidiabetic drug utilization between three different health systems in the same national region. Eur J Clin Pharmacol 1992;42:151-4.
13. Tansella M, Micciolo R. Trends in the prescription of antidepressants in urban and rural general practices. J Affect Disord 1992;24:117-25.
14. DeJong LT, VandenBerg PB, Haaijer-Ruskamp FM, et al. Investigating drug use in pregnancy. Methodological problems and perspectives. Pharm Weekbl Sci 1991;13:32-8.
15. Beghi E, Monticelli ML, Monza G, Sessa A, Zarrelli M. Antiepileptic drugs as "tracers" of disease. A calculation of the prevalence of epilepsy through an analysis of drug consumption. The Group for the Study of Epilepsy in General Practice. Neuroepidemiology 1991;10:33-41.
16. Cohen R, Fontbonne A, Weitzman S, Eschwege E. Estimation of the prevalence of diabetes mellitus in Israel based on hypoglycemic drug supply and consumption. Diabete Metab 1990;16:59-63.
17. Sugarman JR. Hypoglycemia associated hospitalizations in a population with a high prevalence of non-insulin-dependent diabetes mellitus. Diabetes Res Clin Pract 1991;14:139-47.
18. Gran B. Non-pharmacologic methods reduce drug use in the treatment of hypertension. A two-year trial in general practice. Scand J Prim Health Care 1991;9:121-8.
19. Wymenga AB, Hekster YA, Theeuwes A, Muytjens HL, van Horn JR, Sloeff TJ. Antibiotic use after cefuroxime prophylaxis in hip and knee joint replacement. Clin Pharmacol Ther 1991;50:215-20.
20. Fletcher CV, Metzler D, Borchardt-Phelps P, Rodman JH. Patterns of antibiotic use and expenditures during 7 years at a university hospital. Pharmacotherapy 1990;10:199-204.

21. Bergman U, Wessling A, Sjovist F. Validation of observed differences in the utilization of antihypertensive and antidiabetic drugs in Northern Ireland, Norway, and Sweden. Eur J Clin Pharmacol 1985;29:1-8.
22. Baksaas I. Patterns in drug utilization—national and international aspects: antihypertensive drugs. Acta Med Scand 1984;683(suppl):59-66.
23. Aquilonius SM, Granat M, Hartvig P. Utilization of antiparkinson drugs in Norway, Sweden, Denmark, and Finland, 1975–1979. Acta Neurol Scand 1981;64:47-53.
24. Kiivet RA, Bergman U, Sjoquist F. The use of drugs in Estonia compared to the Nordic countries. Eur J Clin Pharmacol 1992;42:511-5.
25. Bjelle A, Mjorndal T. Drug prescription patterns for rheumatic disorders in Sweden. J Rheumatol 1984;11:493-9.
26. Jakovljevic V, Stanulovic M. Extremes in drug utilization patterns. Low prescribing of antihypertensives in the district of Novi Sad, Yugoslavia. Acta Med Scand 1984; 683(suppl):67-9.
27. Gustafsson LL, Boethius G. Utilization of analgesics from 1970 to 1978. Prescription patterns in the county of Jämtland and in Sweden as a whole. Acta Med Scand 1982; 211:419-25.
28. Bergman U, Sjoqvist F. Measurement of drug utilization in Sweden: methodological and clinical implications. Acta Med Scand 1984;683(suppl):15-22.
29. Westerholm B. Drug utilization studies—a valuable tool for optimizing of drug therapy and drug control. J Soc Admin Pharm 1981;1:1-8.
30. Ekedahl A, Lidbeck J, Lithman T, Noreen D, Melander A. Benzodiazepine prescribing patterns in a high-prescribing Scandinavian community. Eur J Clin Pharmacol 1993;44:141-6.
31. McEvoy GK, ed. AHFS drug information. Bethesda, MD: American Society of Health-System Pharmacists, 1997.
32. Capella D. Descriptive tools and analysis. In: Drug utilization studies: methods and uses. Copenhagen: World Health Organization Regional Office for Europe, 1991.
33. Nordic statistics on medicines, 1981–1983. Uppsala: Nordic Council on Medicines, 1985.
34. Hallas J, Nissen A. Individualized drug utilization statistics. Analyzing a populations drug use from the perspective of individual users. Eur J Clin Pharmacol 1994; 47:367-72.
35. International drug benefit/risk assessment data resource handbook. Vol. 1. North America. Prepared by Pharma Corporation and the Degge Group, Ltd. Basel, Switzerland: Ciba-Geigy, 1988.
36. Baum C, Kennedy DL, Forbes MB, Jones JK. Drug use and expenditures in 1982. JAMA 1985;253:382-6.
37. IMS America, Plymouth Meeting, PA.
38. Drug use in office practice—National Ambulatory Medical Care Survey, 1990. Advance Data no. 232. Hyattsville, MD: National Center for Health Statistics, 1993.
39. McCaig LF, Hughes JM. Trends in antimicrobial drug prescribing among office-based physicians in the United States. JAMA 1995;273:214-9.
40. Strom BL, Carson JL, Morse ML, Leroy AA. The Computerized On-line Medicaid Pharmaceutical Analysis and Surveillance System: a new resource for post-marketing drug surveillance. Clin Pharmacol Ther 1985;38:359-64.
41. Fulda TR, Hass SL. Medicaid drug utilization review under OBRA 1990—current issues and future direction. PharmacoEconomics 1992;2:363-70.
42. Kreling DH, Knocke DJ, Hammel RW. The effect of an internal analgesic formulary restriction on Medicaid drug expenditures in Wisconsin. Med Care 1989;27:33-44.

43. Jacobs J, Keyserling JA, Britton J, Morgan GJ, Wilkenfeld J, Hutchings HC. The total cost of care and the use of pharmaceuticals in the management of rheumatoid arthritis: the Medi-Cal Program. J Clin Epidemiol 1988;41:215-23.
44. Kotzan L, Carroll NV, Kotzan JA. Influence of age, sex, and race on prescription drug use among Georgia Medicaid recipients. Am J Hosp Pharm 1989;46:287-90.
45. Sena MM, Pashko S. Drug utilization review using a Medicaid claims database. Clin Ther 1993;15:900-4.
46. Lipowski EE, Collins T. Medicaid DUR programs: 1993—final report to American Pharmaceutical Association Foundation. Washington, DC: American Pharmaceutical Association, 1995.
47. Westerholm B. Data collection in Sweden. In: Bergman U, Grimsson A, Wahba AHW, Westerholm B, eds. Studies in drug utilization. Methods and applications. WHO regional publications. European Series no. 8. Copenhagen: World Health Organization Regional Office for Europe, 1979:63-82.
48. Tognoni G, Liberati A, Pello L, Sasanelli F, Spagnoli A. Drug utilization studies and epidemiology. Rev Epidemiol Sante Publique 1983;31:59-71.
49. Accreditation manual for hospitals. Chicago: Joint Commission on the Accreditation of Healthcare Organizations, 1995.
50. Abrams WB, chair. Proceedings of a Workshop on Drug Utilization Review. Clin Pharmacol Ther 1991;50(suppl):593-640.
51. Crooks J. The concept of medical auditing. Acta Med Scand 1984;683(suppl):47-52.
52. Reilly PM, Pattern MP. An audit of prescribing by peer review. J R Coll Gen Pract 1978;28:525-38.
53. Sartell PE. Retrospective studies: a review for the clinician. Ann Intern Med 1974; 81:381-7.
54. Jick H, Vessey MP. Case–control studies in the evaluation of drug-induced illness. Am J Epidemiol 1978;107:1-7.
55. Herbst AL, Ulfelder H, Poskanzer DC. Adenocarcinoma of the vagina: association of maternal stilbestrol therapy with tumor appearance in young women. N Engl J Med 1971;284:878-81.
56. Jick H, Watkins RN, Hunter JR. Replacement estrogens and endometrial cancer. N Engl J Med 1979;300:218-22.
57. Anderson DW, Bryan FA, Harris BSH III, Lessler JT, Gagnon JP. A survey approach for finding cases of epilepsy. Public Health Rep 1985;100:386-93.
58. Olubadewo JO, Ikponmwamba A Sr. Profile of prescription medications in a pediatric population. Drug Intell Clin Pharm 1988;22:999-1002.
59. Stoller EP. Prescribed and over-the-counter medicine use by the ambulatory elderly. Med Care 1988;26:1149-57.
60. Cassel CK, Rudberg MA, Olshansky SJ. The price of success: health care in an aging society. Health Aff (Millwood) 1992;11:87-99.
61. Ray WA, Griffin MR, Shorr RI. Adverse drug reactions and the elderly. Health Aff (Millwood) 1990;9:114-22.
62. Jörgensen TM, Isacson DGL, Thorslund M. Prescription drug use among ambulatory elderly in a Swedish municipality. Ann Pharmacother 1993;27:1120-5.
63. Melnick SL, Sprafka JM, Laitinen DL, Bostick RM, Flack JM, Burke GL. Antibiotic use in urban whites and blacks: the Minnesota Heart Survey. Ann Pharmacother 1992;26:1292-5.
64. Fillenbaum GG, Hanlon JT, Corder EH, Zigubu-Page T, Wall WE, Brock D. Prescription and non-prescription drug use among black and white community-residing elderly. Am J Public Health 1993;83:1577-82.

65. Hohmann AA, Larson DB, Thompson JW, Beardsley RS. Psychotropic medication prescription in U.S. ambulatory medical care. DICP Ann Pharmacother 1991;25:85-9.
66. Hume AL, Barbour MM, Lapane KL, Carleton RA. Is antidepressant use changing? Prevalence and clinical correlates in two New England communities. Pharmacotherapy 1995;15:78-84.
67. Bjornson DC, Wertheimer AI. Patterns of use: topical and oral acyclovir. J Pharmacoepidemiol 1990;1:49-60.
68. Johnson RE, Mullooly JP, Valanis BG, Andrews EB, Tilson HH. Acyclovir use and its surveillance in a general population. DICP Ann Pharmacother 1990;24:624-8.
69. Grasela TH, Green JA. A nationwide survey of prescribing patterns for thrombolytic drugs in acute myocardial infarction. Pharmacotherapy 1990;10:35-41.
70. Grasela TH, Goodwin SD, Walawander MK, Cramer RL, Fuhs DW, Moriarty VP. Prospective surveillance of intravenous amphotericin B use patterns. Pharmacotherapy 1990;10:341-8.
71. Baum C, Kennedy DL, Knapp DE, Faich GA. Drug utilization in the U.S.—1985: seventh annual review. Rockville, MD: Food and Drug Administration, 1985.
72. Baum C, Kennedy DL, Knapp DE, Juergens JP, Falch GA. Prescription drug use in 1984 and changes over time. Med Care 1988;26:105-14.
73. Wysowski DK, Baum C. Outpatient use of prescription sedative-hypnotic drugs in the United States, 1970 through 1989. Arch Intern Med 1991;151:1779-83.
74. Isacson D, Carsjo K, Bergman U, Blackburn JL. Long-term use of benzodiazepines in a Swedish community: an eight-year follow-up. J Clin Epidemiol 1992;45:429-36.
75. Hense HW, Tennis P. Changing patterns of antihypertensive drug use in a German population between 1984 and 1987. Results of a population-based cohort study in the Federal Republic of Germany. Eur J Clin Pharmacol 1990;39:1-7.
76. Psaty BM, Koepsell TD, Yanez ND, Smith NL, Manolio TA, Heckbert SR, et al. Temporal patterns of antihypertensive medication use among older adults, 1989 through 1992. An effect of the major clinical trials on clinical practice. JAMA 1995;273:1436-8.
77. Gabriel SE, Fehring RA. Trends in the utilization of non-steroidal anti-inflammatory drugs in the United States, 1986–1990. J Clin Epidemiol 1992;45:1041-4.
78. Thompson PL, Parsons RW, Jamrozik K, Hockey RL, Hobbs MS, Broadhurst RJ. Changing patterns of medical treatment in acute myocardial infarction. Observations from the Perth MONICA Project, 1984–1990. Med J Aust 1992;157:87-92.
79. Bjornson DC, Meyer DE, Hiner WO Jr, Tramont EC, Walter Reed Retrovirus Research Group. Prescription drug use patterns of human immunodeficiency virus-infected patients taking zidovudine. DICP Ann Pharmacother 1989;23:698-702.
80. Venturini F, Romero M, Tognoni G. Acute myocardial infarction treatments in 58 Italian hospitals: a drug utilization survey. Ann Pharmacother 1995;29:1100-5.
81. Oster G, Huse DM, Adams SF, Imbimbo J, Russell MW. Benzodiazepine tranquilizers and the risk of accidental injury. Am J Public Health 1990;80:1467-70.
82. Isacsson G, Boethius G, Bergman U. Low level of antidepressant prescription for people who later commit suicide: 15 years of experience from a population-based drug data base. Acta Psychiatr Scand 1992;85:444-8.
83. McLeod DC, Coln WG, Thayer CF, Perfetto EM, Hartzema AG. Pharmacoepidemiology of bleeding events after use of r-alteplase or streptokinase in acute myocardial infarction. Ann Pharmacother 1993;27:956-62.
84. Zito JM, Volavka J, Craig TJ, Czobor P, Banks S, Vitrai J. Pharmacoepidemiology of clozapine in 202 inpatients with schizophrenia. Ann Pharmacother 1993;27:1262-9.

85. Maggini M, Salmaso S, Alegiani SS, Caffari B, Raschetti R. Epidemiological use of drug prescriptions as markers of disease frequency: an Italian experience. J Clin Epidemiol 1991;44:1299-307.
86. Grabenstein JD, Hayton BD. Pharmacoepidemiologic program for identifying patients in need of vaccination. Am J Hosp Pharm 1990;47:1774-81.
87. Weintraub M, Singh S, Byrne L, Maharaj K, Guttmacher L. Consequences of the 1989 New York State triplicate benzodiazepine prescription regulations. JAMA 1991;266:2392-7.
88. Kreling DH, Knocke DJ, Hammel RW. The effects of an internal analgesic formulary restriction on Medicaid drug expenditures in Wisconsin. Med Care 1989;27:34-44.
89. Walker AM, Chan KA, Yood RA. Patterns of interchange in the dispensing of nonsteroidal anti-inflammatory drugs. J Clin Epidemiol 1992;45:187-95.
90. Sclar DA, McCombs JS, Nichol MB. Evaluating the cost–effectiveness and quality of life with retrospective data: a study of sulfonylurea coverage under Medi-Cal. J Pharmacoepidemiol 1990;1:41-60.
91. Capella D, Porta M, Laporte JR. Utilization of antihypertensive drugs in certain European countries. Eur J Clin Pharmacol 1983;25:431-5.
92. Kohn R, White KL. Health care. An international study. Oxford: Oxford University Press, 1976.
93. Moore RD, Stanton D, Gopalan R, Chaisson RE. Racial differences in the use of drug therapy for HIV disease in an urban community. N Engl J Med 1994;330:763-8.
94. Drug utilization bibliography. Copenhagen: World Health Organization Regional Office for Europe, 1989.
95. Drummond MF, Stoddart GL, Torrance GW. Methods for the economic evaluation of health care programs. Oxford: Oxford University Press, 1986.
96. Ware JE, Hays RD. Methods for measuring patient satisfaction with specific medical encounters. Med Care 1988;26:393-402.
97. Dukes MNG, ed. Drug utilization studies. Methods and uses. WHO Regional Publications European Series no. 45. Copenhagen: World Health Organization Regional Office for Europe, 1993.
98. Boethius G. Approaches to assessing the rationality of drug usage in a developed country. Acta Med Scand 1988;721(suppl):21-6.
99. Zimmerman DR, Collins TM, Lipowski EE, et al. Evaluation of a DUR intervention: a case study of histamine antagonists. Inquiry 1994;31:89-101.
100. Soumerai SB, Lipton HL. Computer-based drug utilization review—risk, benefit, or boondoggle? N Engl J Med 1995;332:1641-5.
101. Lipton HL, Bird JA. Drug utilization review in ambulatory settings: state of the science and directions for outcomes research. Med Care 1993;31:1069-82.
102. Ali HN. Problems in assessing rationality of drug utilization in less developed countries. Acta Med Scand 1988;721(suppl):27-30.
103. Briesacher B, DuChane J. Drug utilization review in the managed care environment. Med Interface 1995;8:72-8.
104. Hjort P, Holmen J, Waaler H. The relation between drug utilization and morbidity pattern: antihypertensive drugs. Acta Med Scand 1984;683(suppl):89-93.
105. Westerholm B, Dahlstrom M, Nordanstam I. Relation between drug utilization and morbidity patterns. Acta Med Scand 1984;683(suppl):95-7.

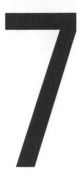

Pharmacogenetic and Biologic Markers of Unintended Drug Effects

Stephen P Spielberg
Denis M Grant

Abstract

This chapter reviews some basic principles of so-called idiosyncratic unintended drug effects (UDEs) and fundamentals of human pharmacogenetics, and provides some examples of pharmacogenetic variants with potential as biologic markers useful in the diagnosis and prediction of drug toxicity risk.

T able 1 provides a comparison of traditional animal toxicology studies with the real world of human patients, as well as the characteristics of patients in preclinical trials and those taking the drugs postmarketing. It is becoming increasingly apparent that the basis for many of the serious unintended drug effects (UDEs) that cause significant patient morbidity and withdrawal or failure of licensing of otherwise useful medications is variability in response to foreign compounds in the heterogeneous human population. The sources of variability include age, gender, disease state, diet, habits (e.g., alcohol, tobacco), drug interactions, and an increasingly recognized role of inherited differences in drug handling and response (pharmacogenetics). Epidemiologic studies, including postmarketing surveillance, can help detect unexpected UDEs, define their incidence, and determine risk factors such as age and drug interactions. Basic investigation of the mechanisms of drug toxicity and of pharmacogenetic factors predisposing to risk has the potential for the development of "biologic markers" that can be used to confirm the diagnosis of complex UDEs, predict who in the population is at risk, and help guide epidemiologic studies. Most progress made in understanding the pathogenesis and decreasing the incidence of UDEs is likely to arise from the collaboration between pharmacoepidemiologists and pharmacogeneticists.

Idiosyncratic Drug Reactions

Idiosyncratic UDEs are not based on the pharmacologic mechanism of the drug in question and typically are unrelated to the dose administered.

Table 1
Preclinical Toxicology, Clinical Trials, and Risk of Unintended Drug Effects

	Preclinical Toxicology and Human Risk	
	Animals	**Humans**
Genetics	inbred	heterogeneous
Environment	defined	heterogeneous
Diet	defined	heterogeneous
Disease	well	sick
Other drugs	none	many
Habits	none	many

	Clinical Trials and Postmarketing Risk	
	Trials	**Postmarketing**
Age	limited	unrestricted
Gender	mostly men	unrestricted
Race	limited	unrestricted
Indication	defined	unrestricted
Other drugs	defined	unrestricted
Habits	defined	unrestricted

As alluded to above, preclinical toxicology studies performed on inbred animals rarely detect or predict human idiosyncratic reactions. Similarly, since the reactions are not related directly to dose or serum concentration, the monitoring of drug serum concentrations will not prevent UDEs. Indeed, one of the main problems with such UDEs is that the usual clinical setting is a patient correctly diagnosed, given the correct drug for the indication, and given the correct dose, and yet a potentially severe UDE unexpectedly develops.

Many of the reactions, including "hypersensitivity reactions," present major diagnostic quandaries. In the absence of confirmatory diagnostic laboratory data, events occurring during therapy such as fever, skin rash, liver function abnormalities, and bone marrow abnormalities could be attributed to a wide spectrum of infectious and autoimmune processes and, with frequent multidrug therapy, to any of the medications. Various approaches to evaluating clinical data (e.g., Bayesian methods) may help in the diagnosis, and large epidemiologic studies may suggest a statistically significant association between the use of a drug and a given event; however, there remains a major need to develop diagnostic tests to confirm both epidemiologic data and the diagnosis. Even with possible drug-induced birth defects, epidemiologic studies can ascertain the relative risk in exposed and unexposed populations, yet individual risk remains undefined. Here, too, the challenge is to understand the pathogenesis of the undesired effect of the drug and to turn understanding of the mechanism into a valid biologic marker of drug effect and susceptibility to toxicity.

In perspective, many idiosyncratic reactions that currently elude our predictive capacity occur with an incidence of less than 1/1000, often less than 1/10 000. This has several consequences when considering possible biologic approaches to help in diagnosis and prediction. Recommendations are given for routine monitoring of liver function tests (serum enzymes and bilirubin) or blood counts for many drugs associated with liver or bone marrow toxicity. When applied to large populations, however, most of the currently available tests exhibit considerable day-to-day variability, with a significant percentage of the population having abnormal values at any given time. In a population of patients taking a specific medication, then, several percent of the patients might reach the criteria for abnormal liver function tests, while only about 1/10 000 would be true drug-induced events. In other words, the vast majority of abnormal screening values represent false positives, and the positive predictive value of such tests is very poor. The consequences of relying on these types of tests to prevent rare UDEs include: diagnostic confusion; pursuit of medically irrelevant laboratory variation; unnecessary discontinuation of medication, with potential exposure of patients to other medications with undefined UDE risk; and substantial costs in laboratory screening and other tests if a value comes back abnormal. In addition, patients may have entirely normal laboratory values, but present with a true UDE several days or weeks later. Routine laboratory tests are very far removed biologically from the mechanism of toxicity of any drug and are rather nonspecific markers of organ function; therefore, it is not surprising that, under most circumstances, such tests are of limited value. The closer a biologic marker is to the approximate mechanisms of toxicity of a compound, the more likely it is to have both diagnostic and predictive utility (see below).

The second issue with respect to relatively infrequent events is that it is intuitively unlikely that risk is distributed evenly throughout the population, just as it is medically unsatisfying to tell a patient that he or she has a 1/10 000 chance of having a specific UDE. We are increasingly recognizing the role of individual differences in the metabolism of and response to drugs based on inherited differences in enzymes and receptors as a basis for many idiosyncratic drug reactions. It is likely that most of the population has essentially no risk of specific UDEs from a specific drug, while a subpopulation is at very high risk. Markers of susceptibility based on pharmacogenetic mechanisms hold the promise of providing individual estimates of risk and predicting such risk, thus decreasing UDEs for both individuals and the population as a whole.

Pharmacogenetics

Pharmacogenetic variants represent a subclass of inborn errors of metabolism. Perhaps their main distinguishing feature is that they are usually "silent" in the absence of exposure to a drug or other foreign chemical. The presence of a variant gene usually is manifest upon exposure to specific chemical structures and can result in (1) functional overdose in patients unable to eliminate an active drug, (2) lack of therapeutic effect in patients unable to convert a prodrug into its active form, and (3) idiosyncratic reactions that often result from overproductions or failure to detoxify a potentially toxic metabolite. Pharmacogenetic traits are divided arbitrarily between rare defects and polymorphism, in which a variant gene product results in a phenotype with a frequency of at least 1% in the population. Similar to other genetic abnormalities, allelic variation is common. It also is common for there to be several variant alleles at a given locus. Finally, it would be expected that gene frequencies for variant alleles will differ among different human populations, and that UDE frequencies thus will vary among different human ethnic and racial groups. The latter considerations have obvious consequences for epidemiologic studies and international drug development.

Pharmacogenetic variants often come to light in the context of investigating variation in drug response in the population. Most well-defined disorders are abnormalities in enzymes responsible for drug metabolism. Unexpected variability in serum concentrations, pharmacologic effect, or unanticipated UDEs may provide the impetus for investigation of the basis for the variability, with family studies used to confirm inheritance. Techniques for study have traditionally included examination of metabolic profiles and clearance of drugs, population and family studies of a specific drug or in vivo test compound, and investigation of drug handling in monozygotic and dizygotic twins. Increasingly, in vitro approaches using human cells to measure specific enzymes and the toxicologic potential of drugs, as well as direct molecular genetic analysis of gene polymorphisms, are being used. The explosive advances of molecular biology in human genetic disease are being applied to pharmacogenetic variants at an ever-increasing rate.

The impact of molecular biology on the utility of pharmacogenetics in the drug development process is most evident in studies on the cytochromes P450.[1-4] It is now possible, through the use of human hepatic microsomes (together with chemical or antibody inhibitors of specific members of the P450 superfamily) and recombinantly expressed P450s, to determine the likely pathways of metabolism of a new chemical entity. If the isoform involved is polymorphic (e.g., CYP2D6 [see below]), the kinetic consequences can be determined early in the clinical development process. Human volunteers can be studied in single-dose experiments to determine whether the polymorphism is likely to have a major or minor impact on the handling of the compound in vivo. If the impact is major, the compound cannot be redesigned to avoid metabolism by a polymorphic pathway, and if the drug is a major therapeutic advance, consideration can be given to a pharmacogenetic prescreen to adjust dosage (or perhaps avoid the drug) in those patients with a pharmacogenetic variant. Assays using small blood samples are becoming even simpler and may be available for use in a physician's office in the not-too-distant future. Similarly, when patients are discovered who are outliers from either an efficacy or toxicity point of view, DNA banked from such subjects can be used to determine the mechanism involved and ultimately to develop screening tools to avoid unwanted outcomes.

Examples of Pharmacogenetic Variants as Possible Markers of UDEs and UDE Susceptibility

Several good reviews of the area of pharmacogenetics are available.[5-12] A few examples are discussed from the vantage point of the possible development of biologic markers of drug toxicity or susceptibility.

THIOPURINE METHYLTRANSFERASE AND UDEs FROM AZATHIOPRINE AND MERCAPTOPURINE

Many drugs undergo metabolism by several pathways mediated by different drug metabolism enzymes. Figure 1 presents the pathways of metabolism of azathioprine and mercaptopurine, drugs used in immunologic disorders and cancer chemotherapy. One of the major adverse effects of the drugs is bone marrow suppression. It has been demonstrated that the enzyme thiopurine methyltransferase (TPMT) is polymorphic in the human population; approximately 0.3% of the population has essentially no TPMT activity, and 11% has intermediate activity.[13-16] Low enzyme activity is inherited as a simple autosomal recessive trait. These studies used peripheral blood erythrocytes for measurement of enzyme activity after proving that enzyme activity in these easily obtained cells correlated with activity in other organs, such as the liver. Furthermore, it has been suggested that low TPMT activity might shunt intracellular metabolism toward 6-thioguanine nucleotides, which might mediate bone marrow toxicity.[17] Using erythrocyte TPMT activity as a marker, researchers have found that patients receiving azathioprine who developed severe bone marrow suppression at conventional doses were in the 0.3% of the population with absent enzyme activity.[18] Furthermore, the concentration of 6-thioguanine nucleotides in their erythrocytes was far higher than among patients who tolerated the drug without excessive myelosuppression.

Several issues are raised by these studies. First, given that the incidence of absent enzyme activity is relatively rare in the population, absent enzyme activity in 5 patients with marrow suppression compared with 16 controls is highly statistically significant. If a rare pharmacogenetic defect is postulated to play a critical role in a given UDE, epidemiologic and clinic ascertainment of only a relatively small number of patients with UDEs is necessary to prove or disprove the hypothesis. Second, for azathioprine or mercaptopurine therapy, it would appear that absent TPMT activity may preclude

Figure 1
Pathways of
Metabolism of
Azathioprine and
Mercaptopurine

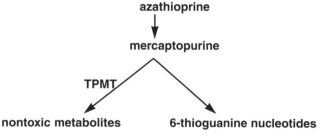

TPMT = thiopurine methyltransferase.

use of the drug. Prescreening patients who might be exposed to the drug may lead to selection of alternative therapy or, if the drugs are used, to dosage adjustments with careful monitoring of intracellular 6-thioguanine nucleotide concentrations. Here, then, is a potential example of a biologic marker of susceptibility to a UDE that could be used in selected patients prior to therapy, coupled with a monitoring technique closely linked to the biologic basis of the UDE to monitor patients during treatment. Third, to be useful, markers must be reasonably simple tests (peripheral blood cells in this example), and correlation must be demonstrated with other potential target tissues in vivo. Finally, drug actions and UDE mechanisms are rarely simple. 6-Thioguanine nucleotides also may be involved in the mechanism of desired action of these drugs as immunosuppressants and cancer chemotherapy agents. Further data are needed to ascertain the importance of the relative balances of the production of different metabolites in determining the overall outcome of therapy. It will also be of considerable interest to fit the gene frequency of TPMT deficiency together with the incidence of marrow suppression from epidemiologic studies to determine whether this abnormality is both necessary and sufficient for a UDE to occur. This may be one of the most interesting aspects of the interaction between drug epidemiology and basic investigation, as each approach generates hypotheses useful by the other discipline.

DEBRISOQUIN OXIDATION POLYMORPHISM

This example illustrates the successful progression, within little more than a decade, from an initial set of clinical observations of variable drug response to an advanced level of understanding concerning its underlying molecular mechanisms. Such knowledge presently is being used to devise tests that will predict UDE risk for compounds metabolized by a specific cytochrome P450 enzyme.

Considering that the majority of lipid-soluble drugs are metabolized at least to some extent through oxidation by members of the liver microsomal monooxygenase (cytochrome P450) enzyme system, it is somewhat surprising that, until the mid-1970s, only a few isolated reports of inherited defects of drug oxidation had been published. This may be due largely to the known multiplicity and overlapping substrate specificity of this enzyme superfamily,[19] implying that for many drugs multiple biotransformation pathways exist. Thus, compensatory metabolism by alternate pathways could prevent the clinical manifestations associated with a defect in a particular metabolic reaction.

The first clear demonstration of polymorphic drug oxidation involving cytochrome P450 was provided during independent studies of the antihypertensive drug debrisoquin[20] and the oxytocic agent sparteine.[21] Mahgoub et al.[20] provided population evidence that previously observed wide inter-patient variations in the dose of debrisoquin required for achieving a hypotensive response were due primarily to genetic differences in the extent to which debrisoquin is hydroxylated to 4-hydroxydebrisoquin. By using a metabolic ratio of the parent drug to its hydroxylated metabolite excreted in urine following a single oral dose, the authors were able to construct a population frequency histogram that was distinctly bimodal, dividing subjects into extensive and poor metabolizers. Further population and family pedigree analyses established that the hydroxylation of debrisoquin was genetically controlled by what appeared to be two alleles at a single autosomal gene locus, with poor metabolizer phenotype frequencies ranging from 6% to 10% in various white populations.

At about the same time, studies of variations in the response to sparteine showed that a similar percentage of subjects in Germany were almost entirely unable to metabolize the compound to its two major metabolites, 2- and 5-dehydrosparteine.[21] Correlation studies subsequently established that defective metabolism of debrisoquin and sparteine is under identical genetic control. Moreover, since these initial observations, the polymorphism has been shown to control, either fully or partially, the rate of oxidation of a number of other drugs as well (Table 2). One of these, dextromethorphan, shows promise as a particularly safe in vivo marker for determining the debrisoquin oxidation phenotype. Simple determination of the urinary excretion of dextromethorphan and its metabolites allows phenotyping of subjects for this polymorphic enzyme.

The clinical consequences of the debrisoquin-type drug oxidation defect have been investigated thoroughly for a number of the affected drugs in Table 2.[22] In this regard, it is important to recognize that, although the biotransformation of each of these compounds is affected by the polymorphism, not all result in UDEs. For example, genetically poor metabolizers experience a greater incidence of excessive beta-blockade and loss of cardioselectivity due to elevated plasma drug concentrations after administration of the beta-adrenergic antagonist metoprolol, but not after closely related propranolol, even though both are linked to the oxidation defect. The reason for this is that propranolol undergoes several additional metabolic pathways that, along with renal elimination, can compensate for defective biotransformation by debrisoquin oxidase.[22] On the other hand, the genetically variable pathway of encainide oxidation gives rise to an active metabolite that is responsible for most of the pharmacologic activity of the drug, so that poor metabolizers respond poorly to the antiarrhythmic effects of this compound.[23] Finally, certain drugs (e.g., quinidine, many neuroleptics) are potent competitive inhibitors of the polymorphic enzyme without necessarily being significantly metabolized by it.[24] Coadministration of these with any of the drugs in Table 2 could lead to potentially significant drug–

drug interactions or even misclassification of normal individuals as having genetically poor drug metabolism.[25]

Much progress has been made in determining the biochemical and molecular mechanisms leading to the occurrence of the poor metabolizer phenotype in human populations. Earlier in vitro studies conclusively established that defective metabolism of debrisoquin and other drugs was related to alterations in the catalytic activity of a specific isozyme of cytochrome P450,[26,27] but two general questions remained to be answered: (1) at the protein level, were the decreases in catalytic activity in affected individuals due to alterations in the quantity of a specific P450 isozyme present or to changes in substrate specificity of a structurally altered variant protein? and (2) at the gene level, what mutations were underlying these enzyme expression characteristics?

Using biochemical, immunologic, and recombinant DNA methods, and with access to liver tissues from individuals whose metabolizer phenotypes could often be determined, researchers obtained the following mechanistic information. With respect to the enzyme protein itself, immunoblotting methods have established that the poor metabolizer phenotype is characterized by a marked decrease in the liver content of a specific isozyme of cytochrome P450, now designated as CYP2D6, rather than a functional difference in an expressed enzyme.[28]

At the genetic level, molecular cloning procedures have resulted in the successful isolation and sequencing of both a full-length complementary

Table 2 Some Drugs Affected by the Debrisoquin-Type Oxidation Polymorphism

Antiarrhythmics	Beta-Adrenergic Receptor Blockers	Tricyclic Antidepressants
Encainide	Alprenolol	Amitriptyline
Flecainide	Bufuralol	Clomipramine
N-Propylajmaline	Metoprolol	Desmethylimipramine
Propafenone	Propranolol	Imipramine
Sparteine	Timolol	Nortriptyline

Neuroleptics	Other Drugs	
Perphenazine	Amiflamine	Methoxyamphetamine
Thioridazine	CGP 15210G	Methoxyphenamine
Zuclopenthixol	Codeine	Paroxetine
	Debrisoquin	Perhexiline
	Dextromethorphan	Phenformin
	Guanoxan	Tomoxetine
	Indoramin	

DNA (cDNA) encoding functional CYP2D6[29,30] and the gene on chromosome 22 (*q11.2-qter*) from which the transcript is produced.[31]

The cDNA probe has been used in southern blot hybridizations to detect restriction fragment length polymorphisms (RFLPs) in human genomic DNA that are associated with the poor metabolizer phenotype,[32] and in northern hybridizations to observe the existence of variant transcripts in livers from polymorphic individuals.[30]

Subsequent genomic cloning studies using DNA isolated from extensive and poor metabolizer subjects have produced a clear picture of the structure, organization, and interindividual variation in what is now known to be a cluster of *CYP2D* genes residing on a contiguous 45-kilobase (kb) region of chromosome 22. Since three of the four possible genes in this cluster (*CYP2D7, CYP2D7′*, and *CYP2D8*) are considered to be nonexpressed pseudogenes,[31] mutations affecting the functional *CYP2D6* gene ultimately determine the expression of the metabolizer phenotype. To date, 25 allelic variants have been detected at the *CYP2D* gene cluster, each of which may be associated with one of four major RFLP patterns detectable by southern hybridization of human genomic DNA.[33]

The *CYP2D6* gene itself may be the functional wild-type allele (*CYP2D6*1A*),[31] or it may contain any one of three different sets of point mutations that impair the expression of CYP2D6: *CYP2D6*3* carries a single nucleotide deletion in exon 5 causing a frameshift[34]; *CYP2D6*4* has a nucleotide substitution that disrupts a 3′ splice site consensus sequence in the third intron[35]; and *CYP2D6*9* possesses a three-nucleotide deletion causing loss of the codon for Lys281 in the *CYP2D6* protein.[36]

Another allelic variant (*CYP2D6*5*) producing the poor metabolizer phenotype is caused by deletion of the entire gene encoding CYP2D6, completely preventing its expression.[37] This information has led to the development of rapid and specific polymerase chain reaction (PCR)–based, allele-specific amplification tests to detect the presence of mutant alleles.[36,38]

By combining these with RFLP analysis, about 95% of all mutant alleles of *CYP2D6* can be identified, allowing for the prediction of more than 90% of poor metabolizer phenotypes.[33] Presumably, the remaining 5% of unaccounted alleles are as-yet-undiscovered mutants. The most common mutation found is *CYP2D6*4*, involving a splice site mutation in the third intron of *CYP2D6* and occurring in more than 75% of all mutant alleles.

As indicated above, the consequences of abnormal metabolism by this polymorphic P450 depend on the compound in question. The outcomes can vary from trivial effects on kinetics, which would be overwhelmed by other sources of variability, to major kinetic perturbation and idiosyncratic reactions by shunting metabolism. For compounds whose metabolism may involve CYP2D6 it should now be possible to include poor metabolizers in early studies to establish how important the polymorphism is for that compound even prior to reported UDEs. When unusual events are noted, it becomes possible to rapidly assess the role of the enzymopathy in causing a specific UDE. If the UDE occurs with high frequency in subjects deficient in the enzyme, prescreening patients for risk potential becomes possible.

ACETYLATION POLYMORPHISM

The story of the acetylation polymorphism lends historical perspective to the field of pharmacogenetics.[39,40] Indeed, it was more than 40 years ago, before the term pharmacogenetics was even formulated, that high inter-individual variations were observed in the urinary excretion of the tuber-culostatic drug isoniazid.[41] This observation was followed by the finding that frequency histograms of plasma isoniazid concentrations after a single oral dose in a normal population were distinctly bimodal, allowing for classi-fication of subjects as "rapid" or "slow" eliminators of the drug.[42] Genetic involvement initially was suggested by (1) a greater concordance among monozygotic than dizygotic twins in isoniazid urinary excretion rates,[43] and (2) an observed ethnic difference in the proportions of the two classes of isoniazid eliminators, with Asian populations displaying a markedly lower frequency of the slow eliminator phenotype than that seen in the white population.[44] Family pedigrees verified this hypothesis and showed that the ability to eliminate isoniazid was controlled by the action of two major alleles at a single autosomal gene locus, with rapid elimination as the apparently dominant trait.[45] Numerous subsequent investigations confirmed these findings and demonstrated that the disposition of a wide variety of drugs and xenobiotics containing a primary arylamine or hydrazine group is under identical genetic control (Table 3).

It soon was established that the basis of the observed population vari-ations was related to differences in the rate of arylamine and hydrazine N-acetylation taking place to a large extent in the liver.[46] The enzymatic reac-tion is now known to be catalyzed by cytosolic arylamine N-acetyltrans-ferase, which uses the essential cofactor acetyl coenzyme A as an acetyl group donor to conjugate primary amino and hydrazino groups with acetate, producing an amide.

Table 3
Some Drugs and Chemicals Affected by the Acetylation Polymorphism

4-Aminobiphenyl	Clonazepam	Nitrazepam
2-Aminofluorene	Dapsone	Phenelzine
Aminoglutethimide	Dipyrone	Procainamide
Amrinone	Hydralazine	Sulfamerazine
Benzidine	Isoniazid	Sulfamethazine
Caffeine	β-Naphthylamine	Sulfapyridine

The clinical toxicologic consequences of the acetylation polymorphism have been studied in considerable detail.[40] For instance, slow acetylators are more prone to develop a drug-induced systemic lupus erythematosus–like syndrome during prolonged therapy with procainamide or hydralazine, hematologic UDEs from dapsone, or polyneuropathy after isoniazid treatment. The slow acetylator phenotype also appears to be one of the predisposing factors in the etiology of sulfonamide-induced idiosyncratic UDEs.[47] In addition, numerous studies indicate that there is an increased incidence of bladder cancer in slow acetylators exposed to carcinogenic arylamines, which presumably are substrates for arylamine N-acetyltransferase. On the other hand, rapid acetylators encounter therapeutic failure more often when receiving isoniazid dosage regimens once weekly. They require higher doses of hydralazine to control hypertension or of dapsone for dermatitis herpetiform. However, reported associations of acetylator phenotype with some apparently unrelated disorders such as Gilbert's syndrome, diabetes, and leprosy require further validation and explanation.

Because of the potential clinical and toxicologic importance of the acetylation polymorphism in determining the response to arylamine drugs and toxins, numerous in vivo methods for determining the acetylator phenotype have been developed. These make use of "probe" drugs that are polymorphically acetylated. Isoniazid was the first drug used for this purpose, and it has been followed by tests using sulfamethazine, procainamide, and dapsone.[40] However, recent observations that the urinary excretion of a caffeine metabolite, 5-acetylamino-6-formylamino-3-methyluracil, is also governed by the acetylation polymorphism have led to the development of a caffeine test for the acetylator phenotype.[48] This test has gained widespread popularity for its safety, simplicity, and sensitivity in the phenotyping of a variety of healthy and patient populations. For example, accurate phenotype determination may be achieved in a single spot urine sample from small children after administration of a caffeinated cola beverage.[47] Moreover, the test is sensitive enough to discriminate the three genotypes of acetylation capacity in human populations,[48,49] a considerably valuable feature for assessing the differential susceptibility of heterozygous and homozygous individuals to toxicity from specific chemicals. Finally, recent in vivo/in vitro correlation studies have verified that the caffeine test specifically and precisely measures only the activity of the genetically polymorphic liver acetylating enzyme.[50]

The underlying mechanism of the acetylation polymorphism has recently been investigated by using similar biochemical and molecular approaches to those applied in the debrisoquin oxidase studies. Three N-acetyltransferase gene loci are now known to exist in humans, one of which (NATP) is a pseudogene.[51]

The two expressed genes, *NAT1* and *NAT2,* are located on chromosome 8 (*pter-q11*), but are separated by at least 25 kb. The intronless protein-coding regions of *NAT1* and *NAT2* share 87% nucleotide sequence identity and encode 290 amino acid proteins, NAT1 and NAT2, which are 81% identical. Expression studies have shown that the human acetylation polymorphism is regulated at the *NAT2* gene locus, since the expressed product of the *NAT2* gene displays kinetic properties[52] that are very similar to those of two human liver *NAT2* isoforms whose content is markedly reduced in phenotypically slow acetylators.[50]

NAT2 shows kinetic selectivity for so-called "polymorphic" substrates (Table 3) whose disposition is affected by the acetylator phenotype in human populations; reduction in the quantity of NAT2 in livers of slow acetylators thus impairs the elimination of such compounds from the body. NAT1, on the other hand, is also expressed in human liver, but selectively metabolizes so-called "monomorphic" substrates, such as *p*-aminobenzoic acid, whose disposition is unaffected by the acetylator phenotype. As of this time, 15 variant *NAT2* alleles that correlate with the acetylator phenotype have been detected in human populations, accounting for nearly 100% of all of the alleles examined.[53]

Each of these alleles possesses a characteristic combination of between one and three nucleotide substitutions occurring within the protein coding region of the *NAT2* gene. Fortunately, all but one of these nucleotide substitutions also leads to an alteration in a naturally occurring restriction endonuclease recognition sequence, providing for straightforward PCR-based restriction digest methods to detect their occurrence in population studies.[54]

The NAT2*4, NAT2*12, and NAT2*13 alleles are associated with the rapid acetylator phenotype, while each of the NAT2*5, NAT2*6, NAT2*7, and NAT2*14 S alleles correlates with the slow acetylator phenotype. From the population studies completed so far, it appears that NAT2*4, NAT2*5, and NAT2*6 are the most prevalent alleles in white subjects, whereas NAT2*5 is very low or absent in the Japanese, accounting for a large part of the interethnic difference in the frequency of the slow acetylator phenotype between white (60%) and Asian (10%) subjects.[55]

This would predict possible interethnic differences in UDE rates in which the acetylation polymorphism plays a major role and provide a direct link with differences in allele frequencies. The mechanisms by which some of these mutant alleles lead to reductions in NAT2 protein content in human liver have also been investigated to a limited extent.[56]

So far, it appears that single amino acid changes in NAT2*6, NAT2*7, and NAT2*14 produce proteins with reduced stabilities, while the *S1B* transcript may have impaired translation efficiency. Thus, similar to the debrisoquin polymorphism, a safe in vivo probe (caffeine) and the molecular tests being developed can be applied to determining acetylator phenotype in patients.

Since neither of the two acetylator phenotypes is rare and many of the UDEs that correlate with phenotype are considerably less frequent than 50% or even 10%, NAT2-dependent acetylation cannot be the only risk factor. However, the fact that N-acetylation is relatively protective against toxicity in certain circumstances can focus basic studies on UDE mechanisms. For instance, although the product of the *NAT1* gene shows kinetic selectivity for compounds whose disposition is unrelated to the classically defined acetylation polymorphism, recent studies[53] have demonstrated that NAT1 expression may also be highly variable in human populations and that variant alleles at the *NAT1* gene locus can indeed be detected. It remains to be determined whether the observed pattern of NAT1 variation is genetically based and related to the occurrence of such variant alleles. If so, these findings may be of considerable clinical and toxicologic significance in light of observations that certain chemicals may be N-acetylated to a significant degree by both NAT1 and NAT2. These include the carcinogenic aromatic amines 2-aminofluorene, benzidine, 4-aminobiphenyl, 3,4-dichloroaniline, and β-naphthylamine.[52,57,58]

Thus, it is conceivable that concurrent variations in NAT1 and NAT2 may be independent contributing factors for predisposition to UDEs. On the other hand, alternate pathways of biotransformation of arylamines may also play a role in producing the UDE. With sulfonamides, for example, slow acetylation by NAT2 appears to be a risk factor for hypersensitivity reactions.[59]

In fact, oxidation of the arylamine to reactive hydroxylamine and nitroso metabolites, with subsequent inherited inability to detoxify (or propensity to further metabolically activate) the latter, may be involved in the pathogenesis.[60,61]

In this case, NAT2-dependent N-acetylation alone would not be an adequate marker of risk, since 50% of the patients would be excluded from using the drugs. However, a combination of markers indicating a "metabolizer profile" might well serve to pinpoint a smaller subset of the general population with a markedly elevated risk. The use of cellular models as markers for diagnosis and prediction is discussed in the context of the aromatic anticonvulsants.

ANTICONVULSANT HYPERSENSITIVITY SYNDROME AND BIRTH DEFECTS

Hypersensitivity reactions to phenytoin and related anticonvulsants can be life threatening, and association with both major and minor birth defects is a major concern in managing pregnancies in epileptic patients. However, it remains striking that the drugs do not cause such toxicities in the majority of patients who are exposed. The precise incidence of hypersensitivity reactions is uncertain, somewhere between 1/1000 and 1/10 000 patients.[62] Similarly, there appears to be approximately a two- to threefold increased risk of major birth defects in pregnancies in epileptic patients taking phenytoin (5–10% of exposed fetuses), with up to a 30% risk of minor abnormalities often classified as the fetal hydantoin syndrome.[63] The challenge, then, is to define the pathogenesis of both the hypersensitivity reactions and fetal effects, and to ascertain whether genetic differences in the handling of or response to the drug determine susceptibility to toxicity.

The hypersensitivity reactions typically are delayed in onset after institution of therapy (often several weeks), and they are characterized by fever, skin rash, lymphadenopathy, and variable involvement of other organs including the liver, kidney, bone marrow, lung, and heart.[62] The pathogenesis appears to involve both direct toxicity to cells and an immunologic response. The reactions might be mediated by cytochrome P450–generated metabolites of the parent drug, possibly arene oxides.[64-67] Current understanding of susceptibility to toxicity is that there is an inherited abnormality in detoxification of such unstable, potentially toxic metabolites. When peripheral blood lymphocytes from patients who have had phenytoin UDEs are exposed to reactive metabolites of phenytoin, the cells exhibit far more toxicity than do normal cells.[65-67] An intermediate pattern of the toxicity of metabolites has been demonstrated in cells from the parents of patients; cells from the siblings are distributed among normal, abnormal, and intermediate responses. The molecular and biochemical bases of the defects are currently under investigation. Prime candidates for the abnormality are mutations in epoxide hydrolase, altering the substrate specificity of the enzyme for reactive metabolites of phenytoin, thereby leading to accumulation of the reactive intermediate, increased covalent binding to cell macromolecules, and resultant cell death and immunologic response to neoantigens (Figure 2).

The decision to use peripheral blood lymphocytes for performing in vitro toxicology experiments depends on the assumption that enzyme ac-

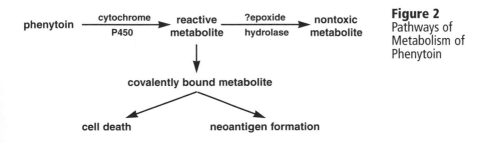

Figure 2
Pathways of Metabolism of Phenytoin

tivities are expressed in this tissue similarly to that in the major organs of xenobiotic biotransformation, such as the liver. However, once this has been established, the method opens up possibilities for aiding in the diagnosis of complex diseases in the face of drug therapy and of prospectively screening patients for possible toxicity. Understanding the molecular defects involved will help in the selection of other anticonvulsant therapy for patients who have had phenytoin UDEs. Studies suggest that the defect in metabolite detoxification is shared in most pedigrees among phenytoin, phenobarbital, and carbamazepine.[67] In other families, the abnormality is somewhat more restricted. Heterogeneity of defects is likely to be the case among most pharmacogenetic variants. Knowledge of the specific defects, the structures of alternative anticonvulsants, and their pathways of metabolism may help in selecting compounds with the least toxicity risk for specific patients and in designing newer, safer anticonvulsants in the future.

The role of anticonvulsants in the etiology of birth defects among mothers with epilepsy is controversial. Phenytoin use has been associated with a two- to threefold increased risk of major defects and a variable risk of minor abnormalities. Regardless of the precise epidemiologic risk, most fetuses exposed to the drug in utero do not have birth defects. In studies on the rate, there was a correlation between birth defects (e.g., cardiac anomalies, cleft palate) and the amount of covalently bound phenytoin metabolites in the fetuses.[68] Inhibition of epoxide hydrolase increased metabolite binding and the yield of malformations. The detoxification ability of peripheral blood lymphocytes was examined in patients exposed to phenytoin in utero who did and did not have birth defects and in their parents.[69] There was a strong correlation between abnormal detoxification (in all cases characterized by an intermediate pattern of detoxification defect) and major birth defects. No correlation was found with minor stigmata of the fetal hydantoin syndrome. For each patient with an abnormality in detoxification, cells from one of the parents were also abnormal. Mothers with intermediate detoxification defects tolerated phenytoin without hypersensitivity reactions.

The results suggest that an inherited abnormality in detoxification of phenytoin metabolites may play a role in the development of birth defects when exposured to the compound. If the intermediate response truly represents a heterozygous state, a single abnormal gene may be sufficient to place a developing fetus at risk for toxicity. Homozygosity is required for hypersensitivity reactions in children or adults. This emphasizes the complex nature of the interaction between developmental processes regulating drug metabolic pathways and inborn errors of metabolism of those pathways. Balances of rates down several potential pathways of metabolism may determine the ultimate outcomes.

In addition, not all effects of a drug such as phenytoin will be mediated by the same metabolites or processes. In our study, we found no correlation between detoxification defects and minor birth defects. In adults, facial coarsening, hirsutism, and gingival hyperplasia are very common events compared with hypersensitivity reactions. Similarly, some of the minor abnormalities associated with phenytoin occur with much higher frequency than major structural birth defects. Once molecular probes are available for pathways critical in phenytoin toxicity, it will become possible to sift through various clinical presentations and determine what abnormalities are and are not related to pharmacogenetic disorders. Ultimately, it may be possible to assign individual maternal–fetal pairs with individual estimates of risk of an abnormal outcome of pregnancy and to ensure a successful outcome for the vast majority of patients.

Summary

Pharmacogenetics is having an increasing impact on our concepts of the pathogenesis of human UDEs. The availability of safe in vivo probes of drug metabolism pathways exhibiting genetic polymorphisms and of cellular models for assaying enzymes and studying drug toxicity in readily available cell types, along with rapid advances in molecular biology, holds great promise for future progress in this area. Biologic markers of susceptibility to UDEs based on pharmacogenetic considerations will be used in early drug development to define outliers in the population and the consequences of polymorphic drug metabolism for new compounds under development. Similarly, the integration of epidemiologic studies and basic pharmacogenetic investigation has the potential for more accurate determination of true UDEs amidst events occurring during therapy (improved diagnosis), prediction of individual as well as population risk, and ultimate UDE prevention.

References

1. Gonzalez FJ, Crespi CL, Gelboin HV. DNA-expressed human cytochrome P450s: a new age of molecular toxicology and human risk assessment. Mutat Res 1991;247: 113-27.
2. Gonzalez FJ. Human cytochromes P450: problems and prospects. TIPS Rev 1992;13: 346-52.
3. Cholerton S, Daly AK, Idle JR. The role of individual human cytochromes P450 in drug metabolism and clinical response. TIPS Rev 1992;13:434-9.
4. Wrighton SA, Stevens JC. The human hepatic cytochromes P450 involved in drug metabolism. Crit Rev Toxicol 1992;22:1-21.
5. Gibaldi M. Pharmacogenetics: part I. Ann Pharmacother 1992;26:121-6.

6. Gibaldi M. Pharmacogenetics: part II. Ann Pharmacother 1992;26:255-61.
7. Kalow W. Pharmacogenetics. Heredity and the response to drugs. Philadelphia: WB Saunders, 1962.
8. Evans DAP. Pharmacogenetics. Am J Med 1963;34:639-62.
9. Propping P. Pharmacogenetics. Rev Physiol Biochem Pharmacol 1978;83:123-73.
10. Vesell ES. Pharmacogenetics. In: Yaffe SJ, ed. Pediatric pharmacology: therapeutic principles in practice. New York: Grune and Stratton, 1980.
11. Roots I, Heinemeyer G, Drakoulis N, Kampf D. The role of pharmacogenetics in drug epidemiology. In: Kewtiz H, Roots I, Voigt K, eds. Epidemiological concepts in clinical pharmacology. Berlin: Springer-Verlag, 1987.
12. Ayesh R, Smith RL. Genetic polymorphism in human toxicology. In: Turner P, Volans GN, eds. Recent advances in clinical pharmacology and toxicology, number 4. Edinburgh: Churchill Livingstone, 1989.
13. Weinshilboum RM, Sladek SL. Mercaptopurine pharmacogenetics: monogenic inheritance of erythrocyte thiopurine methyltransferase activity. Am J Hum Genet 1980;32:651-62.
14. Van Loon J, Weinshilboum RM. Thiopurine methyltransferase biochemical genetics: human lymphocyte activity. Biochem Genet 1982;20:637-58.
15. Woodson LC, Dunnette JH, Weinshilboum RM. Pharmacogenetics of human thiopurine methyltransferase: kidney-erythrocyte correlation. J Pharmacol Exp Ther 1982;222:174-81.
16. Szymlanski CL, Scott MC, Weinshilboum RM. Thiopurine methyltransferase pharmacogenetics: human liver enzyme activity. Clin Pharmacol Ther 1988;43:134-40.
17. Lennard L, Van Loon JA, Lilleyman JS, Weinshilboum RM. Thiopurine pharmacogenetics in leukemia: correlation of erythrocyte thiopurine methyltransferase activity and 6-thioguanine nucleotide concentrations. Clin Pharmacol Ther 1989;46:18-25.
18. Lennard L, Van Loon JA, Weinshilboum RM. Pharmacogenetics of acute azathioprine toxicity: relationship to thiopurine methyltransferase genetic polymorphism. Clin Pharmacol Ther 1989;46:149-54.
19. Gonzalez FJ. The molecular biology of cytochrome P450s. Pharmacol Rev 1988;40:243-88.
20. Mahgoub A, Dring LG, Idle JR, Lancaster R, Smith RL. Polymorphic hydroxylation of debrisoquine in man. Lancet 1977;2:584-6.
21. Eichelbaum M, Spannbrucker N, Dengler HJ. N-Oxidation of sparteine in man and its interindividual differences (abstract). Naunyn Schmiedebergs Arch Pharmacol 1975;287(suppl):R94.
22. Evans DAP. Therapy. In: Kalow W, Goedde HW, Agarwal DP, eds. Ethnic differences in reactions to drugs and xenobiotics. New York: Alan R Liss, 1986.
23. Wang T, Roden DM, Wolfenden HT, Woosley RL, Wood AJJ, Wilkinson GR. Influence of genetic polymorphism on the metabolism and disposition of encainide in man. J Pharmacol Exp Ther 1984;228:605-11.
24. Fonne-Pfister R, Meyer UA. Xenobiotic and endobiotic inhibitors of cytochrome P-450dbl function, the target of the debrisoquine/sparteine type polymorphism. Biochem Pharmacol 1988;37:3829-35.
25. Leeman T, Dayer P, Meyer YA. Single-dose quinidine treatment inhibits metoprolol oxidation in extensive metabolizers. Eur J Clin Pharmacol 1986;29:739-41.
26. Davies DS, Khan GC, Murray S, Brodie MJ, Boobis AR. Evidence for an enzymatic defect in the 4-hydroxylation of debrisoquine by human liver. Br J Clin Pharmacol 1981;11:89-91.

27. Meier PJ, Mueller HK, Dick B, Meyer UA. Hepatic monooxygenase activities in subjects with a genetic defect in drug oxidation. Gastroenterology 1983;85:682-92.

28. Zanger UM, Vilbois F, Hardwick JP, Meyer UA. Absence of hepatic cytochrome P450bufI causes genetically deficient debrisoquine oxidation in man. Biochemistry 1988;27:5447-54.

29. Gonzalez FJ, Vilbois F, Hardwick JP, McBride OW, Nebert DW, Gelboin HV, et al. Human debrisoquine 4-hydroxylase (P450IID1): cDNA and deduced amino acid sequence and assignment of the CYP2D locus to chromosome 22. Genomics 1988;2: 174-9.

30. Gonzalez FJ, Skoda RC, Kimura S, Umeno M, Zanger UM, Nebert DW, et al. Characterization of the common genetic defect in humans deficient in debrisoquine metabolism. Nature 1988;331:442-6.

31. Kimura S, Umeno M, Skoda RC, Belboin HV, Meyer UA, Gonzalez FJ. The human debrisoquine 4-hydroxylase (CYP2D) locus: sequence and identification of the polymorphic *CYP2D6* gene, a related gene, and a pseudogene. Am J Hum Genet 1989;45: 889-904.

32. Skoda RC, Gonzalez FJ, Demierre A, Meyer UA. Two mutant alleles of the human cytochrome P-450db1 gene (*P450C2D1*) associated with genetically deficient metabolism of debrisoquine and other drugs. Proc Natl Acad Sci U S A 1988;85:5240-3.

33. Daly AK, Brockmöller J, Broly F, Eichelbaum M, Evans WE, Gonzalez FJ, et al. Nomenclature for human *CYP2D6* alleles. Pharmacogenetics 1996;6:193-201.

34. Kagimoto M, Heim M, Kagimoto K, Zeugin T, Meyer U. Multiple mutations of the human cytochrome P450IID6 gene (*CYP2D6*) in poor metabolizers of debrisoquine. Study of the functional significance of individual mutations by expression of chimeric genes. J Biol Chem 1990;265:17209-14.

35. Hanioka N, Kimura S, Meyer UA, Gonzalez FJ. The human CYP2D locus associated with a common genetic defect in drug oxidation: a G1934–A base change in intron 3 of a mutant *CYP2D6* allele results in an aberrant 3' splice recognition site. Am J Hum Genet 1990;47:994-1001.

36. Tyndale R, Aoyama T, Broly F, Matsunaga T, Inaba T, Kalow W, et al. Identification of a new variant *CYP2D6* allele lacking the codon encoding Lys-281: possible association with the poor metabolizer phenotype. Pharmacogenetics 1991;1:26-32.

37. Gaedigk A, Blum M, Gaedigk R, Eichelbaum M, Meyer UA. Deletion of the entire cytochrome P450 *CYP2D6* gene as a cause of impaired drug metabolism in poor metabolizers of the debrisoquine/sparteine polymorphism. Am J Hum Genet 1991;48: 943-50.

38. Heim M, Meyer U. Genetic polymorphism of debrisoquine oxidation: analysis of mutant alleles of CYP2D6 by restriction fragment analysis and allele specific amplification. Methods Enzymol 1991;206:173-83.

39. Weber WW. The acetylator genes and drug response. Oxford: Oxford University Press, 1987.

40. Evans DAP. N-Acetyltransferase. Pharmacol Ther 1989;42:157-234.

41. Bönicke R, Reif W. Enzymatic inactivation of isonicotinic acid hydrazide in humans and animals. Arch Exp Pathol Pharmak 1953;220:321-33.

42. Mitchell RS, Bell JC. Clinical implications of isoniazid, PAS, and streptomycin blood levels in pulmonary tuberculosis. Trans Am Clin Chem Assoc 1957;69:98-105.

43. Bönicke R, Lisoba RP. On the inherited basis of intraindividual constancy of isoniazid elimination in man (studies of monozygotic and dizygotic twins). Naturwissenschaften 1957;44:314.

44. Mitchell RS, Riemensnider DK, Harsh JR, Gell JC. New information on the clinical implications of individual variations in the metabolic handling of antituberculous drugs, particularly isoniazid. In: Transactions of the 17th Conference on Chemotherapy of Tuberculosis. Washington, DC: Veterans Administration, 1958.

45. Evans DAP, Manley KA, McKusick VA. Genetic control of isoniazid metabolism in man. Br Med J 1960;2:485-91.

46. Evans DAP, White TA. Human acetylation polymorphism. J Lab Clin Med 1964;63: 394-403.

47. Shear NH, Spielberg SP, Grant DM, Tang BK, Kalow W. Differences in metabolism of sulfonamides predisposing to idiosyncratic toxicity. Ann Intern Med 1986;105: 179-84.

48. Grant DM, Tang BK, Kalow W. A simple test for acetylator phenotype using caffeine. Br J Clin Pharmacol 1984;17:459-64.

49. Gascon M-P, Leeman T, Dayer P. Evaluation d'un test à la caféine pour déterminer le phénotype de la N-acétyltransférase (NAT). Schweiz Med Wochenschr 1987;117: 1974-6.

50. Grant DM, Mörike K, Eichelbaum M, Meyer UA. Acetylation pharmacogenetics: the slow acetylator phenotype is caused by decreased or absent arylamine N-acetyltransferase in human liver. J Clin Invest 1990;85:968-72.

51. Blum M, Grant DM, McBride OW, Heim M, Meyer UA. Human arylamine N-acetyltransferase genes: isolation, chromosomal localization, and functional expression. DNA Cell Biol 1990;9:193-203.

52. Grant DM, Blum M, Beer M, Meyer UA. Monomorphic and polymorphic human arylamine N-acetyltransferases: a comparison of liver isozymes and expressed products of two cloned genes. Mol Pharmacol 1991;39:184-91.

53. Grant DM, Hughes NC, Janezic SA, Goodfellow GH, Chen JH, Gaedigk A, Yu-Plant VL, et al. Human acetyltransferase polymorphisms. Mut Res 1997;376:61-70.

54. Hickman D, Sim E. N-Acetyltransferase polymorphism: comparison of phenotype and genotype in humans. Biochem Pharmacol 1991;42:1007-14.

55. Evans DAP. N-Acetyltransferase. Pharmacol Ther 1989;42:157-234.

56. Blum M, Demierre A, Grant DM, Heim M, Meyer UA. Molecular mechanism of slow acetylation of drugs and carcinogens in humans. Proc Natl Acad Sci U S A 1991;88: 5237-41.

57. Grant DM, Josephy PD, Lord HL, Morrison LD. Salmonella tryphimurium strains expressing human arylamine N-acetyltransferases: metabolism and mutagenic activation of aromatic amines. Cancer Res 1992;52:3961-4.

58. Hewin DW, Doll MA, Rustan TD, Gray K, Feng Y, Ferguson RJ, et al. Metabolic activation and deactivation of arylamine carcinogens by recombinant human NAT1 and polymorphic NAT2 acetyltransferases. Carcinogenesis 1993;14:1633-8.

59. Shear NH, Spielberg SP, Grant DM, Tang BK, Kalow W. Differences in metabolism of sulfonamides predisposing to idiosyncratic toxicity. Ann Intern Med 1986;105: 179-84.

60. Rieder MJ, Uetrecht J, Shear NH, Cannon M, Miller M, Spielberg SP. Diagnosis of sulfonamide hypersensitivity reactions by in vitro rechallenge with hydroxylamine metabolites. Ann Intern Med 1989;110:286-9.

61. Cribb AE, Spielberg SP. Hepatic microsomal metabolism of sulfamethoxazole to the hydroxylamine. Drug Metab Dispos 1990;18:784-7.

62. Thomsick RS. The phenytoin syndrome. Cutis 1983;32:535-41.

63. Kelly TE. Teratogenicity of anticonvulsant drugs: review of the literature. Am J Med Genet 1984;19:413-34.

64. Spielberg SP, Gordon GB, Blake DA, Mellits ED, Bross DS. Anticonvulsant toxicity in vitro: possible role of arene oxides. J Pharmacol Exp Ther 1981;217:386-9.
65. Spielberg SP, Gordon GB, Blake DA, Goldstein DA, Herlong HF. Predisposition to phenytoin hepatotoxicity assessed in vitro. N Engl J Med 1981;305:722-7.
66. Gerson WT, Fine DG, Spielberg SP, Sensenbrenner LL. Anticonvulsant induced aplastic anemia: increased susceptibility to toxic drug metabolites in vitro. Blood 1983;61:889-93.
67. Shear NH, Spielberg SP. Anticonvulsant hypersensitivity syndrome: in vitro assessment of risk. J Clin Invest 1988;82:1826-32.
68. Martz F, Failinger C, Blake DA. Phenytoin teratogenesis: correlation between embryopathic effect and covalent binding of putative arene oxide metabolite in gestational tissue. J Pharmacol Exp Ther 1977;203:231-9.
69. Strickler SM, Dansky LV, Miller MA, Seni M-H, Andermann E, Spielberg SP. Genetic predisposition to phenytoin-induced birth defects. Lancet 1985;2:746-9.

8

Assessing Patient Outcomes of Drug Therapy: The Role of Pharmacoepidemiology

Eleanor M Perfetto
Robert S Epstein
Lisa Stockwell Morris

Abstract

Patient outcomes of pharmaceutical therapy are gaining worldwide attention. While outcomes research is an extension of more traditional approaches, the field rests squarely on the basic principles of epidemiologic research. Thus, it is essential that pharmacoepidemiologists become interested and active in the practice of outcomes research and build upon a clear understanding of its conceptual underpinnings. With the increased emphasis on patient outcomes and the marketplace forces demanding information on the performance of drug therapy in the real world, effectiveness studies have received significant attention. Efficacy trials cannot provide the real-world view as they maximize internal validity at the expense of external validity. On the other hand, the goal of effectiveness studies is to expand the focus to incorporate real-world situations. There are many difficulties in conducting outcomes research and medical effectiveness research. First, there are varying perspectives from which outcomes and effectiveness can be evaluated. Additionally, many methodologic issues arise in these studies. Several of these issues are also faced in epidemiologic research. For example, handling censoring and exposure determination are common concerns in epidemiology. Because of their experiences with these methodologic hurdles, pharmacoepidemiologists could add value to outcomes and medical effectiveness research. The outcomes research movement and the desire for medical effectiveness information can facilitate new roles for pharmacoepidemiologists. Outcomes research can augment the study of unintended drug effects. Additionally, outcomes research shifts the focus to the positive, or intended, effects of treatment. The specialized knowledge of pharmacoepidemiologists, such as drug nomenclature, distribution, use, regulation, and methodologic idiosyncrasies, provides an invaluable resource to a multidisciplinary outcomes research team.

Outline

Pharmaceutical therapy is one of the most common modes of treatment for nearly all clinical conditions. It is not surprising that studies of patient outcomes of pharmaceutical therapy are now gaining worldwide attention. While outcomes research is an extension of more traditional approaches, the field rests squarely on the basic principles of epidemiologic research. Thus, it is essential that pharmacoepidemiologists become interested and active in the practice of outcomes research and build upon a clear understanding of its conceptual underpinnings.

The terms "patient outcomes research" and "medical treatment effectiveness research" are used interchangeably. Both terms refer to the systematic study of relationships between the structure and process of healthcare provision and the ultimate effects on patients, the patient outcomes.[1] An outcomes research focus is generally on the typical use of therapies. Pharmaceutical outcomes research refers to the study of patient outcomes related to alternative therapies when at least one of the available treatments is a pharmaceutical agent.[2]

It is important, therefore, to note that effectiveness is the level of benefit expected when healthcare services are rendered under *ordinary* circumstances by average practitioners to *typical* patients, whereas efficacy is the level of benefit expected when services are rendered under *ideal* circumstances.[3,4] Typically, outcomes research studies are longitudinal in nature, may be retrospective or prospective, and make use of multidisciplinary expertise. Although randomized, controlled trials are routinely used to study efficacy, they are less commonly used to study medical treatment effectiveness because of limiting, design-related features: selective sampling, study-imposed visits and tests, limited generalizability, limited length of follow-up, and related high costs.

The purpose of this chapter is to describe patient outcomes and patient outcomes research, including an expanded role for the applications of pharmacoepidemiology. The history of the outcomes movement is traced and implications for the future are explored. Increased opportunities for pharmacoepidemiologic research, moving far beyond the already widely accepted contributions of the pharmacoepidemiologic study of unintended consequences, are discussed. Specific methodologic challenges regarding outcomes research, particularly involving drug therapy, are addressed.

History of Patient Outcomes/Medical Effectiveness Research

An understanding of the history of patient outcomes/medical effectiveness research provides a conceptual basis for assessing current methodologies for determining outcomes of alternative medical treatments. Three seminal issues are of particular importance: emergence and acceptance of Donabedian's model for assessing quality of care, increased attention to variations in health services use and medical practice, and the shifting emphasis from monitoring efficacy to monitoring effectiveness of care.[3,5-8] Each has considerable impact on the definition of and methodologies used in current assessments of patient outcomes.

Donabedian[5,6] defined patient outcomes in his model for assessing health-care quality. The model places quality measures into three domains: structure, process, and outcome. Structural measures are defined as the material and social instruments used to provide care. Process measures describe how the structural instruments are used. Finally, outcome measures are defined as changes in a patient's health status attributable to the structure and/or process of care.[6] Donabedian stressed that, while structure and process issues are important as care could not be provided without them, the quality of the services provided should ultimately be assessed by how much benefit or harm has been experienced by the patient. In this light, positive, as well as negative, health status changes are important patient outcomes.

Focusing assessments of quality on the outcomes experienced by the patient was further emphasized by Wennberg et al.[9] In studying medical and surgical procedures, Wennberg and Gittelsohn[7,8] found wide variations in rates of use across seemingly similar communities. Wennberg[10] noted, however, that without understanding the relationship between the rate of procedure use and patient outcomes within each community, it is difficult to assess what the "best" rate should be. For example, one community may overuse or another may underuse a treatment compared with the population norm, yet the normative rate may not be the "correct" or most appropriate rate. The rate of use producing the most positive patient outcomes with the fewest negative consequences should be considered correct or most desirable. However, this requires comparison of outcomes for all treatment options, including no treatment, in routine patient care settings. Emphasis was placed on effectiveness, the real-time or real-world nature of the care setting in which care is provided, rather than on efficacy in determining which treatments produce the best outcomes.

Studies of Efficacy Versus Effectiveness

As described earlier in this chapter, efficacy and effectiveness have come to have different meanings to outcomes researchers. As such, the characteristics of efficacy and effectiveness studies differ. Table 1 outlines common differences between studies of efficacy and effectiveness. As indicated in the table, these are not absolute definitions or requirements but they are general tendencies and traditional attributes.

Studies of efficacy are characterized by the traditional randomized, controlled drug trials, in which patients are screened by using explicit inclusion and exclusion criteria and randomized to treatment or placebo

Characteristics	Efficacy	Effectiveness
Design	randomized, controlled trial	randomized, controlled trial, cohort, case–control, and so on
Patient sample	highly selected; strict inclusion/exclusion criteria	characteristic of typical users; population-based
Patient (subject) management	explicit protocol; stringent adherence; intensive management and follow-up	standard care; routine service provision
Setting	academic/tertiary care centers; specialty clinics	real world, usual site of care; primary care settings
Measures	clinical (morbidity, mortality, adverse sequela; physiologic and anatomic measures)	clinical and patient-subjective, plus structure and process; total costs (direct and indirect, individual and social)
Timing of outcomes	short term	short, intermediate, and long term
Comparators	placebo or standard therapy	all available therapies, including non-treatment and nondrug treatment
Control	routinely randomized	randomized (effectiveness trials); statistical, stratify, match, multivariate procedures (quasi-experimental designs)
Providers	specialists; leaders in the field	community based; clinicians providing primary care services
Validity	clinical measures with high internal validity; results with less external validity	clinical measures with less internal validity; patient-subjective measures with high internal validity; results with high external validity
Reliability	high for clinical measures	high for patient-subjective measures
Generalizability	limited to a specific selective population	wide; "average" patients
Data collection	primary; prospective	primary and/or secondary (e.g., claims); prospective and/or retrospective
Investigators	unidisciplinary, generally clinical	multidisciplinary, including clinicians, methodologists, behavioral scientists, economists, and health researchers
Dropouts	withdrawal noted, but little follow-up	intensive follow-up and comparisons whenever possible
Conclusions	causality; cause–effect	causality (effectiveness trials); relationships, associations, estimates (quasi-experimental designs)
Expense	high	relatively low, especially for secondary data; can be high for effectiveness trials

Table 1 General[a] Characteristics Differentiating Efficacy and Effectiveness Research on Pharmaceuticals

[a]Emphasis should be placed on the word "general." These are not absolute definitions or requirements, only general concepts and traditional attributes.

groups.[11] Providers are likely to be leading experts on the condition for which the treatment is being tested. Care is intensively managed with close patient follow-up and is often based in an academic medical center with vast technologic resources. Subjects may be paid to participate, care is likely to be free, drugs and laboratory tests are provided at no charge, and transportation to care sites may be provided to ensure compliance and subject retention. Outcomes of concern are routinely straightforward and short-term measures of clinical effect and safety, collected in rigorous and standardized ways. Necessary sample sizes tend to be smaller. However, efficacy trials are relatively costly to conduct because of patient monitoring. In efficacy trials, internal validity is maximized at the expense of external validity. Results of efficacy studies form the basis for drug approval. In a strict sense, all pharmaceutical clinical efficacy trials are outcomes research; however, in an effectiveness sense, few of them are.

Effectiveness studies have a much broader focus and goal. Both short- and long-term outcome end points should be assessed. Often, results are used in the development of clinical guidelines, for treatment algorithms, or in determination of resource allocation. Because of the multiple potential uses of effectiveness studies, a variety of designs and methodologies are used to conduct them. Controlled trials can be used, but generally effectiveness studies are observational, striving for real-world scenarios. Patients represent the actual population of those having the disease rather than a highly selective sample. Patients are included in the study population and few, if any, inclusion/exclusion criteria are used. Recruitment or patient selection for such studies is often easier. For the condition under study, the care setting should be representative of typical practice. This often means avoiding large tertiary care centers and reaching out to community and primary care providers. Clinicians tend to represent a more heterogeneous group of usual care providers.

Ideally, effectiveness studies compare all therapy options, including nontreatment, to differentiate "what works from what doesn't" in terms of resulting patient outcomes.[1,12] Often, effectiveness studies compare a new program of care versus usual or standard care. While retrospective analyses of secondary databases are common, primary data collection often is used to augment administrative or claims data with patient-subjective outcome measures.[12]

Patients and/or providers may be randomized to various intervention groups in effectiveness trials; however, many effectiveness studies are observational or quasi-experimental, relying on research designs and methodologies from epidemiology. Cohort designs are used often in medical treatment effectiveness research, created retrospectively using secondary data or prospectively with longitudinal data collection. Attempts are made to follow the cohorts for appropriate lengths of time, relative to the condition and outcomes of interest. As in epidemiologic research, relevant characteristics are sought to compare those subjects considered nonresponders or dropouts in an effort to evaluate and address any possible biases created through nonparticipation.

The multitude of potential study designs, ease of patient selection, and ability to use secondary data can result in effectiveness studies being less costly than efficacy trials. However, the expense for naturalistic effectiveness trials using prospective data collection can be quite high, since a larger sample size may be necessary compared with efficacy trials. The design features and types of patients included in effectiveness studies place emphasis on external validity, while possibly compromising internal validity. Results from effectiveness studies may obscure efficacy because of patient noncompliance, variable dosing regimens (e.g., underdosing, high dosing), improper treatment decisions, and less frequently required monitoring.

Although many efficacy trials now incorporate assessments of the quality of life and functional status, most tend to focus on clinical measures of outcome.[13-15] Generally, these clinical measures have undergone extensive validation and reliability testing. Effectiveness studies tend to emphasize patient-perceived outcomes. Since these measures are more subjective and often are perceived as "softer" end points than clinical measures, they are frequently subjected to even more pretesting and validation than are standard clinical measures.

Differences between efficacy and effectiveness studies are not always distinct. Patient consent is generally required in efficacy studies, but may create bias in effectiveness work. A patient enrolled in a prospective effectiveness trial loses the usual "uncontaminated" atmosphere of care simply by signing the consent form. Consenting to a study may create a selection bias, in which those persons willing to enroll in the study are different from those who refuse, a common concern to epidemiologic research. Moreover, both the investigator and patient now know they are in a study, which may encourage them to behave differently than they would have behaved in the real world. An example of a common effectiveness trial design is the large, simple trial that can be considered a hybrid of efficacy and effectiveness research.[16] While the issue of consent may contaminate the real-world focus of an effectiveness trial, it may be an unavoidable obstacle to conducting "pure" outcomes research.

Patient or practitioner consent has not often been a concern in retrospective database studies because specific identifiers, such as names and social security numbers, have not been reported. With the advent of provider profiling and report cards using various claims and other databases, attitudes may change regarding the need for informed consent for database research. The complexities are magnified because of efforts to merge multiple data sources and the determination of ownership of the resulting database.

Results of efficacy and effectiveness studies can be used together for a better understanding of the outcomes associated with certain therapies. For example, the combination of randomized controlled trials and observational epidemiologic studies has enhanced our understanding of the value of cholesterol control in the prevention and treatment of coronary heart disease.[17] Likewise, the relationship of cholesterol concentrations to the development and progression of atherosclerosis, as postulated from epidemiologic studies, has also been identified in randomized controlled trials. In another example, it is important to use information from both efficacy and effectiveness studies, in which surrogate end points have been used to measure efficacy. In efficacy trials, the drug may have a positive effect on the surrogate end point. However, this may not translate to improved health status or decreased mortality. In fact, mortality could be adversely affected.[18]

The purpose of differentiating between efficacy and effectiveness is not to suggest that there are absolute differences or that one is superior. Rather, the purpose is to emphasize that traditional, efficacy-based research constructs serve as a foundation for patient outcomes and medical effectiveness efforts. An outcomes research approach should not force a choice between experimental and quasi-experimental (observational) designs. Instead, it is an opportunity to create and explore innovative research designs that capture widely generalizable real-world patient outcomes in relatively low-cost ways. In addressing most questions of medical treatment effectiveness, researchers must therefore draw from both approaches, most often in combination.

Outcome Measures

The outcomes movement, as Ellwood[19] labeled it, has its roots in health services research, as described in the history section of this chapter. The outcomes movement represents a shift from a focus on structure and process measures of care, such as the number of hospital beds or the presence of a drug utilization review (DUR) program, to patient outcome measures, such as the number of days a patient stays in the hospital or an improved health that is related to drug therapy. Additionally, measurement of outcomes shifted from traditional assessments of change in health status, which have primarily centered on the more apparent or objective measures such as mortality or indicators of morbidity. In general, traditional outcome measures have been those easily derived from administrative data or medical records, including hospitalizations, procedure use, or a laboratory value. Outcomes researchers quickly realized that these measures were only the "tip of the iceberg." While the term "patient outcome measure" is meant to be an umbrella term for all measures indicating a change in health status, recent emphasis is placed on the patient-perceived measures as distinct from traditional, "hard" clinical measures.[20] Various instruments and scales have been developed to assess outcomes, such as changes in functioning, health status, and quality of life.[13,21-23] (For more information, see Chapter 13 on quality of life.)

There is no single, best outcome measure that can be applied universally. The best measures are those most relevant to the condition, treatments, and patient population under scrutiny. Many outcome measures, unless obtained directly from the patient, are proxies for direct health status changes. For example, hospitalizations do not measure health status directly; however, a hospital or long-term-care facility admission suggests a change in health status in a negative direction. In the selection of outcome measures for study, a well-rounded approach that captures relevant, clinical measures, patient-perceived measures, and resource utilization assessments is preferred. With this approach, relationships among various outcome measures, as well as those between treatments and outcomes, can be assessed. A more complete knowledge of the natural history of the condition and of related aspects and outcomes of treatment should result.

While outcomes have become the central focus, structure and process measures are still important. Outcomes of drug therapy cannot be measured in isolation. The researcher must measure and control for structure and process differences that potentially affect therapy provision and outcomes (e.g., confounding). An effective therapy may appear ineffective when inappropriately administered. Hence, it is essential that outcomes evaluations attempt to account for the structure and process under which interventions are used. Assessing multiple outcomes aids in evaluation of structure, process, and outcome relationships by providing a wide range of opportunities to capture change.

Outcomes from Whose Perspective?

When assessing whether a patient's condition has improved or deteriorated, and by how much, researchers must distinguish the perspective from which this judgment is being made. That is what Donabedian[24] referred to as contextual influences defining quality. Changes measured from the patient, clinician, payer, or societal perspective frequently will not be congruent. For example, clinicians may emphasize "objective," physiologic measures of biologic activity while giving less emphasis to "subjective" measures of how the patient may perceive these effects. Physicians often are surprised to find the level of functioning they have reported for a patient is different from that reported by the patient or patient's caregiver.[14,25,26] Also, the perceived value of various outcomes measures is influenced by the perspective.

There often is confusion over the use of the term "outcomes" because of these different players. Differing perspectives can blur the line between outcome and process measures. What one group considers process may be the intended outcome for another, depending on the perspective-influenced overall objectives. For example, the patient hospitalized for infection and treated with an aminoglycoside pays no attention to his/her own peak and trough serum aminoglycoside concentrations. The patient uses care based on personal need and is concerned with such outcomes as feeling better, being discharged from the hospital only when ready, and resumption of normal activities.[27] For the clinician, serum aminoglycoside concentrations are important process indicators that the treatment of choice is being used appropriately. The physician uses other clinical indicators, such as the patient's becoming afebrile and clinically relevant laboratory test results, to decide whether there is adequate response to therapy and when the patient can be discharged.

However, a facility's pharmacy or pharmacokinetic team, responsible for ensuring that patients do not experience adverse consequences due to inappropriate drug use, may view therapeutic serum aminoglycoside concentrations as the intended outcome of the services it provides. To avoid confusion when using the term "outcomes" in the context of healthcare provision, one may find it helpful to differentiate between a patient outcome, referring to health status impacts, and a programmatic clinical outcome such as the scenario described. In the context of Donabedian's model, these kinds of programmatic end points are actually process measures of care quality.

Outcomes from the patient's perspective are those measures providing information on the effectiveness of care in terms of health status, health-related quality of life, symptoms, and satisfaction with care, sometimes referred to as humanistic outcomes.[28] For the clinician, clinical outcomes provide the feedback practitioners are most accustomed to using in their decision-making. Most evaluations of treatment efficacy comprise these objective clinical measures. Payers, however, routinely focus on measures affecting eligibility, coverage, and reimbursement, which ultimately impact their costs, but not on total or societal costs. For example, an insurer may be concerned about the high rate of use for an expensive procedure but not about whether use of that procedure gets the patient back to his/her job.

Often, a "fragmented" perspective has a negative impact on the ability to assess medical treatment effectiveness in totality. For example, the present Medicare program does not cover outpatient prescription drugs, but does reimburse providers for most medical and surgical procedures. To assess the comparative medical treatment effectiveness of a procedure, researchers should include alternative drug therapies and options of the drug therapy used along with the procedure. Since the payer covers only one treatment option, the procedure, data are lacking for comparative assessments. Similarly, carve-out program providers, such as prescription benefit managers and mental health companies, could adversely affect assessment of treatment effectiveness in managed care settings or for self-insured employer groups.

Until recently, the impact of drug alternatives has gone almost unrecognized or has been circuitously addressed for this very reason. Efforts have been made to improve data sources for this purpose as, for example, in the Agency for Health Care Policy and Research (AHCPR)–sponsored patient outcomes research team (PORT), Consequences of Variation in Treatment for Acute Myocardial Infarction. Since the Medicare database does not provide information on thrombolytic, heparin, or other drug use during hospitalization for myocardial infarction, McNeil[29] has turned to other sources as adjuncts to the claims data.

Another example of the hindered ability to assess effectiveness in totality occurs when one of the treatment options is to do nothing, which is rarely captured in a claims database. "Watchful waiting" is the alternative treatment option when the intent is to do nothing but watch the patient closely for disease progression. An example of a study designed to compare this process with surgical intervention is the Veterans Affairs Cooperative Study on prostate surgery.[30] In this study, men with moderate benign prostatic hyperplasia are randomized to receive either watchful waiting or prostatectomy, and they are followed for health outcomes. Beyond effectiveness, the Veterans Affairs wanted to determine whether surgery is cost effective, so an additional subprotocol was added to evaluate the relative cost–effectiveness of the two treatment options, watchful waiting and surgery.

From the perspective of society, total costs, resource allocation, and public health concerns are main issues. Although cost is not a patient outcome, it is an important evaluation end point for society and third-party payers. Costs, charges, and reimbursements often are referred to in the context of economic outcome measures. While medical effectiveness indicates which treatment provides the best patient outcomes in the average care setting, cost–effectiveness refers to the balance between patient outcomes, both positive and negative, and the comparative cost to attain those outcomes from a stated perspective (e.g., payer, patient, society).

It is within the context of the payer or society that outcomes of programs or system changes have become an important focus. A timely example of programmatic changes occurs within the context of a DUR. With implementation of the 1990 Omnibus Budget Reconciliation Act (OBRA) DUR provisions as of January 1, 1993, every state Medicaid program is required to institute prospective and retrospective DURs. For most of these programs, drug use falling outside explicit criteria is considered inappropriate or aberrant. Remedial programs targeted at the outlier provider, prescriber, and/or dispenser are then initiated to improve the quality of drug use.

Similarly, interest in disease- or health-state management programs has also increased. Pharmaceutical manufacturers, prescription benefit managers, managed health care organizations, and disease management companies have all been attempting to alter care behaviors. Some of these programs focus on changing drug use, while others attempt to increase awareness and education. Most of these programs use some cost or use of healthcare resources as a measure of the success of the program. This may assume that a patient who receives less costly services is better managed or has better health outcomes. At this time, most disease management programs focus on financial measures rather than on patient outcomes. For third-party payers, this is the result of the relationship between them and their customers, namely, large employer groups. In the future, it may be necessary to evaluate patient outcomes to measure the success of a disease management program more adequately.

Reductions in the number, percentage, costs, and rate of inappropriate prescriptions dispensed are the measured outcomes of these kinds of efforts.[31-33] Generally, it is assumed that more appropriate drug use will lead to better patient outcomes. However, a measure of more appropriate drug use is not an evaluation of change in any one patient or patient population's health status. Thus, many of these programs assess the improved process of drug provision or the decrease in dollars spent from the pharmacy budget, not patient outcomes. They are referring to programmatic end points, such as changes in drug use resulting from a DUR or disease management program implementation.

The concept of patient compliance or adherence is another example of a process measure often targeted for programmatic leverage.[34,35] Most providers assume that improved patient adherence to a prescribed regimen results in improved patient outcomes. Thus, compliance is often targeted for clinical health promotion activities. However, a change in compliance itself is not a direct measure of a change in health status. If improved compliance results from an organized programmatic effort, it should be considered a process measure, not as a patient outcome. Noncompliance can be viewed as a risk factor; a change in a risk factor should not be confused with a change in outcome.[36]

Thornburg and Fryback[37] provide an example of varying perspectives and measures in their conceptual continuum, hierarchic model of technologic efficacy. While the focus of this model is technology assessment, specifically magnetic resonance imaging, and is intended to be used for appraisal of the literature, it provides the framework for an evolution in thinking about outcome measures and studies. Depending on the point in the continuum and the *perspective* from which the research question is framed, measures of interest will vary. In the model, six tiers of research and measures of interest for each tier are described, beginning with *technical efficacy*, which is comparable to a biomedical foundation. The tiers progress to *diagnostic accuracy efficacy* (sensitivity/specificity, validation) and *diagnostic thinking efficacy* (impact of the application on medical practice). Tier 5 is *patient outcome efficacy;* primary and secondary measures of individual outcomes and costs are evaluated at this tier. Finally, *societal efficacy* goes beyond individual risks and benefits, examining impacts on society as a whole. The authors explain that they used the term "efficacy" for simplicity, fully realizing that effectiveness is the focus of the latter tiers.

This discussion on perspectives is not intended to fuel confusion over, or dictate the correct use of, the term "outcomes." It is intended to encourage researchers to clearly describe their perspective, objectives, and definitions in reporting outcomes assessments. For the purpose of this chapter, the outcomes referred to are patient-oriented (not programmatic) end points, with particular emphasis on patient-perceived measures such as quality of life.

Outcomes Research and Drug Therapy

With reference to the history described, variations and small-area variations research marked the beginning of what has grown into patient outcomes research. These initial studies led to a vast number of hypothesis-testing efforts.[11,12,38] Of particular relevance to pharmacoepidemiology is the work that focuses on patient outcomes associated with drug therapy. The common objective shared by pharmacoepidemiologists focusing on outcomes assessment is to evaluate the impact, positive and negative, of a pharmaceutical intervention on patient health status. Research on patient outcomes of pharmaceutical therapy is conducted by various scientists in many different settings with various long-term objectives. Such research is the focus of clinicians and academicians in evaluating the comparative medical effectiveness of therapies, as well as pharmaceutical industry scientists in product development and safety surveillance.[39] The methods used are as varied as the clinical condition, research question, objectives, and setting dictate to meet the needs of a range of applications.

A principal opportunity for the pharmacoepidemiologist relates to involvement in the planning of clinical trials included in New Drug Applications (NDAs). Outcomes researchers often focus on the gains, maintenance, or decline in the quality of life, health status, or symptom resolution associated with pharmaceutical interventions. In general, these measures have not been used as primary efficacy end points in clinical trials used for

NDAs. The approval of Cognex on the basis of a change in cognitive function is evidence that more attention is and will be given to these measures in the future.[40]

This has led some to speculate on the relative merit of outcomes measures as composite measures of drug safety.[41] That is, perhaps a general quality-of-life assessment is a reasonable way to measure the overall impact of a drug on health status, if the instrument is specific enough to identify adverse drug reactions. If there is no adverse effect on quality of life (i.e., no difference from placebo), then it may be postulated that the drug is causing no demonstrable harm to the subject. This would, however, be an erroneous conclusion for rare events and would lead to considering reporting every change in a quality-of-life questionnaire as an adverse event, which is impractical and somewhat uninterpretable. For example, a change from "some of the time" to "all of the time" when responding to a question about difficulty in walking up a flight of stairs would be a difficult adverse event to interpret. Additionally, single items on a quality-of-life instrument may be difficult to interpret when it is more appropriate to evaluate a change in the domain score.

Anderson and Testa[42] have reported on the area of quality of life and safety reports in clinical trials. These investigators compared standard adverse event reporting with patient-reported symptom distress checklists as a component of quality-of-life measurement and physician checklists for symptoms. As would be expected, patient quality-of-life assessments through the symptom checklist resulted in much higher reporting of most symptoms than serious adverse events reports or physician checklists. For symptoms reported by the patient on his/her checklist, about one-fourth were reported on the physician checklist. Fewer than 7% also appeared in the physician adverse event reports. In related work, efforts to reconcile quality-of-life reports with adverse event reports were found to cost approximately $80 000 per additional adverse event identified, with these events most likely being of mild to moderate severity (personal communication, Marcia A Testa, Harvard School of Public Health, and Ralph R Turner, Phase V Technologic, Inc., August 9, 1996).

Research that provides needed information on patient outcomes and the comparative effectiveness of drug treatments is an integral component of the growing emphasis on cost-effectiveness analyses of pharmaceutical therapy. A prime example is implementation of an Australian regulation in January 1993, requiring submission of formal economic analyses of drug products as part of the application for inclusion onto the Schedule of Pharmaceutical Benefits.[43,44] The Schedule of Pharmaceutical Benefits lists government-subsidized products and is unrelated to marketing approval. However, a product's viability in the marketplace can be dependent on whether the Australian government provides reimbursement for the drug.

Of particular interest are the Australian guidelines established for conducting economic evaluations. Several components of these guidelines are particularly relevant to patient outcomes/medical treatment effectiveness research. Component 1 states that comparator(s) with the new drug should be those most widely used in that country for the relevant condition(s). Component 2 stresses that, in the assessment of relevant outcomes, information should come from trials undertaken under realistic conditions and that, when intermediate outcomes are used, they should directly relate to future patient benefits.[45]

In the 1995 Australian guidelines for conducting economic analyses,[46] additional clarification was provided regarding interpretation of methodologic issues. For example, while the guidelines do not have an absolute requirement for head-to-head randomized trials, there is a preference for this information if it is available. However, the Australian government will accept and give full consideration to economic evidence produced by using other methodologies. Additionally, the guideline contains information regarding the scientific rigor of the various methods used in conducting randomized and nonrandomized trials.

All these efforts, made under the auspices of research and development, regulation, postmarketing surveillance (PMS), healthcare policy, or reimbursement strategy, converge under the umbrella of medical treatment effectiveness research. Pharmacoepidemiologists are making valuable contributions in all areas.

Special Methodologic Challenges in Patient Outcomes Research

Since the methods used in outcomes research involving pharmaceuticals are generally the same as those used in traditional experimental and quasi-experimental (observational) epidemiologic studies, it is not necessary to enumerate and describe them here. However, there are special methodologic challenges of specific relevance to patient outcomes research, particularly involving drug therapies. This section discusses some of these special methodologic challenges.

EXPOSURE INFORMATION

Perhaps one of the key components in studying pharmaceutically related outcomes is adequate measurement of exposure to the pharmaceutical. In a clinical trial, exposure is randomized into specific regimens. Because of the efficacy emphasis on compliance, duration of drug exposure is considered equal to the length of the trial. Patients are either exposed or not exposed to a specific dosage(s) of drug, and categoric variables can be used to capture exposure status. However, in reality, prescribers choose various dosage and treatment regimens, and patients have varying levels of adherence for varying time periods. The challenge is, therefore, to quantify and compare contrasting patient groups and their outcomes.

Short of actually measuring the amount of drug consumed and absorbed by the person using highly technical instrumentation, this information often is gleaned from examining pill counts, numbers of prescriptions filled, self-reports of compliance, and daily diaries. Some companies even market computerized pill container caps that register each time and date the pill container is opened.[47]

In the usual manner of conducting outcomes research studies with administrative data, however, exposure is typically measured by identifying the drug, duration of therapy, dosage, dosing interval (continuous vs. as-needed), and patient compliance. This is, however, a proxy measure for person–time exposure, and whether this indicates the true level of exposure is somewhat controversial.[48-50]

Questions remain as to the most appropriate way to operate and incorporate drug exposure as an independent variable in statistical models of patient outcomes. Drug exposure may be considered a dichotomous, independent variable indicating exposed versus unexposed. When more than one drug therapy is used to treat a particular condition or for comorbidities, the number of drugs has been used as an independent variable, along with other variables, that attempts to capture quantitatively the intensity of drug use (e.g., dosage, duration of use)[51-53] (personal communication, JT Hanlon, Duke University, August 26, 1993). Without capturing information beyond the simple dichotomous variable that indicates that a patient took the drug at some time, valuable information is lost regarding intensity of exposure. Even if the entire duration and dosing are accounted for, statistical handling of the various patterns of exposure (e.g., intermittent dosing) has not been fully explored (personal communication, JM Garrard, University of Minnesota, July 26, 1993; personal communication, JT Hanlon, Duke University, August 26, 1993). For example, Guess[54] identified problems that arise in the behavior of the exposure odds ratio in case–control studies when the hazard function is not constant over time.

VALIDITY OF MEASURES

A controversial issue that has emerged in recent medical literature involves specification of criteria for ensuring validity. That is, what characteristics does an outcome measure require for one to assume that it has been properly validated?[55-57] A proposed schema of the minimum criteria for assessing the validity of an outcomes measure is presented in Table 2, as modified from a model by Kirshner and Guyatt.[56] As illustrated, necessary criteria depend greatly upon the setting in which the outcome measure is used. For example, a measure demonstrating adequate discriminant validity may be useful for cross-sectional surveys, but it may not necessarily be useful for a clinical trial setting, wherein responsiveness (i.e., sensitivity to change) is more important. Individual questions in a questionnaire, for example, may need to be worded differently if their intended purpose is to compare different groups cross-sectionally, rather than to measure change over time within the same group.

Although not illustrated in Table 2, an outcome measure may be validated with one particular patient population, but this may not mean the measure has been validated for use in all diseases or even in all severities of a single disease. Additional validation studies should be conducted to support the use of an outcomes measure in a disease in which it has not been previously studied. Condition- or population-specific modifications to the measure may be required.[55]

MULTIPLE OUTCOMES MEASURES

The rapid increase in outcomes assessment interests has given rise to a proliferation of outcomes measures[41,58] and to the expected situation in which there are now multiple, alternative outcomes measures for many diseases.[55,59,60] This then leads to difficulties in comparing results across studies of the same condition in which alternative measures are used. Additionally, it is difficult to select a measure when there are so many potential options.

One method of selection is to assess the evidence for validity for each of the candidate measures. Another is to conduct a comparative study, deciding the best measure (in terms of validity criteria) in a head-to-head

	Purpose of Study		
Criteria	**Discriminative**[a]	**Predictive**[b]	**Evaluative**[c]
Reproducibility	++	++	++
Responsiveness	+		++
Validity			
content	++	++	+
construct	+	+	++
discriminant	++	++	+

Table 2 Criteria for Assessing the Validity of an Outcomes Measure[56]

+ = moderately important; ++ = very important.
[a]Cross-sectional survey, for example.
[b]Covariate, for example.
[c]Clinical trial, cohort study, for example.

comparison. Instruments may be selected because they capture the most relevant domains or concepts of interest. Finally, many researchers use the measure that has the least respondent burden, will produce the least missing data due to ambiguously worded or potentially sensitive questions, is the simplest for data entry and analysis (e.g., limited, if any, free text), and provides readily interpretable results. For a clinical trial or PMS study in which the outcomes measure is a secondary or tertiary objective, these practical considerations often drive the decision-making.

Also, there is the potential for multiple end points to be assessed as outcomes and, with this, there is the problem of handling statistical multiplicity. For example, many quality-of-life instruments are analyzed as domains of quality of life, and there may be multiple domains per questionnaire. How should these be assessed? Is statistical significance required for each domain separately? If so, there is an assumption that the domains are not correlated, an assumption that is likely to be incorrect. While there is no consensus in the medical literature on how to approach this issue, several recent studies using global statistics show promise.[61] Additionally, there is the opportunity to look at the data multiple times and in multiple ways, particularly with secondary data analyses. This kind of hypothesis-generating search can lead to identification of a significant association that would no longer be significant when adjusted for the number of different subanalyses. Methods for statistical analysis for multiple end points have been identified for use in clinical trials that also may be beneficial.[62,63]

OUTCOMES AVAILABLE AS SECONDARY DATA

Much of outcomes research involving pharmaceutical interventions is conducted using secondary data or data already collected routinely for purposes other than research. In these instances, selection of outcomes is frequently motivated by what is available in the secondary database, and crude measures such as vital status, admission to a healthcare facility, or the use of home healthcare services often are used as proxies for patient outcomes.[49,50] While the events are certainly measurable, discrete, and fairly unambiguous to quantify, their interpretation as outcomes measures from the patient's perspective may be problematic. For example, while one terminally ill patient who is experiencing discomfort may prefer death to surviving in a debilitated and painful state, another in the same state may prefer longer life. Thus, the computation of mortality rates following a given intervention may be misleading, since the outcome of importance may truly be the relief of pain and suffering.

Few secondary data sources currently contain both the patient's self-reported data and data including pharmaceutical interventions. One exception is the growing number of clinicians who are beginning to incorporate health status measures into routine care[14,26] (personal communication, Michael J Goldberg, New England Medical Center, August 26, 1993). However, this is being done on an ad hoc basis, and data are not readily available as secondary data sources. Additional sources of patient-reported data include patient registries, such as the Arthritis, Rheumatism, and Aging Medical Information Systems (ARAMIS) database.[64,65]

COMORBIDITIES AND CONCURRENT THERAPIES

An especially challenging issue in outcomes research is the issue of distinguishing outcomes of a pharmaceutical intervention from other characteristics of the person being studied and from the natural history of the disease for which the intervention is given.[66] That is, unlike efficacy studies in which persons are generally enrolled with few comorbidities, outcomes research studies include persons with multiple medical conditions. This often entails concomitant use of multiple medications, increasing the potential for effect modification or confounding.

Studies based on secondary data often collect data on comorbidities inadequately.[67] Common issues with comorbidities include hierarchic reporting (e.g., space for only 5 diagnoses, with only the "worst" being reported), improper recording,[68] and lack of severity associated with the comorbidity (e.g., the person may have chronic lung disease coded, but that covers a wide range of functional limitations). In studies of pharmaceutical interventions using secondary data, attempts are made to validate the comorbidities (and even the case definition), by retrieving medical records and confirming the accuracy of the data.

A current, ongoing study of Medicare claims is assessing the validity of the data for research purposes.[69] A random sample of 600 acute-care hospitals from across the US have been asked to voluntarily submit copies of medical records for 100 Medicare patients' hospitalizations occurring during 1991 (a list of randomly selected discharges is provided to each hospital). Data from these records are entered into a database by specially trained abstractors who apply the Uniform Hospital Discharge Data Set Coding Clinic Guidelines strictly. No "grouper" software for diagnosis-related groups is being used. This database will be considered the clinical "gold standard."

Data from these discharges will be compared with the corresponding Medicare claims filed by the hospitals. The purpose of the validation study is to identify and assess the amount of error inherent to Medicare claims data. With this information, appropriate statistical adjustments can be made to improve the design and analyses of research using these data. The capability of interpreting results will improve through the use of this study's findings.

EFFECT OF CENSORED FOLLOW-UP ON OUTCOMES MEASUREMENT

A challenge for outcomes research studies, and many other epidemiologic studies, is the issue of censored data. Censoring occurs when the length of follow-up is interrupted, often by death. Thus, not all persons are followed for equal lengths of time, which can lead to problems in analysis and interpretation. For example, if we examine the 12-month effect of two drug therapies on quality of life, one therapy (drug A) may be associated with adverse experiences, poor compliance, and an increase in dropouts as early as 2 months. The other therapy (drug B) may be somewhat better because patients stay on the therapy, but their disease state worsens steadily as the year progresses.

By simply analyzing the difference in quality-of-life change from baseline between drugs A and B, one might think that drug A looks better, because patients left the study before their disease had a chance to deteriorate and because the most recent quality-of-life data are from their last visit. Conversely, although more people remained on therapy, drug B was associated with a continued decline in the disease state, so their last quality-of-life scores may look worse than the last scores for drug A. Which drug was better? Traditional statistical methods to handle unequal follow-up intervals such as this cannot help with extrapolating data for drug A at the end of 12 months. As with mortality trials, which follow up on all randomized patients, extensive follow-up information on every patient is important, regardless of whether that patient remained on therapy.

MORTALITY

The ascertainment of vital status in outcomes research is not as simple as it would appear. Secondary data source errors or idiosyncrasies in coding the occurrence of or date of death are possible. Corroborating evidence of vital status or tests of database validity are important for outcomes research studies that focus on mortality. For example, a date of death field is included in the Medicare database, and it is a verified field. This means that, when a date of death is verified by the Social Security Administration, the actual date of death is entered into the database along with a code denoting verification. When the date of death has not yet been verified, the last day of the month of death is entered in the date of death field, and no code is entered in the verification field. This is for administrative purposes, ensuring that all claims for the month will be paid (personal communication, Kathi A Weis, AHCPR, August 25, 1993). Administrative issues such as this can alter or bias analyses when a relatively short time period between an event and the occurrence of death is expected.

In other administrative databases, identification of death may be even more difficult. For example, in a managed care population, in which death is quite rare, the data may not be tracked well. Managed care members are more likely to terminate benefits because of changing health plans or changing jobs. It is often the responsibility of the employer group to identify changes in enrollment status to the health plan. If the reason for termination of benefits is not provided, then it is impossible to ascertain deaths easily. Anecdotally, there are numerous cases in which managed care continued to pay healthcare costs after the member has terminated benefits, for any reason.

Another issue is the difficulty in interpreting health status assessments that do not include mortality. For example, three of the more prominent assessments do not include a score for those who died (Sickness Impact Profile, Nottingham Health Profile, and Medical Outcomes Study Short Form-36).[21-23] Thus, if one pharmaceutical intervention is associated with greater mortality than another, it may appear to improve health status, since the healthier survivors are left to complete the health status assessment questionnaires. The other intervention may keep more patients alive, but at a lower health status than that of the "healthy survivors." Many of the health status assessments used for utility scoring include methods for weighting death (e.g., the Quality of Well-Being Scale).[55]

LENGTH OF FOLLOW-UP

Another challenge in outcomes research for pharmaceutical studies is to have a biologically plausible period of follow-up in the study. For example, in the examination of the effect of a drug on the development of cancer, it would be rather senseless to examine relatively short time periods of follow-up. However, there is the temptation to do so because many of the secondary data sources have patients who disenroll rather quickly after entering. For example, one study found that 56% of a state's Medicaid recipients disenrolled at the end of a 5-year period.[49] This means that a study that would, for example, require a 20-year follow-up to determine incident cancer rates could not be conducted with this data source, even if the numbers are large and there is the opportunity to show statistical significance with 5 years of follow-up. The 5 years may not be a biologically plausible test of treatment outcome.

Managed care administrative databases also may not have adequate enrollment periods for many studies requiring lengthy follow-up periods. First, very few databases provide extensive longitudinal data. Because the data were generated to pay claims, there was no real incentive to maintain the data over many years. Second, the disenrollment rate for members of these plans varies for certain age groups and certain geographic regions. The average disenrollment has been identified as approximately 20% per year. The turnover in membership may be related to the relatively young population served by managed care, because they are more likely to change jobs. In older age groups, the disenrollment may be less. Thus, the longevity of the longitudinal data and disenrollment pose substantial barriers to using administrative databases for some studies requiring extensive lengths for follow-up.

CLINICAL RELEVANCE OF EFFECT

One of the major challenges to interpretation of outcomes measures is to obtain a clearer understanding of the meaning behind a change in health status. That is, how much change in a measure matters? With the use of large secondary data sources, very small differences can be significant statistically, but their clinical significance is unknown. For example, what is the meaning behind a significant 2-point difference on a 100-point quality-of-life scale?

Various attempts have been made to explore this issue. Lydick and Epstein[70] proposed a taxonomy of methods to assess clinical significance, by dividing methods into either distribution-based or anchor-based approaches. The distribution-based classification includes statistical ways to assess relevance, such as determining the distance of a person's outcome from the status of a reference population by using standard deviation units or percentiles from the norm. Thus, if a person improves the equivalent of 3 standard deviations on an outcomes measure, he/she may be considered to show clinically significant improvement. The anchor-based methods relate the change in an outcome measure to some other measure. For example, if the change in an outcome measure is similar to the change associated with important life events, some researchers feel that a clinically significant change has occurred.[71] There is currently no standard methodology for assigning clinical meaningfulness to quality-of-life measures.

Applications of Outcomes Research: A Role for Pharmacoepidemiology

There are numerous applications of information on outcomes of healthcare provision. These applications range from day-to-day management of individual patients in clinical settings, to reimbursement decisions, or to quality assurance strategies, each offering a range of opportunities for pharmacoepidemiologic insight and methodology. As discussed earlier, perspective often drives the usefulness of the information. Outcomes research evaluations of pharmaceutical interventions, which identify consequences of care such as effectiveness, are often the building blocks for economic evaluations, which incorporate costs and consequences of care. Frequently, economic evaluations involve model-driven, cost-effectiveness analyses that are constructed to aid patients, clinicians, formulary committees, national reimbursement boards, and others in making decisions regarding selection of pharmaceutical treatments. The models themselves are generally epidemiologic and statistically based, using available data sources, published studies, and assumptions, for example, to model the lifelong cost–effectiveness of one therapy versus another. This application of outcomes research is increasing rapidly.

Freund and Dittus[72] have stated, "Ultimately, economic analyses remain models of the anticipated consequences of alternative decisions." Effectiveness research, using epidemiologic techniques, provides the information needed regarding anticipated consequences, particularly regarding their probability or risk of occurrence. Epidemiology and economics are working synergistically in the context of most cost analyses (e.g., cost–effectiveness, utility, minimization).

Study methodology may involve direct drug–drug comparisons. More appropriately, it should include all treatment options, drug and nondrug, and apply epidemiologic strategies to evaluate medical effectiveness. This movement to incorporate comparators other than alternative pharmaceuticals is an innovative area for pharmacoepidemiologic input as part of a multidisciplinary team of outcomes researchers.

Health policy decisions must be balanced between the effectiveness of alternative treatments and efficient resource allocation. When the effectiveness of alternative treatment choices for a disease becomes clearer, more informed decisions about the allocation of healthcare dollars for the treatment of that condition should be possible. Limited resources and economic considerations drive many policy implications of patient outcomes and effectiveness research. A broad epidemiologic approach is one that compares the most widely used treatment alternatives available, including nontreatment, in evaluating patient outcomes of care, and it must provide a rational basis for economic evaluations. This broad epidemiologic approach is one of the pillars of effectiveness research and serves as the basis for these economic considerations.

Another application falls within the realm of outcomes management. Here, results of outcomes research studies are provided to the clinician and/or patient, and presumably the process of care is then affected through this education (Figure 1). Further outcomes research studies are conducted and, again, results are fed back, creating a continuous loop of research and education, which has been termed "outcomes management"; this is literally managing care by reviewing outcomes to determine which treatment is associated with the best results.[19,73] Again, this activity is a multidisciplinary task, often spearheaded within an institution by program administrative groups, cost centers, quality assurance groups, or pharmacy divisions as a new extension of the quality assurance or utilization management efforts of the past.[74] In this context, outcomes research has been included as part of the total quality management and continuous quality improvement movements.[75]

In a broader sense, the loop of education and feedback can extend to the development of treatment guidelines, standards, and review criteria. Results of outcomes research often are evaluated for their application to making general treatment-policy decisions. Studies are rated according to their scientific quality and relevance to the issue under evaluation, and results of examining the weight of the published evidence guide the development of these policy statements.[76] Areas that may be considered include diagnostic strategies, indications for treatment, proper course of therapy, use of concomitant medications, and specification of outcomes to monitor. Outcomes research studies provide valuable information for these guidelines and should be founded upon good epidemiologic science.

Once guidelines, for example, are produced, an educational phase is developed to alter practice. During this phase, an understanding of new gaps in knowledge, more outcomes research, and potential refinements to guidelines emerges. This iterative process incorporates results of outcomes research, as well as results from standard efficacy trials.

With this supporting framework, the pharmacoepidemiologist finds important new roles in the selection, development, validation, application, and interpretation of outcomes measures. Borrowing heavily from the

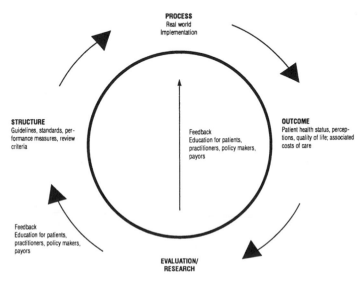

Figure 1
Outcomes
Management
Model

PROCESS
Real world
Implementation

STRUCTURE
Guidelines, standards, performance measures, review criteria

Feedback
Education for patients, practitioners, policy makers, payors

OUTCOME
Patient health status, perceptions, quality of life; associated costs of care

Feedback
Education for patients, practitioners, policy makers, payors

EVALUATION/
RESEARCH

behavioral science and psychology literature, the pharmacoepidemiologist is increasingly addressing questions about the validity and role of patient-perceived outcomes measures in drug development and treatment plans.

Predictive models are being used by clinicians to inform patients of potential risks and benefits and to make choices between treatments. Some of the inputs to these models come from traditional clinical trials, but data from outcomes research studies are increasingly being used for this purpose.[77] Patient education modules that include videodisc technology also are becoming increasingly available.[78-80] Known risks and benefits are presented to the patient in an understandable format, allowing critical patient participation in medical care decisions.

These advancements in outcomes research and its increasing acceptability have many implications for the field of pharmacoepidemiology. As more secondary data sources (clinical and claims) become available, administrative data will be augmented with patient outcomes information. Additionally, outcomes measures will become more refined and acceptable as their use broadens. More extensive validation and reliability testing for specific patient populations and conditions will be necessary. With more data sources and wider outcomes data availability, techniques and strategies for analysis will further address the complex methodologic issues previously detailed.

Where outcomes research affects the regulation of pharmaceuticals is perhaps best envisioned in terms of pre- and postproduct marketing. During the premarketing phase, outcomes measures may be incorporated into standard efficacy drug trials, with the usual requirement to report the results of therapies on these outcomes as well as all others to the regulatory agencies. However, outcomes research studies themselves are not necessarily required for product licensure and are not typically part of the standard NDA package. The studies are helpful for countries that have separate pricing or reimbursement boards (e.g., Australia, Canada). During the postmarketing phase, outcomes research studies are useful in providing information to consumers, physicians, formulary committees, and others, and these data are subject to advertising regulation scrutiny by the Food and Drug Administration.

Implications of outcomes research for regulatory reporting are potentially complex. A preliminary level of knowledge on safety and potential efficacy is clearly needed prior to testing a drug in a large, real-world population. Thus, efficacy trials can be thought of as a test of the pharmacologic mechanism necessary, although not sufficient, for clinical effectiveness. For this reason, it is unlikely that effectiveness studies will replace efficacy and safety study requirements. However, studies that include patient-perceived outcomes of therapy can make a valuable contribution to assessing the impact or value of a drug product.

Thus, patient-perceived measures are incorporated into clinical trials with increasing regularity. This offers both advantages and disadvantages as this embryonic field matures. Table 3 outlines some of the benefits and caveats of these efforts. For example, a patient-perceived outcomes measure provides a direct assessment of health status change that has advantages over the many surrogate measures now used. However, information must be interpreted cautiously, because the instrument is not being applied in the typical, average patient care setting. Results may not be generalizable, or the instrument may lose sensitivity, specificity, or validity in the transfer.

Although they can be viewed as separate and distinct issues, in reality, these applications are interwoven. As shown in Figure 1, information on the outcomes of care forms the basis for clinical practice policies, which include the structure and processes needed for care. This affects patient management, provider education, patient education, the level and intensity of services that are accessible, and, ultimately, costs and resource allocation.

Table 3 Patient-Perceived Outcome Assessment in Clinical Trials	Advantages	Disadvantages
	Direct versus surrogate measure	Measures may not be useful/generalizable to real-world practice
	Increased understanding of the condition's natural history	Increases respondent burden
	Aids in valuing biologic changes	Often difficult to interpret
	Aids in market differentiation	Lack of widespread acceptance
	Some tools can be incorporatedinto economic evaluations	Can be resource and time intensive, particularly if development and training are needed
	Noninvasive	Can be intrusive (personal questions)
	Allows for stratified comparisons within and across studies	Insufficient cross-cultural validation
	Can provide additional safety/tolerability information	Frequently analytically complex
	Illustrates instances where supportive counseling for patients may be needed	Insufficient information on appropriate tools and time intervals for administration

The pharmacoepidemiologist can play an important role throughout the system.

Conclusions: Beyond Unintended Drug Effects

In the past, the major emphasis of pharmacoepidemiology has primarily been the investigation of unintended drug effects (UDEs). A comprehensive annotated bibliography of pharmacoepidemiologic studies, presented in this book and the earlier edition,[81] demonstrated that the large majority of publications described investigation into the adverse effects associated with drug treatment. Outcomes research has given the investigation of UDEs a better numerator. That is, traditional spontaneous reporting of UDEs is notorious for underreporting (thus, an incomplete numerator). However, all persons enrolled in studies that incorporate outcomes measures are requested to supply a response. More complete reporting can provide a well-rounded, albeit less specific, sense of the impact of a pharmaceutical product on patient outcome. Outcomes research can also provide a better denominator than many postmarketing UDE studies, since the denominator (i.e., person–time of exposure) can be more adequately enumerated within a database study than within existing data on a marketed product (which typically provides aggregate and not person-specific information).

Studying all outcomes of a drug treatment provides the opportunity for more direct assessment of drug–effect relationships than is possible with traditional UDE reporting. Outcomes research shifts the focus onto the positive, or intended, effects of treatment. While unintended effects are still of importance, they are but one component of a broad spectrum of outcomes.

Outcomes research has expanded the traditional armamentarium of pharmaceutical study designs beyond randomized efficacy trials or PMS studies. While the former will always play a key role in demonstrating safety and efficacy, the disparity between efficacy and effectiveness in demonstrating improvement in the way patients actually feel has been perceived to be a potentially wide gap. To bridge this gap, outcomes research can be viewed as the way to observe efficacy in the field.

The specialized knowledge of pharmacoepidemiologists with regard to drug nomenclature, distribution, use, regulation, methodologic idiosyncrasies, and other relevant issues provides an invaluable resource to a multidisciplinary outcomes research team. The pharmacoepidemiologist can play a vital role in the growing field of outcomes/medical treatment effectiveness research.

We acknowledge the valuable comments and insights provided by our colleagues. In particular, we recognize the contributions of Ruth Baldwin, Katy Benjamin, Harry A Guess, Eva Lydick, Ira E Raskin, Jane D Scott, and Kathi A Weis, along with those of the editors.

References

1. Raskin IE, Maklan CW. Medical treatment effectiveness research—a view from inside the Agency for Health Care Policy and Research. Eval Health Professions 1991;(June):161-86.
2. Luscombe FA. Data needs and strategies: a view from the pharmaceutical industry. In: Data needs for outcomes research in long term care. Proceedings from a symposium sponsored by the Geriatric Drug Therapy Research Institute, American Society of Hospital Pharmacists, Washington, DC, November 17, 1992:25.
3. Brook RH, Lohr KN. Efficacy, effectiveness, variations, and quality: boundary crossing research. Med Care 1985;23:710-22.
4. Lohr KN. Outcome measurement: concepts and questions. Inquiry 1988;25:37-50.
5. Donabedian A. Evaluating the quality of medical care. Part 2. Milbank Mem Fund Q 1966;44(suppl):166-206.
6. Donabedian A. The quality of medical care. Science 1978;200:856-64.
7. Wennberg JE, Gittelsohn A. Small area variations in health care delivery. Science 1973;182:1102-8.
8. Wennberg JE, Gittelsohn A. Variations in medical care among small areas. Sci Am 1982;246:120-34.
9. Wennberg JE, Bunker JP, Barnes B. The need for assessing the outcome of common medical practices. Annu Rev Public Health 1980;1:277-95.
10. Wennberg JE. Which rate is right? N Engl J Med 1986;314:310-1.
11. Agency for Health Care Policy and Research. Medical treatment effectiveness—PORT IIs. RFA 94-002. NIH guide to contracts and grants. Chap. 22. Rockville, MD: Agency for Health Care Policy and Research, Public Health Service, US Department of Health and Human Services, 1993:6-8.
12. Agency for Health Care Policy and Research. Publications of the patient outcomes research teams (PORTs) as of January 1993. AHCPR Publication. Rockville, MD: Agency for Health Care Policy and Research, Public Health Service, US Department of Health and Human Services, 1993.
13. Boyer JG, Townsend RJ. Quality of life: methodologies in pharmacoepidemiologic studies. In: Hartzema AG, Porta MS, Tilson HH, eds. Pharmacoepidemiology: an introduction. 2nd ed. Cincinnati: Harvey Whitney Books, 1991:207-21.
14. Ware JE. The use of health status and quality of life measures in outcomes and effectiveness research. In: Proceedings of the agenda setting conference on outcomes and effectiveness research. Ann Arbor, MI: Health Administration Press, 1992.
15. Davis KL, Thal LJ, Gamzu ER, Davis CS, Woolson RF, Gracon SI, et al. A double-blind, placebo-controlled multicenter study of tacrine for Alzheimer's disease. The Tacrine Collaborative Study Group. N Engl J Med 1992;327:1253-9.
16. Yusuf S, Collins R, Peto R. Why do we need some large, simple randomized trials? Stat Med 1984;3:409-22.
17. Tyroler HA. Outcomes of cholesterol lowering clinical trials in relation to observational epidemiologic studies. Presented at the Center for Pharmaceutical Outcomes Research, University of North Carolina at Chapel Hill, April 1, 1996.
18. Psaty BM. Establishing appropriate endpoints: surrogate endpoints versus health outcomes. Presented at the Center for Pharmaceutical Outcomes Research, University of North Carolina at Chapel Hill, April 2, 1996.
19. Ellwood PM. Special report: Shattuck Lecture—outcomes management: a technology of patient experiences. N Engl J Med 1988;318:1549-56.

20. Bungay KM, Ware JE. Measuring and monitoring health-related quality of life. In: Current concepts. Kalamazoo, MI: The Upjohn Company, 1993.

21. Bergner M, Bobbitt RA, Carter WB, Gilson BS. The Sickness Impact Profile: development and final revision of a health status measure. Med Care 1981;19:787-805.

22. McEwan J. The Nottingham Health Profile. In: Walker SR, Rosser RM, eds. Quality of life: assessment and application. Lancaster, England: MTP Press, 1988:95.

23. Ware JE, Sherbourne CD, Davies AR, Stewart AL. The MOS short-form general health survey: development and test in a general population. Publication P-7444. Santa Monica, CA: Rand Corp., 1988.

24. Donabedian A. Explorations in quality assessment and monitoring. In: The definition of quality and approaches to its assessment. Vol. I. Ann Arbor, MI: Health Administration Press, 1980:1-31.

25. Najman JM, Levine S. Evaluating the impact of medical care and technologies on quality of life: a review and critique. Soc Sci Med 1981;5:107-15.

26. Meyer K. The quality of my patient's life. Presented at the American Medical Writers Association Eastern Regional Meeting, West Point, NY, June 6, 1993.

27. Hulka BS, Wheat JR. Patterns of utilization—the patient perspective. Med Care 1985; 23:438-60.

28. Kozma CM. Outcomes research and pharmacy practice. Am Pharm 1995;NS35:35-41.

29. McNeil B. AHCPR PORT update. Presented at the annual meeting of the Association for Health Services Research, Washington, DC, June 27, 1993.

30. Wasson JH, Reda DJ, Bruskewitz RC, Elinson J, Keller AM, Henderson WG. A comparison of transurethral surgery with watchful waiting for moderate symptoms of benign prostatic hyperplasia. The Veterans Affairs Cooperative Study Group on Transurethral Resection of the Prostate. N Engl J Med 1995;332:75-9.

31. Soumerai SB, McLaughlin TJ, Avorn JL. Improving drug prescribing in primary care: a critical analysis of the experimental literature. Milbank Q 1989;67:268-317.

32. Lipton HL, Bero LA, Bird JA, McPhee SJ. The impact of clinical pharmacists' consultations on physicians' geriatric drug prescribing. A randomized controlled trial. Med Care 1992;30:646-58.

33. Stergachis A, Fors M, Wagner EH, Simms DD, Penna P. Effect of clinical pharmacists on drug prescribing in a primary-care clinic. Am J Hosp Pharm 1987;44:525-9.

34. Greenfield S. Outcomes, outcomes research, and outcomes assessment: an introduction. In: Research update: does improved medicine compliance improve health outcomes? Presented at the 9th National Conference on Prescription Medicine Information and Education, National Council on Patient Information and Education, Washington, DC, May 6, 1993.

35. Kravitz RL. Linking medication compliance and improved outcomes. In: Research update: does improved medicine compliance improve health outcomes? Presented at the 9th National Conference on Prescription Medicine Information and Education, National Council on Patient Information and Education, Washington, DC, May 6, 1993.

36. Kaplan RM. Behavioral epidemiology, health promotion, and health services. Med Care 1985;23:564-83.

37. Thornburg JR, Fryback DG. Technology assessment—an American view. Eur J Radiol 1992;14:147-56.

38. Agency for Health Care Policy and Research. Study of patient outcomes associated with pharmaceutical therapy. RFA 92-03. NIH guide to contracts and grants, Part I. Chap. 21. Rockville, MD: Agency for Health Care Policy and Research, Public Health Service, US Department of Health and Human Services, 1992:3-6.

39. Testa MA, Anderson RB, Nackley JF, Hollenberg NK. Quality of life and antihypertensive therapy in men. A comparison of captopril with enalapril. The Quality-of-Life Hypertension Study Group. N Engl J Med 1993;328:907-13.

40. Farlow M, Gracon SI, Hershey LA, Lewis KW, Sadowsky CH, Dolan-Ureno J. A controlled trial of tacrine in Alzheimer's disease. The Tacrine Study Group. JAMA 1992; 268:2523-9.

41. Epstein RS, Lydick E. Quality of life assessment: a pharmaceutical industry perspective. In: Dimsdale J, Baum A, eds. Quality of life in behavioral medicine research. Hillsdale, NJ: LEA Publishers, 1995.

42. Anderson RB, Testa MA. Symptom distress checklists as a component of quality of life measurement: comparing prompted reports by patient and physician with concurrent adverse event reports via the physician. Drug Inf J 1994;28:89-114.

43. Mitchell A. Potential for bias in economic analysis (letter). N Engl J Med 1991;325: 1384.

44. Drummond M. Australian guidelines for cost-effectiveness studies of pharmaceuticals: the thin end of the boomerang? Center for Health Economics Health Economics Consortium, Discussion Paper 88. Center for Health Economics, University of York, York, England, 1991.

45. Henry D. Economic analyses as an aid to subsidisation decisions—the development of the Australian guidelines for pharmaceuticals. PharmacoEconomics 1992;1:54-67.

46. Commonwealth Department of Human Services and Health, Commonwealth of Australia. Guidelines for the pharmaceutical industry on preparation of submissions to the pharmaceutical benefits advisory committee. Canberra, Australia: Australian Government Publishing Service, 1995.

47. Eisen SA, Miller DK, Woodward RS, Spitznagel E, Przybeck TR. The effect of prescribed daily dose frequency on patient medication compliance. Arch Intern Med 1990;150:1881-4.

48. Shapiro S. The role of automated record linkage in the postmarketing surveillance of drug safety: a critique. Clin Pharmacol Ther 1989;46:371-86.

49. Ray WA, Griffin MR. Use of Medicaid data for pharmacoepidemiology. Am J Epidemiol 1989;129:837-49.

50. Strom BL, Carson JL. Use of automated databases for pharmacoepidemiology research. Epidemiol Rev 1990;12:87-107.

51. Ray WA, Griffin MR, Downey W. Benzodiazepines of long and short elimination half-life and the risk of hip fracture. JAMA 1989;262:3303-7.

52. Griffin MR, Piper JM, Daugherty JR, Snowden M, Ray WA. Nonsteroidal anti-inflammatory drug use and increased risk for peptic ulcer disease in elderly persons. Ann Intern Med 1991;114:257-63.

53. Ried LD, Johnson RE. Evaluation of the reliability and validity of a measure of anxiolytic drug-use intensity for pharmacoepidemiologic studies. Ann Pharmacother 1992;26:1441-6.

54. Guess HA. Behavior of the exposure odds ratio in a case–control study when the hazard function is not constant over time. J Clin Epidemiol 1989;42:1179-84.

55. Patrick DL, Erickson P. Health status and health policy—quality of life in health care evaluation and resource allocation. New York: Oxford University Press, 1993: 138-41, 370.

56. Kirshner B, Guyatt G. A methodological framework for assessing health indices. J Chronic Dis 1985;38:27-36.

57. Streiner DL, Norman GR, eds. Health measurement scales: a practical guide to their development and use. New York: Oxford University Press, 1989.

58. Schumacher M, Olschewski M, Schulgen G. Assessment of quality of life in clinical trials. Stat Med 1991;10:1915-30.
59. Spilker B, Molinek FR, Johnston KA, Simpson RL, Tilson HH. Quality of life bibliography and indexes. Med Care 1990;28(suppl):DS1-77.
60. Hyland ME. Quality-of-life assessment in respiratory disease: an examination of the content and validity of four questionnaires. PharmacoEconomics 1992;2:43-53.
61. Tandon PK. Applications of global statistics in analyzing quality of life data. Stat Med 1990;9:819-27.
62. O'Brien PC. Procedures for comparing samples with multiple endpoints. Biometrics 1984;40:1079-87.
63. Pocock SJ, Geller NL, Tsiatis AA. The analysis of multiple endpoints in clinical trials. Biometrics 1987;43:487-98.
64. Wolfe F, Fries JF. ARAMIS today: moving toward internationally distributed databank systems for follow-up studies. Clin Rheumatol 1987;6(suppl 2):93-102.
65. Fries JF, McShane DJ. ARAMIS (the Arthritis, Rheumatism, and Aging Medical Information System). A prototypical national chronic-disease data bank. West J Med 1986;145:798-804.
66. Anderson TF, Mooney G. The challenges of medical practice variation. London: The MacMillan Press, 1990.
67. Iezzoni LI, Foley SM, Daley J, Hughes J, Fisher ES, Heeren T. Comorbidities, complications, and coding bias: does the number of diagnosis codes matter in predicting in-hospital mortality? JAMA 1992;267:2197-203.
68. Iezzoni LI, Burnside S, Sickles L, Moskowitz MA, Sawitz E, Levine PA. Coding of acute myocardial infarction: clinical and policy implications. Ann Intern Med 1988; 109:745-51.
69. Weis KA. Study to investigate the accuracy and completeness of data elements in the Medicare claims files. Unpublished protocol. Rockville, MD: Agency for Health Care Policy and Research, Office of the Forum for Quality and Effectiveness in Health Care, 1991. Contract No. 282-91-0073.
70. Lydick E, Epstein RS. Interpretation of quality of life changes. Qual Life Res 1993;2: 221-6.
71. Brook RH, Ware JE Jr, Rogers WH, Keeler EB, Davies AR, Donald CA, et al. Does free care improve adults' health? Results from a randomized controlled trial. N Engl J Med 1983;309:1426-34.
72. Freund DA, Dittus RS. Principles of pharmacoeconomic analysis of drug therapy. PharmacoEconomics 1992;1:20-32.
73. Riesenberg D, Glass RG. The medical outcomes study (editorial). JAMA 1989;262: 943.
74. Payne SM. Identifying and managing inappropriate hospital utilization: a policy synthesis. Health Serv Res 1987;22:709-69.
75. Nash DB. The state of the outcomes/guidelines movement. Decis Imag Econ 1993;6: 11-7.
76. Agency for Health Care Policy and Research. Program note. Clinical guideline development. AHCPR Publication No. OM 90-0086. Rockville, MD: Agency for Health Care Policy and Research, Public Health Service, US Department of Health and Human Services, 1990.
77. Selker HP, Griffith JL, D'Agostino RB. A tool for judging coronary care unit admission appropriateness, valid for both real time and retrospective use—a time-insensitive predictive instrument (TIPI) for acute cardiac ischemia: a multicenter study. Med Care 1991;29:610-27.

78. Weinstein MM. Dr. Video—how best to decide what patients need. New York Times 1992 Dec 13:16.
79. Little L. Interactive videos may help educate patients to make informed decisions. Medical Tribune 1992 Feb 13.
80. Randall T. Producers of videodisc programs strive to expand patient's role in medical decision making process. JAMA 1993;270:160-1.
81. Hartzema AG, McLeod DC. An annotated bibliography on pharmacoepidemiologic studies. In: Hartzema AG, Porta MS, Tilson HH, eds. Pharmacoepidemiology: an introduction. 2nd ed. Cincinnati: Harvey Whitney Books, 1991:357-414.

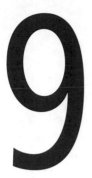

Spontaneous Reporting in the United States

Laurie B Burke
Dianne L Kennedy
James R Hunter

Abstract

Spontaneous reporting is a vital postmarketing surveillance activity that generates important signals of drug-associated adverse events. Even though US regulations require pharmaceutical companies to report certain adverse reactions to the Food and Drug Administration (FDA), the system ultimately relies on the voluntary activities of astute healthcare practitioners. Indeed, this mechanism of surveillance is the only way that some rare adverse events are detected. The FDA established its MedWatch program in 1993 to promote the essential voluntary reporting of important adverse events associated with the use of regulated medical products. Computer automation and international harmonization of regulatory standards and definitions will further increase the effectiveness of spontaneous reporting worldwide.

Outline

Throughout this book, the fundamental premise of pharmacoepidemiology reads: No drug therapy is without risk. However, as explained in Chapter 5, the limited size and selected populations included in premarketing clinical trials ensure that only the most frequent adverse events will be observed and listed in a drug's official labeling when it enters the market. Patients enrolled in clinical trials are rarely representative of the population of individuals who are exposed after marketing, which may include the very old, very young, chronically ill, or those taking a broad array of concomitant medications. There is also rarely enough information in premarketing data to determine a drug's latent toxicities, thereby leaving one more element of uncertainty for prescribers of newly marketed products. Postmarketing surveillance (PMS) is one element of the dynamic process of drug development that seeks to update and to complete knowledge of drug effects. This phase of drug development forms the basis for labeling revisions and other regulatory measures that are designed to facilitate rational decision-making in drug prescribing by healthcare practitioners.

There are many aspects of PMS that can be divided broadly into three major areas. These are the collection and analysis of spontaneous adverse event reports, the measurement of drug use, and the conduct of epidemiologic studies.[1] Drug manufacturers and the Food and Drug Administration (FDA) utilize all three in combination as given situations demand. This chapter focuses on the collection and analysis of spontaneous adverse event reports within the FDA.

History of US Drug Safety Regulation

Regrettably, medical disasters have shaped the history and development of drug safety regulation. The first US drug law came into existence during the 1848 Mexican War, when quinine imported for the US Army was found to have been adulterated.[2] This law outlawed the importation of such drugs. Elixir of sulfanilamide-induced deaths during the 1930s,[3] and chloramphenicol-associated aplastic anemia during the 1950s[3] prompted concern for the collection of postmarketing drug safety information on a national basis. The well-described tragedy of 10 000 birth defects worldwide as a result of in utero exposure to thalidomide[4] was brought to public attention during the same general time period and led the US Congress to address the need for more comprehensive drug regulation. The 1962 Kefauver–Harris Amendments to the Food, Drug, and Cosmetic Act required proof of efficacy before drug approval and marketing; for the first time, drug manufacturers were required to report adverse drug reactions (ADRs) to the FDA.

Through these events, it was recognized that national drug safety surveillance depends on signals that arise from the reporting of ADRs as they are observed by health professionals. The FDA's first system for monitoring these events, the Spontaneous Reporting System (SRS), was modeled after a system designed by the American Medical Association's Committee on Blood Dyscrasias. It served the Agency from 1961 through September 1997. This national system's goal was to collect, automate, evaluate, and generate signals from case reports and to provide new information on drug safety issues to the health industry. With the regulated participation of industry, the SRS rapidly expanded, and the information in the system was included in a database in 1969, the first year for which historical adverse event data can be retrieved. Many countries around the world also began to collect and monitor more systematically adverse event data at approximately the same time.

Moreover, in response to the thalidomide disaster, the World Health Assembly requested that the World Health Organization (WHO) address the safety of pharmaceutical products in international commerce; this resulted in the establishment of the WHO International Drug Monitoring Program. This program, which became operational in 1968,[5] is the only international safety-monitoring effort of its kind. It is currently located at the WHO Collaborating Centre, which is within the Swedish Department of Drugs in Uppsala. The program depends on participation and data contribution by individual countries that have established national systems for spontaneous adverse reaction reporting. The program has been growing steadily since its inception. By 1992, 36 countries regularly submitted reports to the WHO International Drug Monitoring Program. The US was one of the original participants in the WHO's system and continues to provide the largest number of reports per year.

The prompt reporting of serious adverse events by health professionals constitutes the core of drug safety surveillance in the US. Since the beginning of report collection, the majority of healthcare practitioners in the US tend to report adverse events to manufacturers, as opposed to providing reports directly to the FDA. This pattern is not the case in many other countries. Regulations govern how manufacturers are to submit adverse event information to the FDA. In 1985, the US requirements for manufacturer ADR reporting were modified.[6,7] Accompanying guidances were drafted at that time and finalized in 1992.[8,9] Additional regulations for postmarketing reporting of adverse experiences with biological products were promulgated in 1994.[10] Even though these regulations and guidances are directed toward the pharmaceutical industry, familiarity with certain elements of them is instructive and can assist health professionals in making sound decisions in their voluntary reporting.

Regulatory Definitions

In the US, manufacturers of drugs and biologic products have mandatory reporting requirements.[6,7,10] For regulatory purposes, all marketed drugs may be divided into six groups, as defined below. The manufacturers of each drug group have a different set of adverse event reporting requirements. (1) *Grandfathered* drugs are those that were first marketed before the Food, Drug, and Cosmetic Act of 1938; thus, manufacturers of these drugs were not required to submit and do not have approved new drug applications (NDAs). (2) *Investigational new drugs* (INDs) are those that are not yet marketed but for which an application has been submitted to the FDA to allow their study in clinical trials. (3) *NDA* drugs are those approved for marketing by the FDA for the specific indications that appear in the NDA. All prescription drugs first marketed after 1938 have an approved NDA. (4) *Abbreviated new drug application* (ANDA) drugs are the generic, or "me-too," drugs. (5) *New molecular entities* are NDA drugs approved within the past 3 years that contain an active ingredient not previously marketed in the US. (6) *Over-the-counter* drugs are those approved by the FDA that may be purchased by the consumer without a physician's prescription.

The above definitions are not necessarily mutually exclusive. A drug approved for over-the-counter use may also have an approved NDA, be under study for a new indication as an IND, and have a generic version with an ANDA. Such situations are not unusual and can create confusion in interpreting the regulations that govern separate categories of drugs. For example, there are no current reporting requirements for most over-the-counter drugs. However, if an over-the-counter drug has an approved NDA, its reporting requirements are the same as those for a legend drug with an NDA.

Terms Associated with Spontaneous Reporting

Despite the complexities due to varying regulations by drug category, once a new drug is on the market, the following FDA regulatory definition of an *adverse drug experience*[7] applies, regardless of its category:

> *Any adverse event associated with the use of a drug in humans, whether or not considered drug related, including the following: an adverse event occurring in the course of the use of a drug in professional practice; an adverse event occurring from drug overdose, whether accidental or intentional; an adverse event occurring from drug abuse; an adverse event occurring from drug withdrawal; and any significant failure of expected pharmacological action.*

These general elements provide the broad base for categorization of adverse events and ADRs, as does the determination of whether a given event meets the regulatory definition of "serious" (see below) or "severe." Assessment of causality by the reporter or the manufacturer is required for premarketing (clinical investigation) cases but is not necessary or desired for PMS. Causality assessment associated by health professionals of marketed drugs is usually derived from expectations based on known events or patterns of illness, and the purpose of collecting spontaneous reports is to identify signals of potential adverse events. Hence, the utility of such a system is dependent on the reporting of events that represent mere glimmers of suspicion to the reporters.

Serious medical events have always been given the highest priority for review by the FDA. Their importance is codified in FDA regulations requiring that serious events be reported in a more expedited fashion than nonserious events.[7] A serious adverse event is one that results in a death, a life-threatening adverse drug experience, a hospitalization (whether initiated or prolonged by the event), a persistent or significant disability/incapacity, or a congenital anomaly. It also includes important medical events that may not result in one of the above outcomes but may jeopardize the patient and may require medical or surgical intervention to *prevent* one of these outcomes (Table 1[11]). Most adverse events that occur with medications, changes in dosage, discontinuance of drug therapy, or routine treatment with a prescription drug are not considered to be serious.

The FDA regulations consider an "unlabeled" (or "unexpected") adverse event as one that does not appear in the most recent FDA-approved labeling for the product.[7] As new information becomes known about the risks of therapy through PMS, the sponsor of a product either requests FDA approval for a labeling change or is asked by the FDA to change the label to conform with current knowledge about the product.

Regulatory Reporting Requirements

The US adverse event (postmarketing) reporting regulations are summarized in Tables 2 and 3. By regulation, sponsors of all drugs with approved NDAs or ANDAs or of grandfathered prescription drugs are required to report all adverse events of which they are aware to the FDA, providing as much information as possible. The ADR reporting requirements for INDs are substantially different from postmarketing reporting requirements. IND reports are not entered into the SRS. The IND reporting requirements are discussed in Chapter 2. Manufacturers of over-the-counter drugs without NDAs currently are not required to report ADRs.

By regulation, manufacturers forward serious unlabeled events to the FDA within 15 days and all nonserious and serious labeled events to the

FDA periodically (quarterly for new molecular entities and annually for all other approved NDA and ANDA drugs). Manufacturers are not required to submit such periodic reports for grandfathered drugs. They are, however, required to provide follow-up information for all incomplete reports of serious unlabeled events for grandfathered drugs, as well as for all approved NDA and ANDA drugs.

Because drug safety data from other countries are valuable, especially for drugs that may be approved earlier in countries other than in the US, manufacturers of all FDA-approved drugs must also report serious unlabeled ADRs that occur outside the US. The same is true for ADRs detected during the course of any formal study, regardless of that study's location. Manufacturers are also required to survey the international medical literature for reports of serious unlabeled adverse events.

Table 1
Definition of a
Serious Adverse
Event[11]

An event is serious when the outcome is any of the following:

• **Death**
if the patient's death was an outcome of the adverse event

• **Life threatening**
refers to an event in which the patient was at substantial risk of dying at the time of the event; it does not refer to an event that hypothetically might have caused death if it were more severe

• **Hospitalization (initial or prolonged)**
if admission to the hospital or prolongation of existing hospitalization is a result of the adverse event; do not report if a patient in the hospital received a medical product and subsequently developed an otherwise nonserious adverse event, unless the adverse event prolonged the hospital stay

• **Disability**
if the adverse event resulted in significant, persistent, or permanent change, impairment, damage, or disruption in the patient's body function/structure, physical activities, and/or quality of life

• **Congenital anomaly**
if exposure prior to conception or during pregnancy resulted in an adverse outcome in the child

• **Intervention to prevent permanent impairment of damage**
if the adverse event required medical or surgical intervention to preclude one of the outcomes listed above; changes in dosage, discontinuation of therapy, and routine treatment with a prescription medication are not in themselves considered serious

Other Nongovernmental Standards for Reporting

In addition to pharmaceutical industry regulation, there are organizations that facilitate reporting of adverse drug events to the FDA. Hospitals are not required by law or regulation to submit adverse event reports on medications, although the Joint Commission on the Accreditation of Healthcare Organizations (JCAHO) does require for accreditation purposes that a hospital must maintain an adverse drug event reporting system.[12] (Note: Hospitals *are* required by law to report medical device–related deaths and serious injuries to the FDA.[13]) This system must include a working definition of a significant adverse drug event, a written policy and procedure describing the institution's reporting program, and a system in place to regularly review reported ADRs. The American Society of Health-System Pharmacists has also issued guidelines on ADR monitoring and reporting.[14]

Table 2
FDA Requirements for Submission of ADR Reports by Manufacturers[6,7,10]

Type of Drug	Serious Unlabeled Events (15 day)	All Other Events (by quarter for NMEs or by year)	Follow-up of Incomplete Reports
Grandfathered prescription drug	X		X
NDA	X	X	X
ANDA	X	X	X
OTC (non-NDA)			

ADR = adverse drug reaction; ANDA = abbreviated new drug application; FDA = Food and Drug Administration; NDA = new drug application; NME = new molecular entity; OTC = over the counter.

Table 3
Sources of ADRs for Manufacturer Reporting[10]

Source	Serious Unknown (15 day)	Periodic Reports
US	X	X
Foreign	X	
Literature	X	
Study	X	

ADRs = adverse drug reactions.

MedWatch

Reporting of adverse events and product problems by health professionals to the FDA either directly or via the manufacturer is critical to an effective national PMS system. However, individual health professionals are not required by law or regulation to submit such reports to either the Agency or the manufacturer. Moreover, limitations to studies that can reasonably be conducted in the premarketing clinical trials make the reporting of ADRs in the postmarketing period critical to discover previously undetected safety issues. Therefore, the FDA established the MedWatch program in 1993 as a national educational/promotional initiative to educate health professionals about the importance of reporting serious adverse events and important product problems and to facilitate voluntary reporting to the Agency.

MedWatch has four general goals.[15] The first goal is to increase awareness of drug- and device-induced disease and the importance of reporting serious adverse events and product problems. Clinicians are encouraged to consider drugs and devices as possible causes when assessing a problem in a patient and to incorporate that into the process of developing a differential diagnosis. This goal is accomplished through educational outreach, which includes professional presentations, publications, and an active continuing education program, through which the health professional can earn continuing education credits. This continuing education program is accessible via the MedWatch Internet home page (www.fda.gov/medwatch).

The second goal of MedWatch is to clarify what should (and should not) be reported. This is important both to improve the quality of individual reports and to focus on serious ADRs. The essential elements of a quality ADR report are listed in Table 4.[16] It is important to influence health professionals to report only serious adverse events to enable the FDA and the manufacturer to focus on the most potentially significant ADRs. For those manufacturers participating in the FDA's "MedWatch to Manufacturer" program, copies of serious reports submitted directly to the FDA are sent expeditiously to the manufacturer.

Third, MedWatch has made it easier to report adverse events to the FDA. Only one form is necessary for reporting adverse events and product problems with all medications, devices, and special nutritional items (e.g., dietary supplements, medical foods, infant formulas) that are regulated by the Agency. The use of a single form ensures the collection of a standard set of data elements from reporters, regardless of medical product type. The single form, "MedWatch: The FDA Medical Products Reporting Program," replaced all forms previously used by the Agency for reporting on medications and devices.[17] The form is available in two versions (Figures 1 and 2). The postage-paid FDA Form 3500 is used for voluntary reporting (i.e., that not mandated by law or regulation) of adverse events and product problems by health professionals. The second version, FDA Form 3500A, is used for mandatory reporting required of all drug, biologic, and medical device manufacturers, as well as for medical device user facilities and device distributors. These forms are available from the FDA via a toll-free number (1-800-FDA-1088) or can be downloaded from the MedWatch Internet home page.

In addition to mailing the form, voluntary reporters also have the options of faxing their reports (1-800-FDA-0178), calling 1-800-FDA-1088 to give a report verbally, or directly entering a report via the MedWatch home page.

Vaccines are the only FDA-regulated medical products that are not reported on the MedWatch reporting form. Reports concerning vaccines are sent to the vaccine adverse event reporting system (VAERS) on the VAERS-1 form, available by calling 1-800-822-7967.[18,19] The VAERS form is a joint FDA/Centers for Disease Control and Prevention form used for mandatory reporting by physicians of vaccine-related adverse events.

The fourth goal of MedWatch is to provide feedback to health professionals about new safety issues involving medical products. Several methods, including the MedWatch home page and the *FDA Medical Bulletin,* are used to disseminate safety-related information to the broadest possible health professional audience. In addition, MedWatch has a network of more than 120 health professional organizations that have allied themselves with the FDA as MedWatch partners. These partners are used to further disseminate safety notifications to their membership. The FDA's interest in informing health professionals about new safety discoveries is not only to enable them to incorporate new safety information into daily practice, but also to

---

• Product name (if generic, include the name of the manufacturer) • Concise description of the adverse event • Date of onset • Drug start/stop dates • Dose and frequency of administration • Relevant laboratory values • Biopsy/autopsy reports • Patient demographics • Dechallenge and rechallenge information • Confounders (other medical products, medical history, etc.) • Patient outcome	**Table 4** Essential Elements of a Complete ADR Report[16]

ADR = adverse drug reaction.

Figure 1
The FDA Form
3500 for Voluntary
Reporting of
Adverse Events and
Product Problems

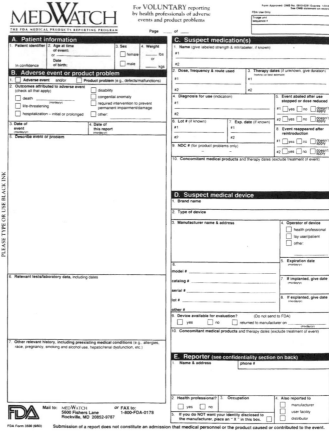

FDA = Food and Drug Administration.

further the development of PMS by reminding them to report medication- and device-induced diseases. The FDA also hopes to demonstrate to health professionals that their spontaneous reports have an impact.

Confidentiality in Adverse Event Reporting

The issue of maintaining confidentiality, both of patients and reporters of ADRs, is one of the FDA's greatest responsibilities. There is no question, and numerous studies over several decades have shown, that healthcare providers are often deterred from reporting because of a fear of litigation should their or their patients' identities be revealed. This fear has frequently been cited as a reason that providers often specifically elect not to

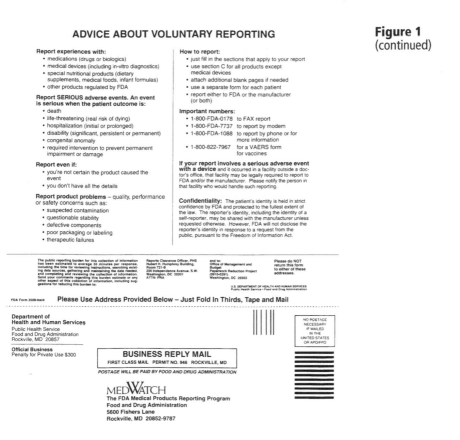

Figure 1
(continued)

ADVICE ABOUT VOLUNTARY REPORTING

Report experiences with:
- medications (drugs or biologics)
- medical devices (including in-vitro diagnostics)
- special nutritional products (dietary supplements, medical foods, infant formulas)
- other products regulated by FDA

Report SERIOUS adverse events. An event is serious when the patient outcome is:
- death
- life-threatening (real risk of dying)
- hospitalization (initial or prolonged)
- disability (significant, persistent or permanent)
- congenital anomaly
- required intervention to prevent permanent impairment or damage

Report even if:
- you're not certain the product caused the event
- you don't have all the details

Report product problems – quality, performance or safety concerns such as:
- suspected contamination
- questionable stability
- defective components
- poor packaging or labeling
- therapeutic failures

How to report:
- just fill in the sections that apply to your report
- use section C for all products except medical devices
- attach additional blank pages if needed
- use a separate form for each patient
- report either to FDA or the manufacturer (or both)

Important numbers:
- 1-800-FDA-0178   to FAX report
- 1-800-FDA-7737   to report by modem
- 1-800-FDA-1088   to report by phone or for more information
- 1-800-822-7967   for a VAERS form for vaccines

If your report involves a serious adverse event with a device and it occurred in a facility outside a doctor's office, that facility may be legally required to report to FDA and/or the manufacturer. Please notify the person in that facility who would handle such reporting.

Confidentiality: The patient's identity is held in strict confidence by FDA and protected to the fullest extent of the law. The reporter's identity, including the identity of a self-reporter, may be shared with the manufacturer unless requested otherwise. However, FDA will not disclose the reporter's identity in response to a request from the public, pursuant to the Freedom of Information Act.

The public reporting burden for this collection of information has been estimated to average 30 minutes per response, including the time for reviewing instructions, searching existing data sources, gathering and maintaining the data needed, and completing and reviewing the collection of information. Send your comments regarding this burden estimate or any other aspect of this collection of information, including suggestions for reducing this burden to:

Reports Clearance Officer, PHS
Hubert H. Humphrey Building,
Room 721-B
200 Independence Avenue, S.W.
Washington, DC 20201
ATTN: PRA

and to:
Office of Management and
Budget
Paperwork Reduction Project
(0910-0291)
Washington, DC 20503

Please do NOT return this form to either of these addresses.

U.S. DEPARTMENT OF HEALTH AND HUMAN SERVICES
Public Health Service • Food and Drug Administration

FDA Form 3500-back   **Please Use Address Provided Below – Just Fold In Thirds, Tape and Mail**

Department of
Health and Human Services
Public Health Service
Food and Drug Administration
Rockville, MD 20857

Official Business
Penalty for Private Use $300

NO POSTAGE
NECESSARY
IF MAILED
IN THE
UNITED STATES
OR APO/FPO

BUSINESS REPLY MAIL
FIRST CLASS MAIL PERMIT NO. 946 ROCKVILLE, MD

POSTAGE WILL BE PAID BY FOOD AND DRUG ADMINISTRATION

MEDWATCH
The FDA Medical Products Reporting Program
Food and Drug Administration
5600 Fishers Lane
Rockville, MD 20852-9787

report ADRs. To encourage reporting of adverse events, FDA regulations offer substantial protection against disclosure of the identities of both reporters and patients. This was further strengthened in 1995, when a new regulation extended this protection to voluntary reports held by pharmaceutical, biologic, and medical device manufacturers.[20] It preempts any state or local law, rule, regulation, or other requirement that requires or permits disclosure/discovery of such identities as might be applied in a lawsuit alleging malpractice or a product liability case. This action, unusual for a government agency, is evidence of the importance that the FDA places on its ability to collect information about safety concerns regarding FDA-regulated products, information that is vital to protect the public health. To facilitate obtaining follow-up information on the MedWatch form, health professionals reporting directly to the FDA are asked to indicate whether they prefer that their identity not be disclosed to the manu-

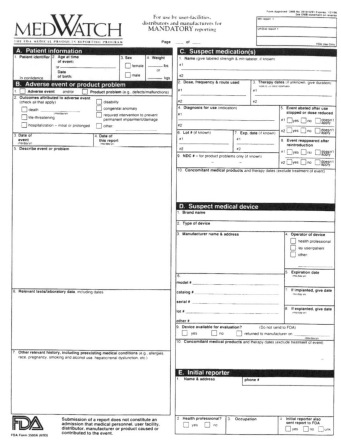

FDA = Food and Drug Administration.

facturer of the product involved in the case being reported. When such a preference is indicated, under no circumstances will that information be shared. Reporters should be aware that it is not necessary to include the specific name of the patient on the reporting form. Patient-identifying codes, known only to the reporting facility, are of value should it be determined that follow-up is necessary.

An Overview of the Spontaneous Reporting System

The trend in the number of ADR reports received by the SRS since 1985 is shown in Figure 3. By the end of 1996, there were more than 1 million reports in the system. Reporting increased dramatically throughout the

Medication and Device Experience Report
(continued)
Refer to guidelines for specific instructions

Submission of a report does not constitute an admission that medical personnel, user facility, distributor, manufacturer or product caused or contributed to the event.

U.S. DEPARTMENT OF HEALTH AND HUMAN SERVICES
Public Health Service • Food and Drug Administration

Figure 2
(continued)

Page ____ of ____   FDA Use Only

F. For use by user facility/distributor–devices only

1. Check one
   [ ] user facility   [ ] distributor
2. UF/Dist report number

3. User facility or distributor name/address

4. Contact person

5. Phone Number

6. Date user facility or distributor became aware of event (mo/day/yr)

7. Type of report
   [ ] initial
   [ ] follow-up #____

8. Date of this report (mo/day/yr)

9. Approximate age of device

10. Event problem codes (refer to coding manual)
    patient code [__]-[__]
    device code [__]-[__]

11. Report sent to FDA?
    [ ] yes (mo/day/yr)
    [ ] no

12. Location where event occurred
    [ ] hospital   [ ] outpatient diagnostic facility
    [ ] home   [ ] ambulatory surgical facility
    [ ] nursing home
    [ ] outpatient treatment facility
    [ ] other: specify

13. Report sent to manufacturer?
    [ ] yes (mo/day/yr)
    [ ] no

14. Manufacturer name/address

H. Device manufacturers only

1. Type of reportable event
   [ ] death
   [ ] serious injury
   [ ] malfunction (see guidelines)
   [ ] other:

2. If follow-up, what type?
   [ ] correction
   [ ] additional information
   [ ] response to FDA request
   [ ] device evaluation

3. Device evaluated by mfr?
   [ ] not returned to mfr.
   [ ] yes   [ ] evaluation summary attached
   [ ] no (attach page to explain why not) or provide code:

4. Device manufacture date (mo/yr)

5. Labeled for single use?
   [ ] yes   [ ] no

6. Evaluation codes (refer to coding manual)
   method [__]-[__]-[__]
   results [__]-[__]-[__]
   conclusions [__]-[__]-[__]

7. If remedial action initiated, check type
   [ ] recall   [ ] notification
   [ ] repair   [ ] inspection
   [ ] replace   [ ] patient monitoring
   [ ] relabeling   [ ] modification/adjustment
   [ ] other:

8. Usage of device
   [ ] initial use of device
   [ ] reuse
   [ ] unknown

9. If action reported to FDA under 21 USC 360(f), list correction/removal reporting number:

10. [ ] Additional manufacturer narrative   and/or   11. [ ] Corrected data

G. All manufacturers

1. Contact office – name/address (& mfring site for devices)

2. Phone number

3. Report source (check all that apply)
   [ ] foreign
   [ ] study
   [ ] literature
   [ ] consumer
   [ ] health professional
   [ ] user facility
   [ ] company representative
   [ ] distributor
   [ ] other:

4. Date received by manufacturer (mo/day/yr)

5. (A)NDA # ____
   IND # ____
   PLA # ____
   pre-1938 [ ] yes
   OTC product [ ] yes

6. If IND, protocol #

7. Type of report (check all that apply)
   [ ] 5-day   [ ] 15-day
   [ ] 10-day   [ ] periodic
   [ ] initial   [ ] follow-up #____

8. Adverse event term(s)

9. Mfr. report number

The public reporting burden for this collection of information has been estimated to average one hour per response, including the time for reviewing instructions, searching existing data sources, gathering and maintaining the data needed, and completing and reviewing the collection of information. Send your comments regarding this burden estimate or any other aspect of this collection of information, including suggestions for reducing this burden to:

Reports Clearance Officer, PHS, Hubert H. Humphrey Building, Room 721-B 200 Independence Avenue, S.W. Washington, DC 20201 ATTN: PRA

and to: Office of Management and Budget Paperwork Reduction Project (0910-0291) Washington, DC 20503

Please do NOT return this form to either of these addresses.

FDA Form 3500A - back

1990s. For example, there were nearly 170 000 reports received in 1996, which was a 17% increase over those in 1995. Approximately 90% were reported through manufacturers, and the remaining 10% came directly to the FDA. Of the approximately 15 000 ADR reports received by the FDA directly from health professionals and consumers in 1996, 46% (n = 7029) were from pharmacists, 19% (n = 2897) from physicians, and 20% (n = 2966) from hospitals without the reporting professional identified. The remainder were from a variety of sources, including consumers, law firms, and sources not specifically identified.

Table 5[21] lists the SRS's reporting frequency distribution of serious ADRs by therapeutic category of the suspect drug. Central nervous system agents were the most frequently reported drug category for serious ADRs. Hormones (and synthetic substitutes) were second and cardiovascular drugs third. These data are interesting but, unfortunately, do not necessarily reflect the frequency of the occurrence of adverse events in patients exposed to products in these classes. They also do not necessarily have any relationship to the relative levels of drug use.

Drug and biologic adverse event reports are entered into the SRS housed within the FDA's Center for Drug Evaluation and Research. Prior to entry into the system, the description of the event itself is coded according to standardized terminology.[22] This allows for future search and more efficient retrieval. The actual report form and all attachments are optically imaged for future retrieval.

After the data are entered into the SRS, every direct report (n = 14 984 in 1996) and all 15-day manufacturers' reports (n = 25 572 in 1996) are given an individual hands-on review by a PMS evaluator who is a health professional. These safety evaluators identify previously unrecognized serious drug/adverse event associations. They monitor new molecular entities more intensively, but continue to follow a drug over its entire marketing lifetime. The nature of the reported events and how well documented the cases are, as well as the previously known safety profile of the drug, are all taken into account in the ascertainment of the report's importance. Strong associations trigger further investigation that eventually may result in regulatory action.

When evaluating a reported event, the safety evaluator looks for documentation of the patient's condition before drug therapy was initiated. Knowledge of the steps taken in diagnosis confirmation is sought in all cases. For example, in a report of Stevens–Johnson syndrome, the presence of biopsy results or a dermatology consult is important. The more objective the data on which the diagnosis was made, the stronger the case. Therefore,

Figure 3
Adverse Drug
Reaction Reports by
Year and Type (Mfr
= manufacturer).

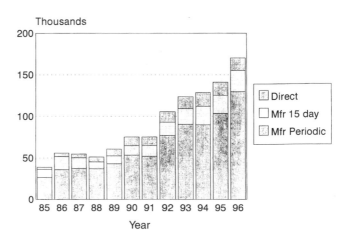

relevant laboratory data describing a patient's condition before, during, and after an event should always be included when available.

One of the most important elements in the evaluation of reports is the clinical pharmacology profile of the drug and how it might interface with the temporal relationship of an adverse event with the use of the drug. Therefore, the reports that are most helpful in evaluations are those that include dose and formulation of the drug administered, therapy dates, or duration of therapy if the exact dates are unknown, as well as information on whether the event abated after the drug was stopped and whether it reappeared when the drug was reintroduced (dechallenge/rechallenge). Rechallenge information is always extremely useful. The value of dechallenge information is less useful in cases in which an event is irreversible (e.g., deafness) or when an event would likely abate on its own (e.g., stroke).

Throughout this process, evaluators look for documentation of plausible alternative explanations for any given event. Such documentation may include concomitant drug and medical device therapy, laboratory data, or other relevant history. For example, in a report of hepatitis, ruling out viral causes is important. In a congenital anomaly case, it is important to know the maternal exposure to both the drug being reported and known teratogens, such as alcohol.

	No.	%
All suspect drug mentions	153 842	100
Central nervous system agents	42 254	28
Hormones and synthetic substitutes	21 173	14
Cardiovascular drugs	15 711	10
Antiinfective agents	14 117	9
Antineoplastic agents	10 191	7
Skin and mucous membrane agents	9115	6
Autonomic drugs	6658	4
Gastrointestinal drugs	5589	4
Unclassified	5436	4
Blood formation and coagulation	3812	2

Table 5
Postmarket ADRs Reported to the FDA by the Top-10-Ranked Classes of Suspect Drugs[21,a,b]

ADRs = adverse drug reactions; FDA = Food and Drug Administration.
[a]The drug classification used was the American Hospital Formulary Service Pharmacologic-Therapeutic Classification (American Society of Health-System Pharmacists, Bethesda, MD, 1996).
[b]Represents the top-10-ranked drug classes associated with the 153 842 suspect drugs computerized from the 130 950 postmarket ADR cases.

Once a serious unlabeled or otherwise important report has been identified, the safety evaluator searches for similar cases in the SRS and in the literature. When there is enough compelling information, the cases are documented and shared with other safety evaluators, medical officers, and epidemiologists for further discussion and determination of whether the event constitutes a safety concern. Sometimes such reviews are sufficient evidence in and of themselves for the FDA to take regulatory action. For example, if reports of death in an unstudied population for an unapproved indication are received within a short time after a new product is marketed, it could be that the product label may not be sufficiently strong to discourage the unapproved use, or it could be that the manufacturer's promotional practices need to be scrutinized. Investigation into such situations is relatively simple, and action can usually be taken quickly. More often, however, reports act as signals of the need for further clinical or epidemiologic investigation.

Signal Follow-up and Risk Assessment

Since the SRS-generated signals are predicated on unexpected events, each investigation requires creativity and analytical techniques to fit the situation. General principles of pharmacoepidemiology used to conduct such investigations are outlined in greater detail in Chapter 19. Common elements typically include the number of reports and how they may or may not reflect the incidence of the event in question, the clinical pharmacology of the drug, previous data from clinical studies, information regarding the population at risk (including the baseline or underlying risk for an event), the extent and distribution of drug use, and how all of these elements do or do not allow for a reasonable estimation of risk. These are not simple data to ascertain or interpret, as confounding and biases cloud risk assessment. Even though interpretation of spontaneous report data represents a gray zone of pharmacoepidemiology, it provides a foundation for risk assessment that contributes to more responsible decision-making and resource allocation in the pursuit of more definitive answers.

The proportion of cases that are reported to the FDA is unknown. Underreporting and variable reporting rates comprise some of the biggest challenges faced in signal follow-up. Many factors determine whether reports reach the FDA. Before an event is reported, it must be observed. It must be considered by a health practitioner that a drug may have had a role in the event's occurrence. That practitioner must actively decide that such may be the case and then consider that perhaps a report to some party is warranted. Such a report must then be generated and actually submitted, which depends on obvious elements of time, incentive, and memory. These and innumerable other factors influence the likelihood of reporting.

The negative influences or disincentives for adverse event reporting include those that have been referred to by Inman[23] as the "seven deadly sins." These are complacency, fear of involvement in litigation, guilt because of perceived harm to a patient caused by the treatment a physician has prescribed, ignorance of how or to whom to report, ambition to collect and publish a personal series of cases, diffidence about reporting mere suspicions that might lead to ridicule, and lethargy—an amalgam of procrastination and lack of interest or time. The most commonly cited positive influences for ADR reporting are those relating to a practitioner's desire to share information that will serve to promote the public health.

For a particular drug, reporting rates (i.e., the likelihood of reporting) are likely to vary over time even if the actual incidence of events with that drug does not. The length of time a drug has been on the market affects its reporting rates; newly marketed products tend to have much more frequent reports of events than older drugs. Publicity about a given drug or adverse event predictably leads to an increase in the reporting of that and similar events. The drug's indication may play a role in the decision to report, as may the population for which it is indicated (or contraindicated). Indications that involve seriously ill patients who are likely to be taking multiple other medications may actually decrease the likelihood of reporting because of inherent confounding within a given case. Marketing and promotion efforts also influence reporting rates. For instance, some manufacturer sales representatives take an active interest in learning about adverse events. These factors play into the evaluation of reports about a given product and complicate any comparisons that one might consider making among similar products.

Other challenges involved in interpreting spontaneous reporting data include the estimation of the population exposed. In most cases, pharmaceutical marketing data are used to estimate the extent of exposure to the drug and, thereby, the importance of the potential public health implications. However, an estimate of risk requires more data than the SRS can provide, even when combined with exposure data.

Risk estimation requires data in all four cells of a 2×2 table, such as is presented in Table 6. For any particular adverse event, accumulated SRS-reported events represent only a fraction of these events that belong in cell a (i.e., those events that occurred in the population treated with the drug of interest). No information from spontaneous reports is available about similar events that may have occurred in nontreated individuals (cell c), about treated patients with no adverse events (cell a), or about the rest of the population who were untreated with no similar events. Clearly then, the incidence rate of an event in the treated or untreated portion of the population and the resultant calculation of the risk associated with exposure cannot be determined by spontaneous reporting. Studies must be designed to measure or estimate risk. The hypotheses and designs of these studies, however, are based on the details received from spontaneous reports. For this reason, again, completeness in reporting is vital for prompt signal follow-up.

Development of a case definition that might be used in collecting information from other data sources beyond the SRS is often based on clinical details that at first seem irrelevant or unrelated to the initial ADR event. Having complete information about the patient and event involved in each case can facilitate ascertainment of the strength of any given drug and event pairing. There are numerous historical examples of a single, very complete report that led to the identification of a significant safety risk associated with a medical product. These cases were often reported after several incomplete reports of what, in retrospect, were nearly identical events but were not identified as such because of the poor quality of the data submitted. Thus, higher-quality data could result in identifying a safety risk even sooner. One such example is Omniflox (temafloxacin), which was associated with a syndrome of hematologic and renal abnormalities that was not identified until all the Omniflox case reports were analyzed collectively.[24] On follow-up, it was discovered that many of the reported cases had indeed experienced the syndrome. (For greater detail of this event and other relevant cases, see Chapter 17, example 9).

All details regarding the temporal sequence of events, delay of onset, dechallenge, rechallenge, any contributing factors, laboratory tests, and elimination of alternative causes are important in the search for population-based patient data that may be accessed to define the risk of the association. Observational studies may be initiated that use data derived from health maintenance organization, Medicaid, or other existing databases. The risk in question often requires an experimental study design that may exist as a sponsor-initiated postmarketing study or may be mounted on an ad hoc basis.

Table 6

	Measurement of Risk		
	No Adverse Event	Event	
Treated	a	b	$a + b$
Nontreated	c	d	$c + d$

Incidence in the exposed $(I_e) = a/(a + b)$

Incidence in the unexposed $(I_u) = c/(c + d)$

Relative risk $= I_e/I_u$

Attributable risk $= I_e - I_u$

Regulatory Actions

After the analysis of all available data and often after consultation with one of the FDA's professional advisory committees, the FDA determines whether regulatory action is necessary. Options available for regulatory actions include the following: (1) changing the product labeling, (2) sending a "Dear Health Professional" letter, (3) restricting the use of the drug product, or (4) withdrawing the drug from the US market. The most common postmarketing regulatory action is a voluntary labeling change by the manufacturer. Two examples of labeling changes prompted by spontaneous reporting are hepatotoxicity associated with flutamide (Eulexin)[25] and pseudotumor cerebri associated with growth hormone (Protropin, Humatrope).[26] If an adverse event is particularly serious, a "boxed" warning may be added to the official labeling. In 1993, a boxed warning of associated hepatotoxicity was placed in the labeling for the injectable benzodiazepine midazolam (Versed).

To notify health professionals of important safety issues that are discovered after marketing, the FDA often requests that the manufacturer send a Dear Health Professional letter or institute an intervention program to warn providers of particular safety issues. This is usually done in combination with a labeling change. In 1988, Roche sent out a national Dear Health Professional mailing followed by an unusually intensive educational campaign to prevent isotretinoin (Accutane) use during pregnancy. In 1993, Burroughs Wellcome sent a letter to physicians regarding lactic acidosis and severe hepatomegaly with steatosis in zidovudine (Retrovir) users.[27] Also in 1993, Marion Merrell Dow sent a letter to healthcare professionals regarding the significant interaction between terfenadine (Seldane) and both macrolide antibiotics and "azole" class antifungals.[28] The FDA also may send out public health advisories, as was done in July 1997, when a letter was sent to healthcare professionals informing them of reports of valvular heart disease in patients receiving concomitant fenfluramine and phenteramine.

The FDA can restrict or ban the use of a product if the adverse reaction associated with a drug product has severe consequences. For instance, fetal abnormalities associated with the use of Accutane, a drug to treat acne, banned its use in women of childbearing age. If serious safety questions remain unanswered, the manufacturer may be asked by the FDA to perform the additional studies needed (often termed Phase IV studies) or to continue Phase III trials beyond their planned stopping date, particularly when a study spans the periapproval time period. Such studies may result in the most severe regulatory action: a request that the manufacturer withdraw a product from the market. For example, results showed that patients taking flosequinan (Manoplax) initially had improved symptoms of congestive heart failure. However, after approval in December 1992, it was found that the treated patients ultimately had both an increased risk of death as well as an increased hospitalization rate.[29] This information led to the withdrawal of the drug from the market in July 1993, 7 months after product launch.

Limitations of Spontaneous Reporting

It is important to understand the use of the SRS as a signaling system. Because it is a compilation of individually observed events that are based solely on the suspicions of the reporting health professional, the signals generated cannot usually imply causality. Neither can the numbers of reported cases be manipulated to create any more than a gross estimate of incidence rates of drug-induced disease that is heavily dependent on estimates of reporting rates for a given event and a given drug. Causality can sometimes be established on the basis of case reports alone, but specific quantification of risk almost always requires formal studies in defined populations.

Estimates of underreporting for one drug-related event do not apply to another drug or even to another event with the same drug. As previously described, reporting varies from drug to drug, depending on the therapeutic class, the patient population exposed, the location of drug use (i.e., hospital or ambulatory care), the time passed since product launch, the publicity surrounding the drug's use, and the manufacturer of the product.

Besides not knowing what proportion of the total number of cases is reported, neither is it known whether the reported cases are representative of all cases. It is possible that health professionals decide to report only the most severe, the most obvious, or the most unacceptable cases (e.g., those occurring in children). Even though the SRS is incapable of detecting the true incidence or the frequency of an adverse event, the signals generated may lead to the design of more directed epidemiologic studies that will provide this information.

Advantages of Spontaneous Reporting

Despite its shortcomings, the SRS is a valuable tool for initiating suspicion and generation of early signals that may warn of unknown safety problems with drugs. It casts a broad net and, thus, has the ability to detect even the rarest adverse event, even though the event is overlooked by other detection mechanisms. The SRS is comprehensive because it covers all drugs marketed in the US. It is relatively inexpensive and does not require the time necessary to assemble an analytical study; therefore, adverse events can be detected more quickly than with other types of surveillance.

There are no limits to patient, provider, drug, or adverse event characteristics that may be detected by the SRS; this is an advantage that cannot be claimed by any other drug safety surveillance mechanism.

Future Directions

In recent years, there has been a significant international effort to standardize pharmaceutical regulatory efforts worldwide. In October 1997, the SRS was replaced by a new computerized science- and analysis-based system that uses powerful software tools and complies with international standards for reporting adverse events.[30] This new system is called the Adverse Event Reporting System (AERS). One purpose of these efforts is to eliminate unnecessary delay in the global development and availability of new drugs while maintaining adequate public health safeguards. The AERS is an automated system that provides for the full life cycle of PMS activities such as information capture, analysis, and dissemination. The AERS features electronic submission of reports, international technical compatibility, international terminology, and automated software tools to assist reviewers in identifying and analyzing safety signals. It provides a more effective tool for both national and international pharmacovigilance.

However, the data that make up the system will still start at the bedside with an astute healthcare practitioner first identifying a potential drug reaction and reporting it to the manufacturer or the FDA. Sound clinical judgment will always remain an integral part of national PMS at the FDA, with AERS facilitating the efficiency of the safety evaluation process.

References

1. Faich GA. Postmarketing surveillance of prescription drugs: current status. Washington, DC: Center for Drugs and Biologics, US Food and Drug Administration, 1986.
2. Davies DM, ed. Textbook of adverse drug reactions. Oxford: Oxford University Press, 1985.
3. Erslev AJ, Wintrobe MM. Detection and prevention of drug-induced blood dyscrasias. JAMA 1962;181:114-9.
4. Schardein JL, ed. Chemically induced birth defects. New York: Marcel Dekker, 1985: 215-59.
5. WHO International Drug Monitoring Program. Uppsala: WHO Collaborating Centre for International Drug Monitoring, 1996.
6. Records and reports concerning adverse drug experiences on marketed prescription drugs for human use without approved new drug applications. 21 CFR 310.305; 1985.
7. Postmarketing reporting of adverse drug experiences. 21 CFR 314.80; 1985.
8. Sills JM, Faich GA, Milstien JB, Turner WM. Postmarketing reporting of ADRs to FDA: an overview of the 1985 guideline. Drug Inf J 1986;20:151-6.

9. Guideline for postmarketing reporting of adverse drug experiences. Rockville, MD: Center for Drug Evaluation and Research, US Food and Drug Administration, March 1992.

10. Postmarketing reporting of adverse experiences. 21 CFR 600.80; 1994.

11. International Conference on Harmonisation. Guideline on clinical safety data management. Federal Register 1995;60(Mar 1):128.

12. Joint Commission on Accreditation of Healthcare Organizations. 1996 Comprehensive accreditation manual for hospitals. Oakbrook Terrace, IL: Joint Commission on Accreditation of Healthcare Organizations, 1995.

13. Medical device reporting. 21 CFR 803;1996.

14. ASHP guidelines on adverse drug reaction monitoring and reporting. Am J Health-Syst Pharm 1995;52:417-9.

15. Kessler D. Introducing MedWatch. JAMA 1993;269:2765-6.

16. Kennedy DL, Burke LB, McGinnis T. National postmarketing drug surveillance and reporting to the MedWatch program. Pharm Times 1995;August:45-54.

17. Form for reporting serious adverse events and product problems with human drug and biological products and devices; availability. Federal Reg 1993;58(June 3):31596-614.

18. Chen RT, Rastogi SC, Mullen JR, Hayes SW, Cochi SL, Donlon JA, et al. The vaccine adverse event reporting system (VAERS). Vaccine 1994;12:542-50.

19. The National Childhood Vaccine Injury Act of 1986, at section 2125 of the Public Health Service Act as codified at 42 USC 300 aa-25 (suppl 1987).

20. Personnel, medical, and similar files, disclosure of which constitutes a clearly unwarranted invasion of personal privacy. 21 CFR 20.63(f);1995.

21. Knapp DE, Robinson JI, Britt ALO. Annual adverse drug experience report: 1995. Rockville, MD: Center for Drug Evaluation and Research, US Food and Drug Administration, 1995.

22. Coding symbols for thesaurus of adverse reaction terms. 5th ed. Rockville, MD: Office of Epidemiology and Biostatistics, Center for Drug Evaluation and Research, US Food and Drug Administration, 1995.

23. Inman WHW, ed. Monitoring for drug safety. 2nd ed. Lancaster, England: MTP Press, 1986.

24. Blum M, Graham D, McCloskey C. Temafloxacin syndrome. Clin Infect Dis 1994;18:946-50.

25. Wysowski DK, Freiman JP, Tourtelot JB, Horton ML. Fatal and nonfatal hepatotoxicity associated with flutamide. Ann Intern Med 1993;118:860-4.

26. Malozowski S, Tanner LA, Wysowski D, Fleming GA. Growth hormone, insulin-like growth factor I, and benign intracranial hypertension. N Engl J Med 1993;329:665-6.

27. Freiman JP, Helfert KE, Hamrell MR, Stein DS. Hepatomegaly with severe steatosis in HIV-seropositive patients. AIDS 1993;7:379-85.

28. Woosley RL, Chen Y, Freiman JP, Gillis RA. Mechanism of the cardiotoxic actions of terfenadine. JAMA 1993;269:1532-6.

29. Higher mortality risk with 100-mg dose of Manoplex. FDA Med Bull 1993;23:3.

30. Nelson RC, Pedersen D, D'Souza TA. U.S. FDA AERS (Chapter) Project. In: Mitchard M, ed. Electronic communication technologies—a practical guide for healthcare manufacturers. Buffalo Grove, IL: Interpharm Press, Inc., 1997.

10

Analytic Strategies for the Evaluation of Pharmacoepidemiologic Studies

Kate L Lapane

Abstract

The rationale for using observational epidemiologic study designs to further our understanding of the unintended and beneficial effects of drugs is given in this chapter. The basic principles of each of the most common epidemiologic study designs are reviewed, and a discussion of the advantages and limitations of each study design is provided. Sources of bias inherent in observational study designs are reviewed. The role of confounding in pharmacoepidemiologic studies is discussed in detail, and methods of eliminating this source of bias in observational studies are explained. Formulas for unadjusted measures of effect for each study design are given. Analytic strategies used to quantify the effect of the drug exposure on the outcome of interest while controlling for confounding are reviewed. A discussion of issues relevant to sample size determination is provided.

The application of epidemiologic methods to the study of the unintended and beneficial effects of drugs provides information that can impact both regulatory policy and public health. The thoughtful use and careful analysis of these study designs can yield meaningful data when clinical trials (Phase III) cannot. Phase III trials evaluate drug effectiveness under conditions that differ from those of actual clinical practice. Phase III trials, by the practical limitations of the design, are unable to detect infrequent adverse effects of drugs. Also, randomized clinical trials are unable to detect the effects of drugs on diseases that do not manifest for many years (i.e., those with long latency periods). A classic example of this is the effect of exposure to diethylstilbestrol (DES) in utero and the increased risk of development of vaginal adenocarcinoma 15 years after exposure.[1]

In addition to identifying unintended effects of drugs, epidemiologic methods are applied to further our understanding of the beneficial effects of drugs in populations systematically excluded from clinical trials. Often clinical trials include highly selected populations with few comorbid conditions. Consider the complex pharmacotherapy of coronary heart disease (CHD) in the frail elderly, with two-thirds of elderly people taking between 5 and 12 drugs per day.[2] While prescribing practice is ideally a function of published research,[3] these trials have generally excluded the frail elderly with comorbid conditions and women of all ages.[4-6] As women comprise the majority of elderly people in the US, clinical trials have not been conducted in the people most likely to present with CHD. As a result, we have the least information on the patients who are most likely to have the disease. Regardless, information from these trials is extrapolated to the daily care of the elderly. Paradoxically, elderly people receive nearly a third of all drugs prescribed in the US, with cardiovascular drugs among the most commonly prescribed.[2] Physiologic changes associated with aging include alterations in pharmacokinetics and pharmacodynamics.[7-8] Therefore, important information regarding the effectiveness of drugs in real-world applications may be derived from observational epidemiologic studies. Using epidemiologic study designs, large automated cross-linked data sets permit the opportunity to investigate the effects of drugs in populations underrepresented, such as the elderly, in both pre- and postmarketing studies.

For these reasons, applying epidemiologic methods to the study of drugs is logical. Disregarding the bias that may be introduced in the design, methods, and analysis can yield misleading results. To provide the background for the description of epidemiologic study designs and the statistical analysis of each, consideration of the key aspects of the randomized clinical trial paradigm is given. Through the elegance of the experimental study design, many sources of bias inherent in observational study designs are not an issue in clinical trials. Understanding the role of each key aspect (randomization, blinding, placebo) will inform the researcher about bias and aid in decision-making regarding minimizing bias in observational studies.

KEY ASPECTS OF CLINICAL TRIALS

Randomization. Randomization in clinical trials refers to the selection of exposure. In experimental studies, the investigator allocates study participants to the exposure group that in drug studies is usually the drug or placebo. In observational studies, the individual selects which drugs he/she is exposed to. The self-selection of a drug may introduce bias in the study if the characteristics that drove a person to seek out and take a drug are associated with the outcome under study. For example, when information from observational studies regarding the potential benefits of hormone replacement therapy was first reported,[9] it was unclear whether the effect of hormone replacement therapy was "real" or whether the women taking the drug were already healthier than women who chose not to take hormone replacement therapy. This noncausal explanation could have explained the beneficial effects of the drug.

When investigators assign study participants randomly to an exposure, each person has an equal chance of receiving each treatment (i.e., drug, placebo). The chance that the person receives a treatment is independent of the chances that other study participants receive a treatment. Given sufficiently large samples, the essential result of this process is that comparable groups are created with respect to all extraneous variables that may distort the effect of the drug on the outcome. The beauty of this process is that, theoretically, randomization creates comparability with respect to all known and *unknown* extraneous variables.

Blinding. To create comparability with respect to the levels of attrition and the quality of the outcome information obtained, blinding is used. Blinding refers to awareness of the treatment regimen and means that the study participants are unaware of their exposure status. Double-blind studies also imply that the investigators are unaware of the participants' exposure status. This aspect of a trial creates comparability of information quality. Interviewers and study personnel cannot differentially probe for symptoms and/or outcomes if they are unaware of the participants' exposure status. Furthermore, the protocol for study follow-up should be identical, regardless of assignment to treatment group. If study personnel more aggressively followed participants assigned to the drug under study (e.g., more reminder phone calls, better tracking of medical records), researchers could, as a result of the aggressive follow-up, determine that subjects taking the drug under study were more likely to have adverse outcomes relative to the placebo group. This finding would not be due to any physiologic effects of the drug, but of the study protocol itself.

Placebo. Another method that provides comparability with respect to the experience of participating in the study is the use of a placebo. The placebo effect is a phenomenon in which study participants report effectiveness of the drug they are taking, even if it is the placebo and cannot possibly have any physiologic effect. Using a placebo further ensures that the only difference between study participants is the actual exposure under study. The underlying principle in the use of the placebo is to create comparability with respect to the study experience.

Each of these key features of a clinical trial creates comparability with respect to every factor, except the particular exposure under study. These features enable investigators to isolate the drug effects on the outcome of interest. The challenge of designing rigorous observational studies lies in the ability to create comparability between the exposed and unexposed groups without the benefit of randomization, blinding, and placebos. Thoughtful application of the underlying principles of these aspects in the design and analysis of observational studies can prevent or limit sources of bias that threaten the validity of these epidemiologic studies.

Observational Study Designs

The two most common observational epidemiologic study designs are cohort studies and case–control studies. Other epidemiologic study designs including ecologic studies, cross-sectional studies, and case series are valuable in describing the patterns of disease occurrence and in forming the epidemiologic hypothesis regarding exposures and disease. Ecologic studies use aggregate data from populations to correlate exposure to disease. These studies are not commonly used in pharmacoepidemiology. Their usefulness in epidemiology is for hypothesis generation. For example, cross-cultural ecologic studies regarding nutrition and cancer have generated a series of hypotheses regarding the value of low-fat, high-fiber diets and decreased risk of breast cancer. Limited availability of descriptive drug use data based on appropriate denominators restricts the use of this study design for hypothesis generation. Cross-sectional studies provide information regarding the individuals' exposure and disease status at the same time. For etiologic research, the limitations of cross-sectional data are clear. With this study design, establishing the temporal sequence of the exposure and disease relation is nearly impossible. In most cases, it is unclear whether the exposure is antecedent to the disease under study or a consequence of disease. Case series are extremely useful in generating hypotheses regarding drug exposures. For example, clinicians developed hypotheses regarding the effect of DES on the risk of vaginal adenocarcinoma based on a case series of seven young women.[1] The remainder of the chapter focuses on the analysis of the two most common study designs for conducting etiologic research: cohort and case–control study designs.

COHORT DESIGN

Detailed information regarding the cohort study design is provided in Chapter 4. We review features of the cohort study to provide background information for the analysis of these studies. A cohort study may be retrospective or prospective, depending on whether the disease has already occurred at the time of the initiation of the study. The distinguishing feature of the cohort study is that the study participants are sampled on their exposure status. Figure 1 depicts the cohort study design. The goal of the study is to compare the occurrence of disease across categories of exposure. Cohort studies may be less subject to bias than are case–control designs, as the temporal sequence of the exposure–disease relation is clear. In addition to being able to study multiple outcomes of interest, direct estimation of disease rates is possible in cohort studies.[10] Moreover, measurement of the drug exposure is unlikely to be related to the outcome under study. Therefore, any error in the classification of the exposure is likely to be random and, as a result, would dilute the measure of effect. However, prospective cohort studies may be costly, are inefficient for rare outcomes such as unintended drug effects (UDEs), and may be subject to bias due to loss to follow-up. If the study attrition is differential with respect to the drug exposure, the validity of the study may have been compromised.

CASE–CONTROL DESIGN

Chapter 4 provides detailed information regarding the case–control study design. In epidemiologic studies of UDEs, the number of case–control studies far exceeds the number of cohort studies. In case–control studies, investigators select study participants on the basis of their disease sta-

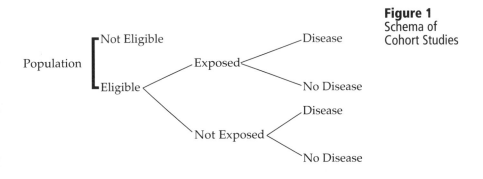

Figure 1
Schema of
Cohort Studies

tus as shown in Figure 2. Once cases and controls are selected, the exposure status is determined. Case-control studies are effficient for the study of rare outcomes and diseases of long duration that are characteristics of studies of UDEs. Furthermore, case–control studies enable the study of multiple drug exposures. Often case–control studies are less expensive than cohort studies. The trade-off for these advantages is the susceptibility of case–control studies to differential bias. Sources of bias particular to case–control studies are discussed below.

The principles in the selection of cases include creating a homogeneous group of newly diagnosed patients whose disease is idiopathic. Critical to the selection of cases is that the diagnosis of the disease is unrelated to the drug under study. For an in-depth discussion of control group selection, the reader is referred to a series of excellent articles on the principles and types of control groups.[11-13] A brief discussion of the thinking behind control group selection is provided here. When evaluating whether a potential control group would be appropriate for the study question, the researcher should ask, *"Would the control have been a case in the study if the person had the disease under study?"* Ensuring that controls and cases have comparability concerning the selection forces that made them eligible for the study and selecting controls that represent the person-time experience with exposure from which the cases came limits biases inherent in case–control studies. The selection of an appropriate control group is critical to limiting bias in case–control studies. Sometimes multiple control groups are used because each control group may limit certain biases, while no one control group reduces all bias. Similar findings within the same study using several control groups may enhance the validity of the study.

Matching may be used in case–control studies to improve the efficiency of the design. However, finding appropriate study participants to match to the cases can be costly as a result of the time involved in finding matching subjects. There are certain situations in which matching may be desirable. For example, matching on siblings may be useful to adjust for genetic and lifestyle similarities. However, given the alternative techniques of handling confounding in the analysis, matching should no longer be used

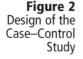

Figure 2
Design of the
Case–Control
Study

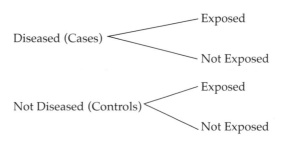

Diseased (Cases) — Exposed / Not Exposed

Not Diseased (Controls) — Exposed / Not Exposed

routinely.[10] By matching on potential confounders, the researcher is actually introducing negative confounding, because selection is based on both the disease and correlates of the exposure.[10] The confounding introduced through matching must be removed analytically, as discussed below.

Sources of Bias

Bias is inherent in observational study designs and can threaten the validity of these studies. However, careful thought in the design and analysis of epidemiologic studies can reduce the role of bias. The impact of bias on the study findings can either dilute or exaggerate the association of interest. There are three main types of bias: information bias, selection bias, and confounding.[10,14] To provide examples of each type of bias, a study of the effects of psychotropic drugs (antidepressants, antianxiety medications) on the risk of developing CHD is examined.[15] Briefly, this is a retrospective cohort study that used information from population-based health surveys cross-linked to hospitalizations and a highly specific CHD morbidity and mortality system. While the data suggested that psychotropic medication use may increase risk of ischemic heart disease, bias may have explained the study results. Examples of each source of bias are provided using this study.

INFORMATION BIAS

Information bias pertains to bias introduced by the manner in which the data are collected. Bias that exists in the measurement of the drug exposure can be differential or nondifferential with respect to the disease under study. Likewise, information bias in the ascertainment of disease may or may not be influenced by the drug exposure. If the error in the classification of disease is uncorrelated to the drug exposure, then the error is nondifferential. This source of bias always attenuates the observed effect.

An example of nondifferential error is provided in the psychotropic drugs and risk of ischemic heart disease study.[15] Information bias in the coding of hospitalizations to the *International Classification of Disease, Ninth Revision, Clinical Modification*[16] (ICD-9), exists because the ICD-9 discharge code assignment may have been influenced by the prospective payment system.[17] The errors in classification were believed to be nondifferential with respect to the exposure, thereby causing a dilution of effect. The authors also used a highly specific standard epidemiologic algorithm as another definition of ischemic cardiac events. The relative risk (RR) describing the effect of antidepressants on the risk of ischemic heart disease was 1.9 (90% CI 1.0 to 3.3) using ICD-9 codes to define the event and 4.0 (90% CI 2.0 to 8.0) using the definition less subject to misclassification.

Information bias, however, is not always nondifferential. In case–control studies, study participants can differentially recall their exposure to the drugs under study. To reduce this source of bias, investigators must create comparability with respect to the data collection methods. The principle in a randomized clinical trial that creates comparability in information gathering is blinding. Regardless of the exposure (or the disease if the study participants are selected on the basis of the disease status, as in a case–control study), information gathering and follow-up must be performed similarly. An example of differential information bias is provided in a study on the relation of male-pattern baldness and acute myocardial infarction.[18] For most of the controls, the ascertainment of the exposure (i.e., baldness) was determined during in-person interviews, whereas most of the cases were released from the hospital before such interviews could be performed. As a result, many of the cases' interviews to determine the extent of baldness were performed over the phone. If men who were interviewed over the phone were more likely to underreport the extent of baldness, this source of information bias could have caused an attenuation of the estimate of the effect of baldness on acute myocardial infarction.

SELECTION BIAS

Selection bias is a type of bias introduced when criteria used to enroll study participants in a study are noncomparable. Case–control studies are more vulnerable to this type of error because study participants are selected on the basis of disease and the exposure has already occurred. When case–control studies of the effect of dexfenfluramine hydrochloride on the risk of primary pulmonary hypertension are performed, selection bias may be an important issue. After the initial reports of the effect of fenfluramine hydrochloride–phentermine hydrochloride on increased risk of primary pulmonary hypertension,[19] knowledge of the possible association is widespread because of the extensive media coverage given to these reports. This may introduce bias in the studies on dexfenfluramine hydrochloride and primary pulmonary hypertension, because women on diet pills may be more likely to see a physician if they are experiencing any symptoms associated with the disease under study, and physicians may be more likely to diagnose primary pulmonary hypertension in patients who exhibit these symptoms while taking dexfenfluramine hydrochloride.

In the study of psychotropic drugs, selection bias could have influenced the study in two ways. First, the data were limited to individuals who sought care for ischemic heart disease, and individuals on prescription medications are more likely to be healthcare system utilizers. While this source of error may have overstated the estimate of effect, a refutation for this argument is that people with diagnostic criteria of ischemic heart disease would have been likely to seek medical attention because of the severity of the symptoms. Second, selection bias could have explained the findings, as people with anxiety attacks often present at emergency departments with symptoms similar to those of a myocardial infarction. However, admission codes did not define the outcome, making this explanation unlikely as well.

CONFOUNDING

Confounding provides the most challenge to epidemiologists performing observational studies. Conceptually, a confounder is a variable that distorts the exposure–disease relationship under study. Confounders are specific to a particular study, because a variable that can cause a mixing of effects in one study may not in another.[20] Confounders can cause the measure of effect to be an overestimate or an underestimate, depending on the direction of the confounding (positive or negative). Three criteria exist for a variable to be a confounder[14]:

1. the variable must be associated with the exposure under study (even among those without the disease);
2. the variable must be associated with the disease under study (even among those not exposed); and
3. the variable must not be in the causal path (i.e., an intermediary variable) of the exposure–disease relationship.

Each of these criteria must be met for the variable to confound the exposure–disease relationship under study.

Thoughtful consideration of potential confounders of the relationship under study must be performed when designing the study. At the design stage, preliminary information regarding which variables may be potential confounders can be determined from (1) reviewing the medical literature about the drug under study and the characteristics of individuals using the drug; (2) reviewing the literature about the disease under study and risk factors for the disease; and (3) reviewing the medical literature of similar studies and identifying potential confounders from previous work. Considering the definition of confounding and reviewing the three sources of information listed above should provide a comprehensive list of potential confounders. It is far better to have collected extraneous information regarding variables that did not confound the relationship under study than wish, after the fact, that information had been collected regarding a potential confounder.

There are several methods to handle confounding in the design and analysis of epidemiologic studies. In experimental studies, randomization creates comparability of the distributions of potential confounders (known and unknown) across the exposure groups. In observational studies, in which randomization is not an option, the investigator can restrict the study sample by introducing eligibility criteria. The variable cannot confound if it does not vary in the study. For example, in a study of the effect of vitamin E and beta-carotene on preventing cancer,[21] neither gender nor cigarette smoking could be confounders because the study included only Finnish men who smoke. Matching and analytic control are two other methods to control for confounding addressed elsewhere in this chapter.

Confounding by indication is a particular challenge to observational pharmacoepidemiologic studies.[22-23] To avoid confounding by indication, one can compare medications within the same class, if the medications within the drug class have the same indication. However, even within drug classes, patients with more severe disease may be channeled to specific agents. Using this approach, a recent cohort study of the effects of beta-agonists and risk of fatal or near-fatal asthma found that bias by confounding by indication may have explained the result that inhaled fenoterol was associated with a higher risk of fatal or near-fatal asthma relative to inhaled salbutamol (albuterol) reported in previous case–control studies.[24] Another suggested method to adjust analytically for confounding by indication when more severe cases are channeled to a particular agent is the use of propensity scores.[25,26] A description of this technique and of the usefulness of this method is discussed elsewhere in this chapter. However, the usefulness of this approach is dependent on available measures that describe the disease severity, which in many analyses may be impractical. An alternative approach, using a case–time–control design, has been proposed to adjust for confounding by indication even when the severity of disease was not measured.[27] This study design permits the adjustment of the severity of disease by using study participants as their own controls within the case–control strategy while adjusting for time trends in drug use.

As many pharmacoepidemiologic studies are derived from large automated cross-linked databases, the availability of data on potential confounders is often lacking. To adjust for confounding, the investigator must have collected the data regarding the potential confounder. It is often impractical to consider collecting information on potential confounders when using data from large automated databases. As a result, investigators are left to argue the hypothesized impact of the potential confounder for which no data exist in the study, based on information in the medical literature. Alternatives to this thought-based method of argument include (1) collecting information regarding potential confounders on a small sample of people in the study and using statistical methods[28] to extrapolate the information to the entire study sample and adjust for confounding analytically, (2) performing "sensitivity analysis" to evaluate the impact of the potential confounder under different scenarios, or (3) using the available data creatively to identify "surrogates" for the confounder. The first alternative is rarely an option because of the protection of individual privacy when using these data sources.

In summary, confounding is a bias in the estimation of the exposure–disease relationship under study and affects the internal validity of the study. It cannot be detected by any statistical test. Confounding is evaluated only by comparing the crude and the adjusted estimates of effect. In the study of the effect of psychotropic drugs on CHD, the most likely source of overestimation was confounding by the indication for the drug. As the authors used existing data to evaluate the hypothesis, there were no direct questions regarding a history of depression or anxiety available. The only variable available for adjustment was a variable indicating whether the medications were being used for a psychiatric condition, which in this case was inadequate.

Crude Analysis

The starting point in the analytic process of pharmacoepidemiologic studies is the estimation of the crude effect of the exposure on the disease. In addition to deriving estimates of effects that have been adjusted analytically for confounding, inferential statistics are needed to evaluate the role of chance as a noncausal explanation of the observed association. In the following sections, the strategies for determining crude estimates of effects and corresponding confidence intervals (CIs) (including formulas) are given.

An overview of the seemingly illogical strategy that underscores *statistical* logic will put the role of statistics in perspective, relative to issues of bias. Hypothesis testing enables researchers to determine the statistical significance of the association under study. To help evaluate the role of chance, or the extent to which sampling variability may explain the study results, we use hypothesis testing. Regardless of statistical significance, what must be of concern is the *clinical relevance* of the association and the magnitude of the association under study.

The hypothesis test begins with a statement of the null hypothesis, which is not even a hypothesis at all but a statement that is contrary to what your true hypothesis is. The null hypothesis would be that there is no association between the exposure and the disease under study, or the RR is equal to 1. This seemingly illogical approach is based on the fact that we can never *prove* anything using statistics. We can only decide, on the basis of the data, to reject or not to reject the null hypothesis. While operationally the specific formulas for hypothesis testing depend on other factors, including the type of data under study and the study design, conceptually, the rhythm of hypothesis testing is similar. First, centering is performed by calculating the absolute difference between the observed and the expected values under the null hypothesis. However, this value is not sufficient to determine whether the difference is "large" enough to warrant rejecting the null hypothesis. Consideration of the underlying variability of the data must be made. The second step, therefore, is to scale the absolute difference by dividing it by the standard error of the effect measure. The standard error is a measure that describes the precision with which we can estimate the true population effect. The standard error depends on the underlying variability of the data in the population and the sample size of the study from which the estimate is derived. This centered and scaled measure is called a standard normal deviate.

Using tables that show the area under the standard normal curve, the result of the hypothesis testing, the investigator can determine the probability or p value. The p value is the probability of obtaining the study result or something more extreme, given that the truth in nature is that there is no association.[29] By convention, researchers claim that, if this probability is small or less than 5% (1 in 20), the result is statistically significant. However, basing the final conclusions of the study on a p value is flawed for several reasons. First, given alone, one cannot tell the direction of the association and the magnitude of it. Also, in the context of a study with an extremely large sample size, the p value is meaningless, because virtually all associations will be statistically significant owing to the small standard error. In the context of a study with more variability due to a relatively small sample size, associations may not yield p values less than 0.05, but they may be providing valuable information that in a larger study would have met the criteria for statistical significance. For these reasons, CIs should be provided instead of a p value.

The CI uses as its base the best estimate of the relation under study, the RR. However, it provides a range of estimates that are also consistent with the data. By examining the 95% CI, one can determine whether the p value was less than 0.05. If the range does not include unity, then the p value must have been less than 0.05, and the association is statistically significant. By definition, if the CI contains 1.0, then the p value is greater than 0.05. The formulas for the RR and corresponding CIs are given in the following sections.

COHORT STUDY

Data from cohort studies can be based on counts (i.e., cumulative incidence) or population-time (i.e., incidence rates). The data layout for a cohort using count data is provided in Table 1. Cumulative incidence is a measure of risk. It is a measure of the proportion of people who become diseased in a specified time period. The range of this measure is from 0 to 1, as the numerator is a subset of the denominator. As the average risk for a population, the cumulative incidence is the probability of developing the disease over a specific time period. Use of cumulative incidence to determine the measure of effect assumes that everyone in the denominator would have survived disease-free to the end of the study period (i.e., no competing risks). To provide an example, data from the study evaluating the risk of ischemic heart disease associated with psychotropic drug use[15] are provided in Table 2.

The following formula estimates the RR in cohort studies and is simply a ratio of the cumulative incidence in the exposed group (numerator) to the cumulative incidence in the unexposed group (denominator):

$$RR = \frac{a/(a+b)}{c/(c+d)} \qquad \text{Eq. 1}$$

So, for the data shown in Table 2, the estimate of effect is computed as:

$$RR = \frac{6/132}{63/5568} = 4.0$$

The RR estimate is interpreted as follows. Antidepressant users were four times more likely to develop ischemic heart disease relative to people who did not use psychotropic drugs.

To compute the 95% CI, follow these four steps:
1. Take the natural logarithm (ln) of the relative risk (ln RR).
   Example: ln RR = 1.39

	Diseased	Not Diseased
Exposed	a	b
Not exposed	c	d

Table 1
Sample 2 × 2 Table for Cohort Study

	Ischemic Heart Disease	Not Diseased
Antidepressant user	6	63
Nonuser	126	5505

Table 2
Relationship Between Antidepressant Use and Ischemic Heart Disease

2. Compute the standard error (SE) of the ln RR:

$$SE_{\ln RR} = \sqrt{\frac{b}{a(a+b)} + \frac{d}{c(c+d)}}$$ Eq. 2

Example:

$$SE_{\ln RR} = \sqrt{\frac{126}{6(132)} + \frac{5505}{63(5568)}}$$

$$= 0.418072$$

3. Determine the lower and upper bounds of the 95% CI on the logarithm scale.
   Lower bound: ln RR $- 1.96SE_{\ln RR}$
   Upper bound: ln RR $+ 1.96SE_{\ln RR}$
   Note: For 90% CIs, the constant used is 1.645 instead of 1.96.
   Example: Lower bound: $1.39 - 1.96(0.418072) = 0.571$
              Upper bound: $1.39 + 1.96(0.418072) = 2.210$
4. Take the antilog to reverse the transformation.
   Example: 4.0 (95% CI 1.8 to 9.1)

In cohort studies, it is often possible to determine the force of morbidity on a population or incidence density. In this time of analysis, the timing of the event is the focus, not just the occurrence of the event. This is calculated as the number of new cases of disease divided by the population-time or person-years (PY) of observation. This measure of disease frequency is a rate and measures the speed of transition from health to disease. Person-time is accumulated until the disease under study occurs, the person withdraws from the study for reasons unrelated to the exposure including loss to follow-up or disenrollment, or the end of the study period. The range of the incidence density rate is from 0 to infinity.

Considering the data in Table 3, the crude RR using population-time (PY) instead of count information is calculated as the ratio of the incidence rate in the exposed group to the incidence rate in the unexposed group (NE):

$$RR = \frac{a/PY_E}{b/PY_{NE}}$$ Eq. 3

Using the data in Table 4 as an example, the RR is calculated as follows:

$$RR = \frac{6/693PY}{63/33\ 995PY} = 4.7$$

	Diseased	Not Diseased
Exposed	a	person-years (PY_E)
Not Exposed	person-years (PY_E) b	person-years (PY_{NE})

Table 3
2 × 2 Format for Incidence Density Data

	Ischemic heart disease	Not Diseased
Antidepressant User	6	693
Nonuser	63	33 995

Table 4
Relationship Between Antidepressant Use and Ischemic Heart Disease (Person-Time Data)

To compute the 95% CI, follow these four steps:
1. Take the ln of the RR.
   Example: ln RR = 1.54156
2. Compute the standard error (SE) of the ln RR:

$$SE_{\ln RR} = \sqrt{1/a + 1/b}$$ **Eq. 4**

   Example: $SE_{\ln RR}$ = 1/6 + 1/63 = 0.427247
3. Determine the lower and upper bounds of the 95% CI on the logarithm scale.
   Lower bound: ln RR – 1.96$SE_{\ln RR}$
   Upper bound: ln RR + 1.96$SE_{\ln RR}$
   Note: For 90% CIs, the constant used is 1.645 instead of 1.96.
   Example:
   Lower bound: 1.54156 – 1.96(0.427247) = 0.70416
   Upper bound: 1.54156 + 1.96(0.427247) = 2.378967
4. Take the antilog to reverse the transformation.
   Example: 4.7 (95% CI 2.0 to 10.8)

CASE–CONTROL STUDY

When using the case–control design (Table 5), one cannot directly estimate the rate of disease because it is fixed through the sampling scheme. Because of this, it is not possible to use the same analytic strategy as cohort studies. Instead, the measure of effect used in case–control studies is the odds ratio (OR), which is approximately equal to the RR when the illness is rare.[30] Whether the OR is a biased estimate depends on the study methods (i.e., control selection, information bias), as described earlier in this chapter. Data from a case–control study to evaluate the association between oral contraceptive use and risk of breast cancer[31] are provided as an example (Table 6).

To quantify the effect of exposure on disease, the following formula is used to estimate the RR:

$$OR = ad/bc \qquad \text{Eq. 5}$$

Example:

$$OR = \frac{118(670)}{269(347)} = 0.85$$

To compute the 95% CI, follow these four steps:
1. Take the ln of the OR (ln OR).
   Example: ln OR = −0.166
2. Compute the SE of the ln OR:

$$SE_{\ln OR} = \sqrt{1/a + 1/b + 1/c + 1/d} \qquad \text{Eq. 6}$$

Example:

$$SE_{\ln OR} = \sqrt{1/118 + 1/269 + 1/347 + 1/670} = 0.128711$$

3. Determine the lower and upper bounds of the 95% CI on the logarithm scale.
   Lower bound: $\ln OR - 1.96 SE_{\ln OR}$

Table 5
2 × 2 Table for Case–Control Studies

	Cases	Controls
Exposed	a	b
Not exposed	c	d

Table 6
2 × 2 Table for a Case–Control Study of the Relationship Between Oral Contraceptive Use and Risk of Breast Cancer

	Cases	Controls Never used oral contraceptives
Used oral contraceptives for ≥5 years	118	269
Never used oral contraceptives	347	670

Upper bound: $\ln OR + 1.96SE_{\ln OR}$
Note: For 90% CIs, the constant used is 1.645 instead of 1.96.
Example:
Lower bound: $-0.166 - 1.96(0.128711) = -0.41835$
Upper bound: $-0.166 + 1.96(0.128711) = 0.086199$

4. Take the antilog of the lower and upper bounds to reverse the transformation.

Example: 0.85 (95% CI 0.7 to 1.1)

MATCHED CASE–CONTROL STUDY

As described earlier in the chapter, matching in a case–control study requires work in both the design and analysis stages. Because negative confounding is introduced by matching in a case–control study, the analytic strategy must be revised to consider the design. Instead of the 2×2 table shown in Table 5, the analysis table should be constructed as shown below. Using the data as shown in Table 7, one computes the matched OR as OR $= b/c$. In multiple regression models used to estimate the effect of exposure on disease, instead of unconditional maximum likelihood estimation, conditional maximum likelihood estimation should be specified to account for the pairing (if 1:1 matching) or other matched sets (if 1:n matching).

Analytic Control of Confounding

Observational pharmacoepidemiologic studies provide particular challenges to overcome, including confounding. Analytic techniques to adjust for confounding include stratified analyses using Mantel–Haenszel methods[32] and multivariable adjustment using statistical models such as logistic regression[33] or survival analysis.[34] Another method that has been used recently in epidemiologic studies[35] is the use of propensity scores.[25,26] Multivariable analysis is often (incorrectly) referred to as multivariate analysis. This is incorrect because a "variate," by definition, is a dependent variable

	Controls	
	Exposed	Not exposed
Cases Exposed	a	b
Not exposed	c	d

Table 7
2×2 Table for Matched Case–Control Studies

or the outcome variable of interest (e.g., disease), whereas a "variable" is an independent variable including confounders and the exposure variable of interest. Therefore, multivariate analyses are actually analyses that simultaneously evaluate multiple diseases or outcomes (e.g., multivariate analysis of variance, Hotellings t-test), whereas multivariable analyses include one outcome variable of interest and multiple independent variables.

The choice of the analytic strategy to handle confounding in pharmacoepidemiologic studies depends on:

- study design
- measure of effect
- number of potential confounders
- sample size
- homogeneity of people receiving the drugs

Regardless of the analytic approach, investigators should have a clear understanding of the potential confounders and the hypothesized effect that they may have on the study estimate prior to performing any of these methods. At each stage in the analysis, the investigator should remain "close" to the data, understanding the impact of each confounder on the exposure–disease relationship under study. Before performing any of these analytic adjustments, the investigator should perform simple analysis to evaluate the distribution of potential confounders by the drug exposure variable. The investigator should never use automated computer-driven algorithms to determine predictive models. Instead, the modeling process should be driven by thoughtful strategy with the purpose of the analysis in mind: to understand the relationship between the exposure and the disease of interest. Given this goal, the investigator does not want to determine the most parsimonious statistical model or the most predictive statistical model; the investigator should attempt to derive the estimate of effect adjusted for confounders. A brief overview of the methods used to achieve this goal and of the reasoning behind the choice of methods is provided in the following.

STRATIFIED ANALYSIS

The purpose of a stratified analysis is twofold. First, the goal is to evaluate and remove confounding by extraneous variables. Second, the purpose is to evaluate and describe effect modification. Effect modification exists when the effect of the exposure on the disease under study is modified, depending on a third variable.[20] If there is no effect modification present, the effect of the exposure on the disease under study is uniform across the strata. Regardless of the study design, the method used to evaluate confounding and effect modification using a stratified analysis is the same. Because the formulas are specific to the study design, each is given. Table 8 shows the organization of the data into homogenous categories by the potential confounder with i levels.

The following steps outline the approach to the stratified analysis.[10]

Step 1: Compute the Crude Estimate of Effect.

$$\begin{array}{cc} \underline{\text{Cohort}} & \underline{\text{Case–Control}} \\ \text{RR} = \dfrac{a/(a+c)}{c/(c+d)} & \text{OR} = ad/bc \end{array}$$

Step 2: Stratify the Data with Respect to the Potential Confounder.

Choose conceptually meaningful categories of the potential confounder. Then, create a separate 2×2 table for each stratum.

Step 3: Compute the Stratum-Specific Estimates of Effect.

Use the formulas given in Step 1 to determine the crude relationship between the exposure and the disease within each stratum.

Step 4: Determine Whether the Effects Are Uniform Across Strata.

In most cases, this is performed by simply "eye-balling" the stratum-specific estimates of effect.[10] Considering prior knowledge of the biologic

Table 8
Organization of Data for Stratified Analysis

i = 1

	Diseased	Not diseased
Exposed	a_1	b_1
Not exposed	c_1	d_1

i = 2

	Diseased	Not diseased
Exposed	a_2	b_2
Not exposed	c_2	d_2

i = *n*

	Diseased	Not diseased
Exposed	a_n	b_n
Not exposed	c_n	d_n

relationship between the variables considered is helpful in determining whether effect modification exists. Effect modification is not specific to a particular study.[20] If the estimates of effect are in opposite directions (and the CIs are not wide), depending on the level of the third variable, effect modification exists. If the estimate of effect is much stronger in one stratum than another, effect modification exists.

Step 5: Calculate the Summary-Deconfounded Estimate of Effect.

Which formula to use depends on not only the study design, but also the determination of effect modification made in Step 4. If the effect of the exposure on disease is uniform across strata, use the formulas provided in A; otherwise, use the formulas in B.

A. If the effect of the exposure on disease is uniform across strata, calculate the Mantel–Haenszel (MH) pooled estimate given by the formulas below. The Mantel–Haenszel pooled estimate pools the data using a weighted average of the stratum-specific estimates.

Cohort

$$RR_{MH} = \frac{\sum a_i(c_i + d_i)/(a_i + b_i + c_i + d_i)}{\sum c_i(a_i + b_i)/(a_i + b_i + c_i + d_i)}$$

Eq. 7

Case–Control

$$OR_{MH} = \frac{\sum a_i d_i/(a_i + b_i + c_i + d_i)}{\sum b_i c_i /(a_i + b_i + c_i + d_i)}$$

Eq. 8

B. If the effects of the exposure on the disease are not uniform across strata, do not use the Mantel–Haenszel formulas given in A. Instead, use the following standardized estimates:

Cohort

$$RR_{Standard} = \frac{\sum a_i}{\sum c_i(a_i + b_i)/(c_i + d_i)}$$

Eq. 9

Case–Control

$$OR_{Standard} = \frac{\sum a_i}{\sum b_i c_i /d_i}$$

Eq. 10

Other options for data presentation when effect modification is present include showing the stratum-specific estimates with corresponding CIs or performing multiple logistic regression.

Step 6: Evaluate Confounding.

The final step in the stratified analysis is to compare the crude estimate of effect as computed in Step 1 with the summary-deconfounded estimate of effect. The summary-deconfounded estimate of effect will either be a Mantel–Haenszel estimate (Equation 7 or 8) or a standardized estimate (Equation 9 or 10). If the crude estimate of effect is similar to the deconfounded estimate of effect, then the extraneous variable did not distort the relation under study. In this case, it is sufficient to report the crude estimate of effect and note that there was no confounding. If the crude estimate of effect differs from the summary-deconfounded estimate of effect, then show the adjusted estimate. How different is different? A rule of thumb is that a variable is a confounder if the adjusted estimate is at least 10% different from the crude estimate. However, several potential confounders may each independently not meet this criterion but together create differences in the adjusted and crude effects. In this case, retain all the variables in the stratification process.

Performing a stratified analysis to control for confounding allows the investigator and the reader to be closer to the data. As a result, a deeper understanding of the relation between the variables under study is attained. However, the usefulness of this approach may be limited by insufficient numbers in all strata. The number of strata required quickly becomes excessive as the number of potential confounders to be considered in the stratified analysis increases. Furthermore, appropriate categorization schemes may be difficult, if not impossible, to determine for variables that are truly continuous. One should always opt for the simplest approach to the data when there are no differences between the adjusted and the crude analyses or no clear advantages to one statistical approach over another.

LOGISTIC REGRESSION

Multiple logistic regression is a statistical technique that is used to derive estimates of effect while simultaneously adjusting for many potential confounders. The rationale for using this method becomes clear when thinking about the number of strata required by the Mantel–Haenszel method to evaluate many confounders with many levels of each variable. While the measure of effect derived from this analytic strategy is an OR, this statistical method is used to analyze both case–control and cohort studies. In the latter studies, the estimate of the OR is interpreted as an RR.[36] The dependent or the outcome variable of interest is a binary variable. The logistic model has the following form:

$$\ln [y/1 - 1] = \beta_0 + \beta_1 X_1 + \beta_2 X_2 + \beta_3 X_3 + \ldots + \beta_n X_n \qquad \textbf{Eq. 11}$$

where $X_1 = 1$ if the individual was exposed to the drug, 0 if otherwise, and $X_2 - X_n$ is the individual's values for the potential confounders.[10]

The estimates of the β coefficients and their corresponding standard errors may be used to calculate the adjusted OR and CIs. In the model described above, $e^{\beta_1} =$ the OR describing the relationship between the drug exposure and disease while holding all other factors in the model constant.

Suggested Analytic Approach

The outlined approach is intended specifically to further the understanding of the relationship between the exposure and the disease. A different modeling approach would be used if the goal were to develop a predictive model.

First, the crude associations between the drug exposure and the outcome of interest should be estimated by using techniques described above. Distributions of potential confounders, exposure variables, and outcome variables must be examined to determine whether any recoding of the data is necessary. Depending on the sample size, potentially confounding variables may be left continuous (if applicable) or recoded to be categorical. Categorical variables with more than two levels should be recoded into dummy variables (with values of 0 or 1); otherwise, a linearity assumption is imposed that may not be appropriate. The number of dummy variables created will be equal to the number of levels of the categorical variable minus one. The choice of the referent group for the categorical variable should be selected first on the basis of conceptually meaningful categories and, if none exists, on the basis of the number of people in each category (with the category with the largest sample serving as the referent group).

Before modeling, one should consider the interrelationship of the independent variables. In pharmacoepidemiologic studies, many of the independent variables may be interrelated. Therefore, the role of multicollinearity with the exposure variable of interest should be considered. Recall that the purpose of the model is to derive a deconfounded estimate of effect. If potential confounders are correlated with each other but not highly correlated with the drug exposure, this may not influence the exposure–disease relationship under study. Regardless, simple correlations between the independent variables should be examined before modeling. If variables are highly correlated (>0.80), consider including only one of the terms in the model or using other statistical methods to account for the collinearity in the model.[37,38]

The logistic model should be developed by using a forward approach (but not using computer-driven algorithms), entering variables sequentially in a conceptually meaningful order (i.e., sociodemographic variables first, clinical variables next) in the presence of the exposure variable of interest. At each step in the modeling process, the parameter estimates should be evaluated and, if the corresponding SEs become inflated, collinearity is present.[39] Each variable should be inserted in the model, and its effect on the variables that characterize the exposure of interest must be evaluated. Regardless of statistical significance, any variable that alters the exposure–

disease relationship under study by more than 10% should be retained in the model. In addition, combinations of variables, each of which may alter the relation slightly, should be evaluated as confounders. The estimate of effect, the OR, can be derived from the final models by exponentiating the beta-coefficients of the exposure variable of interest.

SURVIVAL ANALYSIS USING PROPORTIONAL HAZARDS MODELS

This approach is available for the analysis of longitudinal data collected using a cohort study design. Instead of using "count" data as the outcome of interest, survival models are concerned with the timing of the events. This approach describes the force of morbidity (i.e., the incidence rate) in populations. The model has the following form:

$$\ln [\text{incidence density } (t)] = \beta_0(t) + \beta_1 X_1 + \beta_2 X_2 + \beta_3 X_3 + \ldots + \beta_n X_n \qquad \textbf{Eq. 12}$$

where $\beta_0(t)$ is the baseline incidence rate; $X_1 = 1$ if the individual was exposed to the drug, 0 if otherwise; and $X_2 - X_n$ is the individual's values for the potential confounders.[10]

The measure of effect to be derived from this model is the incidence rate ratio. Conceptually, this method allows the researcher to evaluate differences in the rate of disease onset in different populations while simultaneously adjusting for many potential confounders. While the underlying models can include the exponential, Gompertz, or Weibull models, one can estimate the effect measure by using the Cox partial likelihood method without explicit specification of the probability distribution.[40] Detailed discussion is beyond the scope of this chapter. Other advantages include the ability of Cox regression models to handle censoring, competing risks, and time-varying independent variables. The goal of this discussion is to provide basic understanding of why this approach is used, key features of the strategy, and analytic strategy that may be used to evaluate survival data.

In longitudinal studies, censoring is defined as withdrawal from the study. Reasons for censoring include loss to follow-up and disenrollment (if using health maintenance organization data). Censoring should be non-informative or unrelated to the explanatory variables under study. At the point of censoring, the person no longer contributes to the person-time experience at risk. One can alter the assumptions made by evaluating the study findings, considering that all censored individuals at some point had the event under study. Similarly, one can evaluate the other extreme and consider that none of the censored individuals had the event of interest.

Competing risks are likely to exist in pharmacoepidemiologic studies. An example of competing risk is study participants who may die from other diseases before obtaining the disease of interest. In Cox regression models, the method of handling competing risks is to treat all events as censored except the one of interest to the particular study. While the basic

assumption is that competing risks are noninformative, bias in the estimates derived from models with competing risks can be introduced if this
is not the case. There is no statistical test to evaluate violations of this
assumption, and, unfortunately, in many cases this assumption may be
invalid. Researchers are left to hypothesize the direction and the magnitude of effect that this bias may have had in their study, given the assumptions for handling competing risks are invalid.

Time-varying independent variables enable the model to allow for exposures that may vary over time. This approach may be useful in some epidemiologic studies of drugs. In a study of the effect of beta-blockers after
myocardial infarction on survival, Soumerai et al.[41] treated the exposure
variable, use of beta-blockers, as a time-varying variable within the first 30
days after the acute event to adjust for the real-world experience that medications frequently are adjusted immediately following an acute event.
However, if significant switching of drugs occurs and the switching of
drugs is related to the outcome of interest (i.e., people with more severe
clinical presentation are switched to an agent as a last attempt to prolong
life), this approach may introduce bias that could mask an effect or create
spurious effects.

Suggested Analytic Approach

Before modeling, crude analyses to calculate the incidence density rates
for each outcome by exposure status and the corresponding RR should be
computed. To provide descriptive information, the median survival times
by exposure group should also be computed. Crude survival curves using
methods described by Kaplan and Meier[42] should be plotted. The Kaplan–
Meier method is a nonparametric estimate of survival when all the survival
times may not be known exactly. Comparisons of survival curves for each
exposure group can be made by using the log-rank or Mantel–Haenszel
test.[32,43] This test is appropriate when the hazard ratios are proportionate
over time (i.e., the survival rate in 1 group is consistently higher than the
survival rate in another group, and the ratio is constant over time). Moreover, this method gives equal importance to all deaths within the exposure
groups.

Prior to creating the model, investigators should compare distributions
of potential confounders of people using the drug with those of nonusers
by the use of chi-squared tests or t-tests for categorical and continuous
variables, respectively. The Cox proportional hazards models[40] assume proportional hazards, and an examination of the log–log survival function can
evaluate departures from the proportionality assumption for each model.
Potential confounders should be evaluated by using a forward model-
building (but not computer-algorithm driven) approach. Each variable
should be inserted in the model, and its effect on the variables that charac-

terize the exposure of interest must be evaluated. Regardless of statistical significance, any variable that alters the exposure–disease relationship under study more than 10% should be retained in the model. In addition, combinations of variables, each of which may alter the relationship slightly, should be evaluated as confounders. The goal of this modeling is not to determine the most "parsimonious" model in a statistical sense, but to determine one from which a summary-deconfounded estimate of effect can be derived.[36] Therefore, p values must not be used to evaluate confounding. Estimates of RR and corresponding 95% CIs should be derived from the final models. Graphic displays of the effect of the drug on the rate of disease onset can be obtained by using adjusted Kaplan–Meier curves (product-limit method) for each level of drug exposure using the average value of all potential confounders at baseline.

PROPENSITY SCORES

Another method of dealing with potential confounding is a two-step process that, under certain circumstances, may provide better adjustment than multivariable adjustment procedures.[25,26] An example that demonstrates a scenario in which the use of propensity scores may provide better adjustment is as follows. In an observational retrospective cohort study of people systematically excluded from clinical trials (i.e., frail elderly) to evaluate whether a "new" drug prolongs survival relative to an older drug, the patients who are using the new drug are critically ill and homogeneous with respect to many clinical indices, whereas the people using the existing drug are clinically more stable and represent a heterogeneous group. In this situation, the variances of the potential confounders are unequal across the drug exposure. However, if this is not the case, using propensity scores will provide results similar to those using multivariable adjustment as described previously. Furthermore, this method may be useful if the sample size of the study is limited and if the number of potential confounders is great. In this case, precision is increased by reducing the number of degrees of freedom used in the final model.

This method involves two steps. First, a propensity score is computed that is the conditional probability of assignment to a particular drug, given a set of potential confounders. Operationally, propensity scores are derived from logistic regression models (predicted probability of receiving the drug) that relate the drug choice as the dependent variable to a set of variables that may be related to the selection of drug therapy. Then, the models relating the exposure variable to the outcome of interest include the propensity score as an independent variable, and summary-deconfounded estimates are derived from these models. Again, this method may better control for confounding than adjustment using multivariable analyses when the linear discriminant is not a monotone function of the propensity score and when the variances of the potential confounders are unequal across the type of treatment.

MISSING DATA

Missing data can reduce the total sample available for analysis. Of course, the best way to deal with this problem is to avoid it. When using existing data sources for pharmacoepidemiologic research, this may not be possible. When performing adjustments for confounding using multivariable models, it is essential to be aware of the extent of missing data in the study. Unless methods to deal with missing data are explicitly used, the methods described above are based on the number of study participants with complete information on all the variables considered in the model. In some studies, the sample size for the final analysis (i.e., the analysis from which the final estimate of the drug effect on the disease of interest is derived) can be reduced dramatically by missing data. Therefore, it is essential to report the extent of missing data and the final sample size of the study. There are statistical methods that handle missing data. These include substitution, imputation, and modeling of missing data. As in all analyses, we evaluate the role of missing data by first examining the distributions of all variables that are considered in the analysis. One approach for handling missing data is to create dummy variables to characterize the missing data. This approach does not force any assumptions on the data and allows us to examine the effect of missing data on the outcome of interest. Further discussion of these methods is beyond the scope of this chapter; the reader is referred to the statistical literature for more information regarding this topic.[44-49]

Sample Size Considerations

When designing pharmacoepidemiologic studies, the investigator should consider the sample size of the study to determine whether performing the study is feasible, given the availability of data and resources. Determining the sample size necessary for a study to provide useful information is based on the following factors:

- study design (e.g., case–control, cohort)
- type of effect measure (e.g., RR, OR)
- anticipated size of the effect measure
- analytic strategy (e.g., logistic regression)
- acceptable probability of errors (Type I and Type II) in making the decision

Decisions regarding the *study design* and *type of effect measure* are informed by the issues already discussed in this chapter. Determination of the *anticipated size of the effect measure* may be based on previous research found in the literature, or it is often based on an educated guess. As the sample size is often predetermined as the use of large automated cross-linked databases for pharmacoepidemiologic research becomes common, one can instead determine the minimum effect size detectable, given the "fixed" aspects of the study (i.e., sample size). The *analytic strategy* proposed for the study also determines which sample size formulas should be used to determine the sample size. While methods for calculating sample size based on unadjusted analyses are available for cohort and case–control studies,[50] analyses of pharmacoepidemiologic studies almost always involve analytic adjustment for confounders using methods such as logistic regression. Therefore, determination of sample size must be based on methods that consider the impact of confounding on the study.[51] When calculating a priori the necessary sample size for a study, the *acceptable probabilities associated with the errors* that can be made when making decisions based on statistics must be determined. Figure 3 demonstrates the possible results of decision-making using statistical tests.

A Type I error occurs when the decision, based on the statistical test, is that the exposure is associated with the outcome, and the truth is that no such association exists (i.e., a false alarm). Clearly, the probability of a Type I (α-level) error occurring should be small and is often set to 0.05. A Type II error occurs when the decision, based on the statistical test, is that the exposure is not associated with the outcome of interest when, in fact, there is an association (i.e., missing the boat). The probability of a Type II (β) error is used to calculate the statistical power of the study $(1 - \beta)$. The lack of statistical power may be a valid refutation of studies that fail to show an association between the exposure and the outcome.

The relative severity of making each type of error in the context of a particular pharmacoepidemiologic study must be considered. Consider the following courtroom analogy. A hanging judge, or a judge who, regardless

		"Truth" in Nature	
		Association Between Exposure and Outcome	*No Association Between Exposure and Outcome*
Decision Based on Statistical Test	*Association Between Exposure and Outcome*	Correct decision	Type I error
	No Association Between Exposure and Outcome	Type II error	Correct decision

Figure 3
Results of Statistical Decision-Making

of the evidence, sends all suspects to prison, will be making an abundance of Type I errors. Who benefits from the judge's mistakes? While society will benefit because all the convicts are imprisoned, the innocent people condemned to life in prison do not. Conversely, a lenient judge, who gives all suspects the benefit of the doubt, will continually make Type II errors. The lenient judge will let the guilty person go free. In this scenario, the individual benefits at the expense of society. However, in pharmacoepidemiologic studies, the considerations regarding the relative severity of Type I and Type II errors are not as straightforward. Often the drug under study may have tremendous impact on reducing human suffering from other diseases, and sometimes no other alternative for the drug exists. In a case such as this, the limit set for a Type I error may be extremely small (e.g., 0.01). In general, statisticians begin the process of determining sample sizes with the probability of Type I error (α) equal to 0.05 and the probability of Type II error (β) equal to 0.2.

Depending on these factors, additional information may be needed to determine the sample size, including

- the underlying estimated prevalence of the outcome
- the interrelation of potential confounders to the exposure variable

With both of these, estimates may be derived from the medical literature, from analyses of pilot data, or by an educated guess. Regardless of how the data are estimated, sample sizes and/or the magnitude of effect can be derived for a range of estimates. Often, the most conservative or limiting estimates (i.e., worst-case scenarios) are shown.

For example, during evaluation of whether a sufficient sample size can be derived from a large automated cross-linked database to evaluate a hypothesis, the known quantity is the sample size. For a study on the effectiveness of beta-blocker use in the postmyocardial infarction African-American patient on reducing overall mortality, we first determined the total available sample size (n = 1562). The purpose of performing sample-size calculations in this case was to determine whether sufficient power exists to detect a clinically relevant measure of effect for the study to provide meaningful information. In this case, the study design used was a retrospective cohort study. The measure of effect is an RR that is estimated by using logistic regression to provide a summary-deconfounded estimate simultaneously adjusted for many confounders. Although the measure of effect derived from logistic regression is an OR, analytic adjustment for multiple confounders using logistic regression for cohort studies is common practice. Therefore, the OR derived from the model is interpreted as the RR. Using sample size tables derived by Hsieh,[51] we made assumptions regarding the prevalence of the outcome, the power and α-levels of the study, and the interrelation of the potential confounders to the exposure variable of interest (correlation). Based on a recent study that evaluated the effect of beta-blockers in a population similar in age,[41] we assumed a 2-year mortality rate of 25%. We also set the power of the study to 80% and the probability of a Type I error (α) to 5%. Finally, we performed some preliminary analyses to estimate the multiple correlation coefficient that related the set of potential confounders to the exposure variable of interest. Based on this analysis, the estimated correlation was 0.4. Given these assumptions and using the methodology described by Hsieh,[51] we found the approximate upper bound of the sample size needed to detect an OR of 1.2 to be approximately 1500. Therefore, we had adequate statistical power to perform the study.

Discussion

Increasingly, pharmacoepidemiology is being used to identify unintended and beneficial effects of drugs that cannot be identified in Phase III clinical trials. The field of pharmacoepidemiology is not limited to a specific disease, a specific population, or a specific drug. Furthermore, the questions asked of pharmacoepidemiologists change rapidly as the state of knowledge about drugs increases and the availability of new drugs is continuously changing. An understanding of the basic methods used by pharmacoepidemiologists will enable more comprehensive consideration of the pitfalls and benefits of studies that evaluate UDEs in the medical literature.

The most common study designs used in pharmacoepidemiology are cohort and case–control studies. In the medical literature, the number of case–control studies examining the unintended effects of drugs surpasses the number of cohort studies because of the nature of the study design (i.e., preferable for rare outcomes). The choice of study design is driven by practical considerations including frequency of the event, cost limitations, and purpose of the study (i.e., multiple drug exposures on one type of outcome). However, as pharmacoepidemiologic studies are used to evaluate the beneficial effects of drugs in populations systematically excluded in randomized clinical trials (i.e., the elderly), the number of pharmacoepidemiologic cohort studies in the literature will increase.

The presence of bias in observational studies can alter the study findings dramatically. Careful evaluation of the methods section of articles in the medical literature must be performed to evaluate whether bias has been introduced into the study. Sources of bias include information bias, selection bias, and confounding. Variables that distort the exposure–disease relationship under study are confounders. Potential confounders are associated with the exposure of interest, correlated with the outcome, but not in the causal path of the exposure–disease relationship. Sources of bias in epidemiologic studies can be limited at the design or analysis stage. Methods of reducing or eliminating confounding in pharmacoepidemiologic studies include restriction of the study sample, matching, and analytic strategies. Examples of these sources of bias are provided in this chapter.

While bias threatens the validity of a study, statistical analyses are helpful in determining the precision of a given estimate of effect and in providing mechanisms to adjust analytically for the potentially confounding effects of extraneous variables. However, consider that, in the context of an invalid study from which a grossly distorted estimate of effect is derived, the precision around the estimate of effect derived from statistical methods is almost irrelevant. This chapter provides a discussion of common statistical procedures used to determine both crude estimates of effects given a specific study design and adjusted measures of effect while simultaneously controlling for many potentially confounding variables. This chapter also provides a discussion of the interpretation of these analyses and the thought that drives the decision-making regarding the choice of analytic approach. While an overview of the theoretic assumptions made with each statistical test is given, the reader is referred to the biostatistical literature for more advanced discussions of these techniques.

References

1. Herbst AL, Scully RE. Adenocarcinoma of the vagina in adolescence. A report of 7 cases including 6 clear-cell carcinomas (so-called mesonephromas). Cancer 1970;25: 745-57.
2. Baum C, Kennedy DL, Knapp DE, et al. Drug utilization in the US—1986. Rockville, MD: Food and Drug Administration, Department of Health and Human Services, 1987.
3. Lamas GA, Pfeffer MA, Hamm P, Wertheimer J, Rouleau JL, Braunwald E, for the SAVE Investigators. Do the results of randomized clinical trials of cardiovascular drugs influence medical practice? N Engl J Med 1992;327:241-7.
4. Gurwitz JH, Col NF, Avorn J. The exclusion of the elderly and women from clinical trials in acute myocardial infarction. JAMA 1992;268:1417-22.
5. Mulrow CD, Cornell JA, Herrera CR, Kadri A, Farnett L, Aguilar C. Hypertension in the elderly: implications and generalizability of randomized trials. JAMA 1994;272: 1932-8.
6. Kitler ME. Clinical trials in the elderly. Pivotal points. Clin Geriatr Soc 1993;41:78-84.
7. Hume AL, Owens NJ. Drugs and the elderly. In: Reichel W, ed. Care of the elderly, clinical aspects of aging. 4th ed. Baltimore: Williams & Wilkins, 1995.
8. Kurfees JF, Dotson RL. Drug interactions in the elderly. J Fam Pract 1987;25:477-88.
9. Grady D, Rubin SM, Pettiti DB. Hormone replacement therapy to prevent disease and prolong life in postmenopausal women. Ann Intern Med 1992;117:1016-37.
10. Hennekens CH, Buring JE. Epidemiology in medicine. Boston: Little, Brown, 1987.
11. Wacholder S, McLaughlin JK, Silverman DT, Mandel JS. Selection of controls in case–control studies. I. Principles. Am J Epidemiol 1992;135:1019-28.

12. Wacholder S, Silverman DT, McLaughlin JK, Mandel JS. Selection of controls in case–control studies. II. Types of controls. Am J Epidemiol 1992;135:1029-41.

13. Wacholder S, Silverman DT, McLaughlin JK, Mandel JS. Selection of controls in case–control studies. III. Design options. Am J Epidemiol 1992;135:1042-50.

14. Rothman KJ. Modern epidemiology. Boston: Little, Brown, 1986.

15. Lapane KL, Zierler S, Lasater TM, Barbour MM, Carleton RA, Hume AL. Is the use of psychotropic drugs associated with increased risk of ischemic heart disease? Epidemiology 1995;6:376-81.

16. Department of Health and Human Services. The international classification of diseases, 9th rev., clinical modification: ICD-9-CM. 2nd ed. (DHHS publication no. [PHS] 80-1260) Washington, DC: Government Printing Office, 1980.

17. Assaf AR, Lapane KL, McKenney JL, Carleton RA. Possible influence of the prospective payment system on the assignment of discharge diagnoses for coronary heart disease. N Engl J Med 1993;329:931-5.

18. Lesko SM, Rosenberg L, Shapiro S. A case–control study of baldness in relation to myocardial infarction in men. JAMA 1993;269:998-1003.

19. Abenhaim L, Moride Y, Brenot F, Rich S, Benichou J, Kerz X, et al. Appetite-suppressant drugs and the risk of primary pulmonary hypertension. N Engl J Med 1996;335: 609-16.

20. Rothman K. Causes. Am J Epidemiol 1976;104:587-92.

21. The Alpha-Tocopherol, Beta-Carotene Cancer Prevention Study Group. The effect of vitamin E and beta-carotene on the incidence of lung cancer and other cancers in male smokers. N Engl J Med 1994;330:1029-35.

22. Miettinen OS. The need for randomization in the study of intended effects. Stat Med 1983;2:267-71.

23. Strom BL, Miettinen OS, Melmon KL. Post-marketing studies of drug efficacy: why? Am J Med 1985;78:475-80.

24. Blais L, Ernst P, Suissa S. Confounding by indication and channeling over time: the risks of β_2-agonists. Am J Epidemiol 1996;144:1161-9.

25. Rosenbaum PR, Rubin DB. The central role of the propensity score in observational studies for causal effects. Biometrika 1983;70:41-55.

26. Rosenbaum PR, Rubin DB. Reducing bias in observational studies using subclassification on the propensity score. J Am Stat Assoc 1984;79:516-24.

27. Suissa S. The case–time–control design. Epidemiology 1995;6:248-53.

28. Rosner B, Spiegelman D, Willett WC. Correction of logistic regression relative risk estimates and confidence intervals for measurement error: the case of multiple covariates measured with error. Am J Epidemiol 1990;132:734-45.

29. Ingelfinger JA, Mosteller F, Thibodeau LA, Ware JH. What are p values? In: Ingelfinger JA, ed. Biostatistics in clinical medicine. New York: Macmillan Publishing Co., 1983:160-76.

30. Miettinen O. Estimability and estimation in case–referent studies. Am J Epidemiol 1976;103:226-35.

31. Rosenberg L, Palmer JR, Clarke EA, Shapiro S. A case–control study of the risk of breast cancer in relation to oral contraceptive use. Am J Epidemiol 1992;136:1437-44.

32. Mantel N, Haenszel W. Statistical aspects of the analysis of data from retrospective studies of disease. J Natl Cancer Inst 1959;22:719-48.

33. Hosmer DW, Lemeshow S. Applied logistic regression. New York: John Wiley & Sons, 1989.

34. Elandt-Johnson EC, Johnson NL. Survival models and data analysis. New York: John Wiley & Sons, 1980.

35. Connors AF, Speroff T, Dawson NV, Thomas C, Harrell FE, Wagner D, et al., for the SUPPORT Investigators. The effectiveness of right heart catheterization in the initial care of critically ill patients. JAMA 1996;276:889-97.
36. Kleinbaum DG, Kupper LL, Morgenstern H. Epidemiologic research: principles and quantitative methods. New York: Van Nostrand Reinhold Company, 1982.
37. Diggle PJ, Liang KY, Zeger SL. Analysis of longitudinal data. Oxford: Clarendon Press, 1994.
38. Liang KY, Zeger SL. Longitudinal data analysis using generalized linear models. Biometrika 1986;73:13-22.
39. Pagano M, Gauvreau K. Principles of biostatistics. Belmont, CA: Duxbury Press, 1993.
40. Cox DR. Regression models and life tables. J R Stat Soc (B) 1972;34:187-202.
41. Soumerai SB, McLaughlin TJ, Spiegelman D, Hertzmark E, Thibault G, Goldman L. Adverse outcomes of underuse of β-blockers in elderly survivors of acute myocardial infarction. JAMA 1997;277:115-21.
42. Kaplan EL, Meier P. Nonparametric estimation from incomplete observations. Am Stat Assoc J 1958,53:457-81.
43. Matthews DE, Farewell V. Using and understanding medical statistics. New York: Karger, 1985.
44. Little RJ, Wang Y. Pattern-mixture models for multivariate incomplete data with covariates. Biometrics 1996;52:98-111.
45. Lipsitz SR, Fitzmaurice GM. The score test for independence in R × C contingency tables with missing data. Biometrics 1996;52:751-62.
46. Wu YW. An application of hierarchical linear models to longitudinal studies. Res Nurs Health 1996;19:75-82.
47. Greenland S, Finkle WD. A critical look at methods for handling missing covariates in epidemiologic regression analyses. Am J Epidemiol 1995;142:1255-64.
48. Marshall G, Henderson WG, Moritz TE, Shroyer AL, Grover FL, Hammermeister KE. Statistical methods and strategies for working with large data bases. Med Care 1995;33(suppl):OS35-42.
49. Follmann D, Wu M. An approximate generalized linear model with random effects for informative missing data. Biometrics 1995;51:151-68.
50. Fleiss JL. Statistical methods for rates and proportions. 2nd ed. New York: John Wiley & Sons, 1981.
51. Hsieh FY. Sample size tables for logistic regression. Stat Med 1989;8:795-802.

11

Misclassification in Pharmacoepidemiologic Studies

Abraham G Hartzema
Eleanor M Perfetto

Abstract

This chapter discusses the sources of misclassification of drug exposure (DE) and unintended drug effect (UDE) ascertainment in pharmacoepidemiology. Definitions are provided for the major types of misclassification in cohort and case–control studies. Misclassification can be non-differential or differential and unidirectional or bidirectional. The calculation of sensitivity and specificity is presented as a measure of misclassification. The qualitative and quantitative dimensions of the DE vector are discussed. Drug identification and description, dosage strength, and length of exposure are the major determinants of the DE vector. DE misclassification depends largely on the method used to ascertain the exposure (claims database, completeness of records, survey, interview, recall, prompting technique, and the time span covered). Innovations in dosage, dosage forms, and packaging may also interact with recall. Patient compliance is a major source of misclassification of DE status. Sources of misclassification of UDEs are discussed and related to the study designs used. Precision in diagnostic criteria and error in event ascertainment are major sources of UDE misclassification. Finally, the impact of misclassification of DE and UDE on relative risk and odds ratio estimates is illustrated for cohort and case–control studies with two DE and UDE categories.

Outline

D rug exposure (DE) and unintended drug effect (UDE) misclassification have an important effect on relative risk (RR) estimation in pharmacoepidemiologic studies. Misclassification contributes to a distortion of the relative risk and odds ratio (OR) estimates because of inaccurate ascertainment of DE or UDE. This chapter defines the concept of misclassification in pharmacoepidemiologic studies, outlines potential sources of misclassification, provides a brief overview of the effect size of the misclassification introduced by these sources, and models the effect size of the misclassification introduced by these sources on RR estimators.

Research in drug utilization and outcomes, with emphasis on safety and UDEs, has made extensive use of large computerized data sources.[1,2] These large managerial or billing databases provide the advantage of increased numbers; however, many disadvantages have been described and investigated. The issues that have arisen include patient confidentiality, validity and reliability of the information, cost of data and/or its management, timeliness of retrieval, ability to follow a cohort of patients over time, and differences and difficulties among coding systems.[1]

These databases are predominantly designed for billing purposes. Their sources of information can include the physician's office, the pharmacy, and acute or long-term-care facilities. Because of incontinuities in the care provided, records on a patient's drug use are not always complete. Information may also be gathered directly from the patients by survey or interview and consequently be prone to recall bias. Drugs recorded as being obtained by the patient from a pharmacy may not always be used by that patient, and patient noncompliance with prescription drugs has been estimated to be as high as 90%.[3] Thus, many factors in pharmacoepidemiologic studies utilizing large databases, medical records, pharmacy records, disease registries, death certificates, or specially designed surveys or interviews can introduce misclassification bias.

Previous research on the effect of misclassification in pharmacoepidemiology studies has been conducted by Graham and Smith.[4] These researchers discussed and simulated the impact of misclassification bias on relative risk when both exposure and disease are inappropriately categorized in epidemiologic investigations using a large database. The simulation in their research assumed minimal amounts of exposure misclassification (0.1–1.0%) with varying levels of disease prevalence. The effects of DE misclassification on the risk ratio were found to be large and independent of UDE misclassification. The magnitude of noncompliance as reported in the literature implies that DE misclassification may be higher than the data used in Graham and Smith's simulation and would result in larger effects on estimates of the RR.

This chapter discusses the bias that results from DE and UDE misclassification in pharmacoepidemiologic studies.

Definition of Misclassification in Pharmacoepidemiologic Studies

Misclassification is due to *information bias* and or *ascertainment bias* and has potentially severe consequences. When selection bias occurs, the observed sample is a subset of the target population and external validity is violated. However, when misclassification occurs, a rearrangement of the target population in the 2×2 table results and internal validity is violated.[5] Figure 1 displays the rearrangement due to misclassification.

The individuals truly exposed and truly experiencing the UDE can be misclassified in each of the four cells of the table. The observed classification of a' includes a_{11}, b_{11}, c_{11}, and d_{11}; for b' it includes a_{12}, b_{12}, c_{12}, and d_{12}, and so on, for c' and d'. Only a_{11}, b_{12}, c_{21}, and d_{22} are correctly classified. It can also be concluded from Figure 1 that misclassification can take place for DE, UDE, or both in the same study.

One example of rearrangement due to ascertainment bias is a cohort study that examines the association between estrogen exposure and endometrial cancer. Women receiving estrogen therapy are more likely to have regular medical examinations and, therefore, are more likely to have their cancer diagnosed. Some women who have not taken estrogen are classified as not diseased when actually their disease is undetected. This detection bias results in misclassification: some of the women (b_{22}) in d' belong in cell b.

Another example may be information bias in a case–control study that examines the association between barbiturate use and neural tube defects. Patients diagnosed with neural tube defects (cases) may recall the exposure better than the controls; thus, some of the women (c_{22}) in d' belong in c. The

	Observed **Unintended Drug Effect**	
	Present	Absent
Drug Exposure Exposed	$a' =$ $a_{11} + b_{11}$ $+ c_{11} + d_{11}$	$b' =$ $a_{12} + b_{12}$ $+ c_{12} + d_{12}$
Not Exposed	$c' =$ $a_{21} + b_{21}$ $+ c_{21} + d_{21}$	$d' =$ $a_{22} + b_{22}$ $+ c_{22} + d_{22}$

Drug Exposure Exposed	$a =$ $a_{11} + a_{12}$ $+ a_{21} + a_{22}$	$b =$ $b_{11} + b_{12}$ $+ b_{21} + b_{22}$
Not Exposed	$c =$ $c_{11} + c_{12}$ $+ c_{21} + c_{22}$	$d =$ $d_{11} + d_{12}$ $+ d_{21} + d_{22}$

Figure 1
Rearrangement Due to Misclassification

data source can provide an indication of the expected type of bias and direction. A retrospective, case–control study that uses a claims database may be able to more accurately identify DE (through use of pharmacy claims) than it can UDE due to miscoding. However, a retrospective, case–control study that relies on survey data may have more DE misclassification than UDE misclassification (due to recall bias). Thus, the data source provides clues as to the kinds of biases to anticipate.

TYPES OF MISCLASSIFICATION

A typology of misclassification has been developed. Misclassification bias can be described as differential or nondifferential and as unidirectional or bidirectional.[4,5] This section describes these four types, and Figures 2–5 depict some of the more common arrangements. DE misclassification can be typed as nondifferential when the proportion of error is independent from UDE status (Figure 2). Differential misclassification of exposure occurs when error proportions are different from those with and without the UDE (Figure 3).[5]

Similarly, nondifferential errors in classification of the UDE are the same for those exposed and those not exposed (Figure 4). Nondifferential misclassification can result from a random, systematic, or a mixed measurement error model. Misclassification of the UDE is differential when it

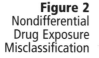

Figure 2
Nondifferential
Drug Exposure
Misclassification

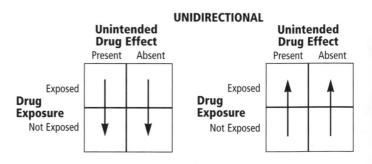

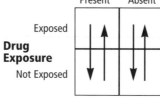

differs among those exposed and those not exposed (Figure 5). Furthermore, misclassification is unidirectional when only one category of a dichotomous DE or UDE variable is affected.[4] It is bidirectional when both categories are affected, equally or unequally (Figure 2).[4]

A 2 × 3 table with three levels of exposure collapsed into two exposure levels can result in nondifferential DE misclassification. Collapsing over categories that have different risks of UDE and different probabilities of UDE classification can induce differential misclassification.[6]

Continuous DE values are often assigned to discrete DE categories in pharmacoepidemiologic data analysis. Such categorization may transform nondifferential misclassification error into differential exposure misclassification.[7] This transformation takes place if the probability of DE misclassification and the probability of UDE vary with true DE within the discrete exposure categories. Homogenous probabilities of UDE within DE categories are unlikely whenever there is a quantitative relationship between DE and UDE (dose–response relationship). The probability of DE misclassification is typically inversely related to the distance from the DE category cut points.

Two approaches taken to address the nondifferential transformation issue are to use quartiles to define DE categories or to examine the impact of misclassification bias by sensitivity analysis. Sensitivity analysis can be performed by adding or subtracting a constant value to or from each category or by multiplying by a constant value and repeating the statistical analysis to examine whether different associations are obtained.[8]

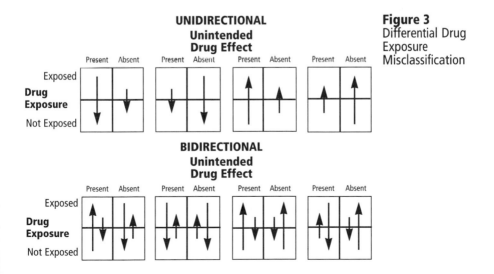

UNIDIRECTIONAL
Unintended
Drug Effect

BIDIRECTIONAL
Unintended
Drug Effect

Figure 3
Differential Drug Exposure Misclassification

SENSITIVITY AND SPECIFICITY

Two parameters are used to establish the probability of correct classification of the cell entries, the sensitivity (Se) and the specificity (Sp). They are commonly used in the evaluation of screening procedures or laboratory tests, and most researchers are familiar with them in that context.

Se and Sp can be calculated for both DE and UDE classification. Se expresses the probability that an individual with the UDE is classified as such, and Sp is defined as the probability that an individual without the UDE will be classified as such.[5] The same definitions can be stated in terms of DE.

Figure 6 shows the calculation of the Se and Sp for both the DE and the UDE. DE and UDE are the correct values; UDE' and DE' are the observed values. Se is calculated as $n_{11}/(n_{11} + n_{21})$; Sp is calculated as $n_{22}/(n_{22} + n_{12})$.

The Se for UDE given exposed is $n_{11}/(n_{11} + n_{21})$ or $400/(400 + 20) = 0.95$. The Sp for UDE given exposed is $n_{22}/(n_{22} + n_{12})$ or $540/(540 + 60) = 0.90$. An Se of 0.95 for UDE given DE implies that a subject who is truly exposed and who has experienced the UDE has a 95% probability of being classified as such. A subject who is truly not exposed and has not experienced the UDE has a 90% probability of being classified as such. The SE for UDE given not exposed is $n_{11}/(n_{11} + n_{21})$, or $19/(19 + 1) = 0.95$. The Sp for UDE given not exposed is $n_{22}/(n_{22} + n_{12})$ or $90/(90 + 10) = 0.90$.

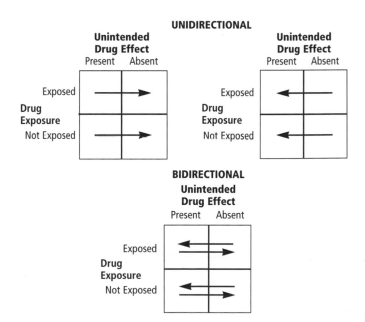

Figure 4
Nondifferential
Unintended Drug
Effect
Misclassification

The Se and Sp estimates can be used to calculate the impact of misclassification on OR and RR estimates. In nondifferential misclassification, the Se and Sp are the same for each DE level or for each level of UDE.[9] The Se (0.95) and Sp (0.90) of UDE, given DE present, must be equal to the Se (0.95) and Sp (0.90) of UDE, given DE not exposed, for misclassification to be considered nondifferential.

In Figure 6, the misclassification of DE is differential; that is, Se UDE present (0.70) does not equal Se UDE absent (0.66), and Sp UDE present (0.69) does not equal Sp UDE absent (0.57). The misclassification for UDE is nondifferential, and Se exposed and Sp exposed are equal to Se not exposed and Sp not exposed, respectively.

True *nondifferential* misclassification of DE exists if true DE Se and Sp are equal; true *differential* misclassification exists if true DE Se and Sp are not equal for cases and controls. A difference has been made between true Se and Sp and apparent Se and Sp. True Se and Sp are obtained from a "gold standard" not prone to misclassification error. Apparent Se and Sp are obtained by another measure that may be the most reliable data available to the researcher, but not necessarily true. For example, DE is obtained for cases and controls by patient interview, a method likely to introduce recall measurement error. Pharmacy records and medical records are pulled for a subsample to examine the validity and reliability of the interview data and to calculate apparent Se and apparent Sp. Knowledge of apparent Se and Sp allows for correcting misclassification in the study population.

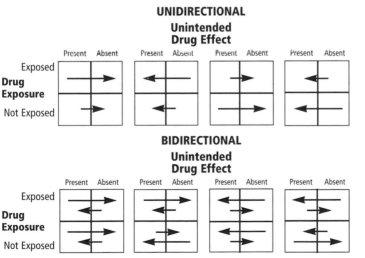

UNIDIRECTIONAL
Unintended Drug Effect

BIDIRECTIONAL
Unintended Drug Effect

Figure 5
Differential Unintended Drug Effect

Another measure is the apparent *relative sensitivity* (relative Se). The apparent relative Se is the ratio of observed case to control DE Se. An apparent relative Se of 1.0 is indicative for nondifferential misclassification, and an apparent relative Se different from 1.0 is usually interpreted as evidence for differential misclassification of DE status.[10] This assumption holds up if the apparent Se and Sp are equal to the true 1.0s.

In the ideal study, true Se and true Sp for both UDE and DE should be 1.0; no misclassification has occurred. The following section addresses the major sources of misclassification.

The Drug Exposure Vector

INFECTIOUS DISEASE VECTOR MODEL

The epidemiologist's earliest endeavors were focused mainly on infectious diseases before other epidemiologic questions came to the foreground. Our knowledge of infectious diseases has increased significantly,

Figure 6 Calculating Sensitivity (Se) and Specificity (Sp)

DRUG EXPOSURE

GIVEN EXPOSED
Unintended Drug Effect

	Present	Absent
Present	400 n_{11}	60 n_{12}
Absent	20 n_{21}	540 n_{22}

Unintended Drug Effect'

Se = 0.95
Sp = 0.90

GIVEN NOT EXPOSED
Unintended Drug Effect

	Present	Absent
Present	19 n_{11}	10 n_{12}
Absent	1 n_{21}	90 n_{22}

Unintended Drug Effect'

Se = 0.95
Sp = 0.90

UNINTENDED DRUG EFFECT

GIVEN UDE PRESENT
Drug Exposure

	Exposed	Not Exposed
Exposed	700 n_{11}	50 n_{12}
Not Exposed	300 n_{21}	90 n_{22}

Drug Exposure'

Se = 0.70
Sp = 0.69

GIVEN UDE ABSENT
Drug Exposure

	Exposed	Not Exposed
Exposed	40 n_{11}	600 n_{12}
Not Exposed	20 n_{21}	800 n_{22}

Drug Exposure'

Se = 0.66
Sp = 0.57

resulting in the initiation of control mechanisms based on epidemiologic knowledge and the introduction of effective new antiinfectives. Later, the focus of the epidemiologist shifted to chronic diseases and, subsequently, it became clear that epidemiology is a powerful tool in making drug therapy safer.

Most infectious or communicable diseases in humans are well described and categorized. Benenson[11] has described and defined the transfer of infectious disease as a causal agent (e.g., bacteria, virus), a reservoir, a mode of transmission, and a resulting disease outcome. Elements identified in describing the vector in the infectious disease model area include the following: identification, occurrence, infectious agent, reservoir, mode of transmission, incubation period, period of communicability, susceptibility, and methods of control.

CHRONIC DISEASE VECTOR

Chronic disease epidemiology is more complex. Most chronic diseases have multiple causal agents and many covariables or modifying variables with interactive effects. In chronic disease etiology, environmental, genetic, lifestyle, and a multitude of other factors play a role. Chronic disease epidemiologists only recently have been able to establish the causes of chronic heart disease and to assess their significance. For most chronic diseases, epidemiologists are still sorting the contributory effects of many of these contributing causes in an effort to quantify them.

Epidemiologists have become more interested in the identification, causes, and distribution of the unintended effects of medications in patient populations. This is distinct from clinical trials, a powerful tool for the evaluation of the efficacy of the intended effects of a drug. Pharmacoepidemiology is different from some other subspecialties in epidemiology (e.g., cancer epidemiology) because it is defined in its exposure, emphasizing the importance of the DE vector. The DE vector is important to pharmacoepidemiology and is discussed in more detail in the following section.

DRUG EXPOSURE VECTOR DEFINED

DE can be modeled as a vector in the transmission of the UDE. The dimension of the DE vector is quite simple: the causal agent is the drug of interest, assuming that a causal association has been established. The methodology to establish a causal association between DE and UDE is discussed in Chapter 5. In Chapter 10, the statistical conditions for such an association are described (Figure 7).

In addition to causality, other dimensions of the DE vector merit attention. These include an accurate definition of the biologic active ingredient, the identification of the characteristics of the exposure, and the description of confounders. Qualifying and quantifying the DE vector are important in cohort and case–control studies to accurately classify DE.

In the most simple approach, a dichotomous exposure level (exposed vs. not exposed) is assumed. In this case, the exposed category is a summary of varying exposure levels. Breaking exposure down into various levels increases statistical power and allows for the testing of a dose–response relationship.[12-16] Defining different levels of DE and UDE, however, may introduce misclassification error, as is discussed later in this chapter. An observed dose–response relationship provides a strong argument for the causal relationship between DE and UDE.

QUALIFYING THE DRUG EXPOSURE VECTOR

The identity of the drug product under scrutiny needs to be defined in the study. The exposing agent is best defined in terms of the biologically active ingredient. Consideration of particular salts and esters can become important. The researcher is faced with the decision of inclusion or exclusion of particular compounds. Although the molecular structure of a drug may be an indicator of its safety profile, the physical and chemical properties of the active ingredient may not always predict its UDE profile. For example, the molecular structures of brompheniramine and zimeldine are similar; however, their patterns of toxicity observed during postmarketing are different.[17]

Many drugs are on the market in different forms and strengths, and the strength of the product may have been changed over time. The daily dose of oral contraceptives has become lower over time, decreasing the strength of exposure, as have the different combinations of estrogen and progesterone. Oral contraceptives also are on the market in many dosage forms, making it difficult to obtain an exact drug identity. Approximately 30 formulations for oral contraceptives have been or are still on the market.[18] In one study, 30% of the women interviewed could not recall the oral contraceptive product by brand name.[19]

Approaches taken in patient interviews to ascertain the product prescribed include the use of a prompting book with photographs of all contraceptives marketed since 1960.[18] An extensive listing of all products (branded, branded generics, and generics), including strengths and dosage

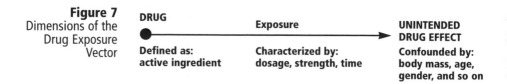

Figure 7
Dimensions of the
Drug Exposure
Vector

DRUG

Exposure

UNINTENDED
DRUG EFFECT

Defined as:
active ingredient

Characterized by:
dosage, strength, time

Confounded by:
body mass, age,
gender, and so on

forms, that contain the active ingredient should be compiled for the study drug. Different coding systems and changes in coding schemes for historical data may be important considerations. The *USAN and the USP Dictionary of Drug Names*[20] contains more than 7700 international nonproprietary names, 3400 brand names, and 3500 investigational drug code designations. The usual or customary strength and recommended daily dose are also important. Properties of the pharmaceutical preparation may alter its UDE profile.[21] In retrospective studies, it may be important to know the time of market introduction for the drug and its different strengths and dosage forms. The latter can verify patient exposure data obtained by survey, interview, or other methods.

Changes in the formularies of health maintenance organizations (HMOs) or Medicaid programs may also be an area of concern. These formularies tend to be modified over time, usually to replace more expensive drugs with less costly ones. Formularies also may limit the covered patient population from exposure to the drug.

QUANTIFYING THE DRUG EXPOSURE VECTOR

The most important dimensions of the DE vector are dosage, strength, and length of exposure (Figure 7). These can become complex issues in measuring the DE vector.

Strength. Different approaches can be taken in assessing the strength of the exposure. Chapter 19 discusses units used to evaluate the strength of the DE. These units can be expressed as prescriptions, dosage, number of dosages, or defined daily doses. If different levels of DE are assessed, it is important to classify the exposure by the most common dosages used. Each level of exposure in the analysis represents a distinct usage pattern. When the dosing of a drug is standard, the length of exposure becomes the major dimension to be considered in the study.

Other approaches may be adapted to assess the strength of the exposure of multiple agents. Such an approach was taken when patients with leukemia were exposed to multiple alkylating agents. To quantify the patient's exposure to these agents, an alkylating agent score was developed on the basis of the total dose/body surface area (mg/m²). A score of 0, 1, 2, or 3 for each agent was given: a 0 for no exposure to the agent and 1, 2, or 3 for the lower, middle, or upper third of the distribution, respectively. These scores are summarized in an alkylator score of the strength of exposure.[22]

Time. Different approaches to quantifying the time dimension are available in the literature. Time can be categorized as length of exposure, time since last use, time since first use, or time in relationship to an event such as pregnancy. In pregnancy, exposure often is related to the trimester in which the exposure has taken place parallel with fetal development. The first trimester, covering early embryogenesis, is most important.[23,24] Also important is the consideration of the timing of the UDE in relationship to the start of DE.[25]

Cumulative Measures. A cumulative measure is achieved by multiplying the time period the subject is exposed, expressed in days, weeks, months, or most commonly years, by the dosing level. For example, 5 years of receiving 250 mg/d is equivalent to 10 years of 125 mg/d. Such a summary measure of DE is the cumulative dose, as used in studies of the association between estrogen replacement therapy and breast cancer. A total milligram-accumulated dose (TMD) can be calculated as the sum of the products of the dose taken in milligrams, the number of days per month it was taken, and the total months of consumption for that dose. Three categories of exposure could be defined: 0 TMD is no exposure, low exposure is less than 1500 TMD, and high exposure is at least 1500 TMD. For instance, 1500 TMD is equivalent to approximately 3 years of daily consumption of 1.25 mg of conjugated estrogens.[26]

Cumulative DE is frequently used as a DE measure in pharmacoepidemiologic studies. However, it is recognized that the imposed symmetry between duration and intensity of exposure is a potential problem. Statistical analysis based on this measure implicitly assumes that duration and dose have equivalent effects on the UDE, the effect of a brief high dose being the same as a long exposure to a low dose. When the UDE is related to an individual's total exposure instead of specific blood concentrations, this approach may be quite reasonable. However, important information may be lost. Understanding the pharmacokinetic and pharmacodynamic properties of the drug assists in the appropriate calculation of exposure level.

A measure frequently used in pharmacoepidemiologic studies is the person-time of exposure or person-time of observation. Person-time for each observation often is used in the calculation of rates for specific outcomes. The duration of time that each individual in the cohort is followed is summed. This value is used as the denominator with the incidence of the event in the numerator, resulting in the incidence density.[5] It is used when the event of interest can occur in one individual more than one time during the period of observation.

This measure also is used when all persons are not followed over the complete time period of the study. This may be due to dropouts, variation in the time periods of individual exposures, or because enrollment has taken place over an extended time period. For example, if 100 individuals were followed for 2 years, 200 person-years of observation would be recorded. This sum also would be obtained if 50 individuals were followed for 1 year and 50 individuals were followed for 3 years: $(50 \times 1) + (50 \times 3)$

= 200 person-years of observation. Cohort studies do not always use person-time of exposure in the denominator of rates of outcomes. They are not used when the observation time period is short or variation is small.

EXPOSURE LAG VALUES OR LAG TIME

Often a lag time or empiric induction period between the DE and the UDE is observed. Such a lag time can even span two generations, such as by mothers exposed to diethylstilbestrol and the increased likelihood of ovarian cancer in their female offspring.[27]

Different approaches can be used in selecting the appropriate lag time. These are a priori defining a lag time based on pharmacologic and toxicologic knowledge, likelihood-based goodness-of-fit statistics, or the highest-estimate criterion. By a highest-estimate criterion, the RR or OR estimates are calculated for different lag times; the lag time with highest-risk estimate is selected in the data analysis. Methodologically, the preference is for defining an a priori lag time based on pharmacologic and toxicologic knowledge or, secondly, through likelihood-based goodness-of-fit statistics.[28]

INTERRUPTION OF EXPOSURE OR ERRATIC DOSING INTERVALS

Certain outcomes may occur because of interrupted or irregular use of a drug; in other words, the hazard function is not constant over time. For example, anaphylactic shock syndrome related to zomepirac sodium may have been precipitated by a patient's irregular use of the drug, producing a hypersensitivity reaction to the product.[29,30] A clear understanding of the use pattern is necessary for the definition of appropriate exposure categories.[30] Only a few pharmacoepidemiologic studies provide an analysis by sequence of drug use or for patterns of drug use.[31] Different statistical methods are proposed to assess the risk of UDE associated with intermittent exposure.[32,33]

Sources for Misclassification of Drug Exposure and Their Relative Magnitude

Many DE data sources are being used in pharmacoepidemiologic studies to classify subjects into those who are exposed or not exposed to a drug. Subjects can be further differentiated according to varying exposure levels. There are four primary sources of DE information. The next section of this chapter presents their inherent contributions to misclassification bias. Figure 8 diagrams the relationship between these sources and exposure misclassification and provides an estimate of the relative magnitude of the misclassification introduced.

PHYSICIANS' OFFICES

Subjects exposed to the drug under study can be identified in the physicians' offices. Such patients often are identified through the use of a double prescription program, in which prescriptions are written by the physician on a prescription pad with carbon copies. The researcher obtains a carbon copy of the prescription. This data collection method is appropriate in prospective case series and cohort studies.

Other approaches to collecting prescribing and disease outcome information are through medical record abstraction or by asking physicians to record information on special forms. This information reflects the mention

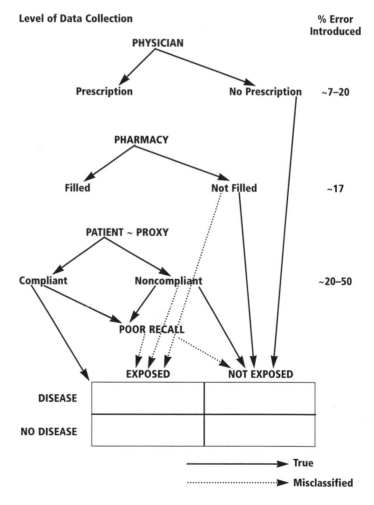

Figure 8
Sources of
Drug Exposure
Misclassification

of drugs or prescriptions written in the physicians' offices. The National Ambulatory Medical Care Survey and the National Disease and Therapeutic Index use this data collection method.[34,35]

Although these appear to be valid ways to identify subjects exposed to a drug, it is obvious that a drug mentioned or a prescription written does not always result in a prescription being filled at the pharmacy. It has been reported that approximately 7% of prescriptions written by physicians are not filled.[36] In a survey conducted for the Pharmacia Upjohn Company,[36] it was found that 19.4% of the patients admitted to not filling at least one prescription given to them by their physician.[37-39] In addition, it does not allow the researcher to establish the diagnosis–drug link to examine for which diagnosis the drug is prescribed; this can be important in ruling out the disease state as a confounder.

Therefore, reliance on physician office data for DE classification can overstate the exposure rate. Establishing DE at the physician level may introduce unidirectional misclassification bias, and 7–20% of the subjects would be classified as exposed who actually are not exposed.

MANAGED ENVIRONMENTS

Hospital and nursing home drug use data can also be valuable sources of DE information (e.g., the Boston Collaborative Drug Surveillance Program).[40] These settings are controlled in the sense that medications are administered under the supervision of medically trained personnel. DE misclassification can result even in these controlled environments. It would be expected that patients receive the drug prescribed because the nursing staff is responsible for drug administration. However, the literature points out that the medication distribution systems in hospitals and nursing homes are not error-free. Medication administration error rates as high as 59.1% have been reported in these settings.[41] Error types that may affect the misclassification of exposure are omissions, unauthorized drugs, wrong dosage, wrong route, wrong dosage form, or wrong time.

Omission, failure to give an ordered drug, is the most prevalent error that occurs in these settings. An unauthorized-drug error takes place when a patient receives a drug that was not ordered. When these two error types occur together, it results in bidirectional misclassification. Those subjects recorded as having received the drug have not. Conversely, those subjects who should not have received the drug have received it.

Omissions can occur for many reasons; medication being unavailable is fairly common. For this reason, it is more likely that omissions will occur more frequently than unauthorized drugs. Therefore, more subjects classified as exposed have not been exposed than vice versa. Misclassification errors are likely to be bidirectional but differential.

The pharmacy dispensing recording system used in these environments may also affect exposure classification.[40] For example, a hospital emergency department may record drugs given there separately from those given after admission. Moreover, records may be inaccurate because what was billed may not necessarily be what was dispensed.

PHARMACY PRESCRIPTION DATA

When a large computerized database is used, prescription billing records are largely the source of DE classification (e.g., Medicaid databases, Group Health Cooperative of Puget Sound, Saskatchewan Health Department computerized database). However, it cannot be assumed that a filled prescription is equivalent to exposure. The prescribed drug may not actually be the dispensed drug. Substitution, particularly therapeutic substitution, may introduce a discrepancy between the drug prescribed, the drug dispensed, and the drug recorded in a database. In collecting prescription data in a sample of pharmacies, researchers found that 4.6% of the prescriptions had escaped detection, resulting in underestimation of the exposure.[42]

In another study,[43] medical records of three staff HMO clinics and central pharmacy records were compared on antihypertensive drug names and dosages dispensed. A high reliability for drug names was observed; for 5–19% of drug name entries in medical records, no pharmacy entries could be identified; otherwise, for 5–8% of prescription files, no medical record entry could be found. Agreement on dosage was somewhat lower (68–70%); 14–21% of entries had nonmatching dosage information, probably reflecting dosage changes on medical records but not in pharmacy records. It is necessary to determine the reliability and validity of the data in any analytic data file prepared for pharmacoepidemiologic studies from a large claims database.

PATIENT COMPLIANCE

Patient interview information can be muddied with issues of noncompliance. Patients often report that they are more compliant than they really are.[44,45] Thus, DE information bias can be created through inaccurate reporting of medication-taking behavior.

Norell[45] found that, of 73 patients interviewed, only 4% reported two or more missed doses during a 1-week period. Objective compliance assessment showed that 33% of the patients missed at least two doses and that 16% missed at least six doses in that time period.

Patient noncompliance with prescribed medications has been estimated to be 20–90%.[3] According to the Schering Laboratories report,[36] 15% of patients stop taking a drug earlier than prescribed, and 32% of patients do not have their prescription refilled. In a large clinical trial, only 33.5% of the individuals in the control group and 32.7% of those in the placebo group took more than 80% of the doses as scheduled.[46] However, compliance may depend on the drug category studied. In examining the rate with oral contraceptives in a prospective cohort, a compliance rate of 91% was measured.[42]

The prescribing decision can be an important modifier of the accuracy of the exposure measure. A study of the effect of multiple daily dosages found compliance rates of 67% for once daily, 50% for twice daily, 44% for three times a day, and 22% for four times a day. Other authors found a high correlation between the daily dosing schedule and compliance: 87% for once daily, 86% for twice daily, 77% for three times a day, and 39% for four times a day.[47] Simpler dosing increases compliance and consequently the accuracy of the exposure estimation.

No correlation has been found between serum concentrations and compliance. Serum concentration determination may be effective only for drugs with a long half-life. Pill counts generally overestimate compliance.[47]

Predominantly, noncompliance is manifested as underuse. This is particularly true for the elderly who report that adverse effects are occurring, that they feel overmedicated, or that the drug was not helping.[48] Those categorized as exposed based on pharmacy prescription dispensing data actually may not be exposed at all or are exposed at a much lower level than assumed. However, for drugs that are abused, the direction of the bias may be reversed; subjects may have additional drug sources and are taking more than prescribed.

PATIENT INTERVIEW

A common approach in pharmacoepidemiology studies is to obtain DE information through interviews. Trained interviewers with a standardized questionnaire can prompt the subject for past exposure to the study drug and/or the UDE. Patient interviews to establish DE may be an important source of recall bias.

Chouinard and Walter[49] examined recall bias in 16 case–control studies with published DE data using a gold standard and interview data. They examined the likelihood of a differential recall bias in cases and controls and an increase in the likelihood of differential recall bias by an increasing difference between the gold standard of DE assessment (pharmacy record, medical record) and a DE interview (recall). No such a relationship was found. For the studies reviewed, no differential recall bias was found between cases and controls, and no recall bias was found as a function of total recall bias.

Significant underascertainment of self-reported DE was found in another study, but little overascertainment was found. This study[50] evaluated the accuracy of recall for the use of nonsteroidal antiinflammatory drugs (NSAIDs) and noncontraceptive estrogens through phone interviews and compared the interview data with the Group Health Cooperative of Puget Sound pharmacy database as the gold standard. Of those with only a single NSAID dispensation, 41% were able to recall any NSAID compared with 85% for those with multiple NSAID prescriptions. Thirty percent recalled the correct NSAID name and 15% the name and dose. For estrogens, 78% recalled the name, but only 26% remembered the name and dose. The drug name was recalled more frequently for exposures stopped 2–3 years prior to interview than for those stopped 7–11 years prior. Sp was high, ranging from 0.92 to 1.0. Phone interviews introduce a significant underestimation of actual DE and only very little overreporting.[48]

Information bias may be created through selective recall if patient interview is the data source.[51] As the length of time between interview and the actual time of taking the drug is increased, the patient's ability to remember accurately declines. The occurrence of a severe UDE will prompt a patient to remember the causative agent. A patient with no UDE is more likely to forget taking the drug. This type of information bias can be bidirectional and differential, and would be additional to the noncompliance misclassification.

As a measure of recall bias, Werler et al.[52] introduced recall sensitivity (Rs), the ratio of exposure reporting accuracy for cases compared with that of controls. Recall bias was recorded for a group of mothers of malformed children versus mothers of children who are not malformed. If the Rs estimate is more than 1, mothers of malformed children are more accurate in recall than mothers of children who are not malformed. The Rs for eight exposure factors was the following: nausea and vomiting, Rs = 0.8; elective abortion, Rs = 1.1; spotting or bleeding, Rs = 1.2; antibiotic or antifungal drug use, Rs = 1.2; history of infertility, Rs = 1.4; urinary tract or yeast infection, Rs = 2.7; and use of birth control after conception, Rs = 7.6. The variation in the Rs values shows the recall biases for the exposure factors and highlights the variability in responses among the exposure factors.[52]

The possibility that severe UDE cases may report exposure systematically different from population controls (recall bias) made some researchers suggest the selection of controls with conditions similar to but sufficiently different from the case group.[53] Selecting "restricted" controls eliminates differential misclassification, but does not eliminate nondifferential misclassification. However, matching for "restricted" controls will introduce selection bias. Drews et al.[54] found that population controls provided observed associations closer to the true association than did "restricted" controls.

Other authors have suggested the appropriateness of stratifying and restricting in case–control studies according to a subject's knowledge of the hypothesis.[55,56] Others have argued that this should be done only when the knowledge would introduce recall bias and that this analysis should be supplemented with one that ignores this strategy.[57]

PROXY RESPONDENTS

Occasionally, it may not be possible to obtain data from patients (e.g., Alzheimer dementia, subarachnoid hemorrhage, postmortem). Then exposure history needs to be obtained from a spouse or other proxy respondent. Spouses are more accurate than nonspouse proxies, with accuracy also depending on the nature of exposure and the time frame for which the exposure history needs to be obtained.[58] Nelson et al.[59] found excellent interclass correlations between patients and proxies for demographic and physical data, as well as cigarette smoking, but lower for medications and hormone preparations (kappa- or interclass correlation range 0.55–0.88). Important bias due to differential nonresponse or differential misclassification (mostly underreporting of exposure) for hormone replacement was observed. It was suggested that studies relying on proxy respondents may require more subjects to offset the effects of nondifferential nonresponse and misclassification on the precision of estimates.

In a case–control study examining the association between paternal occupation and birth defects, the father's report of his own occupation was compared with the mother's report on the father's occupation during a 7-month period around conception. Exact agreement was 59% between the father's and mother's report of the father's occupation. Proxy reports on such a simple fact as the father's occupation appear to be unreliable and need to be validated.[60] DE information obtained from proxies appears to be less valid and reliable than information obtained from patients.

In summary, sources of DE information can introduce misclassification bias resulting from DE recall, drug information recording, medication administration errors, or patient noncompliance with the prescribed or recorded drug regimen. The errors most likely result in an overestimation of the number of exposed patients.

Poor quality data from interviews may also be caused by poor motivation for study participation, preconceptions about disease, the use of proxy responders, or inadequately trained interviewers.[61] Patient interviews do not appear to be reliable in assessing patient exposure or compliance and can result in unidirectional or bidirectional and differential or nondifferential misclassification.

Some of the common considerations in the validation of DE are the use of multiple and independent data sources of drug use information in the study population or a subsample of the study populations (1) to establish the reliability and validity of the data and (2) to obtain true (apparent) Se and true (apparent) Sp. These should include patient interview, medical records, and pharmacy records. Patients or proxies should not be informed about the study hypothesis, and data collection methods for cases and controls should be the same. Interviewers and data abstracters should be blinded to the outcome status of the patient to avoid recall bias or exposure suspicion. In many instances, the interview is the only way to obtain data on DE, although it may not be as reliable as DE information obtained from automated claims databases.

Chapter 23, "An Annotated Bibliography on Pharmacoepidemiologic Studies," presents the operationalization of the DE vector and its validation in the published pharmacoepidemiologic literature.

Misclassification of the Unintended Drug Effect

ASCERTAINMENT OF AN UNINTENDED DRUG EFFECT

Ascertainment bias is a major source of UDE misclassification in pharmacoepidemiologic studies. Differences in the diagnostic criteria used may introduce misclassification and make comparisons among study findings difficult. Even with defined diagnostic criteria ratings, differences may occur. In a review of the rating of 250 temporal artery biopsies, four experienced observers showed interobserver variation that ranged from 4.3% to 13.5% of the cases and intraobserver variation that ranged from 4.4% to 25.6% of the cases.[62] Intra- and interobserver variability are important to consider in UDE misclassification.

Studies may classify histologically confirmed breast cancer as in situ or invasive. Tumor size is measured in length, width, and depth and classified accordingly, small invasive for those up to 1 cm and large invasive for those 1 cm or larger.[62] Other investigators may use a detailed classification scheme to further classify tumors based on cytologic atypia.[63-65] A biopsy confirming epithelial proliferation using a pathologic classification scheme provides additional diagnostic detail.

An accurate case definition can prevent misclassification. In a study[66] of agranulocytosis and aplastic anemia in relation to the use of antithyroid drugs, agranulocytosis is clearly defined, based on the following laboratory values: granulocytes 0.5×10^9/L or less, hemoglobin 100 g/L or more, packed cell volume 0.3 or more, and platelets 100×10^9/L or more.[65] Accurate case definition allows other researchers to replicate study findings. Also, clearly defined diagnostic criteria facilitate the development of evidence tables.

To examine misclassification due to diagnostic uncertainty, Porta et al.[67] developed a diagnostic certainty classification for exocrine pancreatic cancer. It was found that only 52% of the cases fell in the highest diagnostic certainty group. These cases were more likely to be female, showed a longer delay between symptom awareness and first diagnosis (≥1 month), showed a higher proportion of adenocarcinomas, and were more likely to receive radical treatment. Definition of diagnostic certainty classification cutoff points had a significant effect on the level of risk factor exposures: smoking and alcohol use. It was found that the proportion of cases not of pancreatic origin (even if pathologically confirmed) was high enough to cause significant misclassification. The authors suggest that, because past exposure to risk factors may differ among cases with different diagnostic certainty to first include cases that, in spite of lacking pathologic confirmation, have strong clinical evidence supporting the diagnosis. Subsequently, risk estimates should be computed across strata of diagnostic certainty to assess whether heterogenity exists.[68] The potential bias of imperfect Sp (different from 1.0) can also be shown through stratification by level of diagnostic certainty. More restrictive case definitions (increasing Sp) can be expected to produce ORs farther from the null (and closer to the correct ORs).

Misclassification may even occur for a relatively simple-to-establish outcome such as death. Horwitz et al.[31] argue that, for asthmatics, only little difference exists for death and near-fatal asthma and that this difference can largely be explained as a function of the quality of care the patient receives, including early recognition of the symptoms and transfer to an intensive care unit. Classifying near-fatal asthma as being alive, or cases whose lives could be saved with better access to care, as being death, can be considered misclassification in some analyses.

Studies have used survey instruments or patient self-reports for case ascertainment. Solovitz et al.[69] found that patients were able to distinguish UDEs from other extraneous new symptoms. In 75% of identified symptoms, the patients deduced causality. Patient attribution was determined by personal experience, but when the patient education level was high, cognitive factors became more important. In this study, patients were a good information source in the identification of UDEs.

In a study to assess misclassification in a questionnaire survey of the prevalence of varicose veins,[70] a sample of respondents were examined by a surgeon to validate self-reporting of varicose veins. The overall Se (0.92) and Sp (0.93) were good, but the Sp appeared poorer (0.83) among respondents with a family history of varicose veins. Family history of a disease outcome may overestimate its prevalence in the study population.

In the Physicians' Health Study,[71] a randomized trial of physicians aged 40–48 years, a positive response to the questions concerning whether cataract had been diagnosed and date of diagnosis was found to be a good indicator of lens opacification but not a good indicator of an incident, age-related opacity that reduced visual acuity. The authors conclude that additional UDE ascertainment to supplement self-reports should be obtained and strict diagnostic criteria applied to minimize the likely effect of misclassification. Physician self-reports are subject to misclassification bias, as are self-reports by laypeople.

SOURCES FOR THE IDENTIFICATION OF UNINTENDED DRUG EFFECTS

Medical Record Abstraction. Medical records are flawed by recording errors caused by lack of detailed entries by physicians, errors introduced by laboratory and medical personnel, and misinformation from patients. Because of a loss in confidentiality, clinically important but socially sensitive information may not be entered.[72] Despite these flaws, medical records are an important source of UDE information in pharmacoepidemiologic studies.

As part of a British case–control study[73] to investigate the relationship between oral contraceptive use and breast cancer risk, data obtained by interview and medical records were compared. An interview response rating of 72% and 89% were obtained, respectively, for cases and controls, while for 90%, medical records were available. Good agreement between interview and medical record was observed for obstetric history and gynecologic procedures. Medical records were less reliable in documenting use of intrauterine devices, diaphragm, or partner's vasectomy. Only half of the contraceptive use was documented. The authors concluded that, with sole use of medical records, the response rate would have been higher, recall bias eliminated, and data collection costs halved, while associations were the same. However, it would be difficult in Great Britain to rely on medical records for rapid fatal conditions because general practitioners' notes are often destroyed after death of a patient.

In case–control studies, cases often are identified through medical record review and abstraction. Medical record entries are not designed for pharmacoepidemiologic research. Thus, rare UDEs may be omitted because the physician may take a watchful, waiting approach to diagnosis and treatment. A mild, reversible UDE may not be identifiable through records or survey, because it was recognized and the therapy changed by the prescriber without notation.

Alternatively, information obtained through record abstraction may be less biased than that obtained through interview. Subjects who have experienced an adverse effect are more likely to remember it. Subjects may feel that they need to please interviewers by reporting some type of UDE.

Some UDEs may be quite obvious, such as sclerosing peritonitis due to practolol, phocomelia due to thalidomide, or pulmonary hypertension due to aminorex fumarate.[74] Others may be more difficult to detect or identify.

Most UDEs are not unique clinical entities, but are often similar to other conditions prevalent in the general population. An editorial in *Gastroenterology* points out the difficulties in assessing ulcer and gastrointestinal bleeding associated with drugs from the prevalence of this diagnosis in general populations.[75] It cites the example of a 5% prevalence of gastrointestinal problems in the general population, with the incidence of new cases at 0.2% per year. If associated with the drug, the incidence rises fivefold. The prevalence in a control group would be 5.2% and, in the drug-exposed group, 6%, a difference of only 0.8%. The attributable risk of the drug may be small compared with the incidence or prevalence of the condition (disease) in the general population.

In prospective studies, incidence data collected during the length of observation should be used in the analysis instead of prevalence data. Cross-sectional identification of cases or cohort studies with long observation periods may underreport minor, transient, latent, or fatal effects. The bias that results when the evidence of exposure disappears is called Neyman's prevalence–incidence bias.[76]

A distinction needs to be made between induction and latent periods.[77] The period between causal action of the drug and the disease initiation is called the induction period. The period between disease initiation and detection is the latent period. Because it is often difficult to separate these two periods, they are called the empiric induction period (lag time) when combined. Consideration of the empiric induction period is important.

In a study of malignancy following the treatment of rheumatoid arthritis with cyclophosphamide,[78] it was found that the rate of malignancy development was greater after 6 years in the exposed group and that the increased rate persisted even after 13 years. Other researchers found that the risk of gallbladder disease in estrogen users persisted after use of the drug was ceased.[79] Inappropriate considerations about the lengths of the empiric induction period in a pharmacoepidemiologic study can result in nondifferential misclassification and bias toward the null.[76]

An innocent exposure may become suspect if it causes a sign or symptom that precipitates a search for the UDE. Knowledge about a patient's prior exposure may influence both the intensity and the outcome of the diagnostic process. Media publicity may have been used to alert the patient to particular dangers. For example, women exposed to estrogens are encouraged to obtain a medical examination for the detection of endometrial neoplasia. This is called diagnostic suspicion bias.[76]

DATABASES

Misclassification sources in large databases are many. Dick et al.[80] reviewed 289 abstracted records for the diagnosis of non-Hodgkin's lymphoma from two databases. These databases showed a 23.4% disagreement in the diagnosis. The most common errors were coding and problems due to ambiguous terms in the reporting forms.

A review of the Michigan Kidney Register, which collects demographic data and records the diagnosis of endstage renal disease in new cases, shows that there is variation in reporting. Some cases were characterized etiologically (e.g., lead, analgesic, diabetic nephropathy), some were characterized histologically (e.g., glomerulo- or interstitial nephritis), and others were characterized as hypertensive nephrosclerosis with no determination of whether the kidney damage preceded or followed the hypertension.[81-83]

Tennis et al.[84] examined the reliability and validity of the rheumatoid arthritis diagnosis listed in the Saskatchewan hospital separation database as compared with abstracted hospital records. The database showed a reliability of 83.3% with 150 database records confirmed by 125 hospital records. Validity was found lower, with chart documentation for rheumatoid arthritis being greatest for 73 subjects hospitalized by rheumatologists, 69.9% of whom met at least five of the American Rheumatism Association (ARA) criteria for rheumatoid arthritis; 15.1%, fewer than five of the ARA criteria with diagnosis by a rheumatologist; 1.3%, fewer than five criteria with diagnosis of nonrheumatoid arthritis; for 13.7% of the subjects, no diagnosis was found in the records.

Other misclassification errors can be introduced because of a phenomenon called diagnosis-related group "creep." Because of Medicare's prospective payment system for reimbursement, diagnostic and procedure data may be upcoded. The provider is then reimbursed at a higher level. Controversy exists as to whether this is an increase in the accuracy of coding or intentional miscoding.[85,86]

Many sources can be used for case ascertainment. These sources include Medicaid databases, HMO databases, disease registries, death certificates, discharge summaries, autopsy reports, physician office and hospital inpatient records, or direct observations. The method of case ascertainment is important; however, ascertainment of controls can be difficult. Controls should have the same intensity of medical surveillance and diagnostic procedures as cases do.

Direct diagnosis with pathologic evaluation is more accurate than secondary data. To avoid ascertainment bias in prospective cohorts examining the association between estrogen exposure and endometrial cancer, serial endometrial biopsy in cases and controls was proposed, using similar medical surveillance schedules and diagnostic procedures.[87]

CATEGORIZATION OF UNINTENDED DRUG EFFECTS

The diagnostic codes used in medical databases usually are obtained from *The International Classification of Diseases, Ninth Edition* or *Tenth Edition*, or from Common Procedure Terminology (CPT) codes.[88] Other approaches exist in the literature to classify UDEs. For example, Matthews et al.[89] provide a method based on the following organ systems: cardiovascular, dermatologic, endocrinologic, gastrointestinal, hematologic, immunologic, neurologic, ophthalmologic, otologic, pulmonary, renal, and miscellaneous. Within this classification, each UDE is further defined.

Many dictionaries have been developed to facilitate the coding of UDEs. These dictionaries often assign signs, symptoms, and diagnosis the same value. A thesaurus, such as the Food and Drug Administration's COSTART (Coding Symbols for Thesaurus of Adverse Reaction Terms),[90] may collapse terms into large categories for analysis.

In summary, most UDEs have low incidence rates, particularly when the empiric induction period is long. Methods of detection become more important for rare events, including routine examination. Inaccurate diagnostic procedures, measuring devices, interview procedures, or incomplete or erroneous data sources can contribute to UDE misclassification.[76]

Inaccurate diagnostic procedures may lead to under- or overascertainment. Underascertainment may be harder to detect because it implies that all study individuals in which the UDE is not presented have to be examined. Overascertainment is detected more easily because it can be handled by reexamining all cases.

Sackett[76] provides a catalog of biases to be considered in pharmacoepidemiologic research.

Exposure and Outcome Confounders

Confounders are risk factors for UDEs that are distributed unequally among the exposed and the not exposed; thus, they modify the true effect of the exposure on the outcome. To estimate the true effect, the confounder needs to be accounted for. Confounders modify the DE–UDE association by altering the pharmacokinetic and pharmacodynamic parameters and drug metabolism. Age, gender, weight (with respect to lean body weight), and pharmacogenetics are major factors to consider.

Confounding by indication is a source of misclassification of UDE. For example, confounding by indication may occur when a symptom such as persistent ventricular arrhythmia in postmyocardial infarction is treated with propranolol. The drug is associated with adverse outcomes such as sudden death. A UDE may be attributed to the drug when it is actually a manifestation of poor disease outcome.

Confounding by indication does not occur only in patients with poor prognosis. Patients can be selected because they are not as severely ill. In a study in which lidocaine was prescribed prophylactically to prevent death in acute myocardial infarction, it appeared that better-risk patients were chosen to receive therapy.[91] To adjust for confounding by indication, the

Killip–Kimball score was used to stratify the study group according to a commonly used prognostic index of infarct severity.[92] In case ascertainment, the possibility of confounding by indication should be considered.

In the evaluation of the UDE, confounding by indication plays an important role. Those who receive the drug may die, because they receive the drug due to disease severity. The worsening or progression of the disease for which the drug was prescribed is then mistakenly identified as a UDE. Suissa[93] proposed the case–time–control design to handle disease severity as a confounder, because it does not require a measure for disease severity. The case–time–control design differs from conventional case–control design because it uses subjects in the case–control design as their own controls and requires exposure to be measurable at two or more points in time. It adjusts for natural time trends in drug use, thus permitting the separation of the effect associated with the drug from that of disease severity, even if this severity is not measured. Two effects on the OR are observed in the case–time–control design. It produces an OR estimate lower than that of the case–control design. Second, the OR appears less precise than does the corresponding conventional one. This loss in precision results partly from within-subject correlation introduced by the design, which reduces the population size required by the one-to-one matched analysis.

Confounding by indication can lead to ascertainment bias in case selection. Retrospective studies using case–control design are more likely to be biased in this respect. In prospective studies with a control group, DE and symptoms that are attributed to treatment can be more easily confirmed.

The most extensive approach in detecting confounding can be found in the oral contraceptive neoplasm literature. In a case–control study examining the relationship between diethylstilbestrol and clear cell adenocarcinoma, Herbst et al.[27] controlled for the following confounders: use of other hormones, mother's age and pregnancy history, daughter's birth month and weight, age at menarche, use of diethylstilbestrol in pregnancy, and prior spontaneous abortions. In examining the association between oral contraceptive use and breast cancer, other authors have examined up to 25 potential confounders.[18]

In a retrospective cohort study of the association between the use of NSAIDs and upper gastrointestinal tract bleeding,[94] the following confounders were examined: age; gender; state; alcohol-related diagnoses at any time; anticoagulant use at any time; preexisting abdominal conditions; antacid, cimetidine, or steroid exposure; and indication for NSAID therapy. A review of the literature of the UDE under survey may assist in the identification of risk factors that may conclusively link with the UDE.

The use of large databases can restrict the ability to control for confounding. Not all biologically or clinically relevant confounders are captured in the data available. For example, the Quetelet body mass index (height in inches/weight in pounds^2 × 100), which is used to measure obesity, may not be deduced from Medicaid databases.[95] An approach taken in examining confounders not available in a database is to conduct a medical record review for pertinent information on a sample of subjects in the study.[11]

There are several other considerations of misclassification that are beyond the scope of this chapter and, therefore, will be mentioned only briefly. Misclassification of exposure can spuriously introduce effect modification of risk estimates by covariates or confounders.[96] When a confounder has been misclassified, stratification or modeling of a misclassified data set reintroduces confounding in the estimates. Measurement errors in confounders can have serious effects on the risk estimates, even when the measurement error is nondifferential.[97] Adjustment for poorly measured confounders, even when the error or misclassification is independent of exposure, can result in a poorer estimate of the adjusted effect than would be obtained by relying directly on crude estimates.[98] The reader is referred to the literature cited for further discussion of methodologic and statistical considerations in the misclassification of confounders and its effect on risk estimates.

Calculating the Correct Risk Estimate

SIZING THE EFFECT OF MISCLASSIFICATION

Three assumptions are made in further discussions of the effect of misclassification on RR estimates; that is, DE and UDE are dichotomous variables (DE exposed or not exposed, UDE present or absent), a statistically significant association is observed between DE and the UDE, and no confounder is present. There is no bias due to selection or confounding in the data from which the observed risk estimates are calculated. This allows us to illustrate the adjustment procedures for misclassification in the observed population and to demonstrate the effect of misclassification on risk estimates.

Misclassification can be nondifferential or differential and bidirectional or unidirectional in case–control, cohort, and cross-sectional studies. Two parameters, Se and Sp, indicate the misclassification. The following eight probabilities in terms of Se and Sp estimate the misclassification of DE and UDE in a 2 × 2 table:

Se_1, sensitivity for UDE present given DE exposed
Sp_1, specificity for UDE present given DE exposed
Se_2, sensitivity for UDE present given DE not exposed
Sp_2, specificity for UDE present given DE not exposed
Se_3, sensitivity for DE exposed given UDE present

Sp_3, specificity for DE exposed given UDE present
Se_4, sensitivity for DE exposed given UDE absent
Sp_4, specificity for DE exposed given UDE absent

Accordingly, the following conditions can be derived for the major types of misclassification:

1. For no misclassification:
$$Se_1 = Se_2 = Se_3 = Se_4 = 1, \text{ and } Sp_1 = Sp_2 = Sp_3 = Sp_4 = 1$$

2. For UDE nondifferential, unidirectional misclassification:
$$0 \le Se_1 = Se_2 < 1, \text{ and } Se_3 = Se_4 = 1, \text{ and } Sp_1 = Sp_2 = Sp_3 = Sp_4 = 1, \text{ or}$$
$$0 \le Sp_1 = Sp_2 < 1, \text{ and } Sp_3 = Sp_4 = 1, \text{ and } Se_1 = Se_2 = Se_3 = Se_4 = 1$$

3. For UDE nondifferential, bidirectional misclassification:
$$0 \le Se_1 = Se_2 < 1, \text{ and } Se_3 = Se_4 = 1, \text{ and } 0 \le Sp_1 = Sp_2 < 1, \text{ and } Sp_3 = Sp_4 = 1$$

Here, Se_1 and Se_2 or Sp_1 and Sp_2 can but do not need to have the same values.

4. For DE nondifferential, unidirectional misclassification:
$$Se_1 = Se_2 = 1, \text{ and } 0 \le Se_3 = Se_4 < 1, \text{ and } Sp_1 = Sp_2 = Sp_3 = Sp_4 = 1, \text{ or}$$
$$Sp_1 = Sp_2 = 1, \text{ and } 0 \le Sp_3 = Sp_4 < 1, \text{ and } Se_1 = Se_2 = Se_3 = Se_4 = 1$$

5. For DE nondifferential, bidirectional misclassification:
$$Se_1 = Se_2 = 1, \text{ and } 0 \le Se_3 = Se_4 < 1, \text{ and } Sp_1 = Sp_2 = 1, \text{ and } 0 \le Sp_3 = Sp_4 < 1$$

Here, Se_3 and Se_4, or Sp_3 and Sp_4, can but do not need to have the same values.

6. For UDE differential, bidirectional misclassification:
$$0 \le Se_1 \ne Se_2 < 1, \text{ and } Se_3 = Se_4 = 1, \text{ and } Sp_1 = Sp_2 = Sp_3 = Sp_4 = 1$$

7. For UDE differential, bidirectional misclassification:
$$0 \le Se_1 \ne Se_2 < 1, \text{ and } Se_3 = Se_4 = 1, \text{ and } 0 \le Sp_1 \ne Sp_2 < 1, \text{ and } Sp_3 = Sp_4 = 1$$

8. For DE differential, unidirectional misclassification:
$$Se_1 = Se_2 = 1, \text{ and } 0 \le Se_3 \ne Se_4 < 1, \text{ and } Sp_1 = Sp_2 = 1, \text{ and } 0 \le Sp_3 \ne Sp_4 < 1$$

9. For DE differential, bidirectional misclassification:
$$Se_1 = Se_2 = 1, \text{ and } 0 \le Se_3 \ne Se_2 < 1, \text{ and } Sp_1 = Sp_2 = 0, \text{ and } 0 \le Sp_3 \ne Sp_4 < 1$$

10. For misclassification in both DE and UDE, any combination of 2, 3, 6, 7, and 4, 5, 8, 9 can occur.

The values of Se and Sp can be obtained through validation of the DE and UDE classification in the study population. Patient interviews can be validated by secondary and tertiary data sources, such as medical and pharmacy records, by examining the true DE and UDEs in a subsample of the study population, or through use of data from other studies or information published. For example, prescribing information (DE) in a population-based cohort study is obtained from medical records in physicians' offices. It appears that 5% of the individuals do not have their prescriptions filled. This is a nondifferential, unidirectional misclassification with $Se_3 = Se_4 = 0.95$.

Using this information, the researcher can derive the eight Se and Sp probabilities. The true or correct population can be estimated from the observed population.

Given the values for Se_{1-4} and Sp_{1-4} for each category, a general mathematical solution to correct for misclassification is proposed.[5] In matrix terms, this solution is:

$$Y = \mathbf{W}^{-1} \times Y'$$

where $Y = [a, b, c, d]$, the true or corrected cell vector; $Y' = [a', b', c', d']$, the observed misclassified cell entry vector; and $\mathbf{W}$ = the matrix of apparent or true sensitivities and specificities.

$$\mathbf{W} = \begin{bmatrix} Se_1\,Se_3 & (1-Sp_1)Se_4 & Se_2\,(1-Sp_3) & (1-Sp_2)\,(1-Sp_4) \\ (1-Se_1)Se_3 & Sp_1\,Se_4 & (1-Se_2)\,(1-Sp_3) & Sp_2\,(1-Sp_4) \\ Sp_1(1-Sp_3) & (1-Sp_1)(Se_4) & Se_2\,Sp_3 & (1-Sp_2)\,Sp_4 \\ (1-Se_1)\,(1-Se_3) & Sp_1(1-Se_4) & (1-Se_2)\,Sp_3 & Sp_2\,Sp_4 \end{bmatrix}$$

Thus,

$$\begin{bmatrix} a' \\ b' \\ c' \\ d' \end{bmatrix} \times \mathbf{W}^{-1} = \begin{bmatrix} a \\ b \\ c \\ d \end{bmatrix} \qquad\qquad \text{Eq. 1}$$

(observed) (true or correct)

Results of the computation should be evaluated with care. Accurate and realistic probabilities for the Se and Sp parameters are necessary. Negative or erroneous cell values result when the sum of Se_1 or Se_2 and Sp_1 or $Sp_2 = 1$, or when the sum of Se_3 or Se_4 and Sp_3 or $Sp_4 = 1$. This would result in zero denominators, making the formula indeterminate.[5]

In the following section, two examples are presented for establishing the true or correct population from the observed population by using Equation 1.

SIZING THE EFFECT OF NONDIFFERENTIAL CLASSIFICATION

In a hypothetical example of a cohort study, validation of the procedures of medical surveillance and diagnostic ascertainment followed in the study design indicates that an exposed individual showing a UDE has an 0.8 probability of being classified as such and a 0.2 probability of being misclassified. An individual without DE or the UDE has a 0.9 probability of being classified as such and a 0.1 probability of being misclassified. Thus, UDE is misclassified with an Se of 0.8 and a Sp of 0.9.

For the UDE, the following probabilities are derived: $Se_1 = Se_2 = 0.8$ and $Sp_1 = Sp_2 = 0.9$. There is no misclassification for DE in this prospective cohort study, $Se_3 = Se_4 = 1$ and $Sp_3 = Sp_4 = 1$. The misclassification of UDE is the same for those exposed and not exposed and, therefore, for nondifferential and bidirectional. The observed cell entries for the study are shown in Figure 9 (where RR' is the RR for the observed population).

The misclassification rearrangement is reflected in Figure 10. In the notation, UDE represents the true cell entries, and UDE′ is the study's observed classification of the UDEs.

From Figure 10, the relationship between the observed population and the actual or correct population can be observed, as demonstrated in Figure 6. The column marginals for UDE given exposed and UDE not exposed provide the cell entries for the observed population (a' = 310, b' = 690, c' = 170, and d' = 830). The row marginals show the cell entries for the actual or corrected population (a = 300, b = 100, c = 700, and d = 900). Using Equation 1, the researcher can estimate the true or correct cell values as follows:

The observed cell value vector:

$$\begin{bmatrix} a' \\ b' \\ c' \\ d' \end{bmatrix} = \begin{bmatrix} 310 \\ 690 \\ 170 \\ 830 \end{bmatrix}$$

Figure 9
The Observed
Population

	UDE′ Present	UDE′ Absent
Exposed **DE′**	310 a'	690 b'
Not Exposed	170 c'	830 d'

$$RR' = \frac{310/1000}{170/1000} = 1.82$$

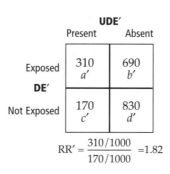

Figure 10
Misclassification
Rearrangement

GIVEN EXPOSED

	UDE Present	UDE Absent	
Present **UDE′**	240	70	310
Absent	60	630	690
	300	700	

GIVEN NOT EXPOSED

	UDE Present	UDE Absent	
Present **UDE′**	80	90	170
Absent	20	810	830
	100	900	

The derived probabilities for Se and Sp:

$Se_1 = 0.8$ $Se_3 = 1.0$
$Sp_1 = 0.9$ $Sp_3 = 1.0$
$Se_2 = 0.8$ $Se_4 = 1.0$
$Sp_2 = 0.9$ $Sp_4 = 1.0$

The matrix of Se and Sp probabilities:

$$
\mathbf{W} = \begin{bmatrix}
0.8 & 0 & 0.1 & 0 \\
0 & 0.8 & 0 & 0.1 \\
0.2 & 0 & 0.9 & 0 \\
0 & 0.2 & 0 & 0.9
\end{bmatrix}
$$

Using Equation 1, the following results are obtained:

$$
\begin{bmatrix} a \\ b \\ c \\ d \end{bmatrix} =
\begin{bmatrix}
1.286 & 0 & -0.143 & 0 \\
0 & 1.286 & 0 & -0.143 \\
-0.286 & 0 & 1.143 & 0 \\
0 & -0.286 & 0 & 1.143
\end{bmatrix}
\times
\begin{bmatrix} 310 \\ 690 \\ 170 \\ 830 \end{bmatrix}'
$$

$a = 300$, $b = 700$, $c = 100$, and $d = 900$.

The RR estimate for the observed population (RR') is 1.82, while the RR estimate for the actual population (RR) is 3.0 (Figure 11). A bias index can be calculated as follows:

$$(RR' - RR)RR = (1.82 - 3)/3 = -0.39$$

SIZING THE EFFECT OF DIFFERENTIAL MISCLASSIFICATION

In the following example, data are represented for a case–control study. Most case–control studies are retrospective in design, making the ascertainment of DE difficult (e.g., patient interview). Therefore, differential DE misclassification will be discussed. Three controls were selected for each case. The observed OR is calculated as 2.39.

Validation studies, in which patient recall of DE is compared with documented DE data, indicate that the exposure misclassification has an Se of 0.7 and an Sp of 0.9 for UDE cases and an Se of 0.6 and an Sp of 0.9 for controls. No misclassification of the UDE is assumed. Thus, $Se_1 = Se_2 = 1$, $Sp_1 = Sp_2 = 1$; $Se_3 = 0.7$, $Sp_3 = 0.9$; $Se_4 = 0.6$, $Sp_4 = 0.9$.

The Se of 0.7 for UDE cases and 0.6 for controls may reflect that cases have better recall differences in compliance or differences in methodology to obtain exposure data. The classification of observed data is as follows.

Figure 12 demonstrates the relationship between the observed cell entries and the true entries. The row marginal shows the observed value of the cell entries ($a' = 290$, $b' = 550$, $c' = 210$, and $d' = 950$; see Figure 13). The column margins show the true cell entries ($a = 400$, $b = 800$, $c = 100$, and $d = 700$; see Figure 14). This relationship is demonstrated in Figure 6.

Based on the identified probabilities for Se and Sp and the observed cell values in Figure 12, the true or correct cell values can be calculated from Equation 1 as follows:

The observed cell value vector:

$$\begin{bmatrix} a' \\ b' \\ c' \\ d' \end{bmatrix} = \begin{bmatrix} 290 \\ 550 \\ 210 \\ 950 \end{bmatrix}'$$

The derived probabilities for Se and Sp:

$Se_1 = 1.0$	$Se_3 = 0.7$
$Sp_1 = 1.0$	$Sp_3 = 0.9$
$Se_2 = 1.0$	$Se_4 = 0.6$
$Sp_2 = 1.0$	$Sp_4 = 0.9$

Figure 11
The Actual
Population
(Nondifferential
Bidirectional)

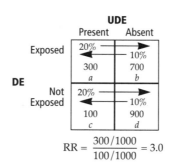

Figure 12
Misclassification
Rearrangement

GIVEN UDE PRESENT

DE

	Exposed	Not Exposed	
Exposed	280	10	290
Not Exposed	120	90	210
	400	100	

DE'

GIVEN UDE ABSENT

DE

	Exposed	Not Exposed	
Exposed	480	70	550
Not Exposed	320	630	950
	800	700	

DE'

The matrix of Se and Sp probabilities:

$$\mathbf{W} = \begin{bmatrix} 0.7 & 0.1 & 0 & 0 \\ 0.3 & 0.9 & 0 & 0 \\ 0 & 0 & 0.6 & 0.1 \\ 0 & 0 & 0.4 & 0.9 \end{bmatrix}$$

Using Equation 1, the following results are obtained:

$$\begin{bmatrix} a \\ b \\ c \\ d \end{bmatrix} = \begin{bmatrix} 1.50 & -0.167 & 0 & 0 \\ -0.5 & 1.167 & 0 & 0 \\ 0 & 0 & 1.8 & -0.2 \\ 0 & 0 & -0.8 & 1.2 \end{bmatrix} \times \begin{bmatrix} 290 \\ 550 \\ 210 \\ 950 \end{bmatrix}$$

with a result of $a = 400$, $b = 800$, $c = 100$, and $d = 700$. The true 2×2 table is shown in Figure 14.

The OR estimate for the observed population (OR') is 2.39, and the OR estimate for the true or corrected population (OR) is 3.5. The bias index can be calculated as follows:

$(OR' - OR)OR = (2.39 - 3.5)3.5 = -0.317$

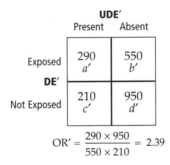

UDE'

	Present	Absent
Exposed **DE'**	290 *a'*	550 *b'*
Not Exposed	210 *c'*	950 *d'*

$$OR' = \frac{290 \times 950}{550 \times 210} = 2.39$$

Figure 13
The Observed Population

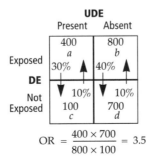

UDE

	Present	Absent
Exposed **DE**	400 *a* 30% ▲	800 *b* 40% ▲
Not Exposed	▼ 10% 100 *c*	▼ 10% 700 *d*

$$OR = \frac{400 \times 700}{800 \times 100} = 3.5$$

Figure 14
The Actual Population (Differential Bidirectional)

Other Issues in Adjusting for Misclassification

Misclassification of DE and/or UDE will bias the risk estimators (e.g., RR, OR). The risk estimator can assume values from zero, indicating a strong negative association, to infinity, indicating a strong positive value. Under the null hypothesis of no association between DE and UDE, the value of the risk estimator is 1, which is called the null value or null.[5]

The direction of the misclassification bias is said to be toward the null if the observed risk estimator is closer than the true risk estimator to the null (closer to 1), on the condition that the true risk estimator and the observed risk estimator are both either larger or smaller than the null. If the bias is toward null, then the observed risk estimator appears to be weaker than it really is. The direction of the bias is away from the null if the observed risk estimator is farther away than the true risk estimator from the null, assuming that both are on the same side of the null. Thus, if the bias is away from null, then the observed effect appears stronger than it really is.

Crossover bias refers to a reverse of the risk estimate. In the discussion of crossover bias, consider the folllowing example. If the observed risk estimator is 2 and the true risk estimator is 0.5, the resulting bias is neither toward nor away from the null. The values are on either side of 1. For crossover bias, DE may be adverse when it is truly protective, or it may appear protective when it is truly adverse. A bias toward or away from the null precludes the possibility of crossover bias.[5] Thus, a bias toward the null implies that the found RR estimate is lower than the true RR and that a bias from the null signifies a RR estimate larger than the true RR.

The following provides some general observations for the direction of bias in case–control studies. In general, nondifferential misclassification produces a bias toward the null. The effect of nondifferential misclassification is a function of Se, Sp, UDE, and DE frequency. In case–control studies, the OR is biased to a greater extent by Sp than by Se.[99] The effect on the RR is largest when the SP decreases from 1.0 to 0.85. If Se and Sp add to 1.0, then the estimate of the RR or OR will become unity (1.0). In case–control studies, the DE Se plays a significant role in the bias of the OR: the less prevalent the DE in cases and controls, the greater the bias. Bias from nondifferential misclassification in case–control studies for three exposure levels depends on risk level, misclassification rate, and exposure distribution. Bias may be toward null or away from null, or crossover bias may occur.[100-103] In cohort studies, the bias is primarily dependent on the Sp and increases with disease rarity. Nondifferential misclassification will generally produce a bias toward the null, although exceptions have recently been discussed with multilevel exposures.

Differential misclassification, which is likely to arise from selective recall in case–control studies, can bias the estimate greatly either toward or away from the null.[16] Dichotomizing a continuous or discrete DE variable may likely introduce differential misclassification. Also, *apparent* misclassification is often differential, even if *true* misclassification in DE is nondifferential.[104] Then, correction procedures for differential rather than nondifferential misclassification should be used.[105] Differential DE misclassification in a case–control study may bias the OR either away from or toward the null value, or not bias at all.

In studies with confounders highly correlated with DE, it becomes important to reduce misclassification. The DE becomes less reliable as the degree of correlation between DE and confounder increases, even when the confounders are measured without error.[97] The use of independent replicated samples helps in adjusting for misclassification in DE and, in confounders, the adjustment procedures will shift the bias from the null and widen the confidence interval of the RR point estimate.

True classification of DE and UDE so that Se and Sp values of 1.0 are achieved is the ideal approach to obtaining valid study outcomes. However, if correct classification cannot be achieved, steps must be taken to adjust for the misclassification and rearrangement of cell entries. The first step in correcting misclassification is to obtain estimates of the Se and Sp of the measures used in DE information and UDE ascertainment. A number of strategies and considerations in achieving correct classification have been discussed.

Estimates of the Se and Sp usually can be determined from previous studies examining comparable populations and the same DE and UDE association. Other approaches include obtaining accurate ascertainment of DE and/or UDE in a subsample of the population, and establishing a gold standard. References from the literature on compliance in similar populations for the same categories of study drugs may also be helpful in assessing misclassification.

Approaches to arrive at Se and Sp are through external validation or internal validation: external validation by comparing a subsample with a gold standard to calculate Se and Sp, and internal validation by multiple independent repeated measures within the study. Confidence intervals using internal repeat measurements are narrower than those using external determinations; both approaches yield approximate correct RR or OR estimators.[105] In terms of precision, it is preferable to correct for misclassification using internal repeat measurements rather than external validation.[106] It should then be reported if the reliability study was conducted on a random subsample of the main study population, the number of subjects in the subsample, and the number of replicate measurements per subject.[107]

These dual DE measurement strategies may eliminate bias or reduce bias if the DE misclassification is truly nondifferential. DE misclassification rates are not always completely independent of measured UDE risk. Even if the misclassification is slightly nondifferential, this can lead to large bias away from the null or to crossover bias.[104] Se analyses are recommended that consider the possible range of misclassification rates as well as the deviation from the nondifferential assumption.[108]

Approaches to obtain estimates of Se and Sp on UDE classification through validation studies are often based on expensive and invasive diagnostic procedures (e.g., angiographic conformation of coronary artery disease). Ethical and practical reasons often do not allow us to obtain this information on those who do not have the disease. Thus, for some, estimates of Se and Sp cannot be obtained. An alternative method to correct risk estimates for nondifferential UDE misclassification may be based on estimates of the positive predictive value. The positive predictive value requires validation of the diagnosis among samples that are classified as having the UDE. The positive predictive value can be calculated as the number of those truly exposed and having the disease multiplied by the Se of the UDE classification among those exposed divided by the number of those exposed with apparent UDE. This correction method based on estimates of the positive predictive value is acceptable when the UDE Se is nondifferential and when the UDE Sp can be either nondifferential or differential.[109] This approach is useful in cohort studies when the UDE is obtained from databases such as cancer registries or vital records, where it is not possible to estimate Se and Sp for the non-UDE cases.

Other authors have questioned the use of Se and Sp as appropriate measures of misclassification. The use of these measures is based on an overestimate of the nondifferential nature of the misclassification, while it is more likely that misclassification is differential. An approach is suggested that also takes into account the degree to which subjects who have been classified by the defective measure are, or are not, correctly classified.[110]

The effect of bias in misclassification on RR and OR estimates is complex. Several different approaches to adjust for misclassification are proposed in the literature.[7,16,111-113] For most approaches, estimates of Se and Sp are needed. The methodology to correct for bias from nondifferential is extensively covered in the literature.[9,16,113,114] A method to correct for bias from differential misclassification in case–control studies for two exposure levels is presented.[115] Correcting for bias in case–control studies with three exposure levels is discussed.[100-102,116] However, preventing misclassification is the surest way to establish reliable risk estimators.

Summary

Misclassification of DE information and UDE ascertainment can introduce substantial bias in estimates of risk. While observational study designs have good external validity, they are often criticized for their lack of internal validity. Misclassification is the most important threat to internal validity in pharmacoepidemiologic studies. Misclassification of DE can be introduced through inappropriate identification of drug product or class. Other errors are due to less-than-optimal consideration of the DE vector with regard to dosage strength and length of exposure. Faulty coding schemes or procedures, unreliable medical or pharmacy records, and patient recall bias contribute to the information bias created by DE misclassification.

Noncompliance is an important source of DE misclassification. Noncompliance is worthy of considerable notation because of its documented prevalence with regard to drug use. Epidemiologic researchers must recognize noncompliance as a considerable source of information bias. Noncompliance can overestimate the number of patients believed to be exposed. This misclassification will most likely be nondifferential and unidirectional and will bias estimates of the RR toward 1, or no difference between exposed and nonexposed.

The misclassification of UDEs can also result in biased risk estimates. The major sources of misclassification of UDEs are implicit and vaguely defined diagnostic criteria, ascertainment bias, prevalence–incidence bias, susceptibility bias, and empiric induction time considerations. Information bias includes medical record entry and coding errors. Most likely, these errors are differential and bidirectional.

The study design, prospective, retrospective, case–control, or cohort study design, has an effect on the type and nature of the misclassification to be considered in the study protocol. Prospective data are preferable to retrospective, since the latter are more subject to measurement errors, such as recall bias that introduce misclassification. Cohort studies are often prospective in design; therefore, disease status ascertainment is a greater problem than exposure ascertainment. Detection bias may be influenced by differential surveillance in exposed and unexposed groups, exposure influence of the diagnostic investigator, or exposure-influenced test interpretation. Exposure ascertainment may be the greatest source of error in case–control studies, because case–control studies are retrospective in design.

Using Se and Sp estimates, the researcher can determine true or correct cell entries for observational studies by using the presented statistical equations. The examples shown use relatively low Se and Sp probabilities that exaggerate the effect of misclassification on the RR and OR estimates.

Misclassification error sources and their effects on RR and the OR deserve consideration in every pharmacoepidemiologic study protocol. These effects, even with Se and Sp probabilities closer to 1, are important. Recent research has pointed out that the effect of misclassification on estimates may be complex and unpredictable. As the extent of pharmacoepidemiologic studies grows, so must the research that evaluates potential biases in DE and UDE outcomes. Prevention may be better than cure, and the use of well-designed instruments, valid data collection techniques, and ensured data quality can prevent misclassification from happening.

References

1. Guess HA. Computer-based medical records linkage systems (lecture). Chapel Hill, NC: University of North Carolina, 1988.
2. Faich GA. Postmarketing surveillance of prescription drugs: current status. Washington, DC: Office of Epidemiology and Biostatistics, Center for Drugs and Biologics, US Food and Drug Administration, 1986.
3. Fincham JE. Patient compliance in the ambulatory elderly: a review of the literature. J Geriatr Ther 1988;2:31-52.
4. Graham DJ, Smith CR. Misclassification in epidemiologic studies of adverse drug reactions using large managerial data bases. Am J Prev Med 1988;4(suppl 2):15-24.
5. Kleinbaum D, Kupper L, Morgenstern H. Epidemiologic research — principles and quantitative methods. New York: Van Nostrand Reinhold Company, 1982:221-41.
6. Wacholder S, Dosemeci M, Lubin JM. Blind assignment of exposure does not always prevent differential misclassification. Am J Epidemiol 1991;134:433-7.
7. Flegal KM, Kegl PM, Nieto FJ. Differential misclassification arising from nondifferential errors in exposure measurement. Am J Epidemiol 1991;134:1233-44.
8. Brenner H. Varied forms of bias due to nondifferential error in measuring exposure. Epidemiology 1994;5:510-7.
9. Bross ID. Misclassification in 2 × 2 tables. Biometrics 1954;10:478-86.
10. Schwartzbaum JA, Setzer RW, Kuper LL. Limitations of relative sensitivity in detecting differential misclassification in case–control studies. Epidemiology 1994;5:315-23.
11. Benenson AS. Control of communicable diseases in man. 16th ed. Washington, DC: American Public Health Association, 1996.
12. Ray WA, Griffin MR, Downey W, Melton LJ III. Long-term use of thiazide diuretics and risk of hip fracture. Lancet 1989;1:687-90.
13. Strom BL, Tamragouri RN, Morse ML, Lazar EL, West SL, Stolley PD, et al. Oral contraceptives and other risk factors for gallbladder disease. Clin Pharmacol Ther 1986;39:335-41.
14. Shy CM, Kleinbaum DG, Morgenstern H. The effect of misclassification of exposure status in epidemiological studies of air pollution health effects. Bull N Y Acad Med 1978;54:1155-65.
15. Gladen B, Rogan WJ. Misclassification and the design of environmental studies. Am J Epidemiol 1979;109:607-16.
16. Copeland KT, Checkoway H, Holbrook RH, McMichael AJ. Bias due to misclassification in the estimate of relative risk. Am J Epidemiol 1977;105:488-95.
17. Agurell S. The research and development of a 5-HT selective reuptake blocker. Acta Psychiatr Scand 1983;308(suppl):19-24.
18. Centers for Disease Control, National Institute of Child Health and Human Development. Oral contraceptive use and the risk of breast cancer, the cancer and steroid hormone. N Engl J Med 1986;315:405-11.
19. Rosenberg L, Shapiro S, Slone D. Epithelial ovarian cancer and combination oral contraceptives. JAMA 1982;247:3210-2.

20. Heller WH, Fleeger CA, eds. USAN and the USP dictionary of international drug names. Rockville, MD: US Pharmacopeial Convention, Inc., 1990.
21. Ellrodt AG, Murata GH, Riedinger MS, Stewart ME, Mochizuki C, Gray R. Severe neutropenia associated with sustained-release procainamide. Ann Intern Med 1984; 100:197-201.
22. Tucker MA, Meadows AT, Boice JD. Leukemia after therapy with alkylating agents for childhood cancer. J Natl Cancer Inst 1987;78:459-64.
23. Mitchell AA, Rosenberg L, Shapiro S, Slone D. Birth defects related to Bendectin use in pregnancy. JAMA 1981;245:2311-3.
24. Resseguie LJ, Hick JF, Bruen JA, Noller KL, O'Fallon WM, Kurland LT. Congenital malformations among offspring exposed in utero to progestins. Olmsted County, Minnesota, 1936–1979. Fertil Steril 1985;43:514-9.
25. Guess HA. Behavior of the exposure odds ratio in a case–control study when the hazard function is not constant over time. J Clin Epidemiol 1989;42:1179-84.
26. Ross RK, Paganini-Hill A, Gerkins VR, et al. A case–control study of menopausal estrogen therapy and breast cancer. JAMA 1980;243:1635-9.
27. Herbst AL, Anderson S, Hubby MM, Haenszel WM, Kaufman RH, Noller KL. Risk factors for the development of diethylstilbestrol-associated clear cell adenocarcinoma: a case–control study. Am J Obstet Gynecol 1986;154:814-22.
28. Salvan A, Stayner L, Steenland K, Smith R. Selecting an exposure lag period. Epidemiology 1995;6:387-90.
29. Strom BL, Carson JL, Morse ML, West SL, Soper KA. The effect of indication on hypersensitivity reactions associated with zomepirac sodium and other nonsteroidal antiinflammatory drugs. Arthritis Rheum 1987;30:1142-8.
30. Levy DB, Vasilomanolakis EC. Anaphylactic reaction due to zomepirac. Drug Intell Clin Pharm 1984;18:983-4.
31. Horwitz RI, Spitzer W, Buist S, Crockcroft D, Ernst P, Habbick B, et al. Clinical complexity and epidemiologic uncertainty in case–control research. Chest 1991;100:1586-91.
32. Feldmann U. Epidemiologic assessment of risks of adverse reactions associated with intermittent exposure. Biometrics 1993;49:419-28.
33. Feldmann U. Design and analysis of drug safety studies, with special reference to sporadic drug use and acute adverse reactions. J Clin Epidemiol 1993;46:237-44.
34. IMS America. National disease and therapeutic index. Plymouth Meeting, PA: IMS America, 1988.
35. Koch M, Campbell W. The collection and processing of drug information. National Ambulatory Medical Care Survey, 1980. National Center for Health Statistics. Vital Health Stat 1982:2(90).
36. Schering Laboratories. The forgetful patient: the high cost of improper patient compliance. Schering Report IX. Kenilworth, NJ: Schering Laboratories, 1987.
37. Upjohn Company. Results of a national prescription buyer survey conducted for the Upjohn Company by Market Facts, Inc., Chicago, IL, 1988.
38. Green LW, Mullen PD, Stainbrook GL. Programs to reduce drug errors in the elderly: direct and indirect evidence from patient education. In: Improving medication compliance. Washington, DC: National Pharmaceutical Council, 1984.
39. Burrell CD, Levy RA. Therapeutic consequences of noncompliance. In: Improving medication compliance. Washington, DC: National Pharmaceutical Council, 1984.
40. Plat R, Stryker S, Komaroff A. Pharmacoepidemiology in hospitals using automated data systems. Am J Prev Med 1988;4(suppl 2):39-47.

41. Allan EL, Barker KN. Fundamentals of medication error research. Am J Hosp Pharm 1990;47:555-67.
42. Persson I, Adami HO, Johansson E, Lindberg B, Manell P, Westerholm B. Cohort study of estrogen treatment and the risk of endometrial cancer: evaluation of method and its applicability. Eur J Clin Pharmacol 1983;25:625-32.
43. Christensen DB, Williams B, Goldberg HI, Martin DP, Engelberg R, LoGerfo JP. Comparison of prescription and medical records in reflecting patient antihypertensive drug therapy. Ann Pharmacother 1994;28:99-104.
44. Evans L, Spelman M. The problem of noncompliance with drug therapy. Drugs 1983;25:63-76.
45. Norell SE. Accuracy of patient interviews and estimates by clinical staff in determining medication compliance. Soc Sci Med 1981;15:57-61.
46. The Coronary Drug Project Research Group. Influence of adherence to treatment and response of cholesterol on mortality in the coronary drug project. N Engl J Med 1980;303:1038-41.
47. Cramer JA, Mattson RH, Prevey ML, Scheyer RD, Ouellette VL. How often is medication taken as prescribed? A novel assessment technique. JAMA 1989;261:3273-7.
48. Cooper JK, Love DW, Raffoul PR. Intentional prescription nonadherence (noncompliance) in the elderly. J Am Geriatr Soc 1982;30:329-33.
49. Chouinard E, Walter S. Recall bias in case–control studies: an empirical analysis and theoretical framework. J Clin Epidemiol 1995;48:245-54.
50. West SL, Savitz DA, Koch G, Strom BL, Guess HA, Hartzema AG. Recall accuracy for prescription medications: self-report compared with database information. Am J Epidemiol 1995;142:1103-12.
51. Austin MA, Criqui MH, Barrett-Connor E, Holdbrook MJ. The effect of response bias on the odds ratio. Am J Epidemiol 1981;114:137-43.
52. Werler MM, Pober BR, Nelson K, Holmes LB. Reporting accuracy among mothers of malformed and not malformed infants. Am J Epidemiol 1989;129:415-21.
53. Louick C, Mitchell AA, Werler MM, Hanson JW, Shapiro S. Maternal exposure to spermicides in relation to certain birth defects. N Engl J Med 1987;317:474-8.
54. Drews C, Greenland S, Flanders DW. The use of restricted controls to prevent recall bias in case–control studies of reproductive outcomes. Ann Epidemiol 1993;3:86-92.
55. Werler MM, Shapiro S, Mitchell AA. Periconceptual folic acid exposure and risk of occurrent neural tube defects. JAMA 1993;269:1257-61.
56. Mitchell AA, Werler MM, Shapiro S. A response to the commentary, "Should we consider a subject's knowledge of the etiologic hypothesis in the analysis of case–control studies?" Am J Epidemiol 1995;141:297-8.
57. Weiss NS. Should we consider a subject's knowledge of the etiologic hypothesis in the analysis of case–control studies? Am J Epidemiol 1994;139:247-9.
58. Lyon JL, Egger MJ, Robison LM, French TK, Gao R. Misclassification of exposure in a case–control study: the effects of different types of exposure in a case–control study: the effects of different types of exposure and different proxy respondents in a study of pancreatic cancer. Epidemiology 1992;3:223-31.
59. Nelson LM, Longstreth WT, Koepsell TD, Checkoway H, Van Bell G. Completeness and accuracy of interview data from proxy respondents: demographic, medical, and life-style factors. Epidemiology 1994;5:204-17.
60. Schnitzer PG, Olshan AF, Savitz DA, Erickson JD. Validity of mother's report of father's occupation in a study of paternal occupation and congenital malformations. Am J Epidemiol 1995;141:872-7.

61. Gordis L. Assuring the quality of questionnaire data in epidemiologic research. Am J Epidemiol 1979;109:21-4.
62. McDonnell PJ, Moore GW, Miller NR, Hutchins GM, Green WR. Temporal arteritis: a clinicopathologic study. Ophthalmology 1986;93:518-30.
63. Kleinerman RA, Brinton LA, Hoover R, Fraumeni JF. Diazepam use and progression of breast cancer. Cancer Res 1984;99:1223-5.
64. Rohan TE, Cook MG, Potter JD, McMichael AJ. A case–control study of diet and benign proliferative epithelial disorders of the breast. Cancer Res 1990;50:3176-81.
65. Rohan TE, Cook MG. Alcohol consumption and risk of benign proliferative epithelial disorders of the breast in women. Int J Cancer 1989;43:631-6.
66. International Agranulocytosis and Aplastic Anaemia Study. Risk of agranulocytosis and aplastic anaemia in relation to use of antithyroid drugs. Br Med J 1988;297:262-5.
67. Porta M, Malats N, Pinol JL, Rifa J, Andrew M, Real FX. J Clin Epidemiol 1994;47: 1069-79.
68. Woolf SH. Manual for conducting systematic reviews. Agency for Health Care Policy and Research, 1996.
69. Solovitz BL, Fisher S, Bryant SG, Kluge RM. How well can patients discriminate drug-related side effects from extraneous new symptoms? Psychopharmacol Bull 1987;23:189-92.
70. Laurikka J, Laara E, Sisto T, Tarkka M, Auvinen O, Hakama M. Misclassification in a questionnaire survey of varicose veins. J Clin Epidemiol 1995;48:1175-8.
71. Christen WG, Glynn RJ, Seddon JM, Manson JE, Buring JE, Hennekens CH. Confirmation of self-reported cataract in the Physicians' Health Study. Ophthalmic Epidemiol 1994;1:85-91.
72. Burnum JF. The misinformation era: the fall of the medical record. Ann Intern Med 1989;110:482-4.
73. Chilvers CED, Pike MC, Taylor CN, Herman C, Crossley B, Smith SJ. General practitioner notes as a source of information for case–control studies in young women. J Epidemiol Community Health 1994;48:92-7.
74. Mann JL. Principles and pitfalls in drug epidemiology. In: Inman W, ed. Monitoring for drug safety. Philadelphia: JB Lippincott, 1980:401-15.
75. Kurata JH, Elashoff JD, Grossman ML. Inadequacy of the literature on the relationship between drugs, ulcers, and gastrointestinal bleeding (editorial). Gastroenterology 1982;82:373-82.
76. Sackett D. Bias in analytic research. J Chronic Dis 1979;32:51-63.
77. Rothman KJ. Induction and latent periods. Am J Epidemiol 1981;114:253-9.
78. Baker GL, Kahl LE, Zee BC, Stolzer BL, Agarwal AK, Medsger TA. Malignancy following treatment of rheumatoid arthritis with cyclophosphamide. Am J Med 1987; 83:1-2.
79. Petitti DB, Sidney S, Perlman JA. Increased risk of cholecystectomy in users of supplemental estrogen. Gastroenterology 1988;94:91-5.
80. Dick FR, VanLier SF, McKeen K, Everett GD, Blair A. Nonconcurrence in abstracted diagnoses of non-Hodgkin's lymphoma. J Natl Cancer Inst 1987;78:675-7.
81. Steenland NK, Thun MJ, Ferguson CW, Port FK. Occupational and other exposure associated with male end-stage renal disease: a case–control study. Am J Public Health 1990;80:153-7.
82. Weller JM, Port FK, Swarz RD, Ferguson CW, Williams GW, Jacobs JF Jr. Analysis of survival of end-stage renal disease patients. Kidney Int 1982;21:78-83.
83. Weller JM, Wu SC, Ferguson CW, Hawthorne VM. End stage renal disease in Michigan. Am J Nephrol 1985;5:84-95.

84. Tennis P, Bombardier C, Malcohm E, Downey W. Validity of rheumatoid arthritis diagnoses listed in the Saskatchewan hospital separations database. J Clin Epidemiol 1993;46:675-83.

85. Steinwald B, Dummit LA. Hospital case-mix change: sicker patients or DRG creep? Health Aff (Millwood) 1989;8:36-47.

86. Horn SD, Horn RA, Sharkey PD, Beall RJ, Hoff JS, Rosenstein BJ. Misclassification problems in diagnosis-related groups. N Engl J Med 1986;314:484-7.

87. Whitehead ML, McQueen J, King RJB, Campbell S. Endometrial histology and biochemistry in climacteric women during estrogen and estrogen/progestogen therapy. J R Soc Med 1979;72:322-7.

88. The international classification of diseases, clinical modification. ICD-9-CM. Ninth ed. Ann Arbor, MI: Commission on Professional and Hospital Activities, 1978.

89. Matthews SJ, Schneiweiss F, Cersosino RJ. A clinical manual of adverse drug reactions. Norwalk, CT: Appleton, Century, Crofts, 1986.

90. US Food and Drug Administration. National adverse drug reaction directory "COSTART." Rockville, MD: Food and Drug Administration, 1970.

91. Horwitz RI, Feinstein AR. Improved observational method for studying therapeutic efficacy: suggestive evidence that lidocaine prophylaxis prevents death in acute myocardial infarction. JAMA 1981;246:2455-9.

92. Killip T, Kimball JT. Treatment of myocardial infarction in a coronary care unit: a two year experience with 250 patients. Am J Cardiol 1967;20:457-64.

93. Suissa S. The case–time–control design. Epidemiology 1995;6:248-53.

94. Carson JL, Strom BL, Soper KA, West SL, Morse L. The association of nonsteroidal anti-inflammatory drugs with upper gastrointestinal tract bleeding. Arch Intern Med 1987;147:85-8.

95. Machado EBV, Gabriel SE, Beard CM, Michet CJ, O'Fallon WM, Ballard DJ. A population-based case–control study of temporal arteritis: evidence for an association between temporal arteritis and degenerative vascular disease. Int J Epidemiol 1989;18:836-41.

96. Greenland S. The effect of misclassification in the presence of covariates. Am J Epidemiol 1980;112:564-9.

97. Kim MY, Pasternack BS, Carroll RJ, Koenig KL, Toniolo PG. Estimating the reliability of an exposure variable in the presence of confounders. Stat Med 1995;14:1437-46.

98. Wacholder S. When measurement errors correlate with truth: surprising effects of nondifferential misclassification. Epidemiology 1995;6:157-61.

99. Goldberg JD. The effects of misclassification on the bias in the difference between two proportions and the relative odds in the fourfold table. J Am Stat Assoc 1975; 70:561-7.

100. Freudenheim JL, Marshall JR. The problem of profound mismeasurement and the power of epidemiological studies of diet and cancer. Nutr Cancer 1988;11:243-50.

101. Birkett NJ. Effect of nondifferential misclassification on estimates of odds ratios with multiple levels of exposure. Am J Epidemiol 1992;136:356-62.

102. Verkerk PH, Buitendijk D. Nondifferential underestimation may cause a threshold effect of exposure to appear as a dose–response relationship. J Clin Epidemiol 1992; 45:543-5.

103. Gullin WH, Bearman JE, Johnson EA. Effects of misclassification in epidemiologic studies. Public Health Rep 1968;83:914-8.

104. Brenner H. Correcting for exposure misclassification using an alloyed gold standard. Epidemiology 1996;7:406-10.

105. Quade D, Lachenbruch PA, Whaley FS, McClish DK, Haley RW. Effects of mis-classifications on statistical inferences in epidemiology. Am J Epidemiol 1980;111: 503-15.

106. Duffy SW, Maximovitch DM, Day NE. External validation, repeat determination, and precision of risk estimation in misclassified exposure data in epidemiology. J Epidemiol Community Health 1992;46:620-4.

107. Willet W. National epidemiology. New York: Oxford University Press, 1990.

108. Brenner H. Inferences on the potential effects of presumed non-differential expo-sure misclassification. Ann Epidemiol 1993;3:289-94.

109. Brenner H, Gefeller O. Use of the positive predictive value to correct for disease misclassification in epidemiologic studies. Am J Epidemiol 1993;138:1007-15.

110. Marshall RJ. Misclassification of exposure in case–control studies: assessment by quality indices. Epidemiology 1994;5:309-14.

111. Duffy SW, Rohan TE, Day NE. Misclassification in more than one factor in one case–control study: a combination of Mantel–Haenszel and maximum likelihood approaches. Stat Med 1989;8:1529-36.

112. Walter SD, Irwig LM. Estimation of test error rates, disease prevalence and relative risk from misclassification data: a review. J Clin Epidemiol 1988;41:923-37.

113. Gladen B, Rogan WJ. Misclassification and the design of environmental studies. Am J Epidemiol 1979;109:607-16.

114. Flegal KM, Brownie C, Haas JD. The effects of exposure misclassification on esti-mates of relative risk. Am J Epidemiol 1986;123:736-51.

115. Flanders WD, Drews CD, Kosinski AS. Methodology to correct for differential mis-classification. Epidemiology 1995;6:152-6.

116. Correa-Villasenor A, Stewart WF, Franco-Marina F, Seacat H. Bias from nondiffer-ential misclassification in case–control studies with three exposure levels. Epide-miology 1995;6:276-81.

12
Meta-analysis of the Pharmacotherapy Literature
Thomas R Einarson

Abstract

Meta-analysis is a statistical approach to the aggregation of independent research studies. Its contribution is the creation of new knowledge synthesized from existing studies. This chapter is intended as an introduction to meta-analysis for healthcare practitioners and students. It provides a stepwise approach to planning and conducting meta-analyses by using two examples. The first illustrates the stepwise approach used in meta-analysis and examines the relationship between fetal abnormalities and Bendectin by using epidemiologic studies. The second demonstrates the analysis of data from clinical trials using published articles on the addition of dexamethasone to ondansetron in the control of vomiting during cancer chemotherapy.

Outline

The literature explosion has resulted in a massive amount of information that must be analyzed and summarized to be useful to practitioners and their patients. Since drug information lies within the domain of pharmacy, it is the responsibility of the pharmacist to evaluate and summarize the literature for use in patient care. It therefore behooves all pharmacists, particularly those specializing in drug information, to be familiar with and use techniques of literature analysis.

Often, conflicting results are produced in different studies of the same topic.[1] Such differences in research outcomes need to be reconciled to provide quality patient care. Resolving such conflict has traditionally been done through narrative review. However, that method has many limitations[2-4] and has probably "outlived its usefulness."[5]

Quantitative methods of integration of research results have been used for many years, but only recently have received a great deal of attention.[6] The quantitative approach to integration of independent research results has been termed "meta-analysis" by Glass in 1976.[3]

Definition

Leviton and Cook[7] have defined meta-analysis as "any systematic method that uses statistical analyses for combining data from independent studies to obtain a numerical estimate of the overall effect of a particular procedure or variable on a defined outcome." Sacks et al.[8] described it as a discipline that "critically reviews and statistically combines results of previous research." Glass[3] introduced the term to describe quantitative aggregation of results. In this case, "meta" refers to the secondary analysis of findings, since the data are derived from previously published (if not published, completed) research. It should be noted that meta-analysis is not a single method, but an approach to summarizing findings. It is an umbrella term that encompasses a great variety of methods and techniques. What these methods have in common is that they are thorough, systematic, and quantitative (i.e., produce a single overall statistic to summarize findings).

At present, meta-analysis is the preferred approach to integration of results from different studies because it incorporates all of the strengths of traditional reviews and further provides (relatively) unbiased quantitative summary estimates. Einarson et al.[2] recommended that it become the standard approach for drug reviews.

Meta-analysis is a legitimate form of research with its own methodology. Its contribution is the creation of new knowledge synthesized from existing studies. Lee[9] has suggested that it be considered as an alternative form of research experience for nurses. The suggestion is equally valid for pharmacy.

Purpose of Meta-analysis

Sacks et al.[8] listed four major purposes of meta-analysis of randomized controlled trials. They were the following: (1) to increase power for primary end points and for subgroups (i.e., where sample sizes in original studies were too small to demonstrate statistical significance), (2) to resolve uncertainty when reports disagree, (3) to improve estimates of effect size, and (4) to answer questions not posed in the original trials.

Other meta-analyses may be concerned with planning new studies, combining results from multicenter trials, or comparing the effectiveness of different types of services or programs. More recently, meta-analysis has been used to provide summary data for input into economic analyses.[10] Thus, this approach to aggregation of findings can be a very useful tool to clinical practitioners, service managers, researchers, and educators alike.

Meta-analysis and Drug Studies

Drug studies may be broadly classified into two main types: clinical studies (i.e., randomized controlled trials) and epidemiologic studies. The former are performed to determine the efficacy of a drug or to compare drugs on the basis of clinical efficacy (or, occasionally, adverse effects). To be used in a meta-analysis, there must be a treatment group and a comparison (i.e., control) group. The comparison group normally receives placebo or standard therapy, depending on the ethics of withholding effective therapy. Occasionally, patients may serve as their own controls, with outcomes compared before and after the patient has been administered the drug.

Epidemiologic studies seek to quantify the relationship between a drug and a given outcome (beneficial or adverse) or to compare two drugs or events with respect to a given outcome. The two main types of comparative epidemiologic studies are *cohort* and *case–control* studies. Cohort studies begin with a group of patients exposed to a drug and a comparison group who are not exposed to the drug and then compare outcome rates. Case–control studies begin with a group of patients having the outcome of interest (e.g., adverse drug effect) and a group of subjects who do not have the outcome (e.g., healthy controls). Records are then examined to determine how many of each group had been exposed to the drug, and rates are then compared. Figure 1 presents a graphic presentation of a 2 × 2 table for epidemiologic studies. That approach may also be taken with clinical drug trials that express outcomes as success/fail or cured/not cured.

Figure 1 2 × 2 Table for Epidemiologic Studies		OUTCOME		
	FACTOR STATUS	**DISEASE**	**NO DISEASE**	**TOTAL**
	Exposure	A	B	n_1
	No exposure	C	D	n_0
	Total	m_1	m_0	N

Whatever the method used, meta-analysis requires results from a treatment group and a comparison group. Such studies form the raw data with which one can produce a statistical summation.

A Brief Overview of Meta-analysis

Meta-analysis is a statistical approach to the integration and summarization of results from independent studies. It is systematic, thorough, objective, and quantitative.

Two different aspects of results may be compared, namely, the magnitude of the difference between groups (i.e., the effect size) and the statistical significance of the difference of the results between groups. The original meta-analyses focused on only one of those aspects. Excellent discussions of the background and statistical methods have been presented by Rosenthal[6] and Hedges and Olkin.[11] A pharmacy example of the use of the effect size has been presented by Einarson et al.[2] Those techniques have become less popular because of the obvious limitation. Techniques have been developed that incorporate both aspects (i.e., effect size and statistical significance) into their calculations.

In fact, a variety of analytical methods is available for use in meta-analysis. Regardless of the method used, all meta-analyses involve three major phases—the three Ps: preparation, performance, and presentation. This sequence is the same as for any other type of research. The project must be planned in advance, then systematically carried out, followed by reporting of results.

Phase I: Preparation

This part represents the planning phase of the project. During this phase, the research design is defined explicitly. It should be noted that the planning takes place *before* any data are collected. It is a serious mistake to collect studies first and then try to analyze. Such a method introduces bias that makes interpretation of results difficult and may be both inaccurate and misleading.

The preparation phase involves four stages: (1) statement of purpose, (2) data definition, (3) data retrieval procedure, and (4) statistical analysis. The first two steps comprise a series of definitions that clarify the research issues. The last two steps describe the analytical procedures to be used. The aim is to answer the research question by finding all possible studies and then methodically analyzing and combining them. Adhering to an established critical protocol serves to enhance the validity of the results.

Table 1 presents a detailed listing of the steps involved in setting up the research protocol, which is discussed below. Examples are provided to illustrate meta-analyses for two different types of pharmacotherapy-related studies.

A STEPWISE APPROACH TO PLANNING META-ANALYSES

This section discusses each of the steps involved in defining the protocol for a meta-analysis. To illustrate these steps, an example that has been published[12] is used. It illustrates a procedure for meta-analysis of epidemiologic studies, but the approach may be used for any type of research project.

To illustrate the computations for meta-analysis of clinical drug trials, a second example is included. In that example, the increase in control of cisplatin-induced emesis from the addition of dexamethasone is quantified. That example will follow the other example, since the same steps are taken, regardless of study type.

Table 1
Steps in Establishing the Protocol for a Meta-analysis

Statement of Purpose: the Research Question	
Data definition	**Data analysis**
Defining acceptable studies	Analysis of individual studies
Inclusion criteria	*Individual effect size*
Exclusion criteria	*Confidence interval or significance*
Defining acceptable patients	Combinability of data
Inclusion criteria	*Statistical analysis*
Exclusion criteria	*Graphical analysis*
Defining acceptable diagnoses	*Identification of moderator*
Inclusion criteria	*variables*
Exclusion criteria	Quality analysis of studies
Defining acceptable treatments	Summary statistics
Inclusion criteria	*Overall effect size*
Exclusion criteria	*Confidence interval or significance*
Defining acceptable comparison	Primary method
groups	Confirmatory method
Inclusion criteria	*Power considerations*
Exclusion criteria	Sample size
Defining outcomes	Publication bias
Inclusion criteria	Subgroup analyses
Exclusion criteria	*Study types*
Data extraction procedure	*Patient types*
Defining search procedure	*Treatment levels*
Defining databases	*Other moderator variables*
Defining search terms	**Interpretation of results**
Identification of acceptable	Analysis of accepted studies
articles	Analysis of rejected studies
Article retrieval	Support of studies
Blinding procedure	Other evidence
Judgment of acceptability	*Animal evidence*
Agreement of judges	*Incidental findings*
Data extraction procedure	Overall conclusions
Blinding procedure	Caveats
Data to be extracted	Implications of findings
Extractor agreement	Economic impact

Step 1. Statement of Purpose: The Research Question.

Every research project is undertaken to address a specific problem. It is absolutely essential that the purpose of a meta-analysis be stated explicitly and unambiguously. Without an explicit statement, it is impossible to judge whether the project accomplished its mission. Consequently, the results could be rendered meaningless.

The statement of purpose must capture the essence of the project, but does not need to include every detail. Subsequent sections define and delimit the problem by supplying operational definitions. Thus, the purpose may be stated in broad terms to allow the reader to understand what problem is being addressed.

> The purpose of the study was to determine whether a relationship exists between maternal consumption of Bendectin during pregnancy and subsequent fetal abnormality.

Step 2. Data Definition.

As stated above, data definition occurs *before* data collection. The purpose of this section is to define variables to clarify the nature of data to be collected and analyzed. It provides operational definitions for the variables under study. These variables include the independent and dependent variables, the sample of studies to be analyzed, and the procedure for finding, verifying, and analyzing the studies.

Like any other form of research, we must carefully and completely define the independent and dependent variables (or their equivalents). Independent variables include, for example, those drugs, forms, doses under study. Dependent variables are the outcomes that are measured, such as decrease in blood pressure, incidences of adverse events, or success rates.

It is essential to identify factors related to the outcome of interest so that only pertinent variables are included in the analysis. Three options are available when mixed results are included in a report: (1) eliminate studies that do not conform to your preestablished protocol, (2) control for factors that influence outcomes, or (3) extract data that do conform. For example, if interest is in the pediatric use of a drug and if a study was found that dealt with a mixture of children and adults, the researcher could eliminate the study as nonconforming, stratify results by age or control for age statistically, or isolate and extract only data from cases that apply to the research at hand. If those data can be extracted, then they should be used.

Defining Acceptable Studies. In this section, the researcher must define the aspects of the study that would be acceptable, including, for example, its research design type, literary presentation, location, and language. As mentioned above, epidemiologic studies may be case–control or cohort types and may be done either prospectively or retrospectively. Some researchers will accept all types, but some may prefer to include only data gathered prospectively that they consider less biased. Intervention studies may be single blind, double blind, or open. Patients may or may not be randomized between treatment and control groups. For example, Sacks et al.[8] analyzed the quality of meta-analyses of randomized controlled trials and found that a wide variety of studies had been used, with varying degress of quality. The researcher must decide beforehand which of the available types of research designs would be acceptable for the meta-analysis.

Literary presentation refers to the type of articles and publications accepted. Consideration must be given to the medium (Will studies published in books be combined with those from journals?), review status (Are nonreviewed articles equivalent to peer-reviewed articles?), prestige of the publication (Are equal weights given to articles in the *New England Journal of Medicine*, which has a panel of biostatisticians on staff, and *Drug Store News*?), article type (Are letters to the editor as valid as "full" articles if they contain sufficient data for analysis?), and time of publication (Is it valid to combine articles published in 1960 with those from 1996?).

Another publication consideration is the language in which the original report is published. Some foreign language journals publish abstracts in English. If the abstract contains adequate information, the data may be usable. However, if a question should arise, there could be a problem with interpretation. Unless you are proficient in other languages and can guarantee a perfect scientific translation, it is preferable to limit your search to studies published in English.

The location of the research study may be important. The analyst must decide in what institutions conditions are sufficiently similar to provide comparable results. For example, types of hospitals may affect results, and at other times the setting may be irrelevant. Teaching hospitals may differ from general, long-term-care, specialty hospitals; clinics; and community or outpatient practice. Also, the country in which the research is done may have an impact on results. Pharmacy, nursing, or medical practice may be different in other countries, which could affect interpretation of results. However, the effectiveness of a drug should not vary unless there are genetic differences to consider, such as differing rates of rapid acetylators in Asian countries.

INCLUSION CRITERIA. Inclusion criteria should list all the requirements for entry into the analysis. All studies should be primary research reports. Subsequent sections below help pinpoint those that will eventually form the source of the data to be analyzed.

This study accepted all research studies published in English that examined the relationship between first trimester Bendectin administration in humans and the presence of malformations in the offspring. Both case–control and cohort studies were accepted, as were prospective and retrospective studies.

EXCLUSION CRITERIA. Exclusion criteria should not repeat the inclusion criteria (i.e., only stating the negative). They should present reasons why studies that do meet inclusion criteria should be subsequently disqualified. The most common criterion is failure to provide adequate data or data that are meaningful to the study.

The exclusion criteria may serve to define variables more precisely than did the inclusion criteria. For example, if the inclusion criteria accepted randomized controlled trials of triazolam in geriatric patients, exclusion criteria could eliminate patients aged younger than 70 years or those older than 90 years. Thus, "geriatric" has been more precisely defined for the purposes of that particular analysis. Another study could focus on adult subjects (inclusion criterion) but reject studies dealing exclusively with geriatrics (exclusion criterion).

Also, exclusion criteria identify confounding variables and how they must be controlled.

> Excluded were studies that did not match or control for confounding factors, including maternal age, parity, diet, smoking, alcohol consumption, concurrent drug use (both prescription and nonprescription), drug abuse, or socioeconomic status, all of which have been shown to be related to adverse fetal outcomes.

Defining Acceptable Patients. When comparing drug studies, there is usually an acceptable range allowable for patients. For example, studies on geriatric patients may include persons older than 60, 65, or even 70 years. Sometimes, the "old-old" (i.e., >80 y, even >90 y) are excluded because of pharmacologic differences in drug effect and disposition. Similar problems occur with pediatric meta-analyses, where it may or may not be permissible to combine results from studies using different ranges of age.

Age is but one consideration. Any patient characteristic or factor that could cause a systematic difference in results needs to be identified. Methods for dealing with systematic differences (e.g., blocking) must be addressed, or such studies may have to be excluded from the analysis. It is therefore necessary for the meta-analyst to decide a priori what types of patients are acceptable for each particular research.

INCLUSION CRITERIA. All adult women aged 18–40 years were accepted.

EXCLUSION CRITERIA. Excluded were women taking drugs, such as anticonvulsants, known to have a risk for malformation. Also excluded were women who had conditions that could cause fetal problems, such as uncontrolled epilepsy.

Defining Acceptable Diagnoses. It is necessary to define precisely the diagnosis. For example, when studying hypertensive patients, the researcher must define what is meant by hypertension (e.g., diastolic >90 mm Hg or >100 mm Hg) and how diagnosis may be determined. It is preferable to have objective measurements to verify the diagnosis (e.g., supine diastolic blood pressure >90 mm Hg).

INCLUSION CRITERIA. For this study, pregnancy was the diagnosis, which is rather straightforward. However, there could be a difference between first, second, or later pregnancies. If so, this must be specified. Twins or multiple births also were accepted.

EXCLUSION CRITERIA. Excluded were women who had already been entered into the study on a previous date. Note that epidemiologic studies often carry on for years; hence, a woman could reenter several times, if allowed.

Defining Acceptable Treatments. The researcher must define the drug used and specify equivalent forms (e.g., tablets, capsules, injectables, suppositories) or products (e.g., brands, generics) that would be accepted as equivalents. The dose and route of administration should be specified (if pertinent) as well as acceptable regimens. If, for example, different doses and regimens alter results, then data may have to be stratified and analyzed separately.

In any primary study, there is a need to verify exposure to the drug, especially in epidemiologic studies or unsupervised settings. There must be a guarantee of exposure to the treatment. Also, patient compliance must be verified.

Adverse reactions to drugs pose a particular problem from the point of view of exposure. Sometimes, a single tablet is adequate to produce the adverse reaction. However, some reactions require prior exposure, and others require prolonged administration or a minimal concentration to produce an effect (e.g., methotrexate).

INCLUSION CRITERIA. The study accepted all mother/child pairs with ingestion/exposure in utero to any amount of Bendectin during the first trimester of pregnancy. Studies that dealt with first-trimester exposure plus other exposure were also included. Bendectin was originally formulated with three ingredients (doxylamine, dicyclomine, and pyridoxine). However, the antinauseant effect was due to the pyridoxine and, in 1976, the antispasmodic dicyclomine was removed. Thus, studies were considered acceptable if they reported on either combination of doxylamine and pyridoxine or doxylamine, dicyclomine, and pyridoxine. Any brand was accepted, including Bendectin, Diclectin, Lenotan, or Debendox.

EXCLUSION CRITERIA. This study excluded articles that examined first-trimester exposure but combined the data with non-first-trimester exposure only. That is, studies were excluded if first-trimester exposure data could not be extracted.

Defining Acceptable Comparison Groups. Most research studies compare a treated group of subjects with a second group. Persons in the second group may receive placebo, standard therapy, or another comparable drug. Other studies may use historical controls or population comparisons, or each subject may serve as his own control (i.e., a pre- and posttest). A valid meta-analysis requires that all comparison groups be either identical or very similar. Otherwise, differences in results could be due to the differences in comparison groups and not due to the drug under investigation. The analyst must decide what constitutes acceptable comparisons. If different types are used, there is the option of performing subanalyses to verify comparability.

INCLUSION CRITERIA. This study accepted only patients who were not exposed to Bendectin during pregnancy as controls. Other antinauseants could be used, provided they did not have a known association with malformations.

EXCLUSION CRITERIA. These criteria were as above for the treatment group.

Defining Outcomes. For each analysis, the acceptable outcomes must be specified. It is not always necessary to have exactly the same method of measuring the outcome or even the same measurement units, as long as the different methods evaluate the same construct. It is important that measurements be objective and replicable.

Where there are categorical outcomes, each must be defined explicitly. For example, outcomes for an antibiotic may be either cured or not cured. Acceptable definitions must be presented for each category (e.g., cure may be microbiologic, clinical, or both).

INCLUSION CRITERIA. There were two possible outcomes: malformed and healthy infants. Malformed included the presence of one or more major malformations or more than one minor malformation as defined by Heinonen et al.[13] Healthy infants were defined as infants not having such malformations.

EXCLUSION CRITERIA. The study excluded case–control comparisons between different types of malformations.

Step 3. Data Extraction Procedure.

The protocol should specify all procedures involved in data extraction including the databases, search words, and methods of extraction. If more than one person is involved, then the tasks of each person should be specified as well as methods for ensuring interjudge agreement.

Defining the Search Procedure. A very important requisite for meta-analysis is a thorough literature review. Glass[3,14] advocated an exhaustive search through published and unpublished sources until all possible articles have been found. The reason is that there may be some articles with differing points of view or different results published in different types of journals. It is essential that all points of view be included and that all possible articles be obtained.

Included sources for a literature search are computerized and printed abstracting services, such as MEDLINE or *Index Medicus*, Embase or *Excerpta Medica, Current Contents,* and *International Pharmaceutical Abstracts*. Dissertations and theses are available from university libraries either bound as books or on microfiche and may be located through Dissertation Abstracts, a computerized service. Current textbooks and handbooks are often sources of original data as well as summaries of studies. Finally, the references of all retrieved articles should be investigated for further information. Additional (unpublished) data may be procured from experts in the field.

Unpublished manuscripts and theses are important. Despite being of high research quality, they may not have been published because they represented unpopular topics or because results may have disagreed with those of others. Often, researchers intend to publish material from their theses, but they never find the time. Consequently, Dissertation Abstracts may be the only place to locate many studies.

Another overlooked source of information is the poster or podium session of scientific meetings. Abstracts are often published for such annual meetings as the American Society of Health-System Pharmacists (ASHP), American College of Clinical Pharmacy (ACCP), or American Association of Colleges of Pharmacy (AACP). Finally, many pharmacy residents or PharmD students perform research projects as part of their program. Those reports are often abstracted or may be located in the libraries of teaching hospitals. As stated above, it is essential to locate all possible articles.

DEFINING DATABASES. In this study, the computerized database of Bibliographic Retrieval Services was searched, using key words listed below. All references from abstracted papers and case reports were investigated. Standard textbooks containing summaries of teratogenicity data, such as those by Schardein,[15] Shepard,[16] and Briggs et al.,[17] were consulted for further undetected references.

DEFINING SEARCH TERMS. Search words are used when trying to locate articles in databases, whether manual or computerized. It is important to search for both independent (i.e., name of drug or service) and dependent (i.e., outcome) variables. Search words should include pertinent key words that are listed in *Index Medicus*. If a drug is being investigated, all trade names and alternate generic names should be used. Generic names may differ in different countries. For example, what most of the world calls salbutamol is referred to as albuterol in the US, and what is meperidine in the US and Canada is called pethidine in Britain. Alternate names may be located in *Martindale's Extra Pharmacopoeia* or from drug information centers. Searches may be limited if alternates are not used.

Search words used in this study included the generic names dox-ylamine and dicyclomine and trade names Bendectin, Debendox, Lenotan, and Diclectin. Also included were the terms antinauseant, birth defect, fetal abnormality, teratogenicity, malformation, and adverse outcome.

Identification of Acceptable Articles. The procedure should be specified here. For example, all articles may be located in the library and photocopied by a research assistant. If more than one person performs the task, it is essential that they all follow the same procedure.

ARTICLE RETRIEVAL. All articles were photocopied by an assistant and assembled for analysis. Selection was done by two blinded data extractors (see below).

BLINDING PROCEDURE. Blinding is done to remove bias due to the perceived importance or prestige of the journal in which the report appeared, of the authors, or of sponsoring agencies. As a result, all identifying marks should be removed, and the articles should be judged solely on their own merit. Sacks et al.[8] recommend that articles be judged on their methods, not results. They suggest copying only the methods section and evaluating suitability based on methods only. Blinding should be done by a person not involved in data analysis in any other way.

Methods sections were photocopied by a third person, and two raters evaluated the methods section based on inclusion and exclusion criteria recorded on a sheet of paper. The two judges evaluated independently.

JUDGMENT OF ACCEPTABILITY. As stated above, acceptability should be based on explicit criteria that are replicable. Other researchers must be able to follow the method and produce similar results. The present meta-analysis was, in fact, independently duplicated by another group of researchers who produced the same results (personal communication, S. Lamm).

Agreement of judges. If more than one person evaluates articles, there should be a test to ensure interjudge agreement. It is essential that different people evaluate in the same fashion, or results could vary substantially. Fleiss[18] presents statistical methods for calculating kappa, the coefficient of agreement for categorical data. Rosenthal[6] discusses the calculation of effective reliability for more than one judge when dealing with continuous data (i.e., data that are measured at interval or ratio level).

In this study, there was agreement on all cases, except one. That case involved animals and hence was excluded after the judges discussed the case. The result was complete agreement on case selection. (Note: Another meta-analyst independently performed the same analysis and arrived at an identical list of studies, thus verifying our results.)

Table 2 lists the studies that were included in this analysis,[13,19-34] and Table 3 lists those rejected, along with reasons for their rejection.[35-42]

Data Extraction. Data extraction refers to the numbers that are derived from the individual studies being analyzed. Included should be the number of observations in each group and summaries of outcomes. If the outcome of interest is a categorical variable (e.g., improved/not improved, success/failure), then frequencies are required for each group. If the variable is continuous, such as blood pressure, then the means and standard deviations for each group should be noted. Also, data describing patients may be collected, if pertinent.

For this study, data were entered for each article into a separate 2 × 2 table. In each table, rows presented data for exposed infants and nonexposed infants, while columns separated malformed infants from healthy infants.

Table 2
Studies of the Teratogenicity of Bendectin Meeting the Inclusion Criteria for Meta-analysis

Reference	Study Type	Data Collection	Malformation
Heinonen et al.[13]	C	P	any major
Eskenazi and Bracken[19]	CC	R	any major
Fleming et al.[20]	C	P	any major
Michaelis et al.[21]	C	P,M	any major
Milkovich and van den Berg[22]	C	P	"severe"
Morelock et al.[23]	C	P	1 major or ≥3 minor
Rothman et al.[24]	CC	R	cardiac
Zierler and Rothman[25]	CC	R	cardiac
Aselton and Jick[26]	C	R	any major
Gibson et al.[27]	C	P	any major
Jick et al.[28]	C	R	any major
General Practitioner Clinical Trials[29]	C	P	any major
Golding et al.[30]	CC	R,M	cleft lip/palate
Greenberg et al.[31]	CC	R,M	any major
Newman et al.[32]	C	R,M	any major
Smithells and Shepard[33]	C	R	any major
Bunde and Bowles[34]	C	R,M	any major

C = cohort; CC = case–control; M = matched control group; P = prospective; R = retrospective.

BLINDING PROCEDURE. Similar to the procedure in acceptance of studies, data extraction may be done by photocopying the results section and tables and by extracting data. This serves to reduce bias and to verify numbers.

DATA TO BE EXTRACTED. A list of data to be extracted should be prepared. In the example, 2×2 tables were prepared for each study to facilitate extraction. Also, criteria for inclusion and exclusion were available to assist in selection or to clarify points of confusion.

EXTRACTOR AGREEMENT. When discrepancies arise, extractors must re-evaluate their findings. It is essential that data be extracted accurately; as a result, there must be agreement. In the present example, two extractors compared data and rechecked where discrepancies existed. In the end, there was total agreement. Table 4 lists the data for accepted articles.

Step 4. Data Analysis.

Once studies have been retrieved and data extracted, the focus shifts to analysis. One must consider the combinability of studies, statistics for individual studies, overall summary statistics, confidence intervals (CIs), and subanalyses.

There are many different ways to analyze data. Rosenthal[6,43] and Hedges and Olkin[11] have presented several statistical methods for combining results from independent studies. It should be noted that all methods are estimates or approximations based on various assumptions. Therefore, there will be variations in results, depending on the methods used. Perhaps the best approach is to use two methods and compare.

Analysis of Individual Studies. To prepare studies for analysis, a table should be prepared listing all accepted studies. Individual statistics should be calculated for each study, including the statistical test, test value, significance, sample size, and effect size.

Reference	Reason for Rejection
Harron et al.[35]	inadequate selection of groups and poor definition of treatment
Nelson and Forfar[36]	reported on dicyclomine only
Cordero et al.[37]	compared specific malformations with other malformations
Mitchell et al.[38]	same as above
Mitchell et al.[39]	same as above
Kullander and Kallen[40]	Bendectin not separated from other antinauseants
Yerushalmy and Milkovich[41]	same as above
Gibson et al.[42]	used animals only

Table 3
Studies of the Teratogenicity of Bendectin Rejected from the Meta-analysis

Table 4
Results of Studies Comparing Outcomes of Fetuses Exposed to Bendectin and Those Not Exposed

Reference	Exposure	Congenital Defect			Chi-Square	p Value
		Yes	No	Total		
Heinonen et al.[13]	yes	79	1090	1169	0.13	0.718
	no	3169	45 944	49 113		
	total	3248	47 034	50 282		
Eskenazi and Bracken[19]	yes	44	78	122	2.67	0.102
	no	659	1634	2293		
	total	703	1712	2415		
Fleming et al.[20]	yes	31	589	620	0.12	0.728
	no	1208	21 149	22 357		
	total	1239	21 738	22 977		
Michaelis et al.[21]	yes	18	856	874	0.00	1.000
	no	19	855	874		
	total	37	1711	1748		
Milkovich and van den Berg[22]	yes	14	614	628	2.80	0.094
	no	343	9234	9577		
	total	357	9848	10 205		
Morelock et al.[23]	yes	31	344	375	0.45	0.503
	no	93	1222	1315		
	total	124	1566	1690		
Rothman et al.[24]	yes	24	46	70	3.92	0.048
	no	366	1208	1574		
	total	390	1254	1644		
Zierler and Rothman[25]	yes	52	121	173	0.13	0.716
	no	240	607	847		
	total	292	728	1020		
Aselton and Jick[26]	yes	2	1362	1364	0.00	0.957
	no	4	3886	3890		
	total	6	5248	5254		
Gibson et al.[27]	yes	78	1607	1685	0.38	0.538
	no	245	5526	5771		
	total	323	7133	7456		

Table 4 (cont.) Results of Studies Comparing Outcomes of Fetuses Exposed to Bendectin and Those Not Exposed

Reference	Exposure	Congenital Defect			Chi-Square	p Value
		Yes	No	Total		
Jick et al.[28]	yes	24	2231	2255	0.20	0.652
	no	56	4526	4582		
	total	80	6757	6837		
General Practitioner Clinical Trials[29]	yes	2	70	72	0.05	0.815
	no	18	571	589		
	total	20	641	661		
Golding et al.[30]	yes	12	9	21	4.91	0.027
	no	184	398	582		
	total	196	407	603		
Greenberg et al.[31]	yes	76	88	164	0.82	0.365
	no	760	748	1508		
	total	836	836	1672		
Newman et al.[32]	yes	6	1186	1192	2.52	0.113
	no	70	6671	6741		
	total	76	7857	7933		
Smithells and Shepard[33]	yes	28	1685	1713	0.07	0.793
	no	31	1682	1713		
	total	59	3367	3426		
Bunde and Bowles[34]	yes	11	2207	2218	2.55	0.110
	no	21	2197	2218		
	total	32	4404	4436		
Total	yes	532	14 183	14 715	184.79	
	no	7486	108 058	115 544		
	total	8018	122 241	130 259		

INDIVIDUAL EFFECT SIZE. For meta-analysis of epidemiologic studies, the odds ratio (OR) is commonly used to express the risk of occurrence of a given outcome following exposure to a drug. Mathematically, it may be stated as:

$$OR_i = A_iD_i / B_iC_i$$

where A_i, B_i, C_i, and D_i are defined in Figure 1. The OR is an estimate of the relative risk of an outcome when an individual is exposed to a drug. An OR of unity (i.e., 1) means that the risks for exposed and nonexposed people are identical. Ratios higher than unity imply a positive association, and ratios less than unity imply a negative association. Thus, an OR of 2 means that a person is twice as likely to experience the outcome than is a person not exposed.

For other studies such as randomized controlled trials, the OR could be used but usually is not. A more usual outcome is the difference in rates of success. The approach to statistical analysis of those studies is presented below. Others, such as the ratio of proportions, P_t / P_c (where P_t = the rate in the treatment group, and P_c = the rate in controls), should not be used.

> This study will use the OR to summarize the risk of teratogenicity from exposure to Bendectin. A ratio statistically more than 1 indicates a positive association and less than 1 indicates no association.

Table 4 presents the data for all of the accepted studies.

CONFIDENCE INTERVALS OR SIGNIFICANCE. Statistical significance of individual tests should be reported. Alternately, the corresponding CI should be reported (or both). The CI is often preferred because it provides a better estimate of the true value than do tests of significance.

Individual significance will be calculated for each study using the Mantel–Haenszel[44] chi-square. Along with the OR, the 95% CI will be calculated.[45] The formula for the Mantel–Haenszel chi-square is:

$$\chi_i^2 = \frac{(N_i - 1)[\,|\,A_iD_i - B_iC_i\,| - N_i / 2]^2}{n_1 \bullet n_0 \bullet m_1 \bullet m_0}$$

where N_i is the total number of subjects in the individual study, and A_i, B_i, C_i, D_i, m, and n are defined as in Figure 1.

Combinability of Data. Glass[3,14] has espoused the theory that all studies on a given topic should be included in a meta-analysis, regardless of flaws (except grossly misleading studies), because there is a kernel of truth in every study. This position is tantamount to stating that all the variation among studies may be considered to be random error, which cancels out in the long run. That position has not been supported by all analysts.

The other extreme, supported by many authors, is that the quality of all articles should be scrutinized and only the very best accepted for analysis.

They contend that differences are mostly due to systematic error and will not cancel out, causing erroneous conclusions when varying studies are aggregated.

Perhaps the real truth lies somewhere in between. Rosenthal[6] recommended testing studies for homogeneity of effect using statistical tests. If there is a difference, he suggests searching for moderator variables that could be responsible for systematic differences. Otherwise, results could be erroneous if combined. He presents several formulas that may be used, depending on the data.

STATISTICAL ANALYSIS. Breslow and Day[45] presented a chi-square formula for analyzing homogeneity of epidemiologic studies. The formula is as follows:

$$\chi^2 = \sum(w_i \bullet \ln^2 OR_i) - [\sum(w_i \bullet \ln OR_i)]^2 / \sum w_i$$

where OR_i is the OR from an individual study and w is the weight:

$$w_i = [(1/A_i) + (1/B_i) + (1/C_i) + (1/D_i)]^{-1}$$

This is a chi-square test with $k - 1$ degree of freedom, k being the number of individual studies analyzed.

Rosenthal[6] has presented methods for detecting heterogeneity of other study types; these methods are also chi-square tests.

> This study used the formula of Breslow and Day[45] to detect heterogeneity. The resultant chi-square was 25.19, df = 16, p = 0.067, indicating no significant differences among studies.

GRAPHICAL ANALYSIS. L'Abbé et al.[46] recommended the creation of a graphical display to detect heterogeneity and to ensure combinability. Outcomes of control and treatment groups are plotted on the x and y axes of a graph, respectively. A regression line can be calculated, and tests can be done to identify outliers.

> Figure 2 presents the data display for this study. Two points were identified as outliers. However, no systematic difference with other studies could be found and, since the statistical test was not significant, the decision was made to include both studies in the final analysis.

IDENTIFICATION OF MODERATOR VARIABLES. If heterogeneity is found on either statistical or graphical tests, a search should be made for moderator variables. Ried et al.[47] detected such a problem and provided an analysis and discussion of how they dealt with the situation.

Quality Analysis of Studies. Chalmers et al.[48] developed a method for assessing the quality of clinical trials based on aspects of research design.

Such a method may be used to assess the quality of studies and then weight results accordingly. Several authors advocate such a procedure.

Since at the time of the analysis, no published checklists for scoring the quality of epidemiologic studies could be found, we modified the method of Chalmers et al. to incorporate the essential elements of research design. Two raters scored each study. However, since the quality scores did not correlate with the effect sizes, we did not use quality weighting in the analysis.

Summary Statistics. The summary statistic provides the overall effect of all studies combined. This statistic answers the research question posed; in other words, this number is the reason for the meta-analysis. This is perhaps one of the easiest steps in the analysis, since all of the numbers have been extracted and analyzed.

OVERALL EFFECT SIZE. The Mantel–Haenszel[44] summary odds ratio (OR_s) is widely used in epidemiology. It weights each study according to sample size and provides a reasonable estimation of the overall risk. The formula is:

$$OR_s = (\Sigma A_i D_i / N_i)/(\Sigma B_i C_i / N_i)$$

where N is the number of subjects in the individual study.

For the 17 studies in this analysis, OR_s was 1.01, which was essentially unity (i.e., 1, which indicates no relationship).

CONFIDENCE INTERVAL OR SIGNIFICANCE. The CI provides a statistical test for the significance of results. If unity (i.e., 1) is in the CI for an OR, then the risk of the outcome in question is not significantly greater than that for con-

Figure 2
Plot of Bendectin Risk Versus Control Risk for Congenital Anomaly Reported

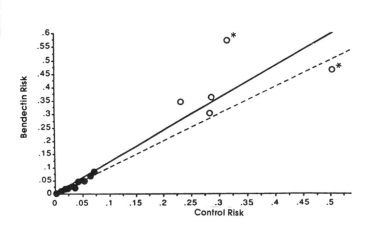

trols. If the lower limit is more than 1, then there is a statistically significant risk. On the other hand, if the upper limit is less than 1, then the exposure is protective against the outcome.

Primary method. Overall significance was tested using the formula of Mantel and Haenszel[44]:

$$\chi^2 = [\Sigma A_i - \Sigma E(A_i) - 0.5]^2 / \Sigma V(A_i)$$

where $\Sigma(A_i) = n_i m_i / N_i$ and $V(A_i) = n_1 \bullet m_1 \bullet n_0 \bullet m_0 / [N_i^2(N_i - 1)]$. The chi-square has 1 degree of freedom that provides a two-tailed result that may be halved for a one-tailed test. The chi-square value was 0.05, which had a two-tailed $p = 0.815$. Since it was not significant, no association was indicated.

Confirmatory method. Rosenthal[6] described the widely used method of Fisher for adding logs. The natural logarithm of the p value for each study is calculated and summed, and this total is multiplied by –2 to arrive at an overall chi-square value that has $2k$ degrees of freedom (where k = the number of studies). Thus, the natural log for the p values in Table 4 was determined. The chi-square value was 39.78 (df = 34; p = 0.228). This result confirmed that of the primary analysis.

POWER CONSIDERATIONS. It is desirable to determine the power or robustness of results. When there are small numbers of studies, results are less conclusive than when there are large numbers. This situation is analogous to the finding of no difference between groups in a clinical trial of two drugs. There may be no difference between groups, or there may have been too few subjects in the study to detect the difference. With a meta-analysis, the same may be true.

Muñoz and Rosser[49] have presented a method for calculating the power of a set of 2 × 2 tables, including those using the Mantel–Haenszel method, and sample size tables. However, that method is rather complex for those who have only a basic understanding of statistics, and help from a biostatistician may be needed to carry out computations. An alternate approach is suggested below under publication bias.

Sample size. The size of the samples in each individual study could have an impact on results. Some authors suggest weighting studies by their sample size or their variance to give more weight to larger studies. That suggestion is based on the premise that studies having larger numbers of subjects are likely to provide a better estimate of the true effect than would small studies.

> Since this study used the Mantel–Haenszel method for combining data, it in fact did weight each effect size (i.e., OR) by its sample size.

Publication bias. Rosenthal[50] identified a tendency in the literature to publish only significant findings. He termed this the "file drawer problem," because it results in the accumulation of unpublished studies in the file drawers of researchers. There is also the case of bias and popularity of topics. For example, Koren et al.[51] have shown that drug studies that indicated a teratogenic effect of cocaine were much more likely to be published than those showing no adverse effect, despite their superior methodologic quality. Therefore, it is recommended that meta-analysts attempt to calculate the impact of potential unpublished reports.

Orwin[52] has published a formula that may be used to determine how many studies would be needed to nullify a given outcome (i.e., effect size) from a meta-analysis. The formula is as follows:

$$N_{fs} = N_0(d_0 - d_c)/(d_c - d_{fs})$$

where N_{fs} is fail-safe N, the number of studies required to raise (or lower, as the case may be) an effect size to any given value; N_0 is the number of studies in the meta-analysis; d_0 is the calculated effect size d; d_c is the desired effect size; and d_{fs} is the effect size of studies "to be added."

> In this analysis, Cohen's d[53] was calculated for each study from its chi-square value and by using the formula:
>
> $$d = [4^2/(N_i - \chi^2)]$$
>
> The overall d was 0.013, which could be described as very small (i.e., not clinically significant). To raise this effect to 0.2, which Cohen would call "small" would require:
>
> $$N_{fs} = 17(0.013 - 0.2)/(0.2 - 0.5) = 10.6$$
>
> or 11 studies having an effect size of 0.5.

Since none of the published studies produced an effect size as large as 0.5 (the largest being 0.007), it would be highly unlikely that one could find 11 unpublished reports (of similar size to those in this meta-analysis) with effect sizes of that magnitude. Similarly, 33 studies having effect sizes of 0.3 would be required. It seems highly improbable that so many studies would have been overlooked on such a contentious issue.

Subgroup Analyses. Subgroups can be divided according to any moderator variables that could influence results. Moderator variables are simply names of groups to which subjects could belong. Examples could be age (e.g., pediatric, geriatric), severity of illness (e.g., mild, moderate, severe), dose of drug given (e.g., high vs. low dose), route given (e.g., iv vs. im or po), gender, or any other factor possibly related to outcomes. Some researchers prefer to use logistic regression that statistically accounts for moderator variables while providing a more accurate estimate of the true results.

> Since Bendectin was marketed in two forms (two-component and three-component), a question naturally arose as to whether the

three-component product could have been problematic, but not the two-component product. Therefore, cohort studies containing only the three-component product were isolated and analyzed. The resultant OR_s was 0.87 (95% CI 0.55 to 1.37), indicating no relationship.

STUDY TYPES. If different types of studies are included, they may provide results that are dissimilar because of the data collection method. For example, case–control studies tend to have very high rates of prevalence of adverse outcomes compared with cohort studies that have low rates but comparable ratios of risk. Thus, it may be wise to separate study types to detect possible discrepancies.

The OR_s for cohort studies was 0.95 (95% CI 0.62 to 1.45), indicating no relationship. For case–control studies, OR_s was 1.17 (95% CI 0.83 to 1.94), again showing no effect. Tables 5 and 6 display the data from these study types.

PATIENT TYPES. The type of patient could influence outcomes. Age, gender, severity of illness, and many more factors could influence outcomes. Therefore, one should determine which factors could be important and analyze data accordingly.

Table 5
Risk Ratios and Confidence Intervals for Cohort Studies Comparing Malformation Risk in Fetuses Exposed and Not Exposed to Bendectin

Reference	Malformation Risk		Risk Ratio	95% Confidence Interval[a]
	Bendectin	Control		
Heinonen et al.[13]	0.068	0.065	1.05	0.84 to 1.30
Fleming et al.[20]	0.050	0.054	0.93	0.65 to 1.31
Michaelis et al.[21]	0.021	0.022	0.95	0.50 to 1.79
Milkovich and van den Berg[22]	0.022	0.036	0.62	0.37 to 1.06
Morelock et al.[23]	0.083	0.071	1.17	0.79 to 1.73
Aselton and Jick[26]	0.001	0.001	1.43	0.26 to 7.78
Gibson et al.[27]	0.046	0.042	1.09	0.85 to 1.40
Jick et al.[28]	0.011	0.012	0.87	0.54 to 1.40
General Practitioner Clinical Trials[29]	0.028	0.031	0.91	0.22 to 3.84
Newman et al.[32]	0.005	0.010	0.48	0.21 to 1.11
Smithells and Shepard[33]	0.016	0.018	0.89	0.54 to 1.51
Bunde and Bowles[34]	0.005	0.009	0.52	0.25 to 1.08
Average	0.030	0.031	0.91	
Standard deviation	0.025	0.022		
Summary odds ratio			0.95	0.62 to 1.45

[a]$CI_i = RR_i \bullet \exp(\pm 1.96 \bullet [(1 - A_i/n_i)/A_i + (1 - C_i/n_{oi}]^{1/2})$, where RR_i = the risk ratio $(A_i/n_{1i})/C_i/n_{oi})$.

In this study, many factors could influence teratogenic outcomes. For example, the age of the mother, alcohol ingestion, smoking, socioeconomic status, have all been linked with adverse outcomes. However, in all of the studies involved, the investigators either matched patients or statistically controlled for all those factors. Therefore, a subanalysis by patient type was not needed.

TREATMENT LEVELS. The amount of drug ingested could affect outcomes. Where possible, data should be separated to determine whether a relationship exists between drug dose and outcome.

A few studies did document the exact number of doses taken, but exact data were difficult to extract. As a result, differences between high exposure and low exposure were not examined.

OTHER MODERATOR VARIABLES. Any other factors (i.e., grouping variables) that could be related to outcomes should be identified and analyzed, if possible. This was not done for this study.

Step 5. Interpretation of Results.

It is necessary to interpret results in the light of the data collected, size of studies, similarity of findings, and study types. The analyst should investigate all aspects of the studies and discuss findings while addressing all concerns. This advice is especially true if controversy exists in the literature.

Table 6
Mantel–Haenszel Estimates of Odds Ratios and Confidence Intervals for Case–Control Studies of Fetuses Exposed and Not Exposed to Bendectin

Reference	AD/N	BC/N	Odds Ratio (AD/BC)	95% Confidence Interval[a]
Eskenazi and Bracken[19]	29.77	21.28	1.40	0.96 to 2.05
Rothman et al.[24]	17.64	10.24	1.72	1.04 to 2.86
Zierler and Rothman[25]	30.95	28.47	1.09	0.76 to 1.55
Golding et al.[30]	7.92	2.75	2.88	1.19 to 6.96
Greenberg et al.[31]	34.00	40.00	0.85	0.62 to 1.17
Total	120.28	102.74	7.94	
Average odds ratio			1.58	
Summary odds ratio			1.17	0.83 to 1.94

A = number of malformed infants who had been exposed to Bendectin; B = number of nonmalformed infants who had been exposed to Bendectin; C = number of malformed infants who had not been exposed to Bendectin; D = number of nonmalformed infants who had not been exposed to Bendectin.

[a] $CI_i = (A_iD_i/B_iC_i) \cdot \exp[\pm 1.96 \cdot (1/A_i) + (1/B_i) + (1/C_i) + (1/D_i)^{-1}]$.

Analysis of Accepted Studies. Of the 17 studies accepted, only two showed a statistically significant relationship between Bendectin exposure and teratogenicity. The ORs were 1.72 and 2.88 and were calculated on 1644 and 603 subjects, respectively. Thus, sample sizes were smaller than the average in those studies. Also, the study by Rothman et al.[24] was questioned because of recall bias that resulted from the method of questioning the mothers. Subsequent analysis showed no relationship.[25] Since the overall OR was not significant, the conclusion is that no relationship exists.

Analysis of Rejected Studies. Rejected studies could not be analyzed, as they did not provide adequate data. Harron et al.[35] did not show exposure to the drug; they merely guessed at the possible number of exposures by dividing the number of tablets dispensed in the country by the estimated number of pregnant women. Results are, therefore, difficult to interpret. Three articles dealt with antinauseants in general, but data for Bendectin could not be separated. Significant problems were not reported in those studies.

This study also did not consider studies that compared specific malformations with other malformations. There were three such studies[37-39] that sought to establish whether Bendectin could have been responsible for a specific syndrome of malformations. None of those studies found a relationship.

Support of Studies. It has been suggested that support of research could influence the results. For example, a study financed by a drug company could tend to produce results favorable to the company.

> In this analysis, eight (47%) were supported by government grants, three (18%) were reports from "research institutions" with support not stated, five (29%) were from physicians affiliated with a university (support not stated), and only one (6%) was supported solely by a pharmaceutical manufacturer. Therefore, there was little evidence of bias due to support.

Other Evidence. Any other evidence, pro or con, should be presented and discussed so that all information may be analyzed. No study in this analysis encountered further evidence of value.

ANIMAL EVIDENCE. Often, animal studies may provide evidence that will confirm or refute human findings. The information from laboratories may help to confirm theories of malformation or drug action that can never be performed on humans. Sometimes, caution must be advised in interpretation of such data or extrapolation to humans. It must be remembered that thalidomide was not teratogenic to rats or mice but, tragically, it is to humans.

None of the animal studies demonstrated a relationship between Bendectin administration and birth defects. This supported our findings in humans.

INCIDENTAL FINDINGS. If any other evidence has been discovered that may have significance to the question under investigation, it should be mentioned. However, it should be noted that those findings were incidental, not planned. Hence, their interpretation may not be straightforward. None was found in this study.

Overall Conclusions. Bendectin was found not to be associated with teratogenicity.

Caveats. Caveats include limitations of the meta-analysis due to method, inclusion and exclusion criteria, or problems encountered. It helps to focus the results by stating limitations. For example, the analyst should state whether a new treatment is more effective than a former one, but must perhaps compare costs. Conclusions may be only suggestions for further research.

Bendectin was not associated with birth defects. However, the product has been removed from the North American market.

Implications of Findings. There should be a discussion of the meaning of the results when extrapolated to the population. Implications may be made in terms of health care, patient status, time saved for professionals, and so on.

Since Bendectin is not teratogenic, cases of litigation have no foundation. As a result, they should cease. Moreover, the only effective treatment for the nausea and vomiting of pregnancy has been removed from the market needlessly. A cost–benefit analysis should be done to determine the economic impact of the drug's removal from the market.

Economic Impact. Sacks et al.[8] have recommended discussion of the impact of new drugs or services because of the climate of cost constraint in health care today.

The impact of not using an antinauseant in pregnancy could affect hospital admissions due to nausea and vomiting of pregnancy, since there is no longer a suitable alternative drug. A study by Neutel and Johansen[54] has shown that this is the case: Hospital admissions have increased for that indication, but cases of teratogenicity have not decreased.

Combining Results from Clinical Trials. The Mantel–Haenszel method is very useful for epidemiologic data. However, the OR is seldom used to describe the results from clinical trials. More often, clinicians are interested in the difference between success rates, rather than their proportion. That difference applies directly to patient care and is readily understood by all.

DerSimonian and Laird[55] have clearly presented a method for combining results from clinical trials. Their method uses the difference between proportions (e.g., success rates) as its effect size. The general approach, including all of the steps listed for the Mantel–Haenszel method, is still followed; the only difference is in the mathematics for calculating summary statistics.

Meta-analysis Example for Clinical Drug Trials

A STEPWISE APPROACH TO UNDERSTANDING CLINICAL DRUG TRIALS

Step 1. Statement of Purpose: The Research Question.

The purpose of this study was to quantify the increase in control of emesis produced by cisplatin by adding dexamethasone to ondansetron therapy.

Step 2. Data Definition.

Defining Acceptable Studies. INCLUSION CRITERIA. Included were randomized, controlled trials of ondansetron and dexamethasone with ondansetron and placebo.

EXCLUSION CRITERIA. Excluded were dose-ranging studies.

Defining Acceptable Patients. INCLUSION CRITERIA. Cisplatin-naïve adults aged 18 years and older receiving cisplatin chemotherapy were included.

EXCLUSION CRITERIA. Excluded were patients receiving concomitant antiemetics and/or psychotropics, or any emetogenic drug; also excluded were patients having other illnesses that could result in emesis (e.g., influenza, Ménière's syndrome).

Defining Acceptable Diagnoses. INCLUSION CRITERIA. Any cancer requiring high-dose cisplatin was eligible for inclusion.

EXCLUSION CRITERIA. Use of multiple chemotherapy regimens was cause for exclusion.

Defining Acceptable Treatments. High-dose (i.e., ≥ 50 mg/m^2) intravenous cisplatin only along with any dose of dexamethasone orally, intravenously, or intramuscularly was an acceptable treatment.

Defining Acceptable Comparison Groups. Similar patients receiving high-dose cisplatin plus placebo, as above, constituted an acceptable comparison group.

Defining Outcomes. INCLUSION CRITERIA. The outcome included complete or major control of emesis (0–2 events in the 24 h after receiving cisplatin).

Step 3. Data Extraction Procedure.
Defining the Search Procedure. DEFINING DATABASES. MEDLINE, Embase, *International Pharmaceutical Abstracts*, and CancerLit were searched, as well as all references.

DEFINING SEARCH TERMS. Terms used included ondansetron, emesis, nausea, cisplatin, dexamethasone, and clinical trial.

Identification of Acceptable Articles. ARTICLE RETRIEVAL. Articles were retrieved by a researcher using the search terms indicated above. Only randomized, placebo-controlled trials were included in the initial search.

BLINDING PROCEDURE. Accepted articles were assigned a random number, and methods sections were photocopied in two sets, eliminating all references to author, journal, title, financial support, date, or location of study.

JUDGMENT OF ACCEPTABILITY. Two blinded judges were given the methods sections and copies of criteria and asked to indicate the acceptability of each study.

Agreement of Judges. Studies accepted by both judges were retained; those with disagreement were arbitrated by a third, unblinded reviewer, whose judgment was binding.

Data To Be Extracted. Data included results for each drug regimen, and results were categorized as either successful (i.e., 2 episodes of vomiting within 24 h of chemotherapy administration) or not successful (i.e., >2 episodes of vomiting). Two other reviewers extracted data into 2×2 tables. Interjudge agreement was adjudicated by a third, unblinded reviewer to reconcile all differences.

In this research, three studies were accepted for the analysis, including those by Roila et al.,[56] Smith et al.,[57] and Smyth et al.[58] Clinical data appear in Table 7.

Step 4. Data Analysis.
Analysis of Individual Studies. INDIVIDUAL EFFECT SIZE. The effect size of interest in this meta-analysis is the difference between success rates. That effect size tells us how much more effective emesis control was when dexamethasone was added to the regimen. For each study, the success rate is calculated for the treatment group (r_t) and for the control group (r_c).

		Rates of Emesis Control		Rate Difference	
Table 7 Clinical Data from Studies Comparing Ondansetron with Ondansetron and Dexamethasone in Cisplatin-Induced Emesis	**Reference**	**Treatment (%)**	**Control (%)**	**(Effect Size)**	**p Value**
	Roila et al.[56]	86/89 (97)	72/89 (81)	0.157	<0.001
	Smith et al.[57]	21/26 (81)	11/24 (46)	0.349	0.011
	Smyth et al.[58]	58/84 (69)	47/84 (56)	0.131	0.055

$$r_t = s_t/n_t \text{ and } r_c = s_c/n_c$$

where s_t = the number of patients in the treatment group who were successfully treated, n_t = the total number of patients who received the treatment, s_c = the number of successes in the control group, and n_c = the total number of patients in the control group. Thus, the effect size R_i for each study = $r_t - r_c$.

Clinical data appear in Table 7. The percentage values are the success rates, r_t and r_c; the effect sizes are also identified.

CONFIDENCE INTERVALS OR SIGNIFICANCE. As for epidemiologic studies, it is possible and often preferable to display effect sizes for each study (see Chapter 10 dealing with CIs). An alternate approach is to determine the statistical significance of findings. With 2×2 tables, one can use Fisher's exact test (which is always the best choice because it is exact), or chi-square, providing all of the requirements for that test are met. To use chi-square, there must be at least 20 observations, no expected frequency can be less than 5 if there are fewer than 40 observations, and no expected frequency may ever equal zero.

The significance of findings for dexamethasone versus placebo appears in the last column of Table 7.

Further Analyses and Identification. STATISTICAL ANALYSIS. Homogeneity of effect sizes was calculated by using the chi-square statistic Q. The finding that Q was not significant ($Q = 2.32$; df = 2; p = 0.31) suggested that the three studies could be combined legitimately.

GRAPHICAL ANALYSIS. Since Q was not significant, graphical analysis was not done.

IDENTIFICATION OF MODERATOR VARIABLES. As above, this was not done. However, one should note the large variation in absolute rates of emesis control, from 69% to 97% in the dexamethasone group and from 46% to 81% in placebo patients. No reason for those differences could be found, but they could reflect differences in measurement.

Quality Analysis of Studies. A quality scoring scheme was developed for this study, adapted from Chalmers et al.,[48] and verified. Studies were weighted by quality, but no difference was found in overall effect.

Summary Statistics. OVERALL EFFECT SIZE. The overall summary effect size is the weighted difference between success rates. In the present example, it tells us how much more control of emesis is produced by the addition of dexamethasone to ondansetron. Results for calculations appear in Table 8. First, the variance (S_i) is calculated for each effect size (R_i):

$$S_i = [r_t(1 - r_t)/n_t] + [r_c(1 - r_c)/n_c]$$

Variances appear in the second column of Table 8. Next, we calculate a weight for each study. The weight (w_i) for each R_i is the reciprocal of the variance:

$$w_i = 1/S_i$$

This step allows us to weight each effect size R_i in proportion to the total number of subjects in that clinical trial. It thereby gives more weight to larger studies, since one would expect larger trials to estimate the true value better than would a trial with fewer patients.

Weights appear in the third column of Table 8. The homogeneity statistic Q is calculated next:

$$Q = \sum w_i(R_i - R_w)^2$$

where $R_w = \sum w_i R_i / \sum w_i$, the weighted average difference in success rates.

Q is actually a chi-square with $k - 1$ degree of freedom, where k is the number of studies being examined. Thus, Q represents a test for the homogeneity of effect sizes.

> The calculation for Q is at the bottom of the fourth column in Table 8. The value for Q of 2.32 (df = 2) is not significant (p = 0.31), which indicates that the effect sizes are not significantly different between studies. These results suggest that the effect sizes may be combined.

If Q were significant, it would indicate that there is a wide range of R values and would cast doubt on the legitimacy of their combination. However, unlike the Mantel–Haenszel method, the DerSimonian–Laird method incorporates Q into its calculations, thereby acknowledging differences between studies, as well as differences within. To do so, we first calculate the amount of between-study variance to be added to the within-study variance that we calculated above:

$$S_b = \max \{0, [Q - (k - 1)] / [\sum w_i - \sum w_i^2 / \sum w_i]\}$$

Table 8
Meta-analytic Calculations for Clinical Trials

$r_t - r_c$	S_i	w_i	w_i^2	$w_i R_i$	$w_i(R_i - R_w)^2$	w_i^*	$w_i^* R_i$
0.157	0.002	475.688	226 278.60	74.827	0.045	332.567	52.314
0.349	0.016	61.281	3755.31	21.409	2.038	58.062	20.284
0.131	0.005	182.539	33 320.47	23.904	0.237	156.667	20.516
Total	$\sum =$	719.507	263 354.38	120.140	2.320	547.296	93.110

Since the value we are seeking is a variance (i.e., the square of the standard deviation), it cannot be negative. Therefore, if the calculation is negative, we assume that finding was a random error, and we ignore it. In other words, when Q is less than $k - 1$, there is no difference between the studies examined; hence, there is no between-study variation, and we will therefore add 0 to the between-study variance. That is called a *fixed-effects model.* Otherwise, we use a *random-effects model* that utilizes the value calculated in the equation below.

For the present data,

$$S_b = [2.320 - (3 - 1)]/(719.507 - 263\ 354.38/719.507)$$
$$= 0.0009$$

An adjusted weight is then calculated for each study:

$$w_i^* = 1/(S_i + S_b)$$

This weight incorporates the within-study variance (S_i) as well as the between-study variance (S_b) into the calculation.

Adjusted weights are presented in the seventh column of Table 8.

Finally, we calculate the summary statistic, which is the overall weighted difference in success rates:

$$R_s = \sum w_i^* R_i / \sum w_i^*$$

For the dexamethasone example:

$$R_s = 547.296/93.114 = 0.170$$

Therefore, the regimen that included dexamethasone had a rate of control of major emesis that was 17.0% greater than that of ondansetron alone.

CONFIDENCE INTERVAL OR SIGNIFICANCE. To construct a CI, we must first calculate the standard error of the summary statistic:

$$SE_{R_s} = (1/\sum w_i^*)^{1/2}$$

For the example:

$$SE_{R_s} = (1/547.296)^{1/2} = 0.043$$

In other words, the standard error of the difference between success rates is 4.3%. Then, we use the standard error to calculate 95% CIs:

$$CI = R_s \pm 1.96^*(SE_{R_s})$$

If 0 lies within the interval, then there is no difference between treatment and control groups. If both limits of the 95% CI are positive, then treatment is superior; if both are negative, then the control group treatment was superior.

For the example:

$$CI = 17.0 \pm 1.96^*(4.3)$$

Therefore, the 95% CI is 8.6% to 25.4%. In other words, the extra benefit due to the addition of dexamethasone lies between those 8.6% and 25.4% limits, with 95% certainty.

It should be noted that, to do a complete meta-analysis, one would have to follow all of the steps outlined in the previous section. This example has been presented to illustrate the calculation method.

Phase II: Performing the Analysis

In performing this phase of the research, the definitions developed in the preparation phase are applied to the available studies. This part of the analysis is straightforward and can be done relatively quickly, especially when using a spreadsheet for calculations. A well-planned meta-analysis, like other types of research, is mostly done when the planning has been completed. Data collection and analysis are quite simple.

Olkin[59,60] recommends that extensive analysis be done when undertaking a meta-analysis. Indeed, one must "worry the data to death," examining all possible aspects so that we have confidence that our results are robust. Such work takes time, but it is time well spent.

Extensive sensitivity analyses should be performed to examine all assumptions and weaknesses. Particular weaknesses are small numbers of observations in 2×2 tables. One approach is to increase and then to decrease all values in a 2×2 table having small numbers and recalculate results for each alteration. If changes produce a substantially different conclusion, then data may be unstable and a firm conclusion may not be made. Additional information would be required before a "bottom line" statement would be valid. That exercise illustrates the dangers of data misclassification, which is not infrequent.

A note of caution must be given with respect to the correlation of data. Results can be inflated if the data are not independent. That may occur when studies are done on the same subjects or when there are confounding variables that are related to one or more independent or dependent variables. Researchers should ensure that they have investigated their data thoroughly to avoid the problem.

Interpretation of results can be a challenge. Authors must consider the context of the analysis, the limitations of the inputs, and the potential impact of the findings. The discussion section should present not only the findings, but also an examination of rejected studies and how they relate to those findings. Often, they may support the conclusions made. Differences must be examined and explained.

Another approach is to exclude each study in turn and to recalculate the results with each study omitted. In that way, the impact of each study can be determined. Those studies that produce dramatic changes require investigation to evaluate their validity.

Suggestions for further research are usually included. The most obvious source of such recommendations is the limitations of the study. For example, the Bendectin study examined only one product, which was an antihistamine. Thus, an examination of all antihistamine use in pregnancy might be warranted. In the dexamethasone example, use of other steroids or other emetogenic drugs could be examined for indications other than cancer.

Phase III: Presentation of Results

As all researchers are aware, no project is complete until results have been presented. For most of us, it means publication in a peer-reviewed journal that reaches the intended audience. However, other suitable means of disseminating such information are available, including books, symposia, or meetings of scientific or professional organizations.

Current Trends and the Future for Meta-analysis

A trend today is toward the use of evidence-based medicine. Meta-analysis is part of that trend.[61] Sackett[62] has discussed the application of meta-analytic results to patient care. A larger movement in that direction has been taken by the Cochrane Collaboration.[63] That group is preparing, storing, and disseminating a database of meta-analyses of randomized, controlled trials that may be used in evidence-based medical decisions. So far, their efforts have been concentrated on randomized controlled trials, and no attempt is being made to do the same for observational (i.e., epidemiologic) studies that have a great deal of potential.

Meta-analysis has become widespread in the literature. However, there are inherent weaknesses, which derive from the original clinical trials they summarize. Droitcour et al.[64] at the US General Accounting Office have begun to develop a new form of meta-analysis that they have termed *cross-design synthesis*. They noted that randomized, controlled trials have limitations on generalizability of results (i.e., external validity), but have excellent control of research design (i.e., internal validity). In contrast, patient databases have excellent generalizability but poor internal controls. As a result, a method has been developed to incorporate the strengths of the two designs into a single meta-analytic framework. The output from such research should prove beneficial to clinicians.

Lau et al.[61] have developed an approach referred to as *cumulative meta-analysis*. They list the studies by year of publication and combine results beginning with the oldest study. The first result presented is the OR and 95% CI for the oldest study, along with the total number of subjects. Next, they combine the results from that study with those from the next oldest and present the combined data for those two studies. Then, they add results from the third study, and so on, until all studies have been included in turn. By presenting results over time, a pattern becomes established (providing there is a sufficient number of studies) in which the OR seems to stabilize near the final estimate of the OR. As the number of subjects increases, the CI becomes more narrow (i.e., the precision of estimate becomes greater), as the CI is based on sample size. That method allows the researcher to determine when statistical significance has been reached. One can readily see the application of such a technique with new drugs. By performing a cumulative meta-analysis, one can determine when an adequate sample has been reached to demonstrate significance, thus preventing the waste of funds in continuing costly research when outcomes are already known.

Anello and Fleiss[65] have suggested another role for meta-analysis when companies are seeking approval for marketing new drugs. Since integrated summaries of data demonstrating evidence of effectiveness for the claimed indication are required, meta-analysis would be an ideal approach.

Since meta-analysis can be used to summarize success rates of new drugs or competing therapies, application may be made in evaluating policy decisions. Rovers et al.[66] used that approach to evaluate the validity of claims for higher doses of clindamycin in treating various infections.

The current emphasis on cost containment has led to a great deal of interest in pharmacoeconomics. As with policy evaluation, meta-analysis is a tool that can provide the inputs for decision-making. Magar et al.[67] used inputs from a meta-analysis to examine the pharmacoeconomics of warfarin in treating atrial fibrillation. Simes and Glasziou[10] predicted that it "will therefore become an essential tool of cost-effectiveness analysis, for determining an unbiased assessment of effectiveness based on all the relevant evidence."

Conclusion

Meta-analysis is a statistical approach to the aggregation of independent research studies. It is an invaluable tool to assist in evaluating the literature to arrive at an overall estimate of effect or of risk. Because it provides a thorough and systematic approach to analysis, it is to be preferred over previous methods. Drug information specialists are urged to adopt this approach to summarizing the literature. It may well become the standard method for drug evaluation in the future. Practitioners are encouraged to become familiar with the concepts involved in meta-analysis to understand and apply results to practice. Students are urged to undertake meta-analyses as research projects. Meta-analysis provides an effective tool for handling drug information.

The second meta-analysis example was extracted from the group project done by Cindy Girvan, Janice Meisner, Krista Pettit, and Lesley Shane as part of the requirements for PHM605 (Critical Appraisal) during their PharmD curriculum at the University of Toronto in 1993.

References

1. Freiman JA, Chalmers TC, Smith H Jr, Kuebler RR. The importance of beta, the type II error, and sample size in the design and interpretation of the randomized control trial. Survey of 71 "negative" trials. N Engl J Med 1978;299:690-4.
2. Einarson TR, McGhan WF, Bootman JL, Sabers DL. Meta-analysis: quantitative integration of independent research results. Am J Hosp Pharm 1985;42:1957-64.
3. Glass GV. Primary, secondary, and meta-analysis of research. Educ Res 1976;5:3-8.
4. Gerbarg ZB, Horwitz RI. Resolving conflicting clinical trials: guidelines for meta-analysis. J Clin Epidemiol 1988;41:503-9.
5. Teagarden JR. Meta-analysis: whither narrative review? Pharmacotherapy 1989;9: 274-84.
6. Rosenthal R. Meta-analytic procedures for social research. Beverly Hills, CA: Sage Publications, 1984:55-8,94-6.
7. Leviton LC, Cook TD. What differentiates meta-analysis from other forms of review? J Pers 1981;49:231-6.
8. Sacks HS, Berrier J, Reitman D, Ancona-Berk VA. Meta-analyses of randomized controlled trials. N Engl J Med 1987;316:450-5.
9. Lee KA. Meta-analysis: a third alternative for student research experience. Nurse Educ 1988;13:30-3.
10. Simes RJ, Glasziou PP. Meta-analysis and quality of evidence in the economic evaluation of drug trials. PharmacoEconomics 1992;1:282-92.
11. Hedges LV, Olkin I. Statistical methods for meta-analysis. Orlando, FL: Academic Press, 1985.
12. Einarson TR, Leeder JS, Koren G. A method for meta-analysis of epidemiological studies. Drug Intell Clin Pharm 1988;22:813-24.
13. Heinonen OP, Slone D, Shapiro S. Birth defects and drugs in pregnancy. Littleton, MA: PSG Publishing, 1977.
14. Glass GV. Integrating findings: the meta-analysis of research. Rev Res Educ 1978;5: 351-79.
15. Schardein JL. Chemically induced drug defects. New York: Marcel Dekker, 1985.
16. Shepard TH. Catalog of teratogenic agents. 5th ed. Baltimore: Johns Hopkins University Press, 1986.
17. Briggs GG, Freeman RK, Yaffe SJ. Drugs in pregnancy and lactation. 2nd ed. Baltimore: Williams & Wilkins, 1986.
18. Fleiss JL. Statistical methods for rates and proportions. 2nd ed. New York: John Wiley & Sons, 1981.
19. Eskenazi B, Bracken M. Bendectin (Debendox) as a risk factor for pyloric stenosis. Am J Obstet Gynecol 1982;144:919-24.
20. Fleming DM, Knox JDE, Crombie DL. Debendox in early pregnancy and fetal malformation. Br Med J 1981;283:99-101.

21. Michaelis J, Michaelis H, Gluck E, Koller S. Prospective study of suspected associations between certain drugs administered during early pregnancy and congenital malformations. Teratology 1983;27:57-64.
22. Milkovich L, van den Berg BJ. An evaluation of the teratogenicity of certain antinauseant drugs. Am J Obstet Gynecol 1976;125:244-8.
23. Morelock S, Hingson R, Kayne H, Dooling E, Zuckerman B, Day N, et al. Bendectin and fetal development. A study of Boston City Hospital. Am J Obstet Gynecol 1982;142:209-13.
24. Rothman J, Fyler DC, Goldblatt A, Kreidberg MB. Exogenous hormones and other drug exposures of children with congenital heart disease. Am J Epidemiol 1979;109: 433-9.
25. Zierler S, Rothman KJ. Congenital heart disease in relation to maternal use of Bendectin and other drugs in early pregnancy. N Engl J Med 1985;313:347-52.
26. Aselton PJ, Jick H. Additional follow-up of congenital limb disorders in relation to Bendectin use. JAMA 1983;250:33-4.
27. Gibson GT, Colley DP, McMichael AJ, Hartshorn JM. Congenital anomolies in relation to the use of doxylamine/dicyclomine and other antenatal factors. Med J Aust 1981;1:410-4.
28. Jick H, Holmes LB, Hunter JR, Madsen S, Stergachis A. First trimester drug use and congenital disorders. JAMA 1981;246:343-6.
29. General Practitioner Clinical Trials. Drugs in pregnancy survey. Practitioner 1963; 191:775-80.
30. Golding J, Vivian S, Baldwin JA. Maternal anti-nauseants and clefts of lip and palate. Hum Toxicol 1983;2:63-73.
31. Greenberg G, Inman WHW, Weatherall JAC, Adalstein AM, Haskey JC. Maternal drug histories and congenital abnormalities. Br Med J 1977;2:853-6.
32. Newman NM, Corey JF, Dudgeon GI. A survey of congenital abnormalities and drugs in private practice. Aust N Z J Gynaecol 1977;17:156-9.
33. Smithells RW, Shepard S. Teratogenicity testing in humans: a method of demonstrating safety of Bendectin. Teratology 1978;17:31-6.
34. Bunde CA, Bowles DM. A technique for controlled survey of case records. Curr Ther Res 1963;5:245-8.
35. Harron DWG, Griffiths K, Shanks RG. Debendox and congenital malformations in Northern Ireland. Br Med J 1980;281:1379-81.
36. Nelson MM, Forfar JO. Associations between drugs administered during pregnancy and congenital abnormalities of the fetus. Br Med J 1971;1:523-7.
37. Cordero JF, Oakley GP, Greenberg F, James LM. Is Bendectin a teratogen? JAMA 1981;245:2307-10.
38. Mitchell AA, Rosenberg L, Shapiro S, Slone D. Birth defects related to Bendectin use in pregnancy. I. Oral clefts and cardiac defects. JAMA 1981;245:2311-4.
39. Mitchell AA, Schwingl PJ, Rosenberg L, Louik C, Shapiro S. Birth defects in relation to Bendectin use in pregnancy. II. Pyloric stenosis. Am J Obstet Gynecol 1983;147: 737-42.
40. Kullander S, Kallen B. A prospective study of drugs and pregnancy. II. Anti-emetic drugs. Acta Obstet Gynecol Scand 1976;55:105-11.
41. Yerushalmy J, Milkovich L. Valuation of the teratogenic effect of meclizine in man. Am J Obstet Gynecol 1965;93:553-62.
42. Gibson JP, Staples RE, Larson EJ, Kuhn WL, Holtkamp DE, Newberne JW. Teratology and reproduction studies with an antinauseant. Toxicol Appl Pharmacol 1968;13: 439-47.

43. Rosenthal R. Combining results of independent studies. Psychol Bull 1978;85:185-93.
44. Mantel N, Haenszel W. Statistical aspects of the analysis of data from retrospective studies of disease. J Natl Cancer Inst 1959;22:719-48.
45. Breslow NE, Day NE. Statistical methods for cancer research. Vol. 1. The analysis of case–control studies. IARC Scientific Publication No. 32. Lyon, France: International Agency for Research on Cancer, 1980.
46. L'Abbé KA, Detsky AS, O'Rourke K. Meta-analysis in clinical research. Ann Intern Med 1987;107:224-33.
47. Ried LD, McKenna DA, Horn JR. Effect of therapeutic monitoring services on the number of serum drug assays ordered for patients: a meta-analysis. Ther Drug Monit 1989;11:253-63.
48. Chalmers TC, Smith H Jr, Blackburn B, Silverman B, Schroeder B, Reitman D, et al. A method for assessing the quality of a randomized control trial. Control Clin Trials 1981;2:31-49.
49. Muñoz A, Rosser B. Power and sample size for a collection of 2×2 tables. Biometrics 1984;40:995-1004.
50. Rosenthal R. The file drawer problem and tolerance for null results. Psychol Bull 1979;86:638-41.
51. Koren G, Graham K, Shear H, Einarson T. Bias against the null hypothesis: the reproductive hazards of cocaine. Lancet 1989;2:1440-2.
52. Orwin RG. A fail-safe N for effect size in meta-analysis. J Educ Stat 1983;8:157-9.
53. Cohen J. Power analysis for the social sciences. New York: Academic Press, 1977.
54. Neutel CI, Johansen HL. Measuring drug effectiveness by default: the case of Bendectin. Can J Public Health 1995;86:66-70.
55. DerSimonian R, Laird N. Meta-analysis in clinical trials. Control Clin Trials 1986;7:177-88.
56. Roila F, Tonato M, Cognetti F, Cortesi E, Favalli G, Marangolo M, et al. Prevention of cisplatin-induced emesis: a double-blind multicenter randomized crossover study comparing ondansetron and ondansetron plus dexamethasone. J Clin Oncol 1991;9:675-8.
57. Smith DB, Newlands ES, Rustin GJ, Begent RH, Howells N, McQuade B, et al. Comparison of ondansetron and ondansetron plus dexamethasone as antiemetic prophylaxis during cisplatin-containing chemotherapy. Lancet 1991;338:487-90.
58. Smyth JF, Coleman RE, Nicolson M, Gallmeier WM, Leonard RC, Cornbleet MA, et al. Does dexamethasone enhance control of acute cisplatin induced emesis by ondansetron? BMJ 1991;303:1423-6.
59. Olkin I. Meta-analysis: reconciling the results of independent studies. Stat Med 1995;14:457-72.
60. Olkin I. Statistical and theoretical considerations in meta-analysis. J Clin Epidemiol 1995;48:133-46.
61. Lau J, Schmid CH, Chalmers TC. Cumulative meta-analysis of clinical trials builds evidence for exemplary medical care. J Clin Epidemiol 1995;48:45-57.
62. Sackett DL. Applying meta-analyses at the bedside. J Clin Epidemiol 1995;48:61-6.
63. Chalmers I. The Cochrane Collaboration: preparing, maintaining, and disseminating systematic reviews of the effects of health care. Ann N Y Acad Sci 1993;703:156-65.
64. Droitcour J, Silberman G, Chelimsky E. Cross-synthesis design: a new form of meta-analysis for combining results from randomized clinical trials and medical-practice databases. Int J Technol Assess Health Care 1993;9:440-9.

65. Anello C, Fleiss JL. Exploratory or analytic meta-analysis: should we distinguish between them? J Clin Epidemiol 1995;48:109-16.
66. Rovers JP, Ilersich AL, Einarson TR. Meta-analysis of parenteral clindamycin dosing regimens. Ann Pharmacother 1995;29:852-8.
67. Magar R, Doucette D, Kassam R, Seto W, Einarson TR. Warfarin atrial fibrillation: a meta-analysis and pharmacoeconomic analysis. Can J Clin Pharmacol 1995;2:109-17.

Appendix I
Reading List

Books

Glass GV, McGaw B, Smith ML. Meta-analysis in social research. Beverly Hills, CA: Sage Publications, 1981.

Hedges LV, Olkin I. Statistical methods for meta-analysis. Orlando, FL: Academic Press, 1985.

Hunter JE, Schmidt FL, Jackson GB. Meta-analysis: cumulating research findings across studies. Beverly Hills, CA: Sage Publications, 1982.

Light RJ, Pillemer DB. Summing up: the science of reviewing research. Cambridge, MA: Harvard University Press, 1984.

Rosenthal R. Meta-analytic procedures for social research. Beverly Hills, CA: Sage Publications, 1984.

Wolf FM. Meta-analysis: quantitative methods for research synthesis. Beverly Hills, CA: Sage Publications, 1986.

Methodologic Articles

DerSimonian R, Laird N. Meta-analysis in clinical trials. Control Clin Trials 1986;7:177-88.

Einarson TR, Leeder JS, Koren G. A method for meta-analysis of epidemiologic articles. Drug Intell Clin Pharm 1988;22:813-24.

Einarson TR, McGhan WF, Bootman JL, Sabers DL. Meta-analysis: quantitative integration of independent research results. Am J Hosp Pharm 1985;42:1957-64.

Gerbarg ZB, Horwitz RI. Resolving conflicting clinical trials: guidelines for meta-analysis. J Clin Epidemiol 1988;41:503-9.

L'Abbé KA, Detsky AS, O'Rourke K. Meta-analysis in clinical research. Ann Intern Med 1987;107:224-33.

Sacks HS, Berrier J, Reitman D, Ancona-Berk VA. Meta-analyses of randomized controlled trials. N Engl J Med 1987;316:450-5.

Teagarden JR. Meta-analysis: whither narrative review? Pharmacotherapy 1989;9:274-84.

Thacker SB. Meta-analysis: a quantitative approach to research integration. JAMA 1988;259:1685-9.

13

Quality of Life: Outcome Assessment in Pharmacoepidemiologic Studies

J Gregory Boyer
Raymond J Townsend
Paul E Stang
H Michael Arrighi

The pharmacoepidemiologist seeks to understand the effects of drug therapy on patient populations. A complete understanding of these effects cannot be achieved without information describing the full range of a drug's impact on those who take it. Clinical data are vital to this study; however, they are insufficient as the sole data source. Data reflecting a drug's impact on patients' physical, social, and emotional functioning, as well as sense of well-being, must be evaluated in concert with the clinical findings if a complete understanding is to be achieved. Quality-of-life assessments offer the pharmacoepidemiologist a convenient and reliable method for documenting both the positive and negative consequences of drug therapy from the patient's perspective. Increasingly, quality-of-life assessments are included in clinical drug studies. The full scope of their usefulness, however, has yet to be realized. It seems certain that quality-of-life assessments will become data sources central to the study of pharmacoepidemiology.

Outline

Many new words and phrases have been added to the vocabulary of the pharmaceutical scientist to describe the ever-expanding field of drug research. Postmarketing surveillance, pharmaceutics, pharmacovigilance, pharmacoepidemiology, pharmacoeconomics, and pharmaceutical outcomes research have been included in the lexicon to describe a particular research activity that evolved into an identifiable and distinct area of study. One of the most recent important additions to this list is the term "quality of life" in pharmaceutical outcomes research. Health-related quality of life is perhaps a more descriptive term for the patient-centered outcomes of medical care. Patrick and Erickson[1] refer to health-related quality of life as the level of well-being and satisfaction associated with events or conditions in a person's life as influenced by disease, accidents, or treatments. Other researchers[2] refer to quality of life as it relates to health as "the qualitative aspects of recovery." It is this health-related component of quality of life that is addressed in this chapter.

Quality-of-life and pharmacoepidemiology data reflect different perspectives on the same patient. Either may be used to provide descriptive data reflecting events occurring following administration of a drug. Quality-of-life data capture subjective, patient-based impressions, whereas pharmacoepidemiologic data reflect the more objective physiologic consequences of drug therapy and are usually based on physician observation or measurement. Quality-of-life assessments seek to capture the patient's own perspective of the consequences and impact of therapy. This perspective is often overlooked in traditional pharmacoepidemiologic studies.

Quality of life has long been used in sociology, economics, public policy, and marketing, but its meaning is not consistent either across or within disciplines.[3,4] Fayers and Jones[5] observed that "the term 'quality of life' and various synonyms are widely used throughout the social, psychological, and medical sciences but definitions are elusive." Depending on the discipline, the objective, and the perspective of the researcher, quality of life can refer to economic components such as income, housing, and working conditions; to the availability of public services; or to those components of a patient's life affected by his or her state of health.[3] Addressing the 1986 conference "Measuring Quality of Life in Clinical and Epidemiology Research," Spitzer[6] commented on the nebulousness of quality of life as it pertains to health care. In reference to quality of life, he noted, "What is said, what is written, and what is done seems to be determined at times by the theme of the conference one attends or the title of the book to which one contributes a chapter." Feinstein[7] expressed similar sentiments when he described quality of life as a kind of umbrella under which are placed many different indices, each having a focus reflecting the user's particular interest.

The impetus for the growth of pharmacoepidemiology arose as part of a regulatory imperative to systematically assess the adverse effects of drugs; quality-of-life research has been borne out of the social scientists' curiosity in the subjective experience of the individual and the need to quantify, validate, and reproduce these data in large groups. A great driver of the momentum to expand research in these areas has been the pharmaceutical industry's seeking to provide additional evidence of efficacy. Although long interested in adverse events, it has not been until recently that the regulatory authorities have professed an interest in quality-of-life findings; however, their interest currently is largely limited to drug-related promotional claims and price justification arguments.

Despite the lack of a universally accepted definition of quality of life within the healthcare arena, much research effort is directed toward its study. Quality-of-life research generally involves the assessment of nonclinical parameters using patient self-administered questionnaires. Face-to-face interviews, telephone interviews, and patient observations are other ways that quality-of-life data are captured. In certain situations, questionnaires completed by a parent, spouse, significant other, or other appropriate proxy for the patient can provide useful information about a patient's quality of life.

Efforts to measure and quantify the subjective end points assessed in quality-of-life evaluations have given rise to an exciting new focus for drug research. Borrowing heavily from the research tools of the social and behavioral scientists, those conducting quality-of-life assessments are expanding the scope of many research projects. Findings from these assessments are changing the mix of attributes considered when prescribing decisions are made.

The Theoretic Framework of Quality of Life

Schipper[8] described the interest in studying quality of life as the result of an evolutionary process that began with the study of the basic sciences and progressed in a stepwise fashion to the study of patient-outcome measures. He observed that "at every level of development the biologic process is studied from a different perspective: the molecule, the cell, the organ, the disease, and the patient." Focusing on the total patient as the unit of analysis, quality-of-life research is the most recent progression on this evolutionary path. The World Health Organization's (WHO's) conceptualization of health is offered by many researchers as the theoretic origin for the study of quality of life as it is influenced by health and medical care.[9-11] In its 1947 constitution, the WHO declared that "health is a state of complete physical, mental, and social well-being and not merely the absence of disease or infirmity."[12] By expanding the definition of health to include total well-being, traditional measures of morbidity and mortality became inadequate as the sole indicators of health status. Morbidity and mortality provide useful benchmarks for evaluating health from some perspectives; however, these aggregations are not adequate as evaluation parameters when other perspectives are taken. When focusing on the health status of one patient or a small group of patients, one must use a multidimensional approach that addresses physical, social, and emotional functioning, and a sense of well-being in their daily lives is the crux of quality-of-life assessments undertaken by pharmaceutical scientists.

The WHO definition of health established a foundation from which researchers have proposed a number of models for conceptualizing quality of life as it relates to health and healthcare interventions. These models differ in complexity, but are linked by a common regard for the multidimensionality and dynamic nature of health. A simple model depicts health as a continuum anchored on one end by death, progressing through negative health to positive health, and anchored by well-being on the opposite end.[1] Ware[13] proposed a more complex model that considers the impact of disease on personal, psychological, and social functioning.

As shown in Figure 1,[13] this model is composed of a series of five concentric boxes, with the center and smallest box representing disease. Progressing outward, the next slightly larger box in the series represents personal functioning. Continuing outward, the three remaining boxes, each one slightly larger than the one preceding it, focus on psychological distress and well-being, general health perceptions, and social role functioning. This model is often referred to as the "rock in the pond" model. The analogy of a rock dropped into a still pond disrupting the entire surface of the water is a good one to convey a similar idea of the impact a disease has on disrupting the entire life, not just the physiologic life, of the entire patient.

Quality-of-life measures may be considered as representing another health dimension apart from those traditionally used in pharmacoepidemiologic research. Traditional pharmacoepidemiologic measures are based on objective criteria, such as blood pressure. Even fewer physiologic measures

Figure 1
Framework for Discussing Disease and Its Impact on Quality of Life[13]

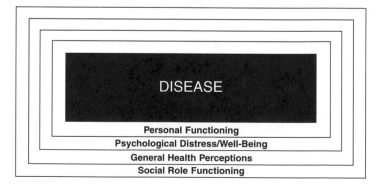

(e.g., socioeconomic status) are based on established objective criteria (e.g., years of education, occupation, income). These traditional, objective measures do not fully explain all the observed differences in health status, which suggests that other, unmeasured health dimensions may be contributing to health. Quality-of-life assessments provide some insight into these currently unmeasured dimensions of health as they directly assess patients for their opinion on their health status. This subjective assessment, in concert with more objective data, provides a more complete framework for the measurement of health status.

Guided by these and other theoretic models depicting health as a multidimensional concept, researchers increasingly became interested in assessing the outcomes or consequences of drug therapy in terms that are traditionally reported anecdotally. It was a logical progression that health assessments of everyday life be included in studies evaluating alternative therapeutic agents. The use of activities of daily living scales, originally developed to assess the level of disability in institutionalized patients and in the elderly, was expanded to include the assessment of physical activities of patients receiving alternative therapies. Used alone, however, activities of daily living scales provide little or no information about the social, psychological, and well-being dimensions of health. A complete evaluation of patient response to treatment is obtained only when the quality-of-life assessment reflects the multidimensionality of health.

The term "quality-of-life assessment" generally has been adopted by the pharmaceutical scientist to refer to the evaluation of the various dimensions of health within a clinical research protocol designed to study patient response to specific therapies. These assessments are increasingly common components of clinical investigations.

The advances in treatment options and the clinical success offered make the findings from quality-of-life evaluations important for prescribers, patients, and policy-makers. Additionally, quality-of-life data are useful to pharmacoepidemiologists as they study the impact of drug therapies on patient populations. Traditionally, epidemiology has been concerned with retrospective analysis of secondary data (e.g., medical records, computer records of diagnoses). For the pharmacoepidemiologists to include quality-of-life assessments in their work, quality-of-life data must be collected prospectively from a patient or a proxy, using repeated measures with the same instrument, and captured in an accessible longitudinal database.

Quality-of-life data provide the pharmacoepidemiologist with the information that often is elusive: the patients' impression of the medication and how they feel it affects their lives. A classic example of this is found in a study by Jachuck et al.,[14] who examined changes in quality of life in 75 hypertensive patients by obtaining questionnaire responses from the physician, patient, and close companion of the patient. All physicians rated their patients as improved (notably, this would have been captured in a study based on the content of the medical record), while 52% of the patients rated themselves as worse or unchanged, and 99% of the close companions rated the patient as worse.

Chronic Diseases and Quality of Life

It is no longer news to report that managing chronic diseases has replaced treating acute infections as the primary activity within health care today.[15-17] The successful treatment of life-threatening infections, the aging population, the lifestyle changes within the population, and the advances in health technology all contribute to the current domination of health care by activities associated with managing chronic diseases. Additionally, although advances in oncology have yielded successful treatments for Hodgkin's disease, testicular cancer, and many childhood cancers, cures remain unavailable for most metastasized solid-tumor malignancies. For many oncology patients, the treatments used make cancer a chronic condition characterized by a series of exacerbations and remissions.[18-20] Managing symptoms, restoring function, and limiting disease progression are the primary objectives of medical care received by patients with chronic maladies.[21]

The General Health Rating Index (GHRI) used in the Health Insurance Experiment[22] demonstrated a relationship with serious physical and/or emotional impairment. Subjects who had a GHRI score in the bottom 10% had a 90% probability of a serious medical or psychiatric diagnosis, while subjects with GHRI scores in the top 10% had only a 10% probability of such diagnoses. Thus, objective measures of health status and diagnoses correlate with subjective general health status measures. These results indicate that the different dimensions, general health status and diagnoses, are related and not coincident. General health status measures reflect some of the underlying individual differences in health status and the individual's perception regarding the impacts of illness and impairments.

The Medical Outcomes Study's 36-item short-form health survey (SF-36) consists of eight quality-of-life subscales: physical functioning, role/physical, bodily pain, general health, vitality, social functioning, role/emotional, and mental health.[23] Among patients with uncomplicated hypertension, a decline in physical functioning, role/physical, and bodily pain is cross-sectionally related to age, while in a 1-year follow-up, a decline was observed in physical functioning, general health, and vitality.[24] These results support the multidimensionality of health status that is not captured by measures of chronologic age and blood pressure alone. Quality-of-life measures are able to further delineate subgroups of the population that may have different responses to therapies. Different quality-of-life scales, incorporating both beneficial and adverse effects, may vary among different diseases or therapies.

Because patients with a chronic illness receive treatment for long periods, quality-of-life assessments can be useful in following their responses to prescribed pharmacotherapy and can help in understanding any disjunction between what the physician can offer and what the patient desires. Quality-of-life assessments, therefore, can have a role to play in finding the optimal therapy for a specific patient by focusing the discussion of treatment on the important aspects of the patient's physical, mental, or social well-being. Patients are unlikely to accept a particular treatment, regardless of its scientific merit, if they perceive it to have no positive impact on their lives.[8] Quality-of-life assessments have the potential to illustrate that positive impact for patients.

In a literature review focusing on quality of life in cancer patients, DeHaes and Van Knippenberg[25] suggest that quality-of-life research is meaningful in three ways. First, findings from quality-of-life studies may provide insight into the patients' reactions to their disease and its treatment. Second, such assessments can provide information needed in the decision process when prescribing therapy. Finally, quality-of-life evaluations may enhance the supportive care provided to patients by family members and medical professionals. These comments are relevant to quality-of-life assessments of patients with other chronic diseases.

Patrick and Erickson[26] also offer uses for quality-of-life findings, including monitoring and assessing patient status, selecting treatments, monitoring the effects of the treatments selected, and developing a shared view of the disease and the treatment outcomes with patients. The usefulness of quality-of-life information in describing patients and evaluating the impact of treatment has been noted by other researchers as well.[17,27,28]

The premise underlying the application of quality-of-life research findings to clinical situations is that this information is important for understanding the full impact of prescribing decisions. Clinical assessment, such as a hemoglobin A1c value, a sedimentation rate, or a white blood cell count, provides invaluable insights into a patient's response to specific pharmacotherapy; however, evaluating only laboratory values cannot provide a complete response profile. By considering quality-of-life findings in conjunction with relevant clinical laboratory results, the clinician is better able to determine the patient's complete response to an intervention. Quality-of-life assessments offer a way for clinicians to capture data in objective and reproducible formats. How and what data to collect depend on the characteristics, the severity, and the prognosis of the conditions being treated.[21,27,29] Characteristics of the patients being studied also must be considered when deciding the format and the content of a quality-of-life assessment.

Capturing Quality-of-Life Data

Karnofsky and Burchenal[30] were early proponents of assessing quality-of-life variables in clinical research. Their 1949 article reporting the use of the Karnofsky Performance Status Scale (KPSS), a 10-point scale for assessing the functional status of cancer patients, is regarded as a significant early contribution to the discipline.[6,10] The 10 levels for assessing performance using the KPSS are detailed in Table 1.[30] Being observation based, the KPSS

	Condition	Performance Status (%)	Comments
Table 1 Karnofsky Performance Status Scale[30]	Able to carry on normal activity and to work; no special care is needed.	100	Normal, no complaints. No evidence of disease.
		90	Able to carry on normal activity. Minor signs or symptoms of disease.
		80	Normal activity with effort. Some signs or symptoms of disease.
	Unable to work. Able to live at home, care for most personal needs. A varying degree of assistance is needed.	70	Cares for self. Unable to carry on normal activities or to do active work.
		60	Requires occasional assistance, but is able to care for most of his or her needs.
		50	Requires considerable assistance and frequent medical care.
	Unable to care for self. Requires equivalent of institutional or hospital care.	40	Disabled; requires special care and assistance.
	Disease may be progressing rapidly.	30	Severely disabled; hospitalization is indicated, although death is not imminent.
		20	Hospitalization is necessary; very sick; active supportive treatment necessary.
		10	Moribund; fatal processes progressing rapidly.
		0	Dead.

has been criticized because it frequently does not yield scores that correlate with the patients' own assessments of their situation and because it fails to address important components of health and well-being.[31] Nonetheless, the KPSS has been used extensively and has been extremely influential.[32]

There have been significant advances in assessing quality of life, in terms of both instruments available and assessments undertaken. An array of quality-of-life scales, indices, and profiles now exists for capturing data. It has been suggested that there may now be too many instruments purporting to measure health status and quality of life.[6] Among the many tools for assessing global quality of life or health status are the Sickness Impact Profile,[33,34] the Nottingham Health Profile,[35,36] the McMaster Health Index,[37,38] and the Duke–UNC Health Profile.[39]

The Medical Outcomes Study-Short Form (MOS-SF) is a global assessment tool that has been used extensively in various iterative forms of quality-of-life research.[40-42] A significant body of literature reporting SF-36 research results is emerging. The SF-36 is the most used tool evolving from the original instrument development work in the Medical Outcomes Study; it contains items that measure physical functioning, social functioning, role functioning, and well-being.[23] Table 2[40-42] contains a brief definition of each of the dimensions measured by the SF-36.

Instruments also are available for assessing quality of life as it is influenced by a specific disease and its treatment. Among these disease-specific instruments are the Functional Living Index—Cancer[18,43] and the Arthritis Impact Measurement Scales.[44-48] A partial listing of disease-specific instruments is found in Table 3.[18,30,44,49-55] A more complete listing can be found in the report by Spilker et al.[56] Assessments undertaken using a combination of disease-specific and general quality-of-life instruments offer the researcher greater insight into a treatment's impact on quality of life than is offered when only a disease-specific or a general quality-of-life tool is used.

Guyatt et al.[57] provide a development sequence to assist the researcher in organizing the activities germane to the development of a disease-specific quality-of-life instrument. Although a number of disease-specific instruments are available, specific questions that investigators want to address may be inadequately covered in existing scales. In these situations, the investigators must develop an instrument to capture the data necessary to answer their questions. The sequence of development steps includes the following: item selection, item reduction, questionnaire formatting, questionnaire pretesting, reproducibility and responsiveness determination, and validity determination. This six-step sequence is also useful to the investigator who must evaluate the appropriateness of existing quality-of-life questionnaires for a particular research project. Reports of instrument development that address each of these six steps assist the investigators in their quest to select well-conceived and rigorously developed assessment tools.

Table 2
Definitions of
Health Concepts
Used in the
Short Form-36
(SF-36)
Instruments[40-42]

Measure	Definition
Physical functioning	extent to which health interferes with a variety of activities (e.g., sports, carrying groceries, climbing stairs, walking)
Role functioning: physical	extent to which health problem interferes physically with usual daily activity
Role functioning: emotional	extent to which health problem interferes emotionally with usual daily activity
Social functioning	extent to which health interferes with normal social activities, such as visiting with friends during the past 4 weeks
Mental health	general mood or affect, including depression, anxiety, and psychological well-being during the past 4 weeks
Health perceptions	overall ratings of current health in general
Vitality	impact of energy level and extent of fatigue during the past 4 weeks
Pain	extent of bodily pain in the past 4 weeks

It was suggested by van Dam et al.[58] that patients are the best judge of their quality of life. Quality-of-life studies use questionnaires self-administered by the patient to collect the data necessary to assess quality of life.

Popular quality-of-life scales included in clinical studies use either a visual analog or a Likert format. These two approaches are most useful because they allow the detection of small changes that may occur during the clinical trial. Using a 10-cm line anchored by the extremes of the item being measured, the visual analog scales allow the respondent to record the response at any point between the two extremes. Modifications of the visual analog scale include capturing the response on a line divided into equal segments[18] and capturing the response in a 10-cm boxed area.[54] It has been suggested that the selection of either the visual analog or the Likert format is appropriate for self-administered questionnaires.[57] Figure 2 provides an illustration of a modified visual analog scale and a Likert scale.

Epidemiology, particularly information on disease natural history, is crucial in placing quality-of-life information into perspective. As many psychological and mood disorders accompany chronic disease, especially depression, understanding the comorbidities and changes in the disease over time may help in the timing of quality-of-life assessments, highlight particular areas of focus for quality-of-life assessments, and aid in the interpretation of quality-of-life results. Population-based epidemiologic data are much more plentiful than population-based quality-of-life data. This is due in part to the difficulties in reconciling data from different sources: epidemiologic measurements of the same event are often acceptable (e.g., myocardial infarction by electrocardiogram evidence vs. symptoms vs. angiogram vs. cardiac enzyme elevations), while quality-of-life measurements by different instruments or surrogates cannot be brought together into a common unit. Language translations and cultural differences to quality-of-life assessments multiply the problem of establishing a common foundation for conducting population-based quality-of-life assessments. Despite the difficulties imposed by languages and cultural variations, much work is progressing to establish valid and reliable translations for existing quality-of-life instruments for use in both research and medical practice.[59-63]

Quality of Life in Clinical Trials

Increasingly, quality-of-life assessments are being included in comparative clinical trials.[10,21] As evidenced by Karnofsky and Burchenal's seminal

Table 3 Partial Listing of Disease-Specific Quality-of-Life Instruments

Disease	Name of Instrument	Reference
Arthritis	Arthritis Impact Measurement Scales	44
Arthritis	Health Assessment Questionnaire disability and pain scales	52
Breast cancer	Breast Cancer Chemotherapy Questionnaire	49
Beast cancer	Linear Analog Self-Assessment Scale	53
Cancer	Functional Living Index—Cancer	18
Cancer	Karnofsky Performance Status Scale	30
Cancer	QL-Index	54
Cancer	Quality of Life Index for Patients with Cancer	55
COPD	Chronic Respiratory Disease Questionnaire	51
Severe burn injury	Burn Specific Health Scale	50

COPD = chronic obstructive pulmonary disease; QL = quality of life.

work,[30] quality-of-life evaluations have been included in cancer research for some time.

Such assessments are becoming commonplace in investigations comparing treatments for coronary artery disease, hypertension, rheumatoid arthritis, and other chronic diseases. Numerous reports of such studies can be found in the medical literature.[47,64-68]

It has been suggested that quality-of-life assessments are not appropriate in all clinical trials. The studies in which these evaluations are most relevant include the following: (1) trials in which the treatments under investigation are anticipated to yield only marginal differences in survival; (2) trials in which one treatment is expected to increase survival while producing severe unintended drug effects compared with alternative therapies; and (3) trials comparing interventions for the lifelong treatment of a chronic disease characterized by mild symptoms.[21,69]

The attribution of causality between event and drug is an integral part of pharmacoepidemiologic research. Often, measures of the strength of the association (i.e., odds ratio, relative risk) are used as evidence that those exposed to the drug are at higher or lower risk of experiencing an event than those who did not receive the drug. Issues regarding time of onset of the event, dose–response, rechallenge, and biologic plausibility are all key concepts in determining whether an effect is attributable to the drug. These issues are particularly difficult to assimilate when the data are obtained outside clinical trials. Quality-of-life data relating to drug therapy are, in contrast, often obtained during the course of a clinical trial in which the environment and all measures are fairly consistent and where the attribu-

Figure 2
Two Formats for Capturing Patients' Responses in Quality-of-Life Studies

Modified Visual Analog Scale

—question from the Functional Living Index—Cancer scale[18]

How much is pain or discomfort interfering with your daily activities?

1	2	3	4	5	6	7

not at all   a great deal

Likert Scale

—question from the Medical Outcomes Study-Short Form[40]

How much bodily pain have you had during the past 4 weeks?

1   *none*
2   *very mild*
3   *mild*
4   *moderate*
5   *severe*

tion of changes in quality of life can be more confidently ascribed to the drug therapy. Changes in quality of life between one period and another may result from a drug's efficacy in treating the illness or managing its symptoms, or quality-of-life changes may result from adverse experiences occurring during the pharmacotherapy.

Reliability, Validity, and Sensitivity of Instruments

Whether selecting a single instrument or a battery of instruments to assess quality of life, the researcher should consider a number of psychometric properties of a given instrument. Unfortunately, there are no published criteria that explicitly state the minimum requirements needed to declare a quality-of-life instrument valid, although the need for such guidelines has been expressed.[10] Nonetheless, failure to consider an instrument's reliability, validity, and sensitivity can render the data collected suspect at best.

RELIABILITY

The reliability of a measurement refers to the proportion of observed variation that is true as opposed to random error.[70] Deyo[71] defines reliability as the ratio of information to random error. Others have defined this term as the extent to which a measuring procedure is free from the effects of random error,[72] the tendency toward consistency of results upon repeated trials,[73] and the degree to which measurements are repeatable.[74] Reliability is a prerequisite for the use of a measurement for any purpose.[75]

The reliability of a quality-of-life instrument is determined by one or more of three possible approaches: internal consistency, test–retest, and interrater. Internal consistency and test–retest reliabilities are reported most often. Interrater reliability usually is provided for instruments designed to capture quality-of-life data through patient observation.

Internal consistency is an estimate of reliability based on the average correlations among items and the number of items in the scale.[76] The general approach used in determining this reliability estimate is known as the split-halves method and involves dividing the instrument into halves and then correlating the half-scale scores. If the original scale is composed of homogeneous items, the two half-scale scores will be highly correlated. A statistical formula, known as Cronbach's coefficient alpha, offers a way to determine the mean reliability coefficient for all possible ways of splitting the instrument into halves. Because it is based on data obtained from a single administration of a scale, internal-consistency reliability is the least expensive and easiest method for determining an instrument's reliability.[26]

The test–retest method correlates data obtained from two administrations of the scale to the same group of respondents under the same conditions. A 2-week interval generally separates these administrations.[75] Because the inherent assumptions of no recall from the first administration and of no change in conditions are weak ones, the test–retest approach is insufficient as the sole determination of an instrument's reliability.

Interrater reliability is an important parameter for instruments designed to capture quality-of-life data by direct observation of individuals. Interrater reliability reflects the degree of agreement among different raters using the same instrument to evaluate the same individuals at the same time.[77]

When selecting an instrument for a quality-of-life study, it is important to understand that reliability coefficients are based on empiric data. These estimates are properties of both the instrument used to capture the data and the population selected to provide the data; the same instrument completed by different populations may give different reliability estimates. It is necessary to consider both the demographic profile and the data collection procedure when evaluating a reported reliability coefficient. Reliability estimates above 0.9 are suggested when making comparisons between individuals. A coefficient between 0.5 and 0.7 allows comparisons between groups.[75] As a rule of thumb, Nunnally[74] suggests that coefficients greater than 0.7 strongly support reliability.

VALIDITY

Random error is not the only threat to accurate measurement. Nonrandom or systematic error can be problematic because of its biasing effect on measurement. The extent to which an instrument is free from nonrandom error is referred to as its validity.[72] Validity is expressed in coefficients that estimate the degree to which an instrument measures what it is intended to measure.[26] Frequent references to content, criterion, and construct validity are encountered in the quality-of-life literature.

Content validity refers to the representativeness of the items included in the instrument. From the domain of all questions that could be asked about a specific dimension of health, only a few make up a quality-of-life scale or subscale targeting that dimension. If the few selected are well representative of this domain, content validity exists. Expert opinion most often serves as the determinant of content validity. Content validity is not empirically based and does not provide sufficient evidence of an instrument's validity.

Criterion validity refers to the extent to which a measure corresponds to some other measure or observation that accurately measures the phenomenon of interest. Traditionally, an agreed-upon gold standard is an assumed prerequisite for determining criterion validity. Since no gold standard exists in the measurement of quality of life,[6,78] determining the criterion validity of quality-of-life instruments uses criteria that are actually related conceptually and provide meaningful empiric tests for a particular clinical application of a scale.[23]

Criterion validity can be determined by assessing the relationship between standard clinical assessments and quality-of-life findings. Examples of this approach to validity assessment are found in reports describing the development of the Arthritis Impact Measurement Scales[44,46-48] and the Chronic Respiratory Diseases Questionnaire (CRDQ).[51] In the Arthritis Impact Measurement Scales development, correlations between the subscale scores and such standard clinical assessments as grip strength and the number of tender joints were reported. In the CRDQ development, scale scores were correlated with forced expiratory volume. For both instruments, logical relationships between scale scores and routine clinical findings were confirmed to support validity claims.

When there is no gold standard, more importance is placed on construct validity, which refers to the strength of the relationship between two or more measurements purporting to measure the same construct. Instruments or subscales within instruments measuring the same construct should be strongly correlated; instruments or subscales within instruments measuring different constructs should be weakly correlated. When data from any independent studies consistently confirm these hypothesized relationships, confidence in a particular instrument's ability to capture information addressing specific constructs is justified. Nunnally[74] suggests that construct validity is established by circumstantial evidence.

SENSITIVITY

The ability to detect either change over time within an individual or current differences among individuals is referred to as sensitivity.[18,71] To be useful, an instrument must be able to detect differences that are meaningful. As with reliability and validity, sensitivity must be addressed empirically. A complete profile of an instrument's reliability, validity, and sensitivity requires data analysis to be approached at both the population and patient levels. Unfortunately, an instrument's ability to detect change within an individual often is investigated inadequately. Because of this deficiency, the psychometric profiles of many quality-of-life instruments lack detailed reports of their sensitivity.

Summary Measures

Because there are very practical applications for quality-of-life assessments in healthcare decision-making, researchers are increasingly exploring ways to combine quality-of-life data with other relevant data such as morbidity and mortality estimates. Healthy year equivalents and quality-adjusted life-years (QALYs) are approaches being developed for valuing outcomes of medical care that combine both quality and quantity of life. There remains much work to be done in this area, and much controversy remains concerning assignment of weights of preference or utilities for various health states or outcomes of care. The work on the Quality of Well-Being Scale, a general quality-of-life instrument addressing symptoms/problems and three dimensions of functional status (mobility, physical activity, and social activity), is a good example of investigators' attempts and interest in developing a summary measure using utility weights derived through population-based research.[79]

The uncertainties surrounding the valuation of health status using quality-of-life data currently limit the usefulness of summary measures such as QALYs. However, a noted researcher in this area writes that for economic analyses of healthcare programs to omit consideration of quality of life in such circumstances because of measurement difficulties would be quite inappropriate.[80] Clearly, we are in the early days of the application of quality-of-life outcome assessments to treatment and policy decisions.

Summary

Quality-of-life assessments in which data are collected by using instruments with acceptable psychometric properties can be useful in the study of pharmacoepidemiology. These evaluations document the outcomes of drug therapy from the patient's perspective. Determining the impact of a pharmaceutical product on a patient's physical, emotional, and social functioning, as well as sense of well-being, is vital to understanding a drug's effects on a patient population.

Several texts are now available that address important issues surrounding quality of life and the instruments developed to evaluate it. These works will assist the pharmaceutical scientists in their efforts to identify questionnaires appropriate and applicable to specific research questions.[72,81-83]

Quality-of-life studies offer the pharmacoepidemiologist a valuable tool for capturing and quantifying the data necessary for a total understanding of a pharmaceutical's effects—those that are beneficial as well as those that are adverse. If quality-of-life data are to be useful in pharmacoepidemiology studies, however, the pharmacoepidemiologist must be involved in designing and conducting prospective research so the necessary quality-of-life data are captured. These data must be captured in such a way as to allow pooling across study sites and across different studies, and they must be captured in a way that allows linkages to the traditional clinical and sociodemographic data routinely used in pharmacoepidemiology studies.

While researchers have been working in the area of quality of life for a number of years, there are still many applications and linkages to other data, such as mortality and morbidity figures, that have not been fully established. Quality-of-life assessment offers pharmacoepidemiologists a valuable tool in documenting and studying the impact of medicines on people's lives.

References

1. Patrick DL, Erickson P. What constitutes quality of life? Concepts and dimensions. Qual Life Cardiovasc Care 1988;4:103-27.
2. Koivukangas P, Koivukangas J. Role of quality of life in therapeutic strategies in brain tumors. Health Policy 1988;10:241-57.
3. Friedman LM, Ferbe CD, DeMets DL. Assessment of quality of life in fundamentals of clinical trials. Littleton, MA: PSG Publishing, 1985:161-71.
4. Mosteller F. Implications of measures of quality of life for policy development. J Chronic Dis 1987;40:645-50.
5. Fayers PM, Jones DR. Measuring and analysing quality of life in cancer clinical trials: a review. Stat Med 1983;2:429-46.
6. Spitzer WO. State of science 1986: quality of life and functional status as target variables for research. J Chronic Dis 1987;40:465-71.
7. Feinstein AR. Clinimetric perspectives. J Chronic Dis 1987;40:635-40.
8. Schipper H. Why measure quality of life (editorial)? Can Med Assoc J 1983;128:1367-70.
9. Katz S. The science of quality of life. J Chronic Dis 1987;40:459-63.
10. Aaronson NK. Quantitative issues in health-related quality of life assessment. Health Policy 1988;10:217-30.
11. Ware JE, Brook RH, Davies-Avery A, Williams KN, Stewart AL, Rogers WH, et al. Conceptualization and measurement of health for adults in the health insurance study: Vol. 1. Model of health and methodology. R-1987/1-HEW. Santa Monica, CA: The Rand Corporation, 1987.
12. The first ten years of the World Health Organization. Geneva: World Health Organization, 1985.
13. Ware JE Jr. Methodology in behavioral and psychosocial cancer research. Conceptualizing disease impact and treatment outcomes. Cancer 1984;53(suppl):2316-26.
14. Jachuck SJ, Brierley H, Jachuck S, Willcox PM. The effect of hypotensive drugs on the quality of life. J R Coll Gen Pract 1982;32:103-5.
15. Read JL. The new era of quality of life assessment. In: Walker SR, Rosser RM, eds. Quality of life: assessment and application. Lancaster, England: MTP Press, 1988:1-8.
16. Najman JM, Levine S. Evaluating the impact of medical care and technologies on the quality of life: a review and critique. Soc Sci Med 1981;15F:107-15.
17. Fletcher AE. Measurement of quality of life in clinical trials of therapy. Recent Results Cancer Res 1988;111:216-30.
18. Schipper H, Clinch J, McMurray A, Levitt M. Measuring the quality of life of cancer patients: the Functional Living Index—Cancer: development and validation. J Clin Oncol 1984;2:472-83.
19. Ganz PA, Rofessant J, Polinsky ML, Schag CC, Heinrich RL. A comprehensive approach to the assessment of cancer patients' rehabilitative needs: the cancer inventory of problem situations and a companion interview. J Psychosoc Oncol 1986;4:27-42.

20. Tannock IF. Treating the patient, not just the cancer. N Engl J Med 1987;317:1534-5.
21. Wenger NK, Mattson ME, Furgerg CD, Elinson J. Overview: assessment of quality of life in clinical trials of cardiovascular therapies. In: Wenger NK, Mattson ME, Furberg CD, Elinson J, eds. Assessment of quality of life in clinical trials of cardiovascular therapies. New York: Le Jacq Publishing, 1984:1-22.
22. Davies AR, Ware JE Jr. Measuring health perceptions in the Health Insurance Experiment. R-2711-HH5. Santa Monica, CA: The Rand Corporation, 1981.
23. Ware JE Jr, Snow KK, Kosinski M, Gandek B. SF-36 health survey manual and interpretation guide. Boston, MA: The New England Medical Center, The Health Institute, 1993.
24. Ware JE Jr, Kosinski M, Bayliss MS, McHorney CA, Rogers WH, Raczek A. Comparison of methods for the scoring and statistical analysis of SF-36 health profile and summary measures: summary of results from the Medical Outcomes Study. Med Care 1995;33(suppl):AS264-79.
25. DeHaes JCJM, Van Knippenberg FCE. The quality of life of cancer patients: a review of the literature. Soc Sci Med 1985;20:809-17.
26. Patrick DL, Erickson P. Assessing health-related quality of life for clinical decision making. In: Walker SR, Rosser RM, eds. Quality of life: assessment and application. Lancaster, England: MTP Press, 1988:9-49.
27. Siegrist J, Junge A. Conceptual and methodological problems in research on the quality of life in clinical medicine. Soc Sci Med 1989;29:463-8.
28. Tarlov AR, Ware JE Jr, Greenfield S, Nelson EC, Perrin E, Zubkoff M. The Medical Outcomes Study. An application of methods for monitoring the results of medical care. JAMA 1989;262:925-30.
29. Fletcher AE, Bulpitt CJ. Measurement of quality of life in clinical trials of therapy. Cardiology 1988;75(suppl 1):41-52.
30. Karnofsky DA, Burchenal JH. The clinical evaluation of chemotherapeutic agents in cancer. In: Macleod CM, ed. Evaluation of chemotherapeutic agents. New York: Columbia University Press, 1949:191-205.
31. Schmale AH. Clinical trials in psychosocial medicine: methodologic and statistical considerations. Part 1. Introduction. Cancer Treat Rep 1980;64:441-3.
32. Selby P. Measuring the quality of life of patients with cancer. In: Walker SR, Rosser RM, eds. Quality of life: assessment and application. Lancaster, England: MTP Press, 1988:181-203.
33. Bergner M, Bobbitt RA, Pollard WE, Martin DP, Gilson BS. The Sickness Impact Profile: validation of a health status measure. Med Care 1976;14:59-67.
34. Bergner M, Bobbitt RA, Carter WB, Gilson BS. The Sickness Impact Profile: development and final revision of a health status measure. Med Care 1981;19:787-805.
35. Hunt SM, McKenna SP, McEwen J, Williams J, Papp E. The Nottingham Health Profile: subjective health status and medical consultations. Soc Sci Med 1981;15A:221-9.
36. Hunt SM, McKenna SP, McEwen J, Backett EM, Williams J, Papp E. A quantitative approach to perceived health status: a validation study. J Epidemiol Community Health 1980;34:281-6.
37. Chambers LW, Sackett DL, Goldsmith CH, Macpherson AS, McAuley RG. Development and application of an index of social function. Health Serv Res 1976;11:430-41.
38. Sackett DL, Chambers LW, Macpherson AS, Goldsmith CH, McAuley RG. The development and application of indexes of health: general methods and a summary of results. Am J Public Health 1977;67:423-8.

39. Parkerson GR Jr, Gehlbach SH, Wagner EH, James SA, Clapp NE, Muhlbaier LH. The Duke–UNC Health Profile: an adult health status instrument for primary care. Med Care 1981;19:806-28.

40. Stewart AL, Hays RD, Ware JE Jr. The MOS short-form general health survey. Reliability and validity in a patient population. Med Care 1988;26:724-35.

41. Wells KB, Stewart A, Hays RD, Burnam MA, Rogers W, Daniels M, et al. The functioning and well-being of depressed patients. Results from the Medical Outcomes Study. JAMA 1989;262:914-9.

42. Stewart AL, Greenfield S, Hays RD, Wells K, Rogers WH, Berry SD, et al. Functional status and well-being of patients with chronic conditions. Results from the Medical Outcomes Study. JAMA 1989;262:907-13.

43. Schipper H, Levitt M. Measuring quality of life: risks and benefits. Cancer Treat Rep 1985;69:1115-35.

44. Meenan RF, Gertman PM, Mason JH, Dunaif R. The Arthritis Impact Measurement Scales. Further investigation of a health status measure. Arthritis Rheum 1982;25: 1048-53.

45. Meenan RF, Pincus T. The status of patient status measures. J Rheumatol 1987;14: 411-4.

46. Meenan RF, Gertman PM, Mason JH. Measuring health status in arthritis. The Arthritis Impact Measurement Scales. Arthritis Rheum 1980;23:146-52.

47. Mason JH, Anderson JJ, Meenan RF. A model of health status for rheumatoid arthritis. A factor analysis of the Arthritis Impact Measurement Scales. Arthritis Rheum 1988;31:714-20.

48. Meenan RF, Anderson JJ, Kazis LE, Egger MJ, Altz-Smith M, Samuelson CO Jr, et al. Outcome assessment in clinical trials. Evidence for the sensitivity of a health status measure. Arthritis Rheum 1984;27:1344-52.

49. Levine MN, Guyatt GH, Gent M, De Pauw S, Goodyear MD, Hryniuk WM, et al. Quality of life in stage II breast cancer: an instrument for clinical trials. J Clin Oncol 1988;6:1798-810.

50. Blades B, Mellis N, Munster AM. A burn specific health scale. J Trauma 1982;22:872-5.

51. Guyatt GH, Berman LB, Townsend M, Pugsley SO, Chambers LW. A measure of quality of life for clinical trials in chronic lung disease. Thorax 1987;42:773-8.

52. Fries JF, Spitz PW, Young DY. The dimensions of health outcomes: the health assessment questionnaire, disability and pain scales. J Rheumatol 1982;9:789-93.

53. Priestman TJ, Baum M. Evaluation of quality of life in patients receiving treatment for advanced beast cancer. Lancet 1976;1:899-901.

54. Spitzer WO, Dobson AJ, Hall J, Chesterman E, Levi J, Shepherd R, et al. Measuring the quality of life of cancer patients: a concise QL-index for use by physicians. J Chronic Dis 1981;34:585-97.

55. Padilla GV, Presant C, Grant MM, Metter G, Lipsett J, Heide F. Quality of life index for patients with cancer. Res Nurs Health 1983;6:117-26.

56. Spilker B, Molinek FR Jr, Johnston KA, Simpson RL Jr, Tilson HH. Quality of life bibliography and indexes. Med Care 1990;28(suppl):DS1-77.

57. Guyatt GH, Bombardier C, Tugwell PX. Measuring disease-specific quality of life in clinical trials. Can Med Assoc J 1986;134:889-95.

58. van Dam FS, Somers R, van Beek-Couzijn AL. Quality of life: some theoretical issues. J Clin Pharmacol 1981;21(suppl):166S-8S.

59. Mathias SD, Fifer S, Patrick DL. Rapid translation of quality of life measures for international clinical trials: avoiding errors in the minimalist approach. Qual Life Res 1994;3:403-12.

60. Ware JE Jr, Keller SD, Gandek B, Brazier JE, Sullivan M. Evaluating translations of health status questionnaires. Methods from the IQOLA project. International Quality of Life Assessment. Int J Technol Assess Health Care 1995;11:525-51.

61. Guillemin F, Bombardier C, Beaton D. Cross-cultural adaptation of health-related quality of life measures: literature review and proposed guidelines. J Clin Epidemiol 1993;46:1417-32.

62. Anderson GF, Alonson J, Kohn LT, Black C. Analyzing health outcomes through international comparisons. Med Care 1994;32:526-34.

63. Berzon R, Hays RD, Shumaker SA. International use, application, and performance of health-related quality of life instruments. Qual Life Res 1993;2:367-8.

64. Croog SH, Levine S, Testa MA, Brown B, Bulpitt CJ, Jenkins CD, et al. The effects of antihypertensive therapy on the quality of life. N Engl J Med 1986;314:1657-64.

65. Bombardier C, Ware J, Russell IJ, Larson M, Chalmers A, Reed JL. Auranofin therapy and quality of life in patients with rheumatoid arthritis. Am J Med 1986;81:565-78.

66. Williams GH, Croog SH, Testa MA, Sudilovsky A. Impact of antihypertensive therapy on quality of life: effects of hydrochlorothiazide. J Hypertens 1987;5(suppl):S29-35.

67. Líang MH, Larson MG, Cullen KE, Schwartz Y. Comparative measurement efficiency and sensitivity of five health status instruments for arthritis research. Arthritis Rheum 1985;28:542-7.

68. Fletcher AE, Hunt BM, Bulpitt CJ. Evaluation of quality of life in clinical trials of cardiovascular disease. J Chronic Dis 1987;40:557-66.

69. Miller L, Dalton M, Vestal R, Perkins JG, Lyon G. Quality of life. 1. Methodological and regulatory/scientific aspects. J Clin Res Drug Dev 1989;3:117-28.

70. Erickson P, Patrick DL. Guidelines for selecting quality of life assessment: methodological and practical considerations. J Drug Ther Res 1988;13:159-63.

71. Deyo RA. Measuring functional outcomes in therapeutic trials for chronic diseases. Control Clin Trials 1984;5:223-40.

72. Alreck PL, Settle RB. The survey research handbook. Homewood, IL: Richard C. Irwin, Inc., 1985:418.

73. Carmines EG, Zeller RA. Reliability and validity assessment. Beverly Hills, CA: Sage Publications, 1988.

74. Nunnally JC. Psychometric theory. 2nd ed. New York: McGraw-Hill, 1978:35-85, 225-99.

75. Ware JE. Methodological considerations in the selection of health status assessment procedures. In: Wenger NK, Mattson ME, Furberg CD, Elinson J, eds. Assessment of quality of life in clinical trials of cardiovascular therapies. New York: Le Jacq Publishing, 1984:87-117.

76. McDowell I, Newell C. Measuring health: a guide to rating scales and questionnaires. Oxford: Oxford University Press, 1987.

77. Van Knippenberg FCE, DeHaes JCJM. Measuring the quality of life of cancer patients: psychometric properties of instruments. J Clin Epidemiol 1988;41:1043-53.

78. Margolese RG. The place of psychosocial studies in medicine and surgery. J Chronic Dis 1987;40:627-8.

79. Coons SJ, Kaplan RM. Cost–utility analysis. In: Bootman JL, Townsend RJ, McGhan WF, eds. Principles of pharmacoeconomics. 2nd ed. Cincinnati, OH: Harvey Whitney Books Company, 1996:102-27.

80. Torrance G. Measurement of health state utilities for economic appraisal: a review. J Health Econ 1986;5:1-30.

81. Walker SR, Rosser RM, eds. Quality of life: assessment and application. Lancaster, England: MTP Press, 1988.
82. Spilker B. Quality of life assessments in clinical trials. New York: Raven Press, 1990.
83. Spilker B. Quality of life and pharmacoeconomics in clinical trials. 2nd ed. Philadelphia: Lippincott-Raven, 1996.

14 Automated Databases in Pharmacoepidemiologic Studies

Jacqueline S Gardner
Byung Joo Park
Andy Stergachis

Abstract

The use of automated multipurpose databases by pharmacoepidemiologists has expanded internationally in the past two decades. These databases contain patient-specific data that were collected in the course of providing routine medical care. The advantages of large linked databases include the availability of data for a large defined population, the minimization of study costs and time to completion, and the rapid identification of potential cases or exposures of interest to the researcher. However, because the data were not collected for research uses, their inherent limitations as well as their strengths must be considered in designing pharmacoepidemiologic studies. These limitations, which include data validity, reliability, and representativeness, are discussed and methods of evaluating data quality are presented.

Outline

A s illustrated amply through the examples in this book, large automated multipurpose databases have been important and effective
tools of pharmacoepidemiology, and they are used routinely in epidemiologic studies and postmarketing drug surveillance (PMS). Of
course, there are many databases used in pharmaceutical research. Among
these, large automated multipurpose databases represent a special and
unique resource. These databases usually consist of information from files
originally developed primarily for nonresearch applications. Through record linkage, it is often possible to create person-based longitudinal files on
an ad hoc basis. For the purposes of this chapter, databases are defined as
exiting data, available by computer through electronic format, which are
complete at the time of the initiation of a pharmacoepidemiologic study.
Ad hoc data collection methods for pharmacoepidemiologic studies are
discussed in Chapter 15.

This chapter groups data sources into multipurpose databases that contain both exposure and outcome data linked at the individual patient level;
databases that contain exposure or drug data only; and databases that contain primarily outcome, disease, or diagnosis information and may or may
not include data about drug exposures. This chapter also discusses several
techniques that are useful in determining the quality of databases used for
pharmacoepidemiologic studies.

Multipurpose Databases and Record Linkage

Record-linkage systems are resources containing longitudinal data
compiled from many sources on individual patients.[1] Multipurpose databases are considered population based if the information contained in the
database consists of or is derived from a population of known size, composition, and geopolitical boundaries. As noted by Roos et al.,[2] several characteristics of databases can facilitate their use in healthcare research:

- the data must be of high quality,
- information on individuals should be linkable across data sets, and
- individuals in the database should be traceable through time to provide longitudinal follow-up.

Generally speaking, the two principal types of files encountered in
multipurpose databases are *administrative records* and *health services files*.
Administrative records of programs or organizations usually include the
enrollment dates and basic demographic data, such as age and gender, of
the enrolled population. The health services databases might include data
on drug exposures, medical visits and diagnoses, and a limited number of
potentially confounding variables (e.g., preexisting or concomitant mor-
bidities). Health services databases can be built on either the basis of individual encounters with the healthcare delivery system or on the basis of
claims submitted by healthcare providers for payment or reimbursement.

Table 1 illustrates the types of data desirable for record-linkage pharmaco-epidemiologic studies.

In some settings, such as the health maintenance organization (HMO) Group Health Cooperative of Puget Sound (GHC) and the Mayo Clinic, automated databases were originally developed as clinical databases for both documenting the process of care and capturing information to facilitate running the organization in an efficient manner.[3,4] Other health services databases, such as Massachusetts General Hospital's computer-stored ambulatory record (COSTAR)[5] and the UK's General Practice Research Database (GPRD),[6] were designed to replace the traditional medical record. Many health services databases have also been developed using insurance claims-based records. For example, the US Medicaid program's claims processing files and data from Canada's Saskatchewan Health plan have been used extensively for pharmacoepidemiologic studies.[7-15]

The use of multipurpose databases in research depends on the ability to integrate files on individuals through *record linkage*. Record linkage is a method for assembling information contained in two or more records and combining the information belonging to the same individual into one record, ensuring that the same individual is counted only once.[16] The concepts underlying record linkage are at least 100 years old,[17] but record-linkage studies first received widespread attention when the Oxford Record Linkage Study was begun in 1962.[18] Here, data on certain health events were abstracted and computerized by using medical records and prescrip-

Table 1
Data Elements Desirable for Pharmacoepidemiologic Studies in Automated Databases

Variable	Database	Data Elements
Exposure	pharmacy dispensing, pharmacy billing	unique patient identifier, drug name, strength, date dispensed, quantity, directions, prescriber, pharmacist
Outcome	hospitalization, ambulatory visit, billing records, disease registries, vital statistics, patient surveys	unique patient identifier, diagnoses (primary and secondary), procedures, reason for visit, date of service, provider, disposition (alive or dead)
Patient characteristics	membership files	unique patient identifier, age, gender, race, tenure in plan
Potential covariates	medical records, patient surveys, selected databases	date of birth, gender, socioeconomic status, marital status, smoking, prior illnesses, concomitant illnesses, family history, reproductive history

tions from the UK's Prescription Pricing Authority for residents of the catchment area of United Oxford Hospitals. In the Oxford Record Linkage Study, automated files were then linked and followed prospectively for the defined population in order to conduct ad hoc research studies and health surveillance activities. Another early example of record linkage is the UK's Royal College of General Practitioners Study,[19] designed to recruit a large group of oral contraceptive users and a comparison cohort and to prospectively follow their morbidity and mortality experiences.

Since that time, concerns about the potential risks of marketed drugs have led to a marked increase in the use of automated record linkage in pharmacoepidemiology. The 1980s saw a wide variety of applications of large automated databases, including their use in cohort studies of specific drugs,[20-22] in case–control studies of events that are possibly drug induced,[23,24] and in cross-sectional studies of possible drug–disease associations.[25] The early 1990s have seen the application of additional databases in pharmacoepidemiology.[26-28]

Exposure Databases

In addition to linked multipurpose databases, there exist database resources that contain only drug information, not necessarily linkable to other data sets, that can nonetheless provide valuable information about patterns of drug use. A growing number of examples of pharmacoepidemiologic studies systematically evaluated only available drug and population data in the formulation or testing of hypotheses to (1) estimate disease prevalence,[29-33] (2) estimate the prevalence of specific exposures in populations,[34-38] and (3) estimate medical care quality and cost.[39-45] Chapter 6 provides an in-depth discussion of research with drug use data.

Specialized Databases and Registries

Other types of databases useful in evaluating drug effects target special diseases or conditions, collect information on only diagnoses or outcomes, or specifically encourage the reporting of adverse drug reactions. The International Medical Benefit/Risk Foundation—Risk Assessment of Drugs–Analysis and Response (RAD-AR) sponsored the compilation of international population-based data resources encompassing registries and morbidity databases, spontaneous reporting systems, and vital statistics records, as well as those containing both drugs and diagnoses, selected drugs or diagnoses, drug data only, and large clinical trials.[46] Information available in these compilations includes contact information, demographics, data-linkage capabilities, researcher access, and references.

REGISTRIES

Population-based disease registries represent a potentially cost-effective data source for observational studies of drug effects, particularly when registry data are linked with drug exposure information. Disease registries have been used for the study of adverse effects of medications in North America,[47-50] as well as in Europe.[51] Adverse effects of medications are also identified through the Toxic Exposure Surveillance System (TESS) of the American Association of Poison Control Centers and the Drug Abuse Warning Network (DAWN). Other registries useful in pharmacoepidemiology are pregnancy and congenital anomaly registries.[52,53] Population-based registry data generally offer the advantage of having diagnostic data of high quality, but exposure information is of variable quality, depending on the information source.

DIAGNOSIS/OUTCOME DATABASES

Through population surveys, claims, or discharge records, data are available that describe the incidence and/or prevalence of specific conditions in identifiable groups within specified time frames. These data resources can be useful in obtaining cases for case–control studies, as well as for estimating the magnitude of hypothesized adverse drug effects (ADEs). Some contain self-reported prescription and nonprescription drug exposures.[54-56] In the US, claims data from Medicare, the national health insurance program for elderly people, have been used by several investigators to investigate rates of fractures as well as ADEs.[57-60] A comprehensive list of US public health databases available for epidemiologic studies was compiled by Gable.[61]

A different approach to outcome databases was reported by French investigators, who compiled published reports of specific drug-induced disorders into computerized databases for use by clinicians and administrators.[62] The utility of these databases—targeting blood disorders, liver and kidney injury, and acute pancreatitis—for testing hypotheses has not been described.

SPONTANEOUS ADVERSE DRUG REACTION REPORTING DATABASES

Spontaneous systems for the reporting of suspected or confirmed adverse reactions to prescribed medications exist in many countries.[46] These systems are maintained by government regulatory bodies as well as by private groups, smaller regional units such as states and provinces, and hospitals. The quality of the systems is variable, and their advantages and disadvantages have been discussed extensively (see Chapter 5 for an in-depth discussion). Generally, however, they are valued for their contribution in alerting to previously unidentified ADEs, particularly those of rare frequency or long latency or that occur primarily in small subgroups of users. Increasingly, pharmacoepidemiologists are reporting methodologic work to improve the utility of spontaneous reports for estimates of disease incidence and prevalence.[63-65]

Advantages of Automated Databases

In carefully designed studies of well-formed hypotheses, automated databases offer a number of advantages: the ability to conduct studies of uncommon diseases or understudied populations with respect to drug exposures; minimization of study costs; reduction in the amount of time required to complete a study; and the opportunity to study large numbers of patients. Each of these advantages will be discussed briefly.

An often-cited limitation of premarketing studies of drug effects is the exclusion of various populations of patients who ultimately use marketed drugs. For example, Gurwitz et al.[66] confirmed that the majority of randomized clinical trials of drug therapies used in the treatment of acute myocardial infarction excluded elderly patients, particularly elderly women. Many large automated databases offer the advantage of including the health records of relevant subpopulations of patients.

Properly used, automated databases can minimize the cost and reduce the amount of time involved in conducting pharmacoepidemiologic studies. Since data are already collected and stored in a computerized format, it is possible to retrieve the data for ad hoc epidemiologic studies. As noted by Faich and Stadel,[67] a major restriction in the conduct of most ad hoc case–control and cohort studies is the time, energy, and expense necessary to assemble the case series or the series of exposed patients. In acknowledging these limitations, the US Food and Drug Administration (FDA) has supported the development of automated linked databases for pharmacoepidemiology (Table 2).[68-73]

Most multipurpose databases offer the distinct advantage of their large size, allowing the accumulation of much larger numbers of patients than were studied during premarketing drug testing. This characteristic permits the study of relatively infrequently used drugs and uncommon drug effects and the determination of more precise incidence rates than is possible through premarketing drug studies. The US Medicaid files, for example, contain automated exposure information for millions of person-years of experience.[3,74] GHC's databases include outpatient pharmacy, hospitalization, and enrollment information on more than 370 000 current enrollees. Saskatchewan Health's insurance databases include records of a wide range of health services provided to a Canadian province of about 1.1 million

Table 2 US Food and Drug Administration Cooperative Agreements and Contracts Using Automated Databases (1996)

Name	Location	Primary Database(s) Used	Representative Published Uses
Boston Collaborative Drug Surveillance Program, Boston University School of Medicine	Lexington, MA	GPRD GHC	68
Vanderbilt University Department of Preventive Medicine	Nashville, TN	Medicaid	7, 20
Kaiser Foundation Hospitals	Portland, OR	Kaiser Permanente Medical Care Program, Northwest Region	69
Harvard Community Health Plan and Harvard Medical School	Boston, MA	HPHC	70, 71
United HealthCare Corporation	Minnetonka, MN	UHC	72
Saskatchewan Health	Regina, Saskatchewan, Canada	Saskatchewan Health	13
IMS America	Plymouth Meeting, PA	NDTI, NPA	37
The Johns Hopkins University School of Medicine	Baltimore, MD	HIV/AIDS Registry, state of Maryland	73

GHC = Group Health Cooperative of Puget Sound; GPRD = General Practice Research Database; HPHC = Harvard Pilgrim Health Care; NDTI = National Disease and Therapeutic Index; NPA = National Prescription Audit; UHC = United HealthCare Corporation.

people.[75] A recent study conducted using VAMP data reported a cohort of more than 33 000 patients who were exposed to sulfonylureas.[76]

With respect to multipurpose databases containing information on prescription drugs, another advantage is that the recorded data are not subject to the limitations of incomplete patient recall or information bias, which are particularly problematic for exposures remote from the index event.[74] Additionally, prescription drug information can also be obtained about deceased or impaired individuals as well as about infants and children. By examining the patterns of dates dispensed, it is possible to examine dose–response and induction period relationships efficiently and the effects of in utero or periconception drug exposures that are less reliably obtained using interview methods.[77]

Problems in Multipurpose Databases

Pharmacoepidemiologic studies based on multipurpose databases are affected by a combination of conceptual and logistical impediments. These include potential limitations in the quality of the data from which they are derived; the lack of automated information on important potential confounders; and inherent limitations in the scope of exposures captured in the databases, such as the effects of drug formularies or other drug restrictions implemented by managed care plans or government insurance programs. In some instances, investigators using large multipurpose databases have had difficulties gaining access to primary medical records of more than just a sample of patients, thereby posing yet another potential limitation.[78] By themselves, multipurpose databases can rarely provide a sufficient basis for comprehensive epidemiologic research. Virtually all pharmacoepidemiologic studies require at least some original data collection from either medical records or patient interviews in order to validate exposure and diagnostic data and to obtain additional information.

Evaluating the Quality of Automated Databases for Pharmacoepidemiologic Studies

While the usual principles for documenting scientifically valid epidemiologic research apply to record-linkage studies,[3] several additional considerations can determine the usefulness of automated databases.

Two components of quality of an automated database are *internal* and *external* quality (Figure 1). Internal quality is the intrinsic quality of the data in the database, which includes comprehensiveness, validity, and reliability of data in the database. External quality means the extent to which the observations in the database are representative of a defined population.

The degree of potential for follow-up of the covered population affects both internal and external quality, depending on the group being studied.

DATABASE COMPREHENSIVENESS

Comprehensiveness of a database can be evaluated by the types of information, such as drug exposure data, outcome or diagnosis data, and covariate data, included in the database or record-linkage system. For instance, a multipurpose database linking prescription and diagnostic data is more comprehensive than databases that contain only drug exposure or outcome data. However, comprehensiveness also includes the completeness of the data coverage, that is, the extent to which all prescriptions filled for patients, all coded diagnoses assigned for outpatient visits and hospitalizations, exposure to nonprescription medications, and potential confounding patient factors appear as variables in the database.

DATA VALIDITY

Several factors can reduce data validity when conducting research with automated databases. For example, if the condition under study is mild, people with the condition may not seek medical attention; if the condition cannot be diagnosed easily by physicians, inaccurate diagnoses may be entered into the database; the compliance of patients with prescribed drug regimens may be poor, compromising exposure estimates that are based on records of prescriptions dispensed.

The validity of drug exposure, outcome, and covariate data can be measured by their *sensitivity* and *specificity*. Database validity can be measured by comparing information found in the database with that ascertained independently.

Figure 1
Components of
Quality of
Automated
Database

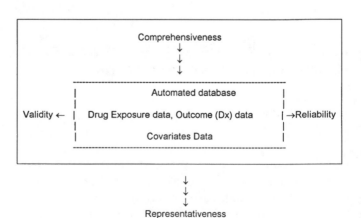

Sensitivity of exposure information is defined as the proportion of all drug exposures (e.g., prescriptions dispensed) in the covered population that appears in the database. Personal interview data have been used as a "gold standard" in evaluating the validity of drug exposure data on the assumption that information on drug exposure can be obtained accurately by personal interview. For example, at GHC, a 1984 survey of 475 randomly selected adult enrollees found that nearly all (99.4%) prescriptions written in the previous 12-month period were filled and obtained from GHC pharmacies.[3,79] A more recent study of the sensitivity of the GHC pharmacy database revealed a slight decrease in the sensitivity of the outpatient pharmacy database over time.[42] There is not universal agreement that personal interview is the most reliable source of exposure data. Stolley et al.[80] found high levels of agreement between prescriber records and patient-reported oral contraceptive histories on the name of the most recently used product. However, patient reports about previous oral contraceptive use were less accurate. Paganini-Hill et al.[81] compared health-related information from multiple sources and found that agreement between data sources for ever/never drug use varied from a low of 68% for the use of barbiturates and related drugs to a high of 87% for the use of antihypertensives. Better correspondence was observed between medical records and interviews than between either medical and pharmacy records or interview and pharmacy records. Using data from the Diethylstilbesterol-Adenosis Project, Tilley et al.[82] reported poor agreement between the mothers' recall and medical records. Kelly et al.[83] measured the reliability of medication exposure reported by hospital patients in structured interviews. Reliability was good for medications used on a regular basis, but medications used intermittently or for minor conditions were reported less reliably. Lau et al.[84] evaluated pharmacy records in comparison with interviews about recent medication use and found 77.6% concordance. Sensitivity of inpatient drug exposures is usually very low, because few automated databases itemize inpatient exposures. However, exceptions have been described by Classen et al.[85] and Xue et al.[86]

Specificity of a database with respect to drug exposure refers to its accuracy in ensuring that patients classified as unexposed to specific drugs are in fact unexposed. For example, studies of the association of nonsteroidal antiinflammatory drugs (NSAIDs) with gastrointestinal bleeding may be compromised by underestimates of nonprescription aspirin used by patients in automated databases.[87] A small-sample study to verify this discrepancy could increase the validity of the overall study results.

The sensitivity of *outcome* information is defined as the proportion of all health outcomes, for example, disease states, encounters such as physician visits or hospitalizations, or deaths, occurring in the covered population that also appear in the database. Quam et al.[26] validated claims-based diagnoses of essential hypertension using medical records and patient surveys, finding high sensitivity (96%) when both medical and pharmacy claims were used but lower sensitivity when either pharmacy claims or medical claims were used alone. Comparisons with vital statistics data have been used to assess the sensitivity of cancer registries[88] and special registries for cardiovascular disease.[89] As part of an evaluation of the Illinois Trauma Registry, Goldberg et al.[90] determined the sensitivity of case reporting by comparing hospital records with the Trauma Registry database. The authors reported a decrease in the sensitivity of reporting to the registry with decreasing severity of injury that would have resulted in misleading conclusions from the uncritical use of the Trauma Registry. Comparisons of cervical cancer diagnoses in the Danish Cancer Registry with a clinical follow-up study showed high sensitivity (97.8%).[91]

Sensitivity also can be estimated by comparing the number of outcome events observed with the number expected. The expected number is determined by applying a known incidence or prevalence rate derived from a population that is demographically similar to the study population.[90] This approach was used by Saxen et al.[92] on a registry of congenital malformations. Another approach to determining sensitivity within a database is simulating patterns of incomplete reporting to examine the possible effects on a specific variable.[90] Patterns of underreporting of burn mortality were studied in this manner by Schork et al.[93]

Specificity of outcomes data refers to the correspondence between the absence of outcomes in the covered population and in the database. After conducting a validation study on the COMPASS database, Carson et al.[94] reported that 44% of hospitalizations due to gastrointestinal bleeding could have been missed without searching for the outpatient diagnoses. Coding system characteristics or coding errors can produce false positive cases, which results in low outcome specificity of a given database.[95] For example, the absence of codes for "rule out" diagnoses in the *International Classification of Diseases*, Ninth Revision, has produced false positive cases.[96]

The sensitivity of a database with respect to *covariates* varies widely according to the classes of covariates. Because research is not the primary purpose of most automated databases, they usually do not contain adequate information on covariates to conduct specific etiologic studies. For instance, data on patient demographic characteristics are usually present because of their common inclusion in the information format for automated databases. However, data on other covariates, such as lifestyle variables and socioeconomic status, are generally absent. The sensitivity of comorbidity data may also be low because of physicians' lack of concern for risk factors, a limited level of detail in the database, variable influence of reimbursement policies, and widespread policies of not including outpatient diagnoses in automated databases.[97]

Jollis et al.[96] found that claims data failed to identify more than half of the patients identified as having prognostically important conditions for ischemic heart disease in a clinical database. However, Roos et al.[97] reported that information on comorbidities obtained from claims data compared with a clinical database showed considerable agreement, ranging from 65% to more than 90%. Iezzoni et al.[98] reported that incomplete coding of secondary diagnoses could bias study results when assessing patients at risk of poor outcome using administrative healthcare databases. VonKorff et al.[99] addressed this issue by using automated pharmacy data to develop a chronic disease score that predicts subsequent mortality and hospitalization rates.

The problem of data quality in medical records[100] and hospital discharge data systems has been the subject of several investigations.[101,102] Claims-based data systems that capture information on diagnoses and procedures have the added disadvantages of the possible influence of reimbursement policies on recording practices.[94] These problems illustrate the need for supplementary data to validate observations in the database.

DATA RELIABILITY

Reliability is the consistency of data within a database. This can be classified as *intramethod* reliability and *intermethod* reliability.[103] Intramethod reliability of an automated database is the degree of agreement between the information repeatedly obtained from the same database. Since information in an automated database is stored on computer disk, cartridge, or magnetic tape, intramethod reliability is almost perfect unless continuous and substantial modification of the input data is occurring among the repeated measurements. Indices of intramethod reliability for discrete variables are *percent agreement, Cohen's kappa,* and the *weighted kappa statistic.*[104]

Intermethod reliability is a measure of the degree of agreement between information obtained from an automated database and from other data sources. This concept of reliability is based on an assumption that no database can be a complete information source. Intermethod reliability can be measured by calculating the agreement between an automated database and other information sources including medical records, personal interview data, or external automated databases.[103] An index of intermethod reliability for continuous variables is the *Pearson correlation coefficient.* For example, if the coefficient is large for a specific variable between an automated database and medical records, reliability of the database is said to be high. The *Spearman correlation coefficient* can be used for calculating intermethod reliability of ordered categorical data.[103]

DATABASE REPRESENTATIVENESS

Representativeness or generalizability of a database can be defined as the degree to which the population covered by the database is representative of the total population. A study is externally valid or generalizable if it can produce unbiased inferences regarding a target population beyond the subjects in the study or an external target population.[16]

Representativeness can be evaluated in either of two ways: (1) by statistical comparison of demographic information (such as age, gender, race, marital status, and socioeconomic staus [including income, occupation, and education level]) between the database population and the target population, or (2) by evaluation of eligibility criteria for enrollment in the organizations that produced the databases. HMOs tend to include a reasonable sampling of the working population but may underrepresent the poor,[57] whereas only medically indigent or disabled people are included in Medicaid databases. Hospital-based databases cover only patients visiting the hospital, which may not represent the surrounding community population. Selection bias can reduce external validity of study results within the database.

If the population covered by a database is not representative of the target population, interpretation of any results obtained in studies using the database should be made very cautiously. For example, Medicaid databases have been frequently used for pharmacoepidemiologic studies in the US because of their strengths (i.e., availability of a large volume of objective and detailed drug exposure information, inexpensiveness, rapidity of obtaining study results). However, demographic characteristics of the databases overrepresent people younger than 15 years and older than 85 years, women, nonwhites, and the poor. Medicaid enrollees not only differ from the general US population, but they also vary from state to state because of differences in eligibility requirements.[7] Thus, results obtained with these databases may not be generalizable to non-Medicaid populations.[105] The geographic location of a particular data resource may also limit the generalizability of results if the sociodemographic profile or standards of medical practice vary considerably from an external target population.

POTENTIAL FOR FOLLOW-UP

One of the most important prerequisites for high-quality pharmacoepidemiologic studies is that individuals in a given database should be traceable through time to permit longitudinal follow-up. The availability of a *unique personal identifier* is very important in correct linkage between different databases, enhancing the possibility of long-term follow-up of individuals. Acheson[18] has suggested that an ideal identification system would fulfill several criteria (i.e., uniqueness, universality, permanence, availability, low cost). A personal identifier should be unique to the person concerned so that each individual can be distinguished from all others in a population. It should also be universal; that is, all members of the defined population should have unique identifiers of similar formats. The identifiers should be permanent from birth to death, and the personal identifiers must be easily available and inexpensive for record linkage.

Currently, personal identifiers consist of a social security number, a unique identifying number assigned by a health plan, or some combination of other types of patient information such as name, birth date, gender, and address. For example, prepaid health plans, such as the GHC, assign a unique medical history number to each enrollee. Once assigned, that number remains with the enrollee, even if the individual disenrolls and rejoins GHC at a later date.[4]

The linkage of databases requires that each individual's unique identifier is common to the data sets that are matched. Errors in correctly identifying individuals within and across databases relate to the accuracy and precision of unique patient identifiers as well as to the quality of the record-linkage methodology. Circumstances that result in underascertainment of database participation include those in which family members share an identifying number with a primary enrollee (e.g., a newborn's sharing its mother's identifying number for a period of time after birth, or an unemployed spouse's sharing the social security number of the primary wage earner). Not only are data unique to these "hidden" enrollees likely to be missed, but data entered for them under the primary enrollee's identifying number will be inaccurate for that member as well.

Having a single unique and permanent identification number greatly facilitates linkage. However, phonetically based methodologies such as Soundex, which uses algorithms based on various combinations of name, gender, and birth date, also have been successfully used to bring together records.[106] The lack of a unique identifying number in the Manitoba Health Services Commission database has been overcome through the use of a combination of family registration number, gender, and birth year.[74] To address the problem of potential lack of uniqueness of identifiers, Neutel and Johansen[107] described two basic approaches to computerized record linkage: *exact* matching and *probabilistic* matching. While exact matching can be accomplished even without a unique identifier through the use of an algorithm, probabilistic matching calculates a ratio of the frequency of agreement of pairs linked through an algorithm and the frequency of agreement of unlinked pairs randomly chosen.

Keeping *loss to follow-up* as low as possible and obtaining information on those not participating are also very important for high-quality research. As noted by Cook and Ware,[75] there are statistical benefits to lengthy follow-up. Some populations represented in automated databases are fairly stable. For example, GHC membership turnover is estimated to be approximately 15% per year, but after 2 years of enrollment, turnover drops to 5% or less.[108] In contrast, the Tennessee and Michigan Medicaid populations experience a 1-year turnover of more than 20% and a 2-year turnover of about 40%, with losses greatest in children and young adults.[7] The rate of turnover is a critical consideration in using automated databases that require eligibility or membership because of the potential for lapses in participation. The nonappearance of pharmacy or medical service entries in the database for an observed time period can be mistaken for nonuse, when in fact it may represent ineligibility for participation during that time period.

Three strategies for dealing with persons lost to follow-up are (1) identification of survival status from external databases, such as the National Death Index in the US or other death certificate access schemes; (2) restriction of subjects to those having a specified minimum period of follow-up or eligibility; or (3) use of a statistical model that calculates person-time at risk and prevents loss of information in analysis (e.g., the Cox proportional hazard model).[109]

Conclusion

The use of automated multipurpose databases by pharmacoepidemiologists has expanded internationally in recent years, as has the methodologic research required to improve the validity of their use. The rapid growth of managed care plans, including pharmacy benefit management companies, offers the potential for new databases for this field. A growing body of literature describes successful applications as well as inappropriate applications of automated databases in pharmacoepidemiologic research. Concern for the impact of national healthcare reform policies on the availability and accessibility of multipurpose databases marks the current decade in many countries. Where these databases continue to be available, there is every indication that their utility will increase as the field continues to grow in sophistication and rigor.

References

1. Bortnichak EA. Coexistence of specialized and multipurpose databases. J Clin Res Drug Dev 1989;3:167-9.
2. Roos LL, Nicol JP, Cageorge SM. Using administrative data for longitudinal research: comparisons with primary data collection. J Chronic Dis 1987;40:41-9.
3. Stergachis A. Group health cooperative. In: Strom BL, ed. Pharmacoepidemiology. New York: Churchill Livingstone, 1989.
4. Fisher LD, Gillespie MJ, Jones M, McBride R. Design of clinical database management systems and associated software to facilitate medical statistical research. Crit Rev Med Inform 1988;1:323-31.
5. Barnett GO. The application of computer-based medical record systems in ambulatory practice. N Engl J Med 1984;310:1643-50.

6. Hall G. Pharmacoepidemiology using a UK database of primary care records. Pharmacoepidemiol Drug Saf 1992;1:33-7.
7. Ray WA, Griffin MR. The use of Medicaid data for pharmacoepidemiology. Am J Epidemiol 1989;129:837-49.
8. Strom BL, Carson JL, Morse ML, LeRoy AA. The computerized on-line Medicaid pharmaceutical analysis and surveillance system: a new resource for postmarketing drug surveillance. Clin Pharmacol Ther 1985;38:359-64.
9. Avorn J, Everitt DE, Bright RA, Gurwitz J, Chown M. AIDS-related diagnoses and drug use among AZT users in New Jersey Medicaid (abstract). J Clin Res Drug Dev 1989;3:203.
10. Carson JL, Strom BL, Soper KA, West SL, Morse ML. The association of nonsteroidal anti-inflammatory drugs with upper gastrointestinal bleeding. Arch Intern Med 1987;147:85-8.
11. Ray WA, Griffin MR, Schaffner W, Baugh DK, Melton LJ 3d. Psychotropic drug use and the risk of hip fracture. N Engl J Med 1987;316:363-9.
12. Malcolm E, Downey W, Strand LM, McNutt M, West R. Saskatchewan Health's linkable databases and pharmacoepidemiology. Post Market Surveill 1993;6:175-264.
13. Spitzer WO, Suissa S, Ernst P, Horwitz RI, Habbick B, Cockcroft D, et al. The use of β-agonists and the risk of death and near death from asthma. N Engl J Med 1992;326:501-6.
14. Ross-Degnan D, Soumerai SF, Fortess EE, Gurwitz JH. Examining product risk in context. Market withdrawal of zomepirac as a case study. JAMA 1993;270:1937-42.
15. Bosco LA, Gerstman BB, Tomita DK. Variations in the use of medication for the treatment of childhood asthma in the Michigan Medicaid population, 1980 to 1986. Chest 1993;104:1727-32.
16. Last JM. A dictionary of epidemiology. New York: Oxford University Press, 1988.
17. In: Lord Herbert, Tulloch A, Farr W. Report on army medical statistics. Parliamentary Paper No. 366. London: 1861.
18. Acheson ED. Medical record linkage—the method and its applications. R Soc Health J 1966;86:216-20.
19. Royal College of General Practitioners. Oral contraceptives and health. London: Pitman Medical, 1974.
20. Griffin MR, Ray WA, Fought RL, Foster MA, Hays A, Schaffner W. Monitoring the safety of childhood immunizations: methods of linking and augmenting computerized data bases for epidemiologic studies. Am J Prev Med 1988;4(suppl):5-13.
21. Jick H, Andrews EB, Tilson HH, Pfanschmidt M, Branche C, Walker AM, et al. Atracurium—a post-marketing surveillance study: methods and US experience. Br J Anaesth 1989;62:590-5.
22. Friedman GD, Ury HK. Initial screening for carcinogenicity of commonly used drugs. J Natl Cancer Inst 1980;65:723-33.
23. Kakar F, Weiss NS, Strite SA. Thiazide use and the risk of cholecystectomy in women. Am J Epidemiol 1986;124:428-33.
24. Strom BL, Carson JL, Morse ML, West SL, Soper KA. The effect of indication on hypersensitivity reactions associated with zomepirac sodium and other nonsteroidal anti-inflammatory drugs. Arthritis Rheum 1987;30:1142-8.
25. Avorn J, Everitt DE, Weiss S. Increased antidepressant use in patients prescribed beta-blockers. JAMA 1986;255:357-60.
26. Quam L, Ellis LBM, Venus P, Clouse J, Taylor C, Leatherman S. Using claims data for epidemiologic research. Med Care 1993;31:498-507.

27. Grabenstein JD, Schroeder DL, Bjornson DC, Hartzema AG. Pharmacoepidemiology and military medical automation: opportunity for excellence. Mil Med 1992; 157:302-7.
28. Herings RMC, Stricker B, Leufkens H, Bakker A, Sturmans F, Urquhart J. Public health problems and the rapid estimation of the size of the population at risk. Torsades de pointes and the use of terfenadine and astemizole in the Netherlands. Pharm World Sci 1993;15:212-8.
29. Gerstman BB, Bosco LA, Tomita DK, Gross TP, Shaw MM. Prevalence and treatment of asthma in the Michigan Medicaid patient population younger than 45 years, 1980–1986. J Allergy Clin Immunol 1989;83:1032-9.
30. Walckiers D. Utilization of drug sales data as a means for estimating the prevalence of drug-treated intraocular hypertension in Belgium (abstract). Post Market Surveill 1993;7:261.
31. Maggini M, Salmaso S, Alegiani SS, Caffari B, Raschetti R. Epidemiological use of drug prescriptions as markers of disease frequency: an Italian experience. J Clin Epidemiol 1991;44:1299-307.
32. Feldman HI, Strom BL. Utilization of drugs for diabetes mellitus. Drug Saf 1991;6: 220-9.
33. dePedro J. Tracers for paralysis agitans in epidemiologic research. V. Prevalence of the disease in Swedish counties. Neuroepidemiology 1986;5:207-19.
34. Petri H, Leufkens H, Naus J, Silkens R, Van Hessen P, Urquhart J. Rapid method for estimating the risk of acutely controversial side effects of prescription drugs. J Clin Epidemiol 1990;43:433-9.
35. Oleen MK, Gardner JS. Survey of the prevalence of long-term use of benzodiazepines (abstract). J Clin Res Pharmacoepidemiol 1990;4:121.
36. Stricker BH, Barendregt M, Herings RM, De Jong van den Berg LT. Ad hoc tracing of a cohort of patients exposed to acitretine (Neotigason) on a nationwide scale. J Clin Pharmacol 1992;42:555-7.
37. Gerstman BB, Gross TP, Kennedy DL, Bennett RC, Tomita DK, Stadel BV. Trends in the content and use of oral contraceptives in the United States, 1964–88. Am J Public Health 1991;81:90-6.
38. Holm M. Prescription of benzodiazepine sedatives in general practice. Ugeskr Laeger 1990;152:2026-8.
39. Petri H, Urquhart J, Herings R, Bakker A. Characteristics of patients prescribed three different inhalational beta$_2$ agonists: an example of the channeling phenomenon. Post Market Surveill 1991;5:57-66.
40. McCombs JS, Nichol MB, Stimmel GL, Sclar DA, Beasley CM Jr, Gross LS. The cost of antidepressant drug therapy failure: a study of antidepressant use patterns in a Medicaid population. J Clin Psychiatry 1990;51:60-9.
41. Soumerai SB, Avorn J, Ross-Degnan D, Gortmaker S. Payment restrictions for prescriptions under Medicaid. Effects on therapy, cost, and quality. N Engl J Med 1987; 317:550-6.
42. Harris BL, Stergachis A, Reid LD. The effect of drug co-payments on utilization and cost of pharmaceuticals in a health maintenance organization. Med Care 1990;8:907-17.
43. Reidenberg MM. Effect of the requirement for triplicate prescriptions for benzodiazepines in New York State. Clin Pharmacol Ther 1991;50:129-31.
44. Weintraub M, Singh S, Byrne L, Maharaj K, Guttmacher L. Consequences of the 1989 New York State triplicate benzodiazepine prescription regulations. JAMA 1991;266: 2392-7.

45. Ferrando C, Herman MC, Corrigan OI. Impact of a nationwide limited prescribing list: preliminary findings. Drug Intell Clin Pharm 1987;21:653-8.

46. Jones JK, Gable C, Floor M, Staffa J, Rajan M. An international survey of data resources for pharmacoepidemiology (abstract). Post Market Surveill 1993;7:222.

47. Weiss NS, Sayvetz TA. Incidence of endometrial cancer in relation to the use of oral contraceptives. N Engl J Med 1980;302:551-4.

48. Strader CH, Vaughan TL, Stergachis AS. Use of nasal preparations and the incidence of sinonasal cancer. J Epidemiol Community Health 1988;42:243-8.

49. Weiss NS. Complementary role of specialized and multipurpose data bases in assessing the safety of prescription drugs. J Clin Res Drug Dev 1989;3:185-90.

50. Brenner DE, Kukull JR, Stergachis AS, Larson EB. The relationship between postmenopausal estrogen replacement therapy and subsequent Alzheimer's disease in a population-based registry case–control study at GHCPS (abstract). Post Market Surveill 1993;7:188-9.

51. Lewis MA, Hannelore L, Allmut H. Drug monitoring in a population-based coronary event register (abstract). Post Market Surveill 1993;7:228-9.

52. Pregnancy outcomes following systemic prenatal acyclovir exposure—June 1, 1984—June 30, 1993. MMWR Morb Mortal Wkly Rep 1993;42:806-9.

53. Kurz X, Leurquin P. Prevalence and reporting of drug use during pregnancy in the EUROCAT registry of congenital anomalies (abstract). Post Market Surveill 1992;6:35.

54. Cornoni-Huntley J, Ostfeld AM, Taylor JO, Wallace RB, Blazer D, Berkman LF, et al. Established populations for epidemiologic studies of the elderly: study design and methodology. Aging Clin Exp Res 1993;5:27-37.

55. Gregoire J-P, Breton MC, Dumas J. Prevalence and correlates of nonprescribed drug use in Quebec (abstract). Post Market Surveill 1993;7:204.

56. Klaukka T, Mäkelä M, Sipilä J, Martikainen J. Multiuse of medicines in Finland. Med Care 1993;31:445-50.

57. Ray WA, Griffin MR, Fought RL, Adams ML. Identification of fractures from computerized Medicare files. J Clin Epidemiol 1992;45:703-14.

58. Fisher ES, Baron JA, Malenka DJ, Barrett J, Bubolz TA. Overcoming potential pitfalls in the use of Medicare data for epidemiologic research. Am J Public Health 1990;80:1487-90.

59. Warren J, McBean AM, Hass SL. Utilization of Medicare data to identify hospitalizations with an adverse event due to digitalis among elderly beneficiaries (abstract). Post Market Surveill 1993;7:262.

60. Weis KA. Using the Medicare database. In: Data needs for outcomes research in long-term care. Alexandria, VA: American Society of Consultant Pharmacists, 1993.

61. Gable CB. A compendium of public health data sources. Am J Epidemiol 1990;131:381-94.

62. Biour M, Moore N, Cheymol G. Hematox—drug-induced blood disorders: an updated database (abstract). Post Market Surveill 1993;7:185.

63. Mann RD, Rawlins MD, Fletcher P, Wood SM. Age and the spontaneous reporting of adverse reactions in the United Kingdom. Pharmacoepidemiol Drug Saf 1992;1:19-23.

64. ARME-P. Methodological approaches in pharmacoepidemiology: application to spontaneous reporting. Post Market Surveill 1993;7:17-171.

65. Hammerstrom T, Tsong Y, Anello C. Comparison of methods for early detection of increased adverse reaction rates (abstract). Post Market Surveill 1993;7:206.

66. Gurwitz JH, Col NF, Avorn J. The exclusion of the elderly and women from clinical trials in acute myocardial infarction. JAMA 1992;268:1417-22.

67. Faich GA, Stadel BV. The future of automated record linkage for postmarketing drug surveillance: a response to Shapiro. Clin Pharmacol Ther 1989;46:387-8.

68. Jick SS, Walker AM, Jick H. Oral contraceptives and endometrial cancer. Obstet Gynecol 1993;82:931-5.

69. Johnson RE, Mullooly JP, Valanis BG, Andrews EB, Tilson HH. Acyclovir use and its surveillance in a general population. DICP Ann Pharmacother 1990;24:624-8.

70. Heckbert SR, Stryker WS, Coltin KL, Manson JE, Platt R. Serum sickness in children after antibiotic exposure: estimates of occurrence and morbidity in a health maintenance organization population. Am J Epidemiol 1990;132:336-42.

71. Hirschhorn LR, Currier JS, Platt R. Electronic surveillance of antibiotic exposure and coded discharge diagnoses as indicators of postoperative infection and other quality assurance measures. Infect Control Hosp Epidemiol 1993;14:21-8.

72. Lanza LL, Walker AM, Bortnichak EA, Gause DO, Dreyer NA. Incidence of symptomatic liver function abnormalities in a cohort of NSAID users. Pharmacoepidemiol Drug Saf 1995;4:231-7.

73. Moore RD, Creagh-Kirk T, Keruly J, Link G, Wang MC, Richman D, et al. Long-term safety and efficacy of zidovudine in patients with advanced human immunodeficiency virus disease. Zidovudine Epidemiology Study Group. Arch Intern Med 1991; 151:981-6.

74. Roos LL, Nicol JP. Building individual histories with registries: a case study. Med Care 1983;21:955-69.

75. Cook NR, Ware JH. Design and analysis methods for longitudinal research. Annu Rev Public Health 1983;4:1-23.

76. Abenhaim L, vanStaa T, Cockburn I. Risk of hypoglycemia in users of oral hypoglycemic agents: a study with the VAMP Health Research database (abstract). Post Market Surveill 1993;7:177.

77. De Jong PCM, Huijsmans AA, Nienhuis HE, Nijdam WS, Zielhuis GA, Eskes TK. Validation of a questionnaire on medical drug use during pregnancy. Am J Epidemiol 1991;134:998-1002.

78. Gerstman BB, Freiman JP, Hine LK. Use of subsequent anticoagulants to increase the predictive value of Medicaid deep venous thromboembolism diagnoses. Epidemiology 1990;1:122-7.

79. Jick H, Walker AM, Watkins RN, D'Ewart DC, Hunter JR, Danford A, et al. Oral contraceptives and breast cancer. Am J Epidemiol 1980;112:577-85.

80. Stolley PD, Tonascia JA, Sartwell PE, Tockman MS, Tonascia S, Rutledge A, et al. Agreement rates between oral contraceptive users and prescribers in relation to drug use histories. Am J Epidemiol 1978;107:226-35.

81. Paganini-Hill A, Ross RK, Tockman MS, Tonascia S. Reliability of recall of drug usage and other health-related information. Am J Epidemiol 1982;116:114-22.

82. Tilley BC, Barnes AB, Bergstralh E, Labarthe D, Noller KL, Colton T, et al. A comparison of pregnancy recall and medical records: implications for retrospective studies. Am J Epidemiol 1985;121:269-81.

83. Kelly JP, Rosenberg L, Kaufman DW, Shapiro S. Reliability of personal interview data in a hospital-based case–control study. Am J Epidemiol 1990;131:79-90.

84. Lau HS, Beuning KS, Postma-Lim E, deBoer A, Porsius AJ. Drug use in the elderly: comparison between interview data and pharmacy records (abstract). Post Market Surveill 1993;7:226.

85. Classen DC, Pestotnik SL, Evans RS, Burke JP. Computerized surveillance of adverse drug events in hospital patients. JAMA 1991;266:2847-51.
86. Xue S, Dai W, LaBraico J. Validation of information on a computerized inpatient record linkage database (abstract). Post Market Surveill 1993;7:264.
87. Lanas A, Sekar MC, Hirschowitz BI. Objective evidence of aspirin use in both ulcer and nonulcer upper and lower gastrointestinal bleeding. Gastroenterology 1992;103: 862-9.
88. Freeman LS. Variations in the level of reporting by hospitals to a regional cancer registry. Br J Cancer 1978;37:861-5.
89. Elmfeldt D, Wilhelmsen L, Tibblin G, Vedin JA, Wilhelmsson CE, Bengtsson C. Registration of myocardial infarction in the city of Gotenborg, Sweden. J Chronic Dis 1975;28:173-86.
90. Goldberg J, Gelfand HM, Levy PS. Registry evaluation methods: a review and case study. Epidemiol Rev 1980;2:210-20.
91. Storm HH. Completeness of cancer registration in Denmark 1943–1966 and efficacy of record linkage procedures. Int J Epidemiol 1988;17:44-9.
92. Saxen L, Klemmetti A, Haro AS. A matched-pair register for studies of selected congenital defects. Am J Epidemiol 1974;100:297-306.
93. Schork MA, Davis DK, Roi LD. Possible effects of case selection on analyses of institutional differences in a registry illustrated by the National Burn Information Exchange. In: Cornell RG, Feller I, eds. EMS system evaluation utilizing a national burn registry. Final Grant Report HS 01906. Washington, DC: Department of Health, Education, and Welfare, 1979.
94. Carson JL, Strom BL, Schinnar R. Do corticosteroids really cause upper G.I. bleeding (abstract)? J Clin Res Drug Dev 1987;1:256.
95. Rawson NS, D'Arcy C. "Validity" and reliability: idealism and reality in the use of computerized health care databases for pharmacoepidemiological research. Post Market Surveill 1991;5:31-55.
96. Jollis JG, Ancukiewicz M, DeLong ER, Pryor DB, Muhlbaier LH, Mark DB. Discordance of databases designed for claims payment versus clinical information systems: implications for outcomes research. Ann Intern Med 1993;119:844-50.
97. Roos LL, Sharp SM, Cohen MM. Comparing clinical information with claims data: some similarities and differences. J Clin Epidemiol 1991;44:881-8.
98. Iezzoni LI, Foley SM, Daley J, Hughes J, Fisher ES, Heeren T. Comorbidities, complications, and coding bias. Does the number of diagnosis codes matter in predicting in-hospital mortality? JAMA 1992;267:2197-203.
99. VonKorff M, Wagner EH, Saunders K. A chronic disease score from automated pharmacy data. J Clin Epidemiol 1992;45:197-203.
100. Burnum JF. The misinformation era: the fall of the medical record. Ann Intern Med 1989;110:482-4.
101. Institute of Medicine. Reliability of Medicare hospital discharge records. Washington, DC: National Academy of Sciences, 1977.
102. Lloyd SS, Rissing JP. Physician and coding errors in patient records. JAMA 1985;254:1330-6.
103. Armstrong BK, White E, Saracci R. Principles of exposure measurement in epidemiology. Oxford: Oxford University Press, 1992.
104. Fleiss JL. Statistical methods for rates and proportions. 2nd ed. New York: John Wiley & Sons, 1981.
105. Carson JL, Strom BL, Morse ML. Medicaid data bases. In: Strom BL, ed. Pharmacoepidemiology. New York: Churchill Livingstone, 1989:173-88.

106. Smith ME, Newcombe HB. Automated follow-up facilities in Canada for monitoring delayed health effects. Am J Public Health 1980;70:1261-8.

107. Neutel CI, Johansen HL. Perspectives on using record-linkage in pharmacoepidemiology. Post Market Surveill 1993;6:159-73.

108. Thompson RS, Michnich ME, Friedlander L, Gilson B, Grothaus LC, Storer B. Effectiveness of smoking cessation interventions integrated into primary care practice. Med Care 1988;26:62-76.

109. Cox DR, Oakes D. Analysis of survival data. New York: John Wiley & Sons, 1984.

15

Hospital Drug Surveillance Networks: Ad Hoc Pharmacoepidemiologic Data Collection Methods

Thaddeus H Grasela, Jr

Abstract

Growing awareness of the prevalence of unintended drug events (UDEs) in hospitals has stimulated the development of monitoring programs to detect and quantify the frequency of such events. The systematic identification of problems, data collection and analysis, and implementation of appropriate action have resulted from changes in the accreditation standards set by the Joint Commission on Accreditation of Healthcare Organizations. Studies of UDEs in the hospital setting are increasingly being performed as formal pharmacoepidemiologic investigations and provide the opportunity to quantitate the incidence of adverse events and to identify patient-specific risk factors. This chapter describes the use of hospital-based drug surveillance networks in general, and the Drug Surveillance Network (DSN) in particular, for pharmacoepidemiologic studies of UDEs in hospitals. Because of the involvement of hospitals of varying bed size, patient population, and drug formularies distributed across wide geographic regions, these networks have the potential to address a number of clinical issues that may not be possible for a single hospital. However, differences in methodologic sophistication, utilization of computer databases, and issues relating to bias and confounding make such studies challenging to implement. The advantages and disadvantages of using hospital-based networks to conduct pharmacoepidemiologic research are explored. The strategies developed by the DSN, as a specific example of a large hospital network, are described.

Outline

H ospitals represent an important setting for the study of unintended drug events (UDEs). Approximately 10% of hospital admissions result from such events, and almost 20% of patients experience an adverse event during hospitalization.[1-4] In 1991, the Harvard Medical Practice Study reviewed 31 429 hospital charts randomly sampled from more than 2.6 million patients admitted to hospitals in New York State in 1984.[5] After extrapolation from the findings of the study, the statewide incidence of adverse events was estimated to be 3.7%, of which 19% were drug related. Thus, UDEs are a major cause of in-hospital morbidity and mortality. Information about the specific nature of these events and possible predictive factors can play a major role in developing mechanisms to minimize their occurrence.

As early as the 1960s, the Boston Collaborative Drug Surveillance Program systematically screened hospitalized patients to determine the incidence of specific adverse events that occurred while patients were in the hospital.[6] That program was unique and revolutionary because trained nurse monitors were specifically responsible for evaluating a defined patient population and for collecting information on specific types and characteristics of adverse events. At that time, there were few concerted efforts to screen for adverse events and little interest in the systematic gathering of this information for large patient populations, in either ambulatory or institutional settings.

Awareness of the value of adverse event monitoring and pharmaco-epidemiologic research in the hospital setting has grown greatly since these first efforts. Over the past 7 years, standards formulated by the Joint Commission on Accreditation of Healthcare Organizations (JCAHO) have shifted the focus of hospital accreditation inspections away from an evaluation of the structure and function of individual hospital departments to evaluation of quality assurance programs affecting the entire institution. Hospitals must now implement a systematic mechanism for identifying problems, collecting and analyzing data, taking appropriate action, and providing evidence of the effectiveness of those actions.[7,8] Important consequences of this shift in accreditation standards have been a greater demand for adverse event monitoring, use of patient outcomes as the basis for evaluating drug utilization, and increased reliance on the principles of epidemiology.

Recognizing that UDEs are of significance in hospitals, the Food and Drug Administration (FDA) actively promotes adverse drug event (ADE) monitoring and encourages the reporting of serious adverse events to the spontaneous reporting system, a database of adverse events maintained by the FDA. An initiative from the Commissioner's Office, referred to as MedWatch, seeks to raise awareness of the need for adverse event reporting by healthcare practitioners. For this purpose, MedWatch uses educational programs, publicity, and feedback mechanisms such as newsletters and journal articles. To conduct research as needed to address evolving issues, the FDA also maintains research contracts with extramural research groups. The extramural contracts have included support for the Drug Surveillance Network (DSN), a hospital network for conducting pharma-coepidemiologic research described below.

A direct result of the JCAHO and FDA initiatives has been an increase in interest and research on the incidence of specific adverse events, the identification of preventable events, and the patient- or drug-related factors that constitute possible screening markers for events.

Hospital Surveillance Networks

In 1987, a cooperative research program responding to the growing interest in hospital pharmacoepidemiology was formed. Assisting hospitals to comply with new JCAHO standards mandating implementation of monitoring programs for UDEs, the DSN performed comprehensive pharmacoepidemiologic investigations to determine the incidence of adverse events and to identify patient-related risk factors. The DSN had the added benefit of being able to achieve larger and more representative population assessments by using data collected from more than 100 hospitals across the US.

This chapter describes the operational issues associated with the use of hospital-based drug surveillance networks. Ad hoc data collection methods used in hospital-based surveillance programs are reviewed, and the advantages and limitations of this approach are presented, followed by a discussion of future developments.

The number and type of hospital-based networks are likely to increase in the coming years because of the accelerating trend for hospitals to form consortia and alliances. Although several hospital networks exist, few have published sufficient information to detail the reliability and validity of the data obtained. Consequently, this chapter presents the DSN as a specific case study of the issues associated with use of hospital-based networks.

Hospital-based networks offer many of the strengths of claims databases for postmarketing surveillance of drugs. By coordinating data collection at a large number of hospitals, hospital-based networks have the ability to rapidly identify large populations of patients and to investigate a wide range of patient types and clinical care settings. Although the populations of patients accessible through these networks do not currently match the sample sizes possible in computer-linked claims databases, the networks have ready access to medical records and the wealth of clinical data collected during a patient's hospitalization. Moreover, when research studies are conducted prospectively, the ability to conduct patient and/or health professional interviews can provide important data on patient outcomes and covariates that are not available with computerized databases.

History of the Drug Surveillance Network

In 1987, clinical pharmacists at over 100 hospitals across the US and Canada were invited to collaborate on the collection of drug utilization and patient outcome information for pharmacoepidemiology research projects. The DSN has since grown to almost 400 actively participating hospitals, and more than 10 000 patients have been studied in the course of approximately 10 prospective cohort studies (Table 1). Participating hospitals are distributed across the US and represent a wide variety of hospital sizes, clinical settings, and organizational types (e.g., nonfederal government hospitals; nongovernment, nonprofit hospitals; for-profit hospitals; and federal government hospitals).

	No. of Patients Enrolled	No. of Institutions
Table 1 Prospective Cohort Studies Completed by the Drug Surveillance Network	**Project Title**	
Antibiotic use in bacterial infection	2310	102
Prospective surveillance of antibiotic-associated coagulopathy[15]	970	54
Antibiotic prescribing patterns and clinical outcomes in patients with bacterial pneumonia[19]	1822	74
Prospective surveillance of intravenous amphotericin B use patterns[20]	397	69
Clinical and economic impact of oral ciprofloxacin as follow-up to parenteral antibiotics[21]	766	54
Antibiotic-associated coagulopathy in critically ill patients[16]	546	97
Patterns of fungal infections and use of antifungal therapy in hospitalized patients		
Part I: results prior to fluconazole marketing[22]	786	69
Part II: results after fluconazole marketing[23]	818	57
Patient risk factors for gram-negative sepsis and complications[13]	1754	80

Ad Hoc Data Collection Methodology

HOSPITAL-BASED NETWORKS IN GENERAL

Pharmacoepidemiologic studies of ADEs require accurate information about the timing of drug exposure, the presence of concurrent illness, the use of concomitant medications, and the occurrence of specific clinical events, including specific patient outcomes and ADEs. Although the use of computer databases has become more prevalent in various hospital departments, such use is generally not at a level of sophistication that would allow automated analyses. Thus, at the present time, hospital-based networks must rely on ad hoc manual data collection procedures, perhaps augmented by use of the pharmacy department database, to identify patients receiving specific medications. Ideally, the ad hoc data collection process would use standardized data forms and on-site personnel trained specifically to monitor drug therapy response and patient outcome concurrently, for example, during the patient's hospital stay. Concurrent monitoring allows for daily assessment of patient outcomes and performance of interviews to obtain necessary data.

Given the reliance on ad hoc data collection procedures, hospital-based network studies generally must focus on narrowly defined patient populations. Eligible patients can be targeted by using the pharmacy department computer database to identify patients receiving specific medications. Patients may also be targeted by the presence of a specific demographic characteristic, for example, elevated serum creatinine, or by diagnosis. This latter criterion can be problematic, however, because diagnosis is generally assigned on discharge of the patient. Therefore, this information would not be available for concurrent monitoring.

THE DRUG SURVEILLANCE NETWORK

The following describes the process by which the DSN designs and executes a study.[9] The impetus for initiating an epidemiologic study can arise from several sources: published case reports of adverse events; the anticipation of UDEs, based on a drug's pharmacologic profile; or case reports submitted to the pharmaceutical company, the FDA, or an individual hospital's adverse event monitoring program. The specific problem is then defined, a hypothesis generated, and the target population identified. The specific type of study design is selected, that is, case–control or cohort study, and a data collection form is designed. Although various epidemiologic methods are available for specific studies, the DSN generally performs prospective cohort studies.

The study protocol and data collection forms are evaluated in a small pilot study at 5–10 institutions before widespread implementation on the network. The form and protocol are then distributed to clinical pharmacists enrolled in the DSN. Hospitals volunteer to participate in a particular study if resources, including time and personnel, are available, and if they have access to the desired patient population. Each hospital is represented by at least one clinical pharmacist who serves as a site coordinator responsible for receiving and distributing study materials to the other participants at the site. Because projects are usually performed as observational studies, thus requiring no change in patient care for enrollment, site coordinators request expedited institutional review of the protocol, a data collection form, and a waiver of the requirement for informed consent.

The focus of a specific project is either drug(s) or disease (unintended effect). At the present time, it is easier to identify patients by specific medications than by specific diagnoses. Although many institutions have computerized pharmacy-dispensing information, few have medical records computerized to the degree that would be helpful in identifying targeted patients.

Participating clinical pharmacists are responsible for collecting information concurrently, that is, during hospitalization of the patient. Depending on the project, monitoring continues for the entire hospital stay or for a shorter, specified time. Although it is possible to obtain follow-up information after patient discharge, this additional level of complexity has not been warranted for the projects completed to date. Concurrent monitoring allows for regular review of the medical record; interviews with nurses, physicians, or patients can be performed as necessary to collect data. The data collection form also allows for abstraction of information on patient demographics, laboratory values, concurrent diagnoses, and medications. The specific outcomes of interest and the parameters for patient monitoring depend on the hypothesis being tested, and influence the design of the data collection forms.

Completed data collection forms are returned to the research center in prepaid envelopes. All forms are reviewed promptly to ensure completeness and consistency of recorded data. If necessary, the clinical pharmacist is contacted for additional information or clarification.

The information on the case report form is then entered into a database, with double data entry ensuring accuracy. Data are analyzed by using the SAS computer software program (SAS Institute, Inc., Raleigh, NC).

Patient confidentiality is ensured by having the participating hospitals assign each patient a sequential study identification number. This number and a hospital identification code (based on the American Hospital Association's *AHA Guide to the Health Care Field*) provide a unique identifier for all patients. Requests for additional data use this study identification number rather than patient-specific information to obtain follow-up information.

A toll-free telephone number facilitates communication with participants, and a quarterly newsletter describes DSN activities and the status of current projects. Site coordinators receive regular updates on their projects and on issues arising during data collection. Participants are also reimbursed for data collection, and the amount of remuneration depends on the duration of patient monitoring and complexity of the data collection process. Additionally, each hospital receives a technical report summarizing the patients enrolled at the hospital as well as an overall summary of the entire study. These reports help hospitals fulfill the accreditation requirements set by the JCAHO.

Advantages of Hospital Networks

When properly coordinated and managed, hospital-based networks can be a unique source of information about drug risks. Access to geographically distributed hospitals having diverse patient populations, formularies, and clinical care characteristics provides a powerful mechanism for investigating therapeutic issues beyond the scope of a single institution.

An important advantage mentioned earlier is that hospital-based networks can access medical records and clinical data, as well as conduct interviews with patients and healthcare professionals, during the patient's hospitalization. This provides information about patient risk factors not available using only computerized databases.

Hospital networks have at least three other advantages. (1) Because the task of fulfilling JCAHO requirements for drug therapy monitoring and ADE monitoring has become the responsibility of the pharmacy department, clinical pharmacists are increasingly familiar with the need for accurate and complete data collection. (2) In addition, patient compliance is not a problem because of the importance of drug administration records maintained by nursing. There is a problem, however, in the study of drugs prescribed on an "as-needed" or emergency basis, because accurate records of drug administration may not be available.[10] Such medications may therefore be more subject to misclassification bias than are regularly scheduled medications. (3) Some medications are primarily used in the hospital setting and can be studied only by using hospital-based monitoring systems.

TIMELINESS

The structure of hospital-based drug surveillance networks allows for rapid development and implementation of projects. Table 2 shows the steps involved in implementing a DSN program and the approximate time required for each step. Projects can be completed in as little as 4–8 weeks, depending on the nature of the project, the frequency of drug use, the availability of patients, and the preparedness of the sites to participate.

ACCESS TO RECORDS (INTERNAL VALIDITY OF DATA)

Because clinical pharmacists are responsible for evaluating drug utilization and monitoring ADEs, they have ready access to medical records. Data collected by hospital-based networks thus represent one of the few sources of information on ADEs and patterns of prescribing drugs within the hospital environment.

Data collection forms can be structured to prompt for the collection of necessary data, and a careful review of the data collection form upon receipt at the research center allows for clarification of missing data. To the extent that the information in the medical record is generated for patient care decision-making, a hospital's quality assurance program (e.g., that performed by the laboratory medicine, microbiology, or pharmacy department) serves to ensure the accuracy of the generated information. It is important to recognize, however, that any subsequent collection of such data could be subject to transcription errors or outright fraud. Transcription errors can be minimized by careful design of the data collection form and redundant capture of essential data. Fraud, on the other hand, can be exceedingly difficult to detect. The quality assurance program for the DSN requires that participating sites provide copies of randomly selected discharge summaries to verify certain key data and the existence of the patient. The information provided on the summaries is frequently incomplete, however, and it is generally not possible to rely on these documents regarding detailed clinical events.

The DSN first compared data collection forms against discharge summaries as part of a nationwide surveillance program evaluating the incidence of bleeding associated with the use of antibiotics.[11] The purpose of this quality assurance measure was to check the quality and completeness

Table 2 Drug Surveillance Network Timetable for Projects	Projects	Months (n)
	Study design	0–1
	Develop and test data collection form	1–2
	Data collection	1–9
	Data processing	1–2
	Analysis and interpretation of data	0–1
	TOTAL	3–15

of the data collected. The final data set represented information collected from 543 patients at 49 hospitals over 1 year. On return, 68% of the data collection forms had been complete, and 98% of those returning incomplete forms had sent additional information on request. According to data collection forms, the incidence of bleeding associated with the use of antibiotics was 10%.

When discharge summaries were requested for comparison, only 55% could be supplied, representing 32 sites and 297 patients. Even though discharge summaries reported that 48 patients (16%) had transfusions and 39 patients (13%) had bleeding, only one discharge summary reported bleeding associated with the use of antibiotics. Furthermore, 90% of bleeding episodes and 95% of transfusions on discharge summaries also appeared on data collection forms, whereas only 39% of bleeding incidents and 29% of transfusions on the data collection forms appeared on the discharge summary. In this study, the prospective data collection approach using data collection forms provided more comprehensive data regarding the incidence of bleeding associated with the use of antibiotics than was available from the discharge summary.

All DSN studies now routinely request 10% of the discharge summaries, selected randomly, to verify information submitted on the data collection form and to minimize fraud.

Disadvantages and Limitations of Hospital Networks

COST–EFFECTIVENESS

The Boston Collaborative Drug Surveillance Program was the prototype for a hospital surveillance program for adverse events monitoring. Nurse monitors searched for adverse events; interviewed patients, physicians, and nurses; and abstracted data from medical records. Although yielding data of unsurpassed quality, the Program was expensive and would be difficult to implement in today's healthcare environment. However, networks utilizing clinical pharmacists, such as the DSN, ultimately constitute a cost-effective mechanism for obtaining answers to relevant questions, certainly when the institution is interested in the question.

EXTERNAL VALIDITY

The voluntary nature of participation in the DSN is an important limitation. The wide variety of site and ownership characteristics makes it difficult to generalize the results to all hospital patients or groups of hospital patients. Ideally, one would identify all eligible patients in a random sample of hospitals. Although this has been attempted in the past, the time required to recruit hospitals renders this approach impractical for most issues.[12]

A related problem concerns the need to minimize selection bias when enrolling patients for study. Selection bias remains a possibility because enrollment of patients often depends on the amount of time available to the pharmacist. Also, the number of patients eligible for a particular study frequently exceeds the number of patients for whom the pharmacist would be able to collect the requisite data.

The DSN has used two procedures for enrolling patients to minimize the risk of selection bias.[13] One procedure consists of enrolling all eligible patients within one area of the hospital, such as an intensive care unit or oncology unit. In the second procedure, eligible patients are identified from the entire hospital population. Then, each site chooses one or more days a week for screening, at which time the patients are screened and a predetermined maximum number enrolled for the study. Use of the last four digits of the hospital identification number ensures sequential enrollment, and the screening of patients and reasons for ineligibility are recorded at each site.

SENSITIVITY OF THE DATA

Identification of patient populations at risk of adverse events can be difficult, particularly if targeted by diagnosis. Diagnosis is generally not available during hospitalization and, even if it were available after discharge, would not be helpful in a prospective study. In general, if studies are performed retrospectively, no data other than those captured in the pharmacy computer and medical record could be used. Another limitation concerns the circumstances of drug use. Obviously, if a drug is not used in a hospital setting, it cannot be studied by using a hospital-based monitoring system. Moreover, if the duration of use of a chronic medication in the hospital is short relative to the time period required for events to occur, it may make little sense to use hospital-based systems. Finally, if a study emphasized data collection from secondary sources, such as medical records, as opposed to direct patient interviews, the ability to obtain crucial information may be impaired. Of course, the latter approach must deal with the problems of recall bias.

CONFOUNDERS

Early researchers in hospital epidemiology quickly realized that evaluating hospital patients could be very complicated because of the presence of several concurrent diseases and simultaneous use of many drugs. The complexity of treating such patients presents difficulties when trying to control for confounding variables and when making a diagnosis with respect to the ADE.

The two important confounding variables in pharmacoepidemiologic studies in hospitals are severity of illness and confounding by indication. Both sources of confounding can be particularly difficult to quantify and control for, either in study design or analysis. Efforts to measure severity of illness have often been less than satisfactory. Although some hospitals use severity scores such as the APACHE III score,[14] this is not done routinely. Determining the severity of illness continues to be a serious problem in any pharmacoepidemiologic study performed in a hospital, and the information required for use of the score must be specifically collected by the data collection form.

BIAS

An additional limitation of hospital-based studies centers on the selection bias that occurs with the use of hospitalized patients, particularly in the conduct of case–control studies. Spurious associations can arise between outcomes and drug exposure because of different probabilities of hospitalization for patients with and without the outcomes and the exposure of interest. A careful evaluation of any given investigation is needed to address the potential effects of selection bias on the study findings.

INTERNAL VARIABILITY

Hospital-based networks rely on the level of sophistication and availability of information systems at each hospital. The ability to perform pharmacoepidemiologic studies is limited by the state of the art of such systems. A 1991 survey performed by the DSN revealed important limitations in using computerized data for pharmacoepidemiologic research in hospitals.[10] Frequent purging or archiving of data without easy retrieval limits the time period during which a hospital pharmacy can conduct its investigation and hampers retrospective evaluations. Also, almost half of the hospitals required programming assistance when generating reports from the database.

CAUSALITY ASSESSMENT

Another important limitation in adverse event surveillance has been the problem of assessing causality. Although numerous algorithms have been helpful in evaluating causality (see Chapter 5), none is fail-safe, and considerable confusion exists regarding the appropriate role of assessing causality in hospital pharmacoepidemiology. Clearly, for the purpose of treating patients, determining the cause of a putative adverse event can be critical. However, in an epidemiologic investigation, events are identified according to a predetermined definition of a "case," and all patients meeting that definition are labeled as such without regard for cause. This practice has been used extensively in computerized database investigations.

Examples of Hospital-Based Surveillance Projects

COAGULOPATHY STUDY

In the 1980s, an ongoing clinical debate centered around the relative importance of patient risk factors (malnutrition and debilitating disease) versus exposure to the N-methylthiotetrazole (NMTT) side-chain in producing coagulopathy associated with the use of antibiotics. As a result, in 1989, the DSN conducted a prospective cohort study at 56 member hospitals to determine the incidence of hypoprothrombinemia in 491 hospitalized patients given parenteral antibiotics.[15] Clinical pharmacists identified eligible patients by screening medical records and prescriptions for antibiotics. All patients selected were then monitored for the duration of antibiotic administration. Case report forms were used to record comprehensive information about patterns of prescribing antibiotics, patient demographics, and selective laboratory data, such as prothrombin time. Hypoprothrombinemia (an increase in prothrombin time of >2 sec) occurred in 29 patients (5.9%). The incidence of hypoprothrombinemia was significantly ($p < 0.05$) higher for patients given a combination of aminoglycoside and an antianaerobic antibiotic than for those given cefoxitin or cefotetan.

To quantify the importance of various risk factors for hypoprothrombinemia, data were subjected to multivariate analysis with stepwise logistic regression. The risk factors evaluated were the presence of liver disease, carcinoma, congestive heart failure, renal dysfunction, or weight loss; the use of cimetidine, ranitidine, subcutaneous heparin, gastrointestinal tract sterilization, or nasogastric suctioning; gender; admission of the patient to the intensive care unit; site of infection (abdomen vs. other sites); serum albumin concentration; age; type and length of antibiotic regimen; and reason for using antibiotics.

The risk of hypoprothrombinemia was found to be significantly higher for patients with liver disease (estimated odds ratio = 3.86) and for those given the combination of aminoglycoside and antianaerobic antibiotic (estimated odds ratio = 2.50). The risk was also inversely related to the estimated creatinine clearance (estimated odds ratio = 0.98).

Because of the higher risk for patients given the aminoglycoside/antianaerobic antibiotic combination and the fact that these patients may have been more seriously ill, the DSN conducted a follow-up study to evaluate more seriously ill patients. The study group consisted of 546 patients at 53 hospitals who had a serum albumin concentration of 3 g/dL or less and required 3 or more days of intravenous antibiotic therapy for certain specified conditions.[16] The study evaluated the incidence of clinical bleeding associated with administration of one of three antibiotic regimens: antibiotics containing the NMTT side-chain; antibiotics not containing NMTT; and the combination of aminoglycoside plus an antianaerobic antibiotic and/or a penicillin. Monitoring for bleeding events consisted of noting entries in the medical record indicating signs of frank bleeding on physical examination or diagnostic testing.

When the conditions warranting antibiotic therapy were analyzed for the risk of bleeding, the frequency of clinical bleeding, which did not differ significantly for the three groups, was 13.7%. Similarly, for those patients for whom a prothrombin time was available, the frequency of hypoprothrombinemia was 26% and was almost identical for the three groups.

ALTEPLASE VERSUS STREPTOKINASE STUDY

Another project also showed the value of widespread hospital participation in drug surveillance projects. In this instance, data collection was retrospective. Clinical pharmacists or physicians at 32 hospitals were asked to review the medical records of 626 consecutive patients given alteplase (recombinant tissue plasminogen activator) or streptokinase to treat acute myocardial infarction.[17] The Carolina Research Group, Inc. (Raleigh, NC), conducted the study, and faculty of the School of Pharmacy, University of North Carolina, Chapel Hill, analyzed the data. Because of its high affinity for fibrin, alteplase was believed to disturb general coagulation to a lesser degree than did streptokinase. However, retrospective review of clinical data did not support this theoretic advantage: no thrombolytic-related differences were found in the incidence or severity of bleeding after the use of these two thrombolytic agents.

Future Directions

Computers are becoming increasingly important in the gathering of healthcare information in hospitals. Some institutions have sophisticated, integrated computer databases that provide a fascinating glimpse into the future of extensively computerized hospital environments.[18] Currently, however, most hospitals have a patchwork of computer systems that do not communicate with each other.

In 1991, the DSN surveyed its membership regarding its level of computerization, the type of data collected in databases, data-querying capabilities, monitoring of ADEs, and evaluations of drug use.[10] The survey found that most of the 166 responding hospitals had begun to computerize various departments. Almost 90% of responding hospitals had computerized pharmacy records, and 75% had computerized medical records. However, of the hospitals having a computerized pharmacy department, only 30% had ready access to computerized medical records from the pharmacy department. Furthermore, of the institutions that did have data access across various departments, few were able to query databases in various departments simultaneously. For example, only 30% of the hospitals could identify patients who had been given an aminoglycoside and also had elevated serum creatinine concentrations, a possible sign of nephrotoxicity.

The survey concluded that several goals would have to be accomplished if hospital databases are to be more helpful in evaluating drug use and monitoring for ADEs:

(1) improved interdepartmental communication among computer systems and databases, implying use of fully integrated computer systems;

(2) more thorough recording of drug administration to specific patients (vendor, lot number, dose);

(3) more comprehensive database information on patient outcome and adverse events;

(4) more responsiveness to the information needs of hospitals by software vendors (i.e., development of interactive programs that provide informative reports and documentation more easily);

(5) training of clinical personnel in the use and interpretation of clinical data in hospital databases;

(6) establishment of patient monitoring programs allowing rapid follow-up of reports generated from hospital databases; and

(7) more active reporting of adverse events to the FDA and pharmaceutical manufacturers by hospitals, so that newly emerging adverse events might be detected more readily.

In recent years, the emergence of vertically integrated healthcare delivery systems holds the promise that comprehensive information sources on both inpatient and outpatient drug use and outcomes might become available. The ability to monitor cost and quality of care is an important motivation for developing the necessary computer systems, while concern over patient privacy rights looms large as an obstacle for this effort. These conflicts will play out over the next several years; if properly managed, these integrated sources can serve as a foundation for the important next development in pharmacoepidemiology research.

Summary

The ability of hospital-based networks to obtain drug-prescribing and patient outcome information from a cross-section of hospitals represents an important mechanism for performing pharmacoepidemiologic research. The development of systematic data collection techniques and the ability to collect comprehensive data about drug exposures, patient outcomes, and covariates permit estimation of the incidence of adverse events in targeted patient populations, as well as determination of risk factors that can then serve as the foundation for preventive programs within the hospital setting.

References

1. Seidl LG, Thornton GF, Cluff LE. Epidemiological studies of adverse drug reactions. Am J Public Health 1965;55:1170-5.
2. Steel K, Gertman PM, Crescenzi C, Anderson J. Iatrogenic illness on a general medical service at a university hospital. N Engl J Med 1981;304:638-42.
3. Ogilvie RI, Ruedy J. Adverse drug reactions during hospitalization. Can Med Assoc J 1967;97:1450-7.
4. Seidl LG, Thornton GF, Smith JW, Cluff LE. Studies on the epidemiology of adverse drug reactions. III. Reactions in patients on a general medical service. Bull Johns Hopkins Hosp 1966;119:299-315.
5. Brennan TA, Leape LL, Laird NM, Hebert L, Localio AR, Lawthers AG, et al. Incidence of adverse events and negligence in hospitalized patients. Results of the Harvard Medical Practice Study I. N Engl J Med 1991;324:370-6.
6. Slone D, Jick H, Borda I, Chalmers TC, Feinleib M, Muench H, et al. Drug surveillance utilising nurse monitors. An epidemiological approach. Lancet 1966;2:901-3.
7. Roberts JS, Coale JG, Redman RR. A history of the Joint Commission on Accreditation of Hospitals. JAMA 1987;258:936-40.
8. Joint Commission on Accreditation of Healthcare Organizations. Accreditation manual for hospitals, 1991. Chicago, IL: Joint Commission on Accreditation of Healthcare Organizations, 1991.
9. Grasela TH Jr, Schentag JJ. A clinical pharmacy-oriented drug surveillance network: I. Program description. Drug Intell Clin Pharm 1987;21:902-8.
10. Grasela TH, Walawander CA, Kennedy DL, Jolson HM. Capability of hospital computer systems in performing drug-use evaluations and adverse drug event monitoring. Am J Hosp Pharm 1993;50:1889-95.
11. Goss TF, Walawander CA, Grasela TH. Quality assurance in a prospective data collection network with comparison to hospital discharge summaries. J Clin Res Pharmacoepidemiol 1990;4:118-9.
12. Townsend TR, Shapiro M, Rosner B, Kass EH. Use of antimicrobial drugs in general hospitals. I. Description of population and definition of methods. J Infect Dis 1979;139:688-97.
13. Conboy K, Welage LS, Walawander CA, Duffy LC, Welliver RC, Zielezny MA, et al. Sepsis syndrome and associated sequelae in patients at high risk for gram-negative sepsis. Pharmacotherapy 1995;15:66-77.
14. Knaus WA, Wagner DP, Draper EA, Zimmerman JE, Bergner M, Bastos PG, et al. The APACHE III prognostic system. Risk prediction of hospital mortality for critically ill hospitalized adults. Chest 1991;100:1619-36.
15. Grasela TH Jr, Walawander CA, Welage LS, Wing PE, Scarafoni DJ, Caldwell JW, et al. Prospective surveillance of antibiotic-associated coagulopathy in 970 patients. Pharmacotherapy 1989;9:158-64.

16. Goss TF, Walawander CA, Grasela TH Jr, Meisel S, Katona B, Jaynes K. Prospective evaluation of risk factors for antibiotic-associated bleeding in critically ill patients. Pharmacotherapy 1992;12:283-91.

17. McLeod DC, Coln WG, Thayer CF, Perfetto EM, Hartzema AG. Pharmacoepidemiology of bleeding events after use of r-alteplase or streptokinase in acute myocardial infarction. Ann Pharmacother 1993;27:956-62.

18. Classen DC, Pestotnik SL, Evans RS, Burke JP. Computerized surveillance of adverse drug events in hospital patients. JAMA 1991;266:2847-51.

19. Grasela TH Jr, Welage LS, Walawander CA, Timm EG, Pelter MA, Poirier TI, et al. A nationwide survey of antibiotic prescribing patterns and clinical outcomes in patients with bacterial pneumonia. DICP Ann Pharmacother 1990;24:1220-5.

20. Grasela TH Jr, Goodwin SD, Walawander MK, Cramer RL, Fuhs DW, Moriarty VP. Prospective surveillance of intravenous amphotericin B use patterns. Pharmacotherapy 1990;10:341-8.

21. Grasela TH Jr, Paladino JA, Schentag JJ, Huepenbecker D, Rybacki J, Purcell JB, et al. Clinical and economic impact of oral ciprofloxacin as follow-up to parenteral antibiotics. DICP Ann Pharmacother 1991;25:857-62.

22. Grasela TH, Goodwin SD, Pasko MT, Walawander CA, Raebel MA. Use of antifungal therapy in hospitalized patients I. Results prior to the marketing of fluconazole. Ann Pharmacother 1994;28:252-60.

23. Grasela TH, Pasko MT, Goodwin SD, Walawander CA, Blackwelder N, Bruder-Holt RJ. Use of antifungal therapy in hospitalized patients II. Results after the marketing of fluconazole. Ann Pharmacother 1994;28:261-70.

16

Community Pharmacy Networks in Pharmacoepidemiology

Ron MC Herings
Hubert GM Leufkens

Abstract

This chapter describes and discusses the organization and structure of community pharmacy networks as a resource for drug exposure information. Pharmacy networks should be organized as modular patient-tracking systems to facilitate collection of additional data through record linkage techniques. First, several issues are discussed relevant to the validity and completeness of drug exposure information obtained from pharmacy-based networks, such as prescription handling, organization and structure of pharmaceutical care, and coding standards. Next, problems and methods pertaining to the use of pharmacy records as a source of drug exposure information are discussed. Attention is focused on methods for estimating exposure measures and several causes of drug exposure misclassification bias. Finally, the clinical relevance of pharmacy networks is discussed with respect to risk management, cohort tracing, case–cohort studies, prescription sequence analysis, and causes of selective drug prescribing. Accurate drug exposure assessment is of crucial importance to pharmacoepidemiologic studies. Even with the most extensive validation of morbidity, pharmacoepidemiologic studies are of little value without proper definition and assessment of exposure.

Outline

D rug exposure information can be collected by patient surveys or by extracting information from large administrative physician-, pharmacy-, or claims-based databases. Each of these methods has strengths and limitations in defining drug exposure explicitly.[1,2] When drug exposure information is obtained from large administrative databases, the accessibility and quality of data are defined by administrative processes embedded in the organization of health care and society. Without standard drug-coding schemes, data become virtually inaccessible. The completeness of drug exposure information is thwarted if such information is scattered over multiple physicians' offices, pharmacies, or hospitals and when linkage of these different resources on an individual patient level is impossible. The validity of estimating exposure on a patient-based level is sensitive to local differences in protocols for entering data and largely depends on the level of administration where data are collected. Claims-based databases record what is claimed for reimbursement, pharmacy-based databases record what is dispensed, and physicians' databases record what is prescribed.

The availability and high quality of computerized pharmacy records have contributed to a strong focus of pharmacoepidemiologic research on drug exposure characterization in the Netherlands.[3-10] Characterization of drug exposure is needed to answer the question, "What patient got which drugs, when, and in what doses?"[11] Furthermore, accurate characterization of drug exposure allows for a strong pharmacologic perspective in the analysis of pharmacoepidemiologic data, because drug effects relate most often to dosage, timing, and the length of exposure. The temporal sequence of drug exposure/effect is therefore basic to the inference of causality. It is also important to have accurate dose-timing information of multiple drug use. Drug–drug interactions and prevailing underlying diseases are just two examples of factors that are important in the evaluation of the benefit and risk associated with the use of a particular drug. Detailed characterization of drug exposure is therefore essential to detect and study the causal or noncausal mechanisms related to adverse reactions to drugs.

This chapter discusses the organization and structure of community pharmacy networks as a resource for drug exposure information. First, we discuss the organization and structure of pharmacy networks in which the focus is on data quality. Later, we discuss several topics and methods related to drug exposure characterization.

Organization of Pharmacy Networks

Community pharmacy-based networks have developed in several countries throughout the world (e.g., Portugal, Denmark, the Netherlands,

Canada, Poland). These networks have little in common, however, because the access, completeness, and validity of drug exposure data depend largely on the organization of the national or regional drug-dispensing process. As an example of the influence of the organization of the drug-dispensing process on the quality of drug exposure data, we describe the Dutch situation.

PRESCRIPTION HANDLING IN THE DUTCH COMMUNITY PHARMACY

In the organization of pharmaceutical care, Dutch community pharmacies play a central role. These pharmacies are typically three to four times larger than their counterparts in other western European countries or North America, having 8000–14 000 patients per pharmacy. In small, remote villages, drugs are dispensed through physician-based pharmacies. On the average, each Dutch inhabitant is within 3–5 miles of the nearest pharmacy.

The assortment of products dispensed in Dutch pharmacies includes all prescription drugs, some medical devices (e.g., incontinence pads), and several over-the-counter (OTC) products. Today, virtually all Dutch pharmacies are automated. Each time a patient presents a prescription order in the pharmacy, patient, prescriber, and medication information is updated and stored for monitoring and billing purposes in patient-based, drug-dispensing histories. Before dispensing medication and filing information, the pharmacist routinely checks new prescriptions with reference to the patient's drug history for drug–drug interactions, double medications, contraindications, or other inconsistencies. If potential medication errors are detected, the pharmacist might communicate these with the prescriber, eventually resulting in substitution or cancellation of the prescription or dosage adaptations. Pharmacists may also change the total number of prescribed units to available standard package sizes or may substitute name brands with generic drugs (e.g., Tagamet with cimetidine). These procedures depend on individual or collective agreements with prescribers or insurance companies. After these checking procedures, the dispensing information is used for reimbursement purposes. Today, for more than 90% of all Dutch inhabitants, these bills are sent directly to health insurance companies for reimbursement. In the event that a patient fills a prescription at other than the designated pharmacy, he or she must pay cash. Because of these economic incentives, Dutch pharmacy drug-dispensing histories are virtually complete in documenting drug use over time.

ORGANIZATION AND STRUCTURE OF PHARMACY NETWORKS

A pharmacy network should be viewed as a modular concept in which each pharmacy represents a single module. For each pharmacy, dispensing data are converted to a standard format and are subsequently included in a central database for research purposes. This information covers all dispensed drugs, independent of the type of prescriber (e.g., family practitioner, medical specialist, midwife, dentist), that are actually dispensed to patients in a defined population. All drugs are identified with unique product codes that are maintained in a large drug reference database. This database is also used by health insurance companies to verify the reimbursement for each product. Linkage to these databases also enables selection of drugs, groups of drugs, chemical entities, product types (e.g., drugs, incontinence pads), drug formulations (e.g., tablets, solutions), and route of administration. Problems in risk assessment and comparison may occur when coding or classification schemes are not uniformly defined.[3,7] For example, to identify drugs, the World Health Organization (WHO) Anatomical-Therapeutical Chemical Classification (ATC) coding is often used.[12] However, this coding system is frequently and irregularly updated, which might bias longitudinal analyses of drug exposure. Angiotensin-converting enzyme inhibitors formerly coded as C02DE and C02LM have been coded as C09 since 1996. Drug use statistics therefore no longer match and require cumbersome reanalyses each time the ATC coding system is updated.

Patient information is stored in a separate patient file for each patient, with a unique identification code. This code is an alphanumeric identification number that can be used by the pharmacist to track additional information in the pharmacy or general practitioner's office that is not routinely collected. Unfortunately, there is no incentive to eliminate patients who are deceased or have relocated; consequently, these patients' files are not suitable to define denominators. This problem, however, can be corrected by using local vital statistics, as is the case in the PHARMO record linkage system.[7] To protect confidentiality, patient information is accessible only through the pharmacists. Procedures to collect additional information by contacting general practitioners of patients have been used several times. Furthermore, patient information (e.g., date of birth, gender, family practitioner) is used to link pharmacy data to hospital data using probabilistic record linkage algorithms.[7]

Whenever pharmacy networks are set up, they should preferably be organized as patient information tracking systems. Such systems consist of a core database with drug information online, thus enabling the collection of clinical and other information from hospitals, general practitioners' offices, or other registrations on an ad hoc basis. Drug use and associated events of individual patients can therefore be followed over time. Such automated linkage with morbidity data is necessarily important for rapid response to acute drug-associated health hazards (postmarketing risk management).[13] The PHARMO system is designed to facilitate postmarketing risk management and postmarketing studies and is, in fact, a patient-tracking system, with the pharmacy network as a high-quality source of drug exposure information. From 1986 through 1995, the network had collected data on more than 600 000 persons. The data are collected once or twice a year and are linked on the patient level with the hospital discharge diagnoses of more than 10 hospitals. The linkage process uses probabilistic record linkage techniques based on several patient characteristics and other dispensing process-related information. Validation of approximately 10 000 patient records showed that both databases (pharmacy and hospital) were linked, with a sensitivity and specificity exceeding 95%.[4,14] The hospital diagnoses are standardized codes according to the WHO *International Classification of Diseases,* Ninth Revision, Clinical Modification, coding system and have a high validity, because coding of diagnoses is performed by central trained faculties in each hospital in the Netherlands. In Figure 1, an integrated drug-dispensing and hospital admission history of a fictitious 77-year-old woman is presented.

DATA QUALITY

With a growing interest in using data from medical and pharmaceutical information systems for epidemiologic research, evidence has indicated the great need for quality assessment of such data.[15] The quality of drug-dispensing histories in pharmacy-based databases is explained by several incentives for pharmacists to maintain accurate and complete drug-dispensing histories and for patients to designate a single pharmacy to fill their prescriptions.

When using existing pharmacy networks for research purposes, researchers must control for the eligibility of each patient for filling prescriptions.[1] If a patient moves, dies, or becomes institutionalized (e.g., hospital, nursing home), he or she cannot fill prescriptions at the pharmacy. Unfortunately, information on the exact entry and exit of a patient in a particular pharmacy is to some extent incomplete. Therefore, when performing epidemiologic studies, researchers must use additional eligibility criteria to demonstrate that patients are present and alive during the study period. A frequently used approach defines patients eligible for filling prescriptions between the dates of the first and last recorded encounter in the databases. When eligibility is not defined, it is impossible to distinguish between truly unexposed patients and those who were not eligible for filling prescriptions because they had already died, had moved, or had been admitted to a nursing home.

A small percentage (3–5%) of drug prescriptions is missed because patients sometimes must fill prescriptions in pharmacies other than the designated one. Several studies demonstrated that this occurs when patients need drugs outside working hours and weekends when their regular pharmacy is closed. These prescriptions mainly concern treatment of acute diseases with, for example, analgesics and antibiotics. As in almost every large

Figure 1
Dispensing History
of a Fictitious
Patient.
Projected Are the
Date and Duration
of an Admission.

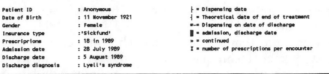

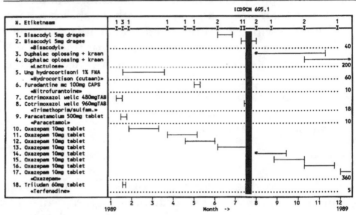

LEGEND

No.	Product	ATC code	Drug Product Name	No.units	Dose	Duration	UPD	Disp.Date	Prescriber
1.	243264	A06AB02	Bisacodyl 5mg dragee	40.000	2T ZN	20	2.00	07-06-89	1
2.	243264	A06AB02	Bisacodyl 5mg dragee	40.000	2T ZN	20	2.00	15-07-89	1
3.	028673	A06AD11	Duphalac oplossing + kraan	3000.000	1D30ML	100	30.00	05-08-89	2
4.	028673	A06AD11	Duphalac oplossing + kraan	3000.000	1D30ML	100	30.00	13-10-89	2
5.	264520	D07AA02	Ung hydrocortisoni 1% FNA	60.000	2D DA	60	1.00	19-01-89	1
6.	215007	G04AC01	Furadantine mc 100mg caps	40.000	4D10Z	10	4.00	06-05-89	1
7.	400483	J03BA01	Cotrimoxazol welic 480mgtab	30.000	2D2T	8	4.00	10-01-89	1
8.	412856	J03BA01	Cotrimoxazol welic 960mgtab	20.000	2D1T	10	2.00	20-07-89	1
9.	244716	N02BE01	Paracetamolum 500mg tablet	20.000	2D1T	10	2.00	19-01-89	1
10.	443980	N05BA04	Oxazepam 10mg tablet	90.000	2D1T	45	2.00	10-01-89	1
11.	443980	N05BA04	Oxazepam 10mg tablet	90.000	2D1T	45	2.00	24-03-89	1
12.	443980	N05BA04	Oxazepam 10mg tablet	90.000	2D1T	45	2.00	21-04-89	1
13.	443980	N05BA04	Oxazepam 10mg tablet	90.000	2D1T	45	2.00	07-06-89	1
14.	443980	N05BA04	Oxazepam 10mg tablet	90.000	2D1T	45	2.00	05-08-89	2
15.	443980	N05BA04	Oxazepam 10mg tablet	90.000	2D1T	45	2.00	01-09-89	1
16.	443980	N05BA04	Oxazepam 10mg tablet	90.000	2D1T	45	2.00	13-10-89	1
17.	443980	N05BA04	Oxazepam 10mg tablet	90.000	2D1T	45	2.00	04-12-89	1
18.	440426	R06AX12	Triludan 60mg tablet	10.000	2D1T	5	2.00	19-01-89	1

No	Prescription ID number
Product	KNMP trade product code
ATC code	Anatomical Therapeutical Chemical Classification
No.units	Total amount of units dispensed
Dose	Dose regimen (2D1T = 2 tablets a day)
Duration	Theoretical stop date medication
UPD	Number of units to be used per day
Disp. date	Dispensing date (Day-month-year)
Prescriber	1 = General practitioner, 2 = medical specialist

database, OTC drug use is also not recorded or is incompletely recorded in drug-dispensing histories. The percentage of missed OTC use depends largely on whether patients regularly frequent pharmacies for prescription drugs. The need to obtain drugs in nonpharmacy outlets declines with the number of prescriptions filled. The elderly, who use large numbers of prescription drugs, almost never use OTC drugs.[16] The largest number of incomplete drug histories is observed for nonresidents who fill prescriptions incidentally. These patients are most often easy to detect because they lack a valid date of birth or have been prescribed drugs by unknown prescribers.

EXTERNAL VALIDITY

Pharmacy networks typically comprise a sample of pharmacies in different geographic regions. With respect to external validity, two issues need discussion: the geographic distribution of the network pharmacies and the representation of the patient population. A major challenge of pharmacy networks is to produce statistics on individual drugs and groups of drugs that are representative for a particular region or nation. The provision of pharmaceutical services from Dutch pharmacies is population based. Specific populations (e.g., the very poor, the unemployed) are therefore not excluded from pharmaceutical services. However, as medical practice, marketing activities, prescribing habits, availability of drug formularies, and product package deals with wholesalers may vary considerably in a particular region or country, careful geographic selection of urban and rural community pharmacies to enroll in a network is required. Even in a reasonably large network comprising information on hundreds of thousands of patients, the size of the population exposed to a particular drug is sensitive to questions of validity. Especially in the first few years of marketing, seeding trials or other activities might result in biases in estimating the number of patients exposed to a particular drug when using pharmacy-based networks. In such a case, validation using other sources of drug information is always required.

Focus on Drug Exposure

DEFINITION OF DRUG EXPOSURE

Defining drug exposure for individual patients is important for risk estimation in pharmacoepidemiologic study designs (e.g., follow-up, case–control). Incorrect exposure estimates may cause exposure misclassification. To characterize exposure, six dimensions are identified: the assessment level of exposure (e.g., prescribing, dispensing, adminstration); identification of the drug (e.g., composition, strength); route of administration (e.g., oral, parenteral, topical); timing and duration of exposure (e.g., start, duration); dosing (e.g., milligrams, international units); and the indication for exposure (e.g., symptoms, complaints, diagnoses). Discussions of the procedures relevant for proper ascertainment of drug exposure follow.

EXPOSURE ASSESSMENT LEVELS

Over the past decades, large computerized databases have become available to identify drug exposure in individual patients and large populations. Most of these registrations are based on prescription, dispensing, or reimbursement data. "True" exposure cannot, however, be easily assessed in these population-based registrations, although they may give a fairly good approximation. Prescribed drugs may not have been filled or dispensed, or reimbursed drugs may have been used incompletely or not at all. Furthermore, as discussed in other chapters, databases are not always complete in documenting the exposure status of the patient. Pharmacy data are then a welcome substitute for patient data as they are very close to the ultimate process of individual drug use. However, sample validation of drug exposure data is recommended.

Exposure estimates obtained at different levels of the healthcare system may not be comparable. For instance, a general practitioner–based prescription registration in the Netherlands would miss, for some patients, up to 80% of all prescriptions, because these are prescribed by medical specialists or other prescribers. When comparing data originating from population surveys, wholesalers, pharmacies, or general practitioners, it is not surprising that population drug exposure estimates may vary considerably.

POPULATION DRUG EXPOSURE MEASURES

Estimations and comparisons of the frequency of disease or exposure are the sinew of observational epidemiologic studies.[17] To express the extent of drug exposure at a population level, several units of measurement have been used throughout the years (e.g., defined daily dose [DDD]/1000 inhabitants/day, ever users/1000 inhabitants/year, prescriptions/1000 inhabitants/year). Which of these measures should be used depends on the research questions and the availability of data. For example, for expressing the frequency of drug use in DDD/1000 inhabitants/day, the availability of data on an individual patient level is not required. The DDD-based statistic is therefore widely used in drug utilization studies and is useful when comparing population drug use among different regions where detailed information is not available. The basic comparison unit of these calculations is the DDD. Although the DDD often equals the recommended daily dose, it is best described as an "exchange rate" to compare drug use among different regional settings.[12] The DDD/1000 inhabitants/day is calculated by first converting the total amount of milligrams into DDDs. By dividing the total number of DDDs by the size of the population and the number of days the drug is used, the number of DDDs/1000 inhabitants/day can be calculated. Suppose, in a fictitious country with 50 million inhabitants, 400 kg of temazepam were sold in a period of 1 year. With temazepam 20 mg defined as 1 DDD, we can calculate the use of temazepam as 11 DDDs/1000 inhabitants/day. This method can also be used to measure the extent of use of drug groups, for example, all benzodiazepines. For every benzodiazepine, the total number of milligrams is first converted to DDDs and subsequently summarized to calculate the number of DDDs/1000 inhabitants/day.

Besides the advantage of the DDD-based statistics through their wide applicability, this statistic is sensitive to a wide variety of biases. Dosing may, for instance, differ by age, gender, weight, or local prescribing habits; hence, demographic differences between two regions may result in unpredictable biases when comparisons are based on the DDD/1000 inhabitants/day measure. A major limitation of the applicability of the DDD-based statistic in epidemiologic studies is that this measure is a very crude approximation of the number of individuals exposed to a single drug or drug group. For instance, the exposure prevalence[18] of benzodiazepines in the Netherlands in 1992 was estimated as 36 patients per 1000 inhabitants; thus, 36 of 1000 inhabitants of the Netherlands use benzodiazepines on a daily basis. The use of benzodiazepines based on the DDD statistic was estimated in the same data set as 47/1000 inhabitants/day. The difference between the two measures is to a large extent explained by the fact that 10% of the patients who use benzodiazepines were using two benzodiazepines concomitantly (e.g., temazepam 20 mg once daily and oxazepam 10 mg three times daily).

HAZARD FUNCTIONS

Timing of exposure is crucial in risk assessment. Risk is a dynamic, not static, concept and should therefore be considered as a function of exposure time, a hazard function.[19] One of the first hazard functions was published in the late 1960s and shows the time relationship between ampicillin exposure and occurrence of rash.[20] Ampicillin-associated rash is most likely to occur within 10 days of initiation of exposure. The hazard function therefore represents a probability distribution of the adverse reaction relative to drug exposure. Some adverse effects might occur instantly (e.g., accidental falls), whereas other effects might occur several days, months, or even years after discontinuation of exposure (e.g., cancer). Unfortunately, the hazard function is rarely known, and observational and clinical information should be used to define a theoretic model.

To define a hazard function, precise determination of the exposure duration is important. There is, however, no single accurate method to estimate the duration of exposure by using databases. In general, two methods are used: a *fixed-duration* and a *time-window* approach.[21] In the fixed-duration method, the legend duration of exposure is estimated as a fixed period of 30 or 60 days. The legend duration of exposure is derived from standards in pharmacy practice. However, other fixed periods are also possible (e.g., a fixed exposure time of 8 d for antibiotics). The time-window approach is more flexible and estimates the legend duration of exposure by dividing the total number of dispensed tablets by the number of tablets to be used per day (e.g., 60 tablets ÷ 3 tablets daily = 20 d). As the legend duration of exposure is a time window for possible events, errors in estimating the period of exposure are sensitive to information bias. The magnitude and direction of the bias are determined mainly by the shape of the hazard function. If single exposure is associated with a lifelong increased risk for cancer, either method can be used. In the case of events that occur only while exposed, the fixed-duration method may cause substantial nondifferential misclassification bias.[21] If dosing information is available, the time-window approach is preferred (see also Figure 1). However, both methods are approximations of the actual exposure time; they are inaccurate in estimating the exposure of as-needed drug therapy (e.g., some antiasthmatic, H_1-antihistamine, or analgesic medications) or in situations of poor compliance. As better information is often not available, sensitivity analyses to explore the presence and direction of misclassification bias should have high priority. Pharmacy dispensing data provide useful information to explore several definitions of duration, dosing, and timing of exposure and to evaluate the effects of these on risk estimates using sensitivity analyses.

OVER-THE-COUNTER DRUG MISCLASSIFICATION

In claims-, prescriber-, and pharmacy-based registrations, no or limited information is available concerning exposure to OTC medications. If one of these OTC preparations is associated with the adverse effect studied, misclassification in, for example, a case–control study might invalidate risk estimates. Suppose a case–control study is conducted to assess the risk of gastrointestinal bleeding and exposure to nonsteroidal antiinflammatory drugs (NSAIDs). Suppose further that acetylsalicylic acid preparations and ibuprofen are available as OTC preparations. If the same proportion of cases and controls is exposed to one or both of these OTC drugs, the misclassification is nondifferential and the odds ratio does not change. In most studies addressing this exposure relation, such nondifferential misclassification is tacitly assumed. If, however, the proportion of cases and controls exposed to these OTC drugs differs, the misclassification may be differential. Hence, the odds ratio is under- or overestimated. Such a situation occurs if exposure to OTC preparations is related to exposure of NSAIDs, which is plausible in situations of differences in reimbursement status of the two drug classes. Elderly patients in the Netherlands and heavy users of prescription drugs use fewer OTC drugs compared with relatively healthy elderly persons who may be selected as controls in case–control studies.[16]

A second problem results from changing prescription drugs to OTC status. If drugs change to an OTC status, risk assessment of any adverse effect is very difficult and rather impossible using pharmacy-based networks. The availability of H_1-antihistamines, as well as other potent drugs, through nonpharmacy outlets will have a substantial impact on the conduct of postmarketing studies in this area, because no registers of use of such drugs are commonly available. Prospective and retrospective monitoring for adverse effects or drug–drug interactions (e.g., erythromycin interactions[22]) would become impossible. Especially when new chemical entities are introduced, potential life-threatening drug–drug interactions are difficult to detect.

Clinical Relevance of Pharmacy Networks

The use of pharmacy-based networks has two implications. It supports the role of the pharmacy as a professional discipline through the clinical information it provides, and it fosters pharmacoepidemiology as a scientific discipline.[2] Pharmacy networks can be used to answer important scientific and clinical questions. In the next paragraphs, several examples are discussed.

RISK MANAGEMENT

When signals emerge from voluntary adverse drug reaction (ADR) reporting systems or the literature, there is an urgent need to assess whether the suspected unintended drug effect (UDE) is an isolated case or represents a real health hazard. Often, at that time, the association is unproven, and the incidence of the adverse reaction and the exposure prevalence are unknown. Because such information is not readily available, the impact of the ADR in a population is unknown. We used community pharmacy networks to assess the extent of a possible public health problem after the US Food and Drug Administration expressed concern about the safety of terfenadine (Seldane, Triludan). It was suggested that concomitant use of erythromycin, ketoconazole, or cimetidine increased blood concentrations of terfenadine, thereby elevating the risk of torsade de pointes. The PHARMO network was searched for patients exposed to terfenadine and other H_1-antihistamines to estimate the extent of exposure on a national level and the attributive risk of the mentioned interactions. The results showed that the number of expected cases of torsade de pointes due to the risk factors of overprescribing and interactions was less than three patients per year.[13] Although the causality of the potential interaction is, of course, not studied, the maximum size of the population at risk can be estimated. Thus, it is important for health authorities to set priorities for further action.

COHORT TRACING

Pharmacy networks may be used to trace and subsequently warn or study patients exposed to a particular drug.[23] Adverse reactions can be monitored either by linkage to clinical databases or by collecting information from patients or prescribers. Prospective cohort tracing of recipients of drugs is important for postmarketing surveillance and risk management and should be further developed, with appropriate safeguards of patient privacy. An example of cohort tracing has been conducted by Stricker et al.[24] who traced patients exposed to isotretinoin after a warning for possible teratogenic effects occurring long after exposure took place. This UDE was thought to result from the pharmacokinetic properties of the drug.[8,24] The pharmacist can also act as an intermediary between researchers and physicians. Coded and sealed envelopes were used for the exchange of information, making it feasible to validate drug exposure information with medical data provided by general practitioners.[25] Although identification and tracing of patients are feasible through pharmacy networks, each endeavor should be balanced with respect to privacy regulations.

CASE–COHORT STUDIES

In situations in which both exposure and adverse reactions are rare, for instance in the first few years after marketing, follow-up and case–control designs fail to provide reliable risk estimates. New approaches to quantify these "rare-to-rare" problems have been developed over the past years. van der Klauw et al.[26] used a case–cohort design to quantify the risk of developing anaphylaxis associated with the use of the analgesic glafenine. All hospitalizations due to anaphylaxis in 1987–1988 were identified in a national morbidity register in the Netherlands. Diagnoses were validated by an audit committee of medical specialists. The causative agent was identified in the medical charts, and the extent of exposure was ascertained on the basis of 1987–1988 dispensing information derived from a representative network of 28 community pharmacies throughout the Netherlands. The relative risk of anaphylaxis due to glafenine was compared with that of other drugs. Relative to all other drugs, a relative risk of 168 was calculated (95% CI 63 to 446). The high relative risk was a major reason why glafenine was withdrawn from the Dutch and several other European markets in 1992.

PRESCRIPTION SEQUENCE ANALYSIS

In contrast to many other substantive areas of interest in epidemiology (e.g., cancer, nutritional epidemiology), the exposure to a drug may reflect the morbidity treated. Many times, this source of confounding poses serious difficulties in epidemiologic designs. However, one could take advantage of this when a drug is prescribed to treat a (iatrogenic) disease caused by a previously prescribed, different drug. This principle was used by Petri et al. (1990)[27] to develop a population-based method to study drug-induced effects. The method, called prescription sequence analysis, is in fact a follow-up study with drug use as both exposure and outcome. This method was used to study the association between flunarizine and depression. In a network of computerized pharmacies, 1284 users of flunarizine were identified. Of these, 180 (14%) had, at one time or another during the study period, also been prescribed an antidepressant. If, as postulated, flunarizine did trigger depression, one would have expected to see an increase of antidepressant prescribing following flunarizine exposure. The data showed only a small, marginally significant increase in the use of antidepressants. The prescription sequence analysis method is a welcome alternative for outcomes research when morbidity data are not available.

SELECTIVE DRUG PRESCRIBING

Pharmacoepidemiology has a major, single characteristic that is typical of many problems that occur when using analytic pharmacoepidemiologic designs: Exposure to a drug under investigation is not randomly distributed in populations. If confronted with a particular symptom, even a poorly trained prescriber may make a structured decision to prescribe a particular drug. By this decision process, the prescriber might introduce several types of selection bias into the study base that, in turn, may cause several exposure-related problems such as confounding by indication, channeling, or depletion of susceptibles.

Confounding by indication might occur if the disease for which the drug is prescribed is causally related to an increased or decreased risk to develop the studied drug-induced effect. Consequently, the observed relative risk is prone to be over- or underestimated. This type of confounding is difficult to control for, because patients with the same indication and characteristics and who are not treated with the drug in question are rare. Confounding by severity of disease is, in fact, a special form of confounding by indication. The issue of disease severity as a determinant of drug therapy outcomes has been addressed extensively following the controversy over the mortality risk attributed to the use of beta-agonists: Patients with more severe asthma are more likely to use or abuse inhaled medication.[28,29]

The problem of channeling occurs when drugs with more or less identical pharmacology and indications are used by different risk groups of patients. Here, preferential prescribing might be related to a wide variety of risk factors for ADRs. Marketing of products to patients with typical characteristics is a major source of channeling, especially when prompting physicians to choose a new product with strong claims of safety or efficacy. Pharmacy networks provide data for identifying such biases in the treatment of asthma and the prescription of NSAIDs.[30,31] New products are also susceptible for selective prescribing for other reasons. In many countries, there is growing resistance to the use of new pharmaceutical products, mainly because of economic reasons. This resistance is not uniformly felt throughout the community of prescribers. As a result, the adoption of new drugs tends to occur in selective groups of prescribers and their patients. These adoption patterns deserve pharmacoepidemiologic analysis for the proper assessment of the efficacy and safety of newly marketed drugs.

Another type of selective prescribing might occur when a particular drug, known for causing an adverse reaction, is in time prescribed less frequently to patients at risk. Consider a study to assess the risk of depression among users of beta-blocking agents. This problem received considerable attention, and it is not unlikely that, today, patients at risk of developing depression are prescribed lipophilic beta-blocking agents. Those "risk susceptible" patients are thus depleted in time. Hence, the relative risk of developing depression when on propranolol would be much lower than it was several years ago. This selection bias phenomenon, known as depletion of susceptibles, is described in detail by Moride.[32]

Selective prescribing of drugs needs to be identified and understood in pharmacoepidemiologic studies. Whether termed confounding by indication, channeling, or depletion of susceptibles, selective prescribing emphasizes one of the basic questions in pharmacoepidemiology: Did the drug bring the problems to the patient, or did the patient bring the problems to the drug?

Conclusion

The increasing availability of large computerized databases opens new possibilities for better definitions and assessment of exposure in epidemiologic designs. In this chapter, several possibilities and problems, typical for drug-dispensing data from pharmacy networks, are discussed, although the mechanisms may be valid for other data sources as well. Shapiro[33] has criticized the often invalid definition or assessment of exposure. It is noteworthy that most of the efforts in pharmacoepidemiologic studies so far are directed toward case descriptions and validation of morbidity.[33,34]

Exposure assessment has not received much attention because, at least in our perception, exposure data are often considered wrongly as valid and reliable data. Although we discussed only a selected number of exposure-related problem areas, we have illustrated that pharmacoepidemiologic studies, even with the most extensive validation of morbidity, are of little value without proper definition and assessment of exposure. Pharmacy networks represent one resource, if not a very powerful one, to strengthen the development of better ways to ascertain "true" exposure.

References

1. Stergachis AS. Record linkage studies for postmarketing drug surveillance: data quality and validity considerations. Drug Intell Clin Pharm 1988;22:157-61.
2. Hartzema AG, Martini N. Pharmacoepidemiology: the role of the clinical pharmacist. Contemporary pharmacy issues. Kalamazoo, MI: Upjohn, 1991.
3. Leufkens HGM. Pharmacy records in pharmacoepidemiology. Studies on antiinflammatory and antirheumatic drugs (thesis). Utrecht: Utrecht University, 1990.
4. Petri H. The prescription drug history in pharmacoepidemiology (thesis). Maastricht: 1992.
5. de Jong-van den Berg LTW. Drug utilization studies in pregnancy: what can they contribute to safety assessment? (thesis). Groningen: University of Groningen, 1992.
6. Hoes AW. Non-potassium sparing diuretics and sudden cardiac death in hypertensive patients: a pharmacoepidemiologic approach (thesis). Rotterdam: Erasmus University, 1992.
7. Herings RMC. PHARMO. A record linkage system for postmarketing surveillance of prescription drugs in the Netherlands (thesis). Utrecht: Utrecht University, 1993.
8. Sturkenboom MCJM. A field-oriented postmarketing surveillance study on the teratogen acitretin. Groningen: University of Groningen, 1995.
9. Heerdink ER. Clustering of drug use in the eldery. Population-based studies into prevalence and outcomes. Utrecht: Utrecht University, 1995.
10. Ottervanger JP. Pharmacoepidemiology of sumatriptan: cardiovascular adverse reactions to a new antimigrainous drug. Rotterdam: Erasmus University, 1996.
11. Urquhart J. Time to take our medicines, seriously (inaugural lecture, University of Limburg, April 3, 1992). Pharm Weekbl 1992;127:769-76.
12. WHO Collaborating Centre for Drug Statistics Methodology. ATC classification and DDD assignment. Oslo: World Health Organization, 1996.
13. Herings RMC, Stricker BHCh, Leufkens HGM, Bakker A, Sturmans F, Urquhart J. Public health problems and the rapid estimation of the size of the population at risk. Pharm World Sci 1993;15:212-8.
14. Herings RMC, Stricker BHCh, Nap G, Bakker A. Pharmacomorbidity linkage: a feasibility study comparing morbidity in two pharmacy-based exposure cohorts. J Epidemiol Community Health 1992;46:136-40.
15. Feinstein AR. Quality of data in the medical record. Comput Biomed Res 1970;3: 426-35.
16. Heerdink ER, Leufkens HGM, Kopperdraaijer C, Bakker A. Information on drug use in the elderly: a comparison of pharmacy, general practitioner and patient data. Pharm World Sci 1995;17:20-4.
17. Grisso JA. Making comparisons. Lancet 1993;342:157-9.
18. Rothman KJ. Modern epidemiology. Boston: Little, Brown, 1986.
19. Collet JP, Boivin JF, Spitzer WO. Bias and confounding in pharmacoepidemiology. In: Strom BL, ed. Pharmacoepidemiology. 2nd ed. Chichester: John Wiley & Sons, 1994:609-28.
20. Shapiro S, Slone D, Siskind V, Lewis GP, Jick H. Drug rash with ampicillin and other penicillins. Lancet 1969;2:969-72.
21. van Staa TP, Abenheim L, Leufkens HG. Selective prescribing of non-steroidal anti-inflammatory drugs—implications for postmarketing surveillance. Postmarket Surveill 1992;5:339-49.

22. Monahan BP, Ferguson CL, Killeavy ES, Lloyd BK, Troy J, Cantillena LR. Torsade de pointes occurring in association with terfenadine use. JAMA 1990;264:2788-90.
23. Borden EK, Lee JG. A methodologic study of postmarketing drug evaluation using a pharmacy-based approach. J Chronic Dis 1982;35:803.
24. Stricker BH, Barendregt M, Herings RM, de Jong-van den Berg LT, Cornel MC, De Smet PA. Ad hoc tracing of a cohort of patients exposed to acitretine (Neotigason) on a nation-wide scale. Eur J Clin Pharmacol 1992;42:555-7.
25. Leufkens HG, Ruter EM, Ameling CB, Hekster YA, Bakker A. Linkage of pharmacy data on heavy users of nonsteroidal anti-inflammatory drugs to information from general practitioners. J Pharmacoepidemiol 1991;2:67-77.
26. van der Klauw M, Stricker BHCh, Herings RMC, Cost WS, Valkenburg HA, Wilson JHP. A population based case–cohort study of drug-induced anaphylaxis. Br J Clin Pharmacol 1993;35:400-8.
27. Petri H, Leufkens HG, Naus J, Silkens R, van Hessen P, Urquhart J. Rapid method for estimating the risk of acutely controversial side effects of prescription drugs. J Clin Epidemiol 1990;43:433-9.
28. Petri H, Urquhart J. Channeling bias in the interpretation of drug effects. Stat Med 1991;10:577-81.
29. Ernst P, Habbick B, Suissa S, Hemmelgarn B, Cockcroft D, Buist AS, et al. Is the association between inhaled beta-agonist use and life-threatening asthma because of confounding by severity? Am Rev Respir Dis 1993;148:75-9.
30. Petri H, Urquhart J, Herings R, Bakker A. Characteristics of patients prescribed three different inhalational beta-2 agonists: an example of the channeling phenomenon. Postmarket Surveill 1991;5:57-65.
31. Leufkens HG, Urquhart J, Stricker BHCh, Bakker A, Petri H. Channeling of controlled release formulation of ketoprofen (OSCOREL) in patients with history of gastrointestinal problems. J Epidemiol Community Health 1992;46:428-32.
32. Moride Y. Exposure characterization and risk assessment in pharmacoepidemiology: nonsteroidal anti-inflammatory drugs and gastrointestinal bleeding (thesis). Montreal: McGill University, 1992.
33. Shapiro S. The role of automated record linkage in the postmarketing surveillance of drug safety: a critique. Clin Pharmacol Ther 1989;46:371-86.
34. Guess HA. Limitations of available sources of data on prescription drug safety. In: Horisberger B, Dinkel R, eds. The perception and management of drug safety risks. Berlin: Springer-Verlag, 1989:51-6.

17

Drug Safety, Pharmacoepidemiology, and Regulatory Decision-Making

Robert C Nelson

Abstract

The safety or risk assessments of a pharmacotherapeutic agent begin early in product development and continue throughout marketing and use cycles. The practice of pharmacoepidemiology is the art of using the science and the tools of science to generate information about pharmaceutical outcomes, including associated risks, in the postmarketing environment. A pharmacoepidemiologist must be capable of functioning within a matrix constructed of three components: a knowledge base, a conceptual framework, and an interpretive framework. From this perspective, one can establish surveillance schemes or understand a posed research question, select strategies, apply methodologies, and interpret the results of purposeful investigations. When conveyed to the risk manager, appropriately interpreted results of a properly conducted risk assessment can be used in regulatory decision-making. Eleven case studies are presented as pragmatic examples of this approach.

T herapeutic intervention with modern pharmaceutical agents is a mainstay of medical practice. The multiple levels of required premarket testing are very effective in identifying and eliminating potential drugs that are markedly toxic. However, every known physiologically active exogenous agent also possesses an adverse consequence profile, the components of which can remain hidden until the drug is being marketed and used in a broader population than experienced in the preapproval clinical trials. This chapter provides an introductory view of the way pharmacoepidemiologic principles are conceptualized and have been applied to drug and therapeutic biologic product postmarketing safety issues within the regulatory environment of the Food and Drug Administration (FDA).

A set of conceptual and methodologic approaches is presented, some that were developed in an effort to conduct meaningful epidemiologic research at the FDA. To illustrate these approaches, many unpublished but public citations have been noted. The reader is encouraged to review these public citations, which are available through a Freedom of Information Act request, and to consult the references included in the other chapters of this book for the standard references in pharmacoepidemiology.

This chapter proposes a functional framework for pharmacoepidemiology and proceeds to practical application. The latter is a set of examples in which pharmacoepidemiologic approaches were used to address drug safety concerns. A distinction is made between the function of risk assessment and decision-making risk management within the FDA.

Background

The safety or risk assessment of a pharmacotherapeutic agent is a complex task, requiring a multidisciplinary synthesis of information. This synthesis should take place early in the development of the agent and continue throughout its use cycle. Conventionally, postmarketing risk assessment for pharmaceutical agents is limited to the identification of iatrogenic morbidity (the adverse consequences of legitimate pharmacotherapy). However, because our modern society is afflicted with pharmacophilia, a complete assessment also must include the unintended drug effects (UDEs) associated with the nonmedical use of legal drugs.

Adverse drug experience[a] is currently (a new definition is contained in the Postmarketing Regulations Rewrite under consideration at the FDA, as of this writing) defined in US federal regulation 21 CFR (Code of Federal Regulations) 314.80 as follows:

---

[a]For the purpose of uniformity, UDE is used throughout.

any adverse event associated with the use of a drug in humans, whether or not considered drug related, including the following: an adverse event occurring in the course of the use of drug product in professional practice; an adverse event occurring from drug overdose whether accidental or intentional; an adverse event occurring from drug abuse; an adverse event occurring from drug withdrawal; and any significant failure of expected pharmacological action.

Figure 1 diagrams a conceptual framework for the UDEs of drug use intentionally consumed for therapy. UDEs may be direct or mediated by an interaction with another factor. The latter factors include other concomitant medication, specific foods, the presence or absence of food, age, gender, genetics, and comorbid conditions.

UDEs directly attributable to the administration of a pharmacotherapeutic agent may manifest acutely as allergic or idiosyncratic reactions, as dose-related toxicities to organ systems, or chronically due to accumulation of the agent or its metabolites in the body.

A more complex framework for the consequences of nontherapeutic drug use, which is divided as to the motive of consumption (i.e., unintentional or intentional consumption of the nontherapeutic dose of the drug), is shown in Figure 2. Unintentional nonmedical consumption includes the erroneous acute ingestion of a drug, the chronic ingestion of an excessive amount, or the accidental acute poisoning episode. The intentional nontherapeutic ingestion of a drug is an abuse situation. The intentional ingestion for self-destruction, whether a suicide gesture or attempt, is included here as a component of a drug's safety profile. The capacity for a drug to produce psychic effects and/or induce psychological dependence or to

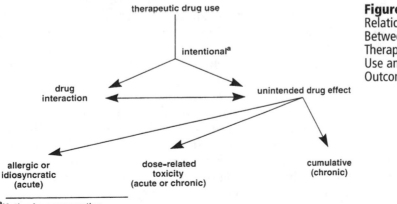

Figure 1
Relationship Between Therapeutic Drug Use and Adverse Outcomes

[a]Motive for consumption.

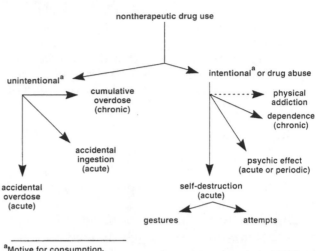

Figure 2
Relationship
Between
Nontherapeutic
Drug Use and
Adverse Outcomes

[a]Motive for consumption.

lead to a physical dependence is indicative of a drug's abuse potential and must be considered in risk assessment. This component of a drug's safety profile is particularly pertinent for psychoactive drugs.

The intentional consumption in a nontherapeutic mode model has undergone a revision to include use for "physical enhancement." The anabolic steroids and, most recently, human growth hormone are two such agents. It is important to understand that all UDEs associated with the use of legal pharmaceutical products fall within the regulatory mandate of the FDA.

The potential limitations of the UDE data obtained from clinical trials have been discussed extensively in the literature[1,2] and are addressed by Rogers in Chapter 5. The UDE rates derived from clinical trial data are reported to be more conservative than those derived from formal Phase IV studies for the more common and generally less serious reactions and, therefore, are usually not useful for low-incidence reactions.[3] However, these clinical trial data are used in the FDA-approved final printing labeling (i.e., the product package insert), which accompanies the drug product to the healthcare marketplace. All industry-generated advertising of the product, whether verbal (i.e., through professional sales representatives) or written, must conform to this approved labeling. Because most practicing physicians learn about new drug products from the manufacturer, the importance of the labeling information is evident. The labeling can be revised when new UDEs are detected and assessed in postmarketing surveillance.

Prescription drug labeling may lag behind the practice of medicine for beneficial new events (i.e., indications) because inclusion is contingent on demonstration by the drug's sponsor of substantial evidence of both safety and efficacy in an amendment to the new drug application (NDA). The labeling usually is more current for new UDEs. That is not to say that the addition of a UDE to a product label is easy and straightforward. The detection of a UDE and its attribution to a drug product are more difficult in the postmarketing period than during premarketing. Confounders abound in the open or uncontrolled environment. A UDE may be due to the drug product, the indicated underlying disorders, a spontaneously generated disorder, genetic differences in metabolism, irrational prescribing, a patient compliance problem, an interaction with food or another drug product, or an individual variation. Clearly, the relationship between a drug and a UDE often appears to be casual rather than causal.

The preceding chapters in this text have explained the breadth and scope of pharmacoepidemiology, as well as the history of drug regulation and the discipline of spontaneous reports by the FDA (Chapter 9). The reader has also been introduced to theory, algorithms, and the wide variety of data sources that can or could be tapped for study. However, the conversion of data into information and the proper weighting of abstract knowledge into a decision-making equation concerning the safety of a pharmacotherapeutic agent currently defy predictive modeling. Skill, logic, a healthy dose of ingenuity, and a degree of pragmatism are required, especially if one is forced to function within a regulatory environment with its inherent time lines. Safety issues are not absolute; they must be evaluated in light of competing risks, benefits associated with the drug's approved indication(s), and competing benefits from other forms of therapy.

The FDA's Regulatory Mandate

The FDA shares with the product manufacturer the responsibility for the initial and continual assessment of drug safety. The Agency's authority to affect the conditions of marketing for drugs and therapeutic biologic products comes from the Food, Drug, and Cosmetic Act (1938) as amended, the Public Health Service Act (1904) as amended, and Section 201 of the Controlled Substances Act (1971). The FDA's regulatory role is placed in the proper perspective when one understands that the FDA does not approve drugs or "biologics." Rather, these cited US statutes and regulations provide the basic requirements for determining the safety and efficacy of new drug *products*. The process includes the development of safety and efficacy data during the investigational new drug (IND) phase and the submission of these data in support of a marketing application (the NDA). The FDA approves a drug product or a biologic for a specific indication if adequate and well-controlled clinical trials support its safety and efficacy for the specific indication.

The Division of Pharmacovigilance and Epidemiology (DPE) (formerly the Division of Epidemiology and Surveillance) within the Center for Drug Evaluation and Research (CDER) is the FDA's functional pharmacovigilance and pharmacoepidemiology unit (i.e., the *risk assessors*). This Division houses the new Adverse Event Reporting System (AERS) (formerly the Spontaneous Reporting System), which contains UDE data from FDA MedWatch Form 3500(A) (and, historically, Form 1639). The DPE also manages a program of cooperative agreements for extramural sources for epidemiologic data (see Chapter 14) and employs epidemiologists and other health professionals to assess drug safety in the postmarketing arena. Interaction with the regulatory component of the CDER is vital. The 13 new drug product review divisions within the Offices of Drug Evaluation I through V (ODE I–V) are the functional regulatory decision-making units, that is, the *risk managers*.

In addition to informal communication pathways, the main forum for interaction is the monthly safety conference. Key individuals of the DPE risk assessment team meet separately with each of the 13 drug product review divisions to discuss issues of safety. The three general areas for discussion at these safety conferences are any important new UDE signals received through the AERS, consultations from or areas of regulatory concern to the ODE divisions, and recent literature reports and relevant epidemiologic studies. Normally, an individual from the DPE, referred to as a *reports evaluator*, identifies and researches a new UDE, which, if of clinical substance, is then referred to as a signal. The strength of this signal is contingent upon both the quantity and quality of the AERS reports. Usually, two or three well-documented reports make up the minimal data set. In a rare case, causality may be attributable from a single well-documented report, particularly in the case of positive rechallenge.[4]

The data supporting this new signal are then presented to the regulatory divisions either for their information or as an action item, depending on the strength of the case series. The DPE staff, as advisors and consultants to the ODEs, prepare epidemiologic reports on areas of regulatory concern and present these results at the safety conferences. The goal is, whenever possible, to narrow the breadth of a regulatory decision gap with a well-conducted safety assessment. Although it is generally recognized that the most concentrated postmarketing effort should be directed toward the detection and verification of new, unexpected, and serious reports, such reports functionally comprise only a small portion of the total amount of safety and relative safety issues that arise.

The FDA must address all the safety issues brought to its attention and make a decision as to the action necessary; the actual research questions are varied in nature and importance. High-quality and accessible data sources used by well-skilled reports evaluators increase the likelihood of reliable and timely risk assessments.

When an application for a new drug product enters the FDA review process, it receives a priority designation based on its chemical uniqueness and a prediction of its eventual medical use. In an ideal situation, the DPE epidemiology staff monitor the in-house premarketing progress of priority NDAs. When the situation warrants, formal Phase IV programs should be planned by the ODE staff, with close and in-depth consultation from the DPE staff, as early in the drug development process as possible. The DPE staff obtain advance information (usually a copy of the NDA approval "action package") on the new molecular entities and other designated drug products of special interest from the reviewing division before they are marketed, so that an efficient and effective postmarketing surveillance (PMS) effort can be set into place. If residual concerns about safety remain at the potential approval point, a formal Phase IV safety study can be negotiated with the manufacturer. In either case, the postmarketing risk assessor requires full knowledge of the drug product—including the drug's pharmacokinetic profile, the UDE profile seen in the Phase III clinical trails, data from foreign marketing experience, and knowledge of the UDE profile of pharmacologically similar marketed drugs—to increase the probability of predicting the problems that may occur in the marketplace. The ideal goal of PMS is to bring the time of discovery of a major proportion of new information as close to the time of marketing the new drug as possible.[5]

Functional Frameworks

Pharmacoepidemiology, an epidemiologic specialty, requires a synthesis of multidisciplinary information; its practice is the use of the sciences and the tools of science to generate information about pharmaceutical outcomes. The practice of pharmacoepidemiology in a regulatory environment is the art of using the science and the tools of science to generate information that is then used as part of the basis for regulatory decisions that impact the public health by their effect on drug therapy.

A pharmacoepidemiologist must be capable of functioning within a matrix constructed of three components: a knowledge framework made up of the information on drugs and disease states, as well as clinical and general medical care principles; a conceptual framework for understanding, orientation, and direction, which includes the epidemiologic principles and methodologies; an interpretive framework that relies heavily on logic and elimination of alternative explanations. Knowledge and understanding of the availability and validity of data sources are required across all parts of the matrix.

The conceptual framework is discussed most extensively in this section. When referring to the UDEs of drug use, one can envision a five-segment continuum in the pharmacoepidemiologic approach: (1) the detection of an event (often referred to as a signal or signaling), (2) generation of a hypothesis, (3) description, (4) assessment of the strength of an association, and (5) testing of a hypothesis.

These segments appear in Table 1, with the latter two segments distinguished by the validity of underlying statistical assumptions. The conceptual framework for pharmacoepidemiologic techniques as presented in Table 1 has been modified from the frameworks developed by Jones.[5,6] This framework allows one to organize the many approaches and data sources available for the study of drug effects. The two main conceptual categories, ascertainment by drug and by event, were originally described by Finney,[7] but are presented here in a revised and modified form. The strategies in each category are those in current use and are not an exhaustive listing.

Table 1
Conceptual Framework for Pharmacoepidemiologic Techniques

	Detection or Signaling	Hypothesis Generation	Description	Strength of Association	Hypothesis Testing
Ascertainment by drug					
A: monitoring (without controls)	A-1 yes	A-2 yes	A-3 no	A-4 no	A-5 no
B: numerator analysis across events (without controls)	B-1 yes	B-2 yes	B-3 yes	B-4 no	B-5 no
C: cohort studies (with controls)	C-1 no	C-2 no	C-3 no	C-4 yes	C-5 yes
Ascertainment by event					
D: numerator analysis—event-specific (without denominators, without controls)	D-1 yes	D-2 yes	D-3 yes	D-4 no	D-5 no
E: single drug–event analysis (with denominator, without controls)	E-1 no	E-2 yes	E-3 yes	E-4 no	E-5 yes[a]
F: comparative proportional analyses (with internal controls)	F-1 no	F-2 yes	F-3 no	F-4 yes	F-5 no
G: case–control study design (with controls)	G-1 no	G-2 yes	G-3 no	G-4 yes	G-5 yes

[a]With external or historical controls.

These two conceptual categories differ in directionality, in the time lapse until functional, and in use. Each category contains a number of strategies or methods used either in a surveillance mode or in addressing a specific research question. The ascertainment by drug category begins with the drug, and then identifies and evaluates the adverse pharmaceutical outcomes. These address the question: What UDEs are associated with this drug? In a larger sense, this is not limited just to UDEs, but includes new, beneficial ones. This concept is similar to the one that underlies the practice of clinical epidemiology: the evaluation of the consequences of therapeutic intervention. The *ascertainment by drug* category has three components that vary in function: monitoring, numerator analysis across events, and the cohort study design. The first two do not have the advantage of controls.

The primary surveillance mode (i.e., monitoring) is practiced through the use of the FDA AERS (which includes the direct spontaneous report data that come through the MedWatch program) and the medical literature. In general, this large-scale operation is used to detect new events or signals. When the signal is an unexpected one from the perspective of biologic plausibility, or one for which the interpretation is controversial, additional confirmation is necessary, and a hypothesis is generated. A numerator analysis (across events without a denominator and without controls) can present a qualitative and a quasiquantitative description of the drug's safety profile. For example, reported UDEs can be plotted across physiologic body systems, and then at a finer level, across diagnostic terms within a body system. The comparison of these profiles among drugs within a pharmacologic class often is informative and may lead to new signals and/or new hypotheses. The formally designed prospective cohort study with a control group can be used to assess the strength of an association or as a formal test of a hypothesis.

A reversal of directionality yields *ascertainment by event*. This addresses the question: What are the pharmaceutical risk factors for this UDE? The four methods in this conceptual category are the following: numerator analysis (event specific, without denominators, and without controls), single drug–event analysis (with denominators, without controls); comparative proportional analyses (with denominators, internal control); and the case–control study design. The event-specific numerator analysis can be used to examine which drugs have been associated with a specific UDE (e.g., hepatotoxicity). The single drug–event analysis can examine the context in which the events occur through a content analysis of the data. Comparative proportional analyses assess the strength of associations relative to other members of a comparable drug group. The formally designed case–control study can be used to generate hypotheses, but it is most valuable when used to test a hypothesis. The integration of existing data sources into this conceptual framework is illustrated in the next section.

The interpretive framework concerns interpretation, use, and decision-making. An axiom of empiric research says that the more well controlled and internally valid the study design, the more straightforward, statistically valid, and less judgmental the interpretation of results. At best, a properly designed, analytic, epidemiologic study, which is based on observational data that did not have the benefit of random allocation and other design features of prospective controlled trials, is difficult to interpret. The open research methods often used to address pharmacoepidemiologic questions contain most, if not all, of the threats to internal validity listed by Campbell and Stanley.[8] Interpretation of such results usually requires the use of additional outside sources of information, such as multiple databases, to eliminate or assess the relative likelihood of alternative explanations. The most important source of information used in the interpretation of pharmacoepidemiologic findings is the previously described knowledge framework. Overall, this medicologic form of interpretation could be called the art of epidemiologic diagnosis.

Utilization of the results of epidemiologic research requires information dissemination. The DPE staff submits in-house reports on its risk assessment efforts to become part of the NDA (the official administrative record) and to the ODE divisions for regulatory decision-making and elective dissemination in regulatory media. For selected issues, collaborative publication in the medical literature is also sought.

The phrase "regulatory decision-making" is used in this context to differentiate it from scientific, or clinical, decision-making. Scientific decision-making includes decisions concerning what to study and how to study it and then infers deductive logic and the refutation of the null hypothesis through formal testing. The diagnosis and treatment of the individual based on a well-established knowledge framework characterize the sphere of clinical decision-making. Regulatory decision-making, like the forms discussed above, often occurs in the environment of uncertainty. In the postmarketing arena, the decision gap, that is, the difference between the amount of information one has and the amount required for a comfortable determination regarding drug safety, may be quite large. The interpreted pharmacoepidemiologic results are of regulatory value to the extent that they serve to narrow this gap for the risk component of the risk/benefit decision, a decision that must be made in a timely manner to protect the public health.

To establish an effective postmarketing system for the evaluation of drug safety, a network of data sources must be supported and maintained. Selection of the appropriate types of sources is contingent upon a clear understanding of need and goals. Early detection and reliable and valid assessment are the general goals. The assessment goal, however, often is elusive because of the many forms a drug safety research question can take.

Application of Pharmacoepidemiology Strategies

The first line of defense, now commonly referred to as pharmacovigilance, is ascertainment by drug through active use of the passive case report monitoring system, the AERS, and published reports in the medical literature. Use of spontaneously submitted case reports can be considered both an inherently limited and abundantly useful endeavor. Proper use of the submitted reports is somewhat like panning for gold; that is, valuable nuggets can be found among the massive quantities of common matter, but diligent panning by the DPE staff can actualize the potential of spontaneous UDE reporting. Pending changes in the UDE reporting regulations, expected to be in effect early in 1998, should increase the efficiency of this mining process.[9] Also, the receipt of complete and well-documented serious reports (via MedWatch Form 3500) from health professionals can increase the potential.

The next challenge for the pharmacoepidemiologist is to find strategies that maximize the quality and value of a comprehensive risk assessment, given a signal and/or a specific research question. At this point, the strategies for functioning within the conceptual framework (Table 1) can be integrated with the methods and data sources that are available. Many of the currently available data sources are described in Chapter 14. Some of those sources represent specific research methods and a variety of research methods used with the FDA AERS database and are listed in Table 2. The annotations in the primary and secondary function columns in Table 2 refer to the cells in Table 1. It is readily apparent from the tables that the primary function of many of these methods is detection of UDEs or signaling (cell A-1). It is fortunate that their value often is not limited to these indicated functions.

Alerting, now referred to by the DPE as monitored adverse reaction (a MAR), implies the hands-on review by an in-house health professional of a 15-day (i.e., serious and unlabeled) or a direct (from healthcare provider) MedWatch report. Formal algorithms for causality assessment are *not* used by DPE risk assessors, as a proper knowledge framework allows evaluation by global introspection.

Automated surveillance refers to the computer-controlled screening of all received reports. Five levels of pharmacovigilance screening have been programmed into the FDA's new AERS.

An AERS safety profile refers to numerator analysis of all events, clustered by a meaningful unit of examination (e.g., a body system) reported for a specific drug. Such profiles are informative and more so when they are compared with those of the other drugs in a pharmacologic or therapeutic class.

A standardized event rate (SER) type of analysis is a form of comparative proportional analysis. Essentially, it examines whether the observed reporting rate for a specific drug–event pairing is greater than would be expected in a set of comparable drugs, given that it is an event reported with use of the compared drugs. No causality assessment is conducted here. The SER is used to examine the relative strength of an association by using the reporting event rates for the comparable drugs as an internal control.

Registries, such as the national ophthalmology and dermatology registries, are ascertainment-by-event vehicles used to describe the spectra of drugs reported to be associated with the outcome events of emphasis. Occasionally, a new drug–event pairing is detected from these sources.

The medical literature is a rich but often underused source of data and information. The information available in the medical literature ranges from single case reports of UDEs (usually in the form of letters to the editor), through the formal reporting of the results of an epidemiologic or randomized investigation, to relevant research results from other disciplines and sciences, especially those that shed light on the pharmacokinetics or pharmacodynamics of a drug of interest or the pathogenesis of the disease under treatment as well as the one being characterized as the UDE.

Also available to the FDA is a program of extramural cooperative agreements, several of which are described in Chapter 14. Billing records from the US Medicaid system form the largest, but probably the most complex

Table 2 Relationship of Current Databases and Methods to the Conceptual Framework

Database or Method	Primary Function	Secondary Functions
"Alerting"	A-1	A-2
Automated surveillance	A-1	B-3, A-2
AERS "safety profile"	B-3	B-1, B-2
SER-type analyses	F-4	F-2
Registries	D-3	D-1
Medical literature	A-1	C-5, G-5
Medicaid	C-4	B-2, G-4
Puget Sound (BCDSP)	G-5	C-5, E-3
DAWN	A-1	B-3, F-4
SEU	G-2	G-5

AERS = Adverse Event Reporting System; BCDSP = Boston Collaborative Drug Surveillance Program; DAWN = Drug Abuse Warning Network; SER = standardized event rate; SEU = Slone Epidemiology Unit.

and confounded, source of pharmacoepidemiologic data available to the Agency. Although the most common use of these data is for formal cohort studies, case–control studies have been conducted by using them. Broad-based screening by drug also has been attempted with these data.

Components of the medical database at the Puget Sound health maintenance organization are under the management of the Boston Collaborative Drug Surveillance Program. This arrangement provides data linkage suitable for a variety of study methodologies, especially the case–control design.

The Drug Abuse Warning Network (DAWN), currently managed by the Substance Abuse and Mental Health Administration, is one of a few useful drug abuse indicator systems. These data have been used to describe the abuse situations associated with specific psychotropic drugs and to perform a variety of comparative proportional analyses. The Slone Epidemiology Unit in Boston maintains a case–control surveillance program to generate hypotheses about drug–event associations and to test specific research questions.

Monitoring through ascertainment by drug is an effective means of detection or signaling; however, the nature of the research question, the nature of the drugs of interest, the availability of data sources, and the working time frame determine the optimal research methods used for risk assessment. Less than a full understanding of any of these factors can lead to a flawed and misleading evaluation.

Case Examples

This section illustrates the varied nature of drug safety research questions and demonstrates the impact some recent epidemiologic risk assessments have had on regulatory decision-making. The case example format provides a pragmatic approach. Full details of the methods used are contained in the literature referenced for the cited unpublished documents.

It is important to understand that the regulatory actions cited in the case examples were not taken solely from the results of the postmarketing risk assessments. New findings are added to the existing knowledge database, and the risk/benefit equation is recalculated or more correctly rejudged by the risk manager. Decisions are based on consideration of the aggregate information available.

Each of the cases is, by necessity, presented in abbreviated format. The relationship of the three underlying frameworks, while present, may not be readily apparent as a consequence of this brief outline format. However, the importance of the frameworks in organizing and conducting inquiries in response to drug safety research questions cannot be overstated.

CASE EXAMPLE 1—AMOXAPINE TOXICITY FROM OVERDOSE

Signal. A literature report based on poison control center data signaled a greater likelihood of lethality from an amoxapine overdose relative to the tricyclic antidepressants. More seizures were also reported.[10]

Purpose. Support or refute the conclusions of the literature report. Assess the relative toxicity and seizure profile of the marketed antidepressants from overdose.

Data Sources. FDA AERS, DAWN, Poison Control Center data, National Disease and Therapeutic Index (NDTI), National Prescription Audit (NPA), and medical literature.

Methods. Relative case fatality rates were calculated for each marketed antidepressant from a number of the above databases. For example, a DAWN case fatality rate was estimated as DAWN medical examiner (DAWN-ME) mentions per 1000 DAWN emergency room (DAWN-ER) mentions. They then were rank-ordered and compared. Consistent support was obtained from similar calculations performed independently on data from the National Poison Center and FDA AERS databases. Therapeutic ratios also were calculated, after a content analysis of blood concentration data in the AERS reports, and compared.

Results. No substantial difference in lethality on overdose was found between amoxapine and the standard tricyclic antidepressants. However, amoxapine was found to differ in the clinical manifestations of overdose, most notably the presence of intense seizure activity. A potential selection bias was alleged for the local Poison Control Center data used in the original literature reports.[11]

Action. No regulatory action was considered necessary regarding the relative lethality issue. The overdose section of the amoxapine label was revised to mention the presence of seizures as a major symptom and recommended an aggressive course of treatment. Physicians were encouraged to contact their local Poison Control Center for the latest overdose treatment advice.

Follow-up. Monitor and reassess periodically.

Comment. Strategies from Table 1 used in this case included cells D-3, E-2, E-3, and F-4. The consistencies in results on multiple measures across multiple databases provide a sufficient level of certainty for decision-making. However, all the event measures were from invalidated data sources; therefore, continual reassessment and external validation were considered necessary.

CASE EXAMPLE 2—TRAZODONE: OVERDOSE TOXICITY VERSUS PRIAPISM

Signal. The continuing concern over a previous signal regarding priapism and the contrasting allegations that trazodone was less toxic on overdose than other drugs (e.g., the tricyclic antidepressants used to treat depression).

Purpose. The regulatory division was weighing the need to recommend, via the labeling, that trazodone use be considered second-line because of the occurrence of priapism. The DPE was asked to assess the risks associated with trazodone overdose relative to its pharmacologic class and to contrast that with the risk of the unique reaction of priapism.

Data Sources. AERS, National Poison Control Center, DAWN, NDTI, NPA, and medical literature.

Methods. Similar to that used in Case Example 1 but on a more recent time frame.

Results. Overdoses with trazodone appeared less likely to be lethal in this initial analysis. Seventy percent of the overdose episodes were in women. Priapism in men is estimated to occur about once per 7000 trazodone exposures.[12]

Action. Labeling was modified with new information. A second-line drug status was not conferred upon trazodone, although use in men was recommended only with a clear understanding of the risk for priapism.

Follow-up. Periodically monitor and reassess the overdose profile.

Comment. When this analysis was conducted, trazodone had been marketed for a brief time. Confirmation was needed. However, the suggestion that it may be less likely to be lethal on overdose was sufficient to retain its full indication.

CASE EXAMPLE 3—MAPROTILINE AND SEIZURES

Signal. Seizures had been mentioned as a concern by the British Committee on the Safety of Medicines (CSM), FDA AERS, and the medical literature.

Purpose. Seizures have been reported with the use of most antidepressants. However, the British signal suggested a higher frequency with maprotiline exposure. The DPE was asked to assess whether seizures that occur while on therapy are more strongly associated with maprotiline than with comparable antidepressants.

Data Sources. AERS, NPA, NDTI, and the medical literature.

Methods. SERs were calculated for a comparison of events for maprotiline, amoxapine, and trazodone. Seizures in an overdose situation were excluded from the analyses.

Results. Seizure events were associated more strongly with maprotiline than with therapy with comparable antidepressants.[13]

Action. Label was modified. A "Dear Doctor" letter was required.

Follow-up. Two hypothesis-testing studies using Medicaid data were commissioned. Those results were inconclusive. External support for these findings appeared in a subsequent literature report.[14]

Comment. Strategies from Table 1 included cells D-3 and F-4. This innovative analysis was used to test for substantial differences in a specific event across a group of comparable drugs. It addresses a manufacturer's claim that all drugs in a class are associated with a specific event already in the labeling. Proper use requires the acceptance of a set of assumptions and adjustment for known biases in the AERS database.

CASE EXAMPLE 4—PIROXICAM AND UPPER GASTROINTESTINAL REACTIONS

Signal. Multiple signals, from the British CSM, AERS, Health Research Group's Citizen Petition, and the medical literature, of a possible excess of upper gastrointestinal reactions with piroxicam.

Purpose. To assess whether piroxicam was more strongly associated with upper gastrointestinal events than the other drugs in the nonsteroidal antiinflammatory drug (NSAID) group. The initial signal was seen for the older age group.

Data Sources. FDA AERS, NPA, NDTI, medical literature, Boston Collaborative Drug Surveillance Program, and Vanderbilt University's Medicaid database.

Methods. SER calculation adjusted for the variable secular reporting trend over the past decade.

Results. When adjusted for known biases and trends in the AERS database and then adjusted for drug use, an SER analysis showed that piroxicam was not substantially different from other NSAIDs for gastrointestinal-associated morbidity and mortality. Results from the other cited databases supported this finding.[15]

Action. The Health Research Group's petition was denied.

Follow-up. Continual monitoring.

Comment. This was the most extensively researched drug safety question of the early 1980s. Some of the extramural data sources supported by the FDA were consulted with high priority because of the high visibility of this issue. Their input supported the SER analysis performed by in-house staff. The usefulness of large automated databases was substantial.

CASE EXAMPLE 5—HUMAN GROWTH HORMONE AND CREUTZFELDT–JAKOB DISEASE

Signal. Three spontaneous case reports of Creutzfeldt–Jakob disease were submitted to the FDA for the National Institutes of Health–sponsored treatment IND.

Purpose. To assess whether these three reports of this very rare neurologic disorder were more than expected.

Data Sources. National Center for Health Statistics mortality data and exposure data from the IND phase.

Methods. The observed rate was compared with the expected rate to test the hypothesis of no difference.

Results. A rate of 3 per 10 000 exposed was significantly greater than could be expected in the population.[16]

Action. The production and distribution of pituitary-derived human growth hormone were halted. The NDA for a recombinant product received FDA priority, under orphan drug status, and was thereafter approved for use in human growth hormone–deficient conditions. A Health and Human Services task force was created to identify and monitor the balance of the exposed individuals.

Follow-up. A Health and Human Services task force monitored and conducted a National Death Index–based study, which confirmed the initial findings.

Comment. A simple but innovative analysis was sufficient to allow a confident decision. This analysis is best described as a special case of strategy E-5 (Table 1), with a firm denominator and external control from the National Center for Health Statistics data.

CASE EXAMPLE 6—IMPACT OF NALOXONE ON PENTAZOCINE ABUSE

Signal. Follow-up on an earlier concern that was raised by an internal FDA request from the Agency's drug abuse staff over the increase in abuse of the tablets of pentazocine.

Purpose. To assess the impact of a regulatory action taken about 3 years prior, when the narcotic antagonist naloxone was added to the oral tablet formulation of pentazocine.

Data Sources. DAWN, NPA, medical literature, and FDA AERS.

Methods. A hypothesis-testing trends analysis of DAWN emergency department and medical examiner data over NPA retail prescription data that compared data before and after the addition of naloxone to the oral tablet dosage form of pentazocine.

Results. There was a significant decrease in the number of drug abuse mentions per reporting quarter in each of the DAWN system parameters since the addition of naloxone.[17]

Action. No additional regulatory action was warranted. The intervention appears successful to date.

Follow-up. Analysis to be repeated if a new signal requires another examination.

Comment. The strategy is a special case of cell E-5 (Table 1) using a historical control to test the hypothesis of no change in trend. This assessment of prior regulatory action clearly demonstrated a public health impact. The original agreement to add naloxone illustrated a constructive spirit of cooperation between industry and government (FDA, Drug Enforcement Administration, National Institute on Drug Abuse).

CASE EXAMPLE 7—WITHDRAWAL SEIZURES WITH ALPRAZOLAM

Signal. Seizure reports to FDA AERS.

Purpose. To describe the condition under which seizures occur and to assess whether they are more strongly associated with any specific benzodiazepine anxiolytic.

Data Sources. FDA AERS, medical literature, NPA, NDTI.

Methods. Content analysis of FDA AERS reports.

Results. Seizures secondary to withdrawal from benzodiazepine anxiolytics are rare events. They are reported most frequently for the potent benzodiazepines alprazolam and lorazepam. The data were plotted as dosage against duration of therapy. Risk appeared to be dependent on sufficient exposure to produce a physical dependence state. For alprazolam, higher doses appear to decrease the time to risk. These data support the pharmacologic theory of cumulative exposure.[18] The data on lorazepam were insufficient to draw a defensible conclusion. Analyses of these data were presented to an FDA advisory committee in the fall of 1989.

Action. A dosage-tapering regimen was added to the product label to minimize the potential for withdrawal sequelae.

Follow-up. Continued AERS and literature monitoring.

Comment. Strategies D-2 and D-3 were used (Table 1). A comparative proportional analysis could not be conducted because the NDTI data demonstrated that alprazolam had a unique usage pattern (i.e., more often prescribed by psychiatrists for affective and panic disorders). Therefore, there were no comparable drugs. Additionally, an appropriate denominator for this contingent event was not available. The generated hypothesis awaits testing. The conduct of confirmatory studies will be difficult, however, because these types of data are outside the scope of all the usual postmarketing databases.

CASE EXAMPLE 8—ISOTRETINOIN AND BIRTH DEFECTS

Signal. Although this issue was discussed on a number of earlier occasions, this particular review was prompted by a Centers for Disease Control (CDC) December 1987 communication to the FDA based on a cluster of reports from the New Jersey Birth Defects Surveillance Program.

Purpose. To quantitate the magnitude of the occurrence of this previously documented drug–outcome relationship.

Data Sources. CDC, FDA AERS, Medicaid, NDTI, NPA, and the National Health and Nutrition Examination Survey (NHANES).

Methods. This multidatabase evaluation[19] included an estimate (obtained via NHANES) of severe cystic acne in women of childbearing age, an estimate (via NPA, NDTI) of drug use and prescriber information, a risk estimate (via Medicaid) in a population, a content analysis, and an estimate of the degree of underreporting in spontaneous reports (via FDA AERS). Foreign experience, literature reports, and estimates of contraceptive failure also were important data sources.

Results. Use of this potent teratogen was 15–20 times greater than the estimate of severe recalcitrant cystic acne in women. This disease is 4–5 times more prevalent in men. Between 70% and 85% of isotretinoin was prescribed by dermatologists. Medicaid data illustrated that exposure of isotretenoin by pregnant women was not uncommon. An extrapolation of these data provides an estimate of 900–1300 severe birth defects that have occurred since the 1982 introduction of isotretinoin (Accutane; Hoffmann-LaRoche, Nutley, NJ). The FDA AERS, however, had only about 90 reports. The CDC estimated that 25% of all pregnancy exposures, if brought to term, would produce birth defects.

Action. The most extensive product relabeling and repackaging effort ever requested of a drug manufacturer were mandated. In addition, an extensive prescriber and consumer education campaign, plus an intervention assessment survey, was launched.

Follow-up. The FDA formed an internal multidisciplinary Accutane Monitoring Group to monitor compliance with the new regulatory action, the epidemiologic data, and the progress of the intervention assessment efforts. The manufacturer was required to submit a quarterly update on all components of the program and then to meet with the Accutane Monitoring Group to review and discuss the findings. A long-term follow-up study, sponsored by Hoffmann-LaRoche, is ongoing by the Slone Epidemiology Unit in Boston. Publications from that study indicate a lower pregnancy exposure rate than expected. Very few exposed mothers brought their pregnancies to term.[20] Multiple reasons for that finding could be offered, given the study design.

Comment. Soon after marketing began in 1982, reports of congenital defects were received by the FDA. The FDA conducted a limited epidemiologic evaluation at that time. This topic was discussed at public advisory committees in 1983 and 1984. Professional labeling was modified to include a boxed warning regarding the association of the drug with human birth defects. After receipt of the CDC query in 1987, the FDA DPE began a comprehensive epidemiologic assessment of the issue. The strength of those results was the basis for the May 1988 regulatory action.

This case illustrates the importance of an in-depth comprehensive multidatabase assessment that includes the use of natural history and drug use data. In addition, the formation of an active monitoring group that will continually assess this issue and the success of the regulatory interventions will prevent this important public health issue from once again losing priority.

CASE EXAMPLE 9—TEMAFLOXACIN AND UNUSUALLY HIGH INCIDENCE OF SERIOUS ADVERSE REACTIONS

Signal. Soon after the launch of the quinolone antibacterial agent temafloxacin in February 1992, both the FDA AERS and the manufacturer received increased reports of serious adverse events (acute renal failure, severe hypoglycemia, acute hepatic damage, anaphylactic reactions, and hemolytic anemia) associated with the use of the drug.

Purpose. To assess whether temafloxacin was more strongly associated with these adverse events, some of which were totally unanticipated, in terms of both experience with other quinolones and with regard to the performance of temafloxacin in premarketing trials in which treatment was withdrawn from less than 4% of the patients involved.

Data Source. FDA AERS.

Methods. The FDA's Division of Antiinfective Drug Products, DPE, and the manufacturer looked closely at the spontaneous reports in the AERS database and were convinced that there was a problem with temafloxacin.

Results. A syndome of hemolysis, thrombocytopenia, and liver and kidney failure was described.[21]

Action. Addition of hemolytic anemia and hypoglycemia was proposed in the labeling for temafloxacin in late May 1992. Then on June 5, 1992, in consultation with the FDA, the manufacturer voluntary recalled the product from the world market.

CASE EXAMPLE 10—TERFENADINE DRUG INTERACTIONS

Signal. A single case of torsade de pointes in a patient at a Washington, DC, teaching hospital.

Purpose. To verify this signal and to explore the reasons why and under what circumstances this reaction occurred.

Data Sources. FDA AERS, literature, and directed clinical pharmacology studies.

Results. The AERS had many similar reports. Upon content analyses, most of these reactions occurred in the presence of terfenadine and either ketaconazole or erythromycin. The clinical pharmacology studies were directed at the metabolic enzymes in the liver. Terfenadine is an inactive prodrug that required activation by a metabolic step. Ketaconazole, and less so erythromycin, had stronger affinity for this required enzyme and competitively blocked the activation. The parent molecule therefore accumulated in the blood and produced these noted toxicities.

Action. A "Dear Doctor" letter was issued in 1990. In 1992, mailgrams were sent by the manufacturer to health professionals warning of these drug–drug interactions. Labeling was changed to contraindicate the concomitant use of these drugs.

Follow-up. In 1996 the Agency began its action to remove the drug from the market. However, the manufacturer has replaced terfenadine in the product line with a product composed of its active metabolite.

Comment. This case demonstrates the need to apply multiple sciences toward the resolution of a drug safety question. Here, clinical pharmacology and pharmacovigilance worked hand in hand.

CASE EXAMPLE 11—TRAMADOL AND SEIZURES

Signal. Six months after marketing of tramadol tablets in the US, spontaneous reports of seizures in patients taking recommended doses were received by the AERS system. Tramadol was labeled for seizure risk at excessive single oral doses.

Purpose. To assess the risk factors surrounding the occurrence of seizures in patients taking therapeutic doses of tramadol.

Data Sources. FDA AERS, medical literature, manufacturer's foreign marketing data, and IMS-NDTI.

Methods. At 6-month, 9-month, and 1-year intervals after marketing, the DPE and the manufacturer looked closely at the spontaneous reports and foreign tramadol product postmarketing experiences. The reporting numbers of seizure compared with the total number of reports, reporting trend by month, outcome of the reports, and reporting rate were analyzed. The seizure reports were clinically evaluated to establish the temporal relationship to tramadol administration, to identify the pattern of seizure risk, and to make necessary recommendations.

Results. Reports of seizure including fatalities constituted more than 10% of the total reports, and they had been persistently increasing at 6, 9, and 12 months of postmarketing. Seizure had occurred after a single dose or after multiple therapeutic doses, or overdose, with or without seizure history in all age groups. Concomitant use of multiple medications, such as monoamine oxidase inhibitors, selective serotonin-reuptake inhibitors, or tricyclics, may predispose patients toward increased seizure risk due to drug interaction with tramadol that results in lowering the seizure threshold.

Action. Revision of the labeling to include stronger warning statements regarding seizure risk was made in September 1995 and March 1996. A "Dear Doctor" letter was issued in March 1996 by the manufacturer.

Follow-up. Continue close monitoring of the seizure reports and reassess the need for even stronger labeling revision should reports continue. The DPE is conducting an observational cohort study within its cooperative agreements to further clarify the risk and risk factors.

Comment. Tramadol is an effective analgesic medication with wide uses. The incidence rate on seizure risk using spontaneous data cannot be calculated. Tramadol caused seizure in preclinical work-ups, and seizures were noted in clinical trials at high doses. A Phase IV epidemiologic postmarketing study recommended and initiated at approval may have been able to better define the seizure risk, given the residual concerns at the time of approval.

Summary

Risk assessment of a new drug is a continual process. Pharmacoepidemiologic risk assessment is the postapproval stage of the drug development continuum. Postmarketing risk assessment strategies should be guided by the cumulative experience with the new drug to that point. Phase IV safety studies should address specific residual concerns. Rare and unexpected reactions are the forte of the pharmacovigilance tool of spontaneous reporting systems.

Responsibilities for assessing postmarketing risks and for the application of these to the risk management and regulatory functions exist in different organizational components of the FDA. The postmarketing decision-makers are the same functional units who worked with the drug throughout its entire development process.

The practice of pharmacoepidemiology is not amenable to a standardized or cookbook approach. This chapter explains the concepts and foundations of the art in pharmacoepidemiology so that thinking, creative individuals can apply them as the research questions warrant. It is important to reemphasize that each new research question requires an individualized approach, and that there are more exceptions than methodologic rules. The only valid rules in this field are those of research logic. The need for mastering a conceptual framework and a solid knowledge base cannot be stressed too strongly. Diverse data sources are required to address the breadth of potential questions that arise in this field. Because of the secondary and imprecise nature of most of the available data, multiple data sources should be examined for each research question so that consistent and confirmatory findings are generated. Unfortunately, current extramural databases are used only on a limited scale to address FDA-initiated research questions, and only limited funds are available to maintain and develop such valuable sources. Clearly, there remains much room for improvement. Each question posed to the FDA must be addressed in a timely manner. However, not all questions can currently be answered, and additional data sources are needed.

Epidemiologic data on drug safety in the postmarketing arena are valuable in the regulatory environment only when they can be used to form an interpretable risk assessment that can narrow the often large decision gaps and aid rational regulatory decision-making. Regulatory adjustments made by the FDA impact public health by affecting patient care through prevention and/or minimization of unsafe drug therapy.

The sponsors bear responsibility for identifying and characterizing actual and potential safety issues associated with the use of their products in the postapproval environment, as well as prior to approval. The new drug sponsors need to develop pharmacoepidemiologic capabilities so they can meet their responsibility. The FDA views pharmacoepidemiologic assessment of risk as a necessary component of its public health mission — a mission that does not end when an approval (to market) letter is issued.

The FDA will continue to refine its program and will assess risks by using the best techniques and data sources possible. The FDA is also collaborating with the European community, Japan, and the World Health Organization (WHO) to harmonize pharmacovigilance standards, because drug safety issues have no national boundaries. Better sources of vigilance and epidemiologic data will increase the probability that the decision the FDA has to make on safety issues will be rational and correct.

An earlier version of this chapter was presented at the 4th International Conference on Pharmacoepidemiology, September 1987, and was published in its proceedings.

The valuable assistance of my FDA colleagues, David Graham MD MPH, Min Chen RPh, Szed Rizwan Admad MD MH, and Anna Szarfman MD PhD, in formulating some of the case examples is gratefully acknowledged.

References

1. Gross FH, Inman WHW, eds. Drug monitoring. New York: Academic Press, 1977:1-16, 79-89.
2. Faich G. Adverse drug reaction monitoring. N Engl J Med 1986;314:1589-92.
3. Rossi AC, Knapp DE, Anello C, O'Neil RT, Graham CF, Mendelis PS. Discovery of adverse drug reactions. A comparison of selected Phase IV studies with spontaneous reporting methods. JAMA 1983;249:2226-8.
4. Temple R, Jones JK, Crout JR. Adverse effects of newly marketed drugs (editorial). N Engl J Med 1979;300:1046.
5. Jones JK. Broader uses of post-marketing surveillance. In: Wardell WM, Velo G, eds. Drug development, regulatory assessment and post-marketing surveillance. New York: Plenum Press, 1981:203-16.
6. Jones JK. Regulatory use of adverse drug reactions. In: Skandia International Symposia. Detection and prevention of adverse drug reactions. Stockholm: Almqvist & Wiksell International, 1984:203-14.
7. Finney D. Statistical logic in the monitoring of reactions to therapeutic drugs. Methods Inf Med 1971;10:237-45. Revised and updated. In: Inman WHW, ed. Monitoring for drug safety. Lancaster: MTP Press, 1980:383-400.
8. Campbell DT, Stanley JC. Experimental and quasiexperimental designs for research. Boston: Houghton Mifflin, 1963:5-6.
9. US Code of Federal Regulations, Part 314.80, as amended.
10. Litovitz TL, Troutman WG. Amoxapine overdose: seizures and fatalities. JAMA 1983; 250:1069-71.

11. Nelson RC. Amoxapine toxicity on overdose. Unpublished report. Rockville, MD: Food and Drug Administration, Office of Epidemiology and Biostatistics, 1984.

12. Baum C, Nelson RC. Trazodone toxicity on overdose. Unpublished report. Rockville, MD: Food and Drug Administration, Office of Epidemiology and Biostatistics, 1985.

13. Nelson RC. Maprotiline and seizures. Unpublished report. Rockville, MD: Food and Drug Administration, Office of Epidemiology and Biostatistics, 1984.

14. Jabbari B, Bryan GE, Marsh EE, Gunderson CH. Incidence of seizures with tricyclic and tetracyclic antidepressants. Arch Neurol 1985;42:480-1.

15. Rossi A, Hsu JP, Faich GA. Ulcerogenicity of piroxicam: an analysis of spontaneously reported data. Br Med J 1987;294;147-50.

16. Piper J. HGH & CJD. Unpublished report. Rockville, MD: Food and Drug Administration, Office of Epidemiology and Biostatistics, 1984.

17. Baum C, Hsu JP, Nelson RC. Impact of the addition of naloxone on the abuse of pentazocine tablets. Public Health Rep 1987;102;426-9.

18. Nelson RC, Barash D, Graham D. Intense abstinence syndromes and the newer benzodiazepine anxiolytics. Unpublished report. Rockville, MD: Food and Drug Administration, Office of Epidemiology and Biostatistics, 1985.

19. Graham D. Maternal exposure to Accutane. Unpublished report. Rockville, MD: Food and Drug Administration, Office of Epidemiology and Biostatistics, 1988.

20. Mitchell AA, Van-Bennekom CM, Louic C. A pregnancy prevention program in women of childbearing age receiving isotretinoin. N Engl J Med 1995;333:101-6.

21. Blum MD, Graham DJ, McCloskey CA. Temafloxacin syndrome: review of 95 cases. Clin Infect Dis 1994;18:946-50.

18

Collateral Uses of Pharmacoepidemiology
Olav M Bakke

Abstract

An overview is presented of the different settings and situations in which data on the use and effects of drugs are of particular interest and relevance. The role of the pharmaceutical industry and the use of clinical trial data, postmarketing surveillance, and other types of epidemiologic research for commercial purposes are discussed. Drug registration and reimbursement issues are often controversial and have considerable political as well as socioeconomic connotations. Likewise, pharmacoepidemiologic data are often part of legal arguments. Prospective pharmacoepidemiologists should be aware of the potential for various types of collateral uses and interpretations of data and be prepared to deal with problems that require insight into many other fields.

Outline

1. Introduction
2. Background attitudes
3. Commercial uses
    Pharmacoeconomic studies
    Postmarketing surveillance studies
    Creative promotional epidemiology
    Biases and fallacies
4. Pharmacopolitics
    Social image of drug makers
    Drug regulations
    Legal issues
5. Summary
6. References

P
harmacoepidemiology is a multidisciplinary area involving professionals from academia, drug regulatory agencies, the pharmaceutical
industry, and international organizations.[1,2] All these people have a
common aim of developing and applying scientific methods to the
study of the use and effects of drugs. However, since they are a mixed
crowd, other objectives may differ among individual workers.

Drug effects and adverse reactions are of great interest to the general
public and to various sectors of society. Pharmacoepidemiologists must
therefore be prepared to see many different uses of their data. Sometimes
they will also find themselves involved in intricate political situations and
legal questions. Pharmacoepidemiology is therefore not for timid souls, and
it is definitely not a field in which the so-called learned professionals can
easily hide in their "ivory towers."[1]

In this pluricultural setting, the term "collateral uses" is not necessarily pejorative. It is used in this context only to alert students and prospective pharmacoepidemiologists to the fact that they must be prepared to
play roles and tackle problems that go far beyond their basic training and
specialized skills. They will also discover that, in the real world, science is
not as pure, objective, and unselfish as one would wish.

Background Attitudes

Personal background and attitudes often determine how different individuals or groups of people interpret and use results of medical research.
Pharmacoepidemiologists have an important role to play as communica-
tors to bring their message to other people. Unless properly argued and
sustained, scientific premises and reserve are sometimes lost or forgotten in
the process. Awareness of these aspects is essential if one wants to avoid
misunderstanding or abuse of pharmacoepidemiologic data or evidence by
other sectors of society.

There is plenty of room for cultural collisions when scientists interact
with decision-makers either within the drug industry or in public life. It is
often difficult for a statistician or an epidemiologist to explain the concept
of hypothesis testing and the meaning of p values to the top management
of a pharmaceutical company or to health service administrators. In their
ears, it must sound strange when scientists brought up on Popperian refu-
tationism are reluctant to reject the null hypothesis of no difference and to
accept the alternative (and often more attractive) option until efforts have
been made to disprove it. Moreover, managers are used to making judgments that are much more daring and adventurous than that implied by
the conventional limits for risks of type 1 and type 2 errors, which are usually as low as 1–5% and 10–20%, respectively.

Decision-makers usually want clear answers that scientists, at least in the field of clinical research and epidemiology, can seldom provide without feeling uneasy or compromised. Somehow, in the industry, scientifically sound reserve and skepticism are often viewed as being counterproductive and unwanted. Spilker[3] has described a condition labeled "negative disease" that affects individuals in the pharmaceutical industry who allegedly find it safer to "raise objections" than to "agree or take a realistic approach." Many successful academicians would probably be flattered and proud to exhibit such personality features, but apparently they would not fit in with the culture of the pharmaceutical industry.

Admittedly, many scientists are not aware of the economic and political realities. They are therefore often, quite understandably, considered by senior managers as being both vague and naive. Successful collaboration within a drug company requires considerable effort on the part of the research and development staff to overcome this obstacle to mutual respect.

Pharmacoepidemiologists will also discover that there is considerable latitude of judgment within their own profession. An example is the different views and philosophies of the "observational" type of pharmacoepidemiologists and the "clinical trialists."[4,5] Sometimes the general public does not appreciate these differences and regards discrepancies among experts as "tribal feuds" that do not contribute to solving socially relevant problems. However, professional controversy is undoubtedly sound for further progress and, fortunately, there is a middle road on which both kinds of professionals can meet.

Conflicts regarding the confidentiality and the right to publish industry-sponsored research are commonplace. Investigators will normally wish to publish their results as soon as possible to promote their own careers and for the "sake of science." On the other hand, the sponsoring firms may want to delay the publication of certain data to coincide with their marketing campaigns or to censor the results.[1]

Other problems may arise when pharmacoepidemiologic data are released prematurely without prior publication in peer-reviewed journals. Early publicity of overoptimistic interpretations of results that, at most, are "hypothesis-generating" is a by-product of the competition for funds and prestige. Journalists and scientists sometimes form an "unholy alliance," and "all sorts of people want to get their message out through the newspapers for all sorts of reasons."[6,7] Early release or carefully timed disclosure of preliminary data may also be a way of boosting stock prices.[8]

The consequences are particularly serious in the field of therapeutic research, where thousands of patients suffering from incurable diseases and their relatives are clinging to the hope that new active medicines will appear. In this situation, people are just too eager and willing to believe in any breakthrough, even if it might be hype.[7,9]

Commercial Uses

Clinical trials and pharmacoepidemiology in general are important commercially for various reasons.

1. They provide information on the efficacy and safety of drugs in different patient populations.
2. The data can sometimes be analyzed in economic terms to show that society can save money when using drugs.
3. Postmarketing surveillance (PMS) studies and clinical trials help the prescribing physicians get acquainted with new drugs.
4. Any study or activity that permits the sales representatives to get close to the physicians can be useful for promoting drugs.

The first point is a pure necessity for the registration of new drugs, and it is obviously also true that well-documented products sell better than poorly sustained ones. The second point is of importance for the social acceptance of drugs and for price negotiations and the reimbursement of pharmaceutical products by government schemes. The latter two points refer to aspects of increasing commercial involvement and usefulness as marketing tools for the promotion of drugs.

PHARMACOECONOMIC STUDIES

Economic evaluation of drug therapy is an important marketing device.[10] Pharmacoepidemiologists should be aware that even studies intended just to focus on "hard" efficacy and safety variables may be used collaterally in an economic context.

Efficacy and quality-of-life variables, when translated into economic terms, are open to many "soft" or subjective interpretations.[10,11] More variation is introduced when the economic dimension is added, and the statistical premises (e.g., the sample size) that appear to be adequate for the efficacy variables may no longer be appropriate. Properly designed clinical trials that from the outset include an economic evaluation are less likely to be biased or open to random errors.

POSTMARKETING SURVEILLANCE STUDIES

As pointed out by professionals from different quarters, Phase IV or postmarketing studies carried out by the pharmaceutical industry in the past have been rather disappointing as a way of identifying important safety hazards.[12-14] In principle, the large-scale observational cohort studies involving a large number of patients early after the launch of a new drug make sense, particularly if they include control groups.[13-18] Once a new drug is on the market, it is feasible to collect data from a large number of patients undergoing medical treatment. PMS studies are sometimes recommended or requested by the drug regulatory agencies. Moreover, in many countries, the ethical constraints and formal requirements for carrying out purely observational studies are minimal, provided they do not involve confidential patient information.

However, in the field of PMS, there is often only a short step from the observational to the experimental (or "pseudoexperimental") situation. First, there are no safeguards to ensure that the patients are not selected before the decision to administer a treatment is made. Second, payments for completed case record forms, selective and convincing promotional information, and free samples may represent a strong inducement for the physician to actively recruit patients. In such circumstances, the requisite of an observational study that "the act of observing does not modify what is being observed" is often not fulfilled.[13,14,18,19] The study may then be biased or become a pseudoexperimental "seeding trial," which leading professionals in and outside the pharmaceutical industry regard as scientifically unjustified, dishonest, or unethical.[14,19-21]

The British quadripartite guidelines on PMS (1988)[17] address the problem of the commercial abuse of such activities in their Point 14, which reads, "Company representatives should not be involved in such a way that the study can be seen as a promotional exercise." The Pharmacoepidemiology Section of the American Society for Clinical Pharmacology and Therapeutics[18] has also generated a position paper. Although this document takes issue with marketing studies undertaken without a "valid scientific reason," it does not explicitly mention the role of the sales representatives. In the real-life situation, however, it is difficult or sometimes even impossible to collect data from tens of thousands of patients without using the sales organization as a vehicle. Hence, the new British guidelines for company-sponsored safety assessment of marketed medicines (1993)[22] have taken a more realistic approach.

The enormous resources that drug firms worldwide invest in poorly designed, uncontrolled PMS studies can be explained only in terms of the collateral benefits of such borderline "seeding trials." By the looks of it, clinical trials must be good marketing, but most authors of textbooks and organizers of courses on pharmaceutical marketing seem to avoid covering the subject in any depth. This leads to the obvious conclusion that even the pharmaceutical industry admits that this activity is not "kosher" from a scientific and social point of view.

As pointed out in an editorial in *Pharmaceutical Medicine*,[13] the time has come to reconsider PMS studies. Apart from improving the design and the logistics of the studies, it has been suggested that the multifocus approach should be replaced by more emphasis on specific safety issues identified from preclinical studies, premarketing trials, or postmarketing experience (e.g., spontaneous adverse reaction reporting).[12,13]

CREATIVE PROMOTIONAL EPIDEMIOLOGY

The pharmaceutical industry is pioneering not only drug discovery and development, but also innovative marketing. One often gets the impression that the industry's marketing departments will carry out any kind of "pharmaco-whatever-it-takes" study that permits its representatives to get close to the physicians and establish a dialogue.

Even drug utilization studies and merely descriptive epidemiologic surveys can be used for promotional purposes. In some countries where commercial Phase IV seeding trials are made difficult by recent legislation or professional or public attitudes, these have been replaced by purely descriptive studies. Curiously, but not surprisingly, the presentation of results to participating physicians of, for example, the incidence of a particular disease or the pattern of utilization of a certain therapeutic group of drugs usually coincides with the launch of a new and related medicine.

The healthcare industry also helps in the creation of "disease awareness" as well as other novel concepts and potentially treatable new nosologic entities or "diseases." There is a remarkable coincidence between the resurrection of the value of lowering cholesterol to reduce the incidence of cardiovascular morbidity and the introduction of the new generation of lipid-lowering "statins" in the late 1980s. Benign age-related memory disturbance is currently struggling for recognition as a disease entity, while the drug industry is spending billions of dollars on finding new therapeutic remedies, which by all tokens will, at most, be marginally efficacious.

BIASES AND FALLACIES

Sometimes there seems to be a long distance between the department of research and development and the marketing group within the same drug company. Some years ago, a pharmaceutical firm promoted an antihypertensive drug with lipid-lowering properties by distributing programmed calculators to assess the risk of cardiovascular diseases from blood cholesterol concentrations and other relevant prognostic factors, allegedly using data from the time-honored Framingham Study as a basis. Given the opportunity, any qualified epidemiologist or clinical investigator within or outside the company would probably have advised against taking advantage of the more-than-obvious fallacy of assuming that normalizing blood cholesterol at a mature, adult age would transfer people to the lower risk group of individuals who have always had normal concentrations.

The collateral use, or even misuse, of pharmacoepidemiologic data is not necessarily intentional or deceitful. As already discussed, management and marketing personnel live in a different culture with a more "positive" attitude than do those whose job it is to generate or assess data in a department of research and development. They are therefore easily carried away by favorable and useful or usable information.

For the sake of fairness, it must also be admitted that the medical profession has always used the placebo effect to give added value to its therapies. Even the most well-trained physician and clinical trialist may never have been properly initiated into the mysteries of the ubiquitous "regression toward the mean." This is particularly sad since more than 100 years have gone by since Galton[23] first noticed that the mating of two tall pea plants produced offspring that were, on the average, shorter than either parent plant. This phenomenon, together with the placebo effect, different biases, and other circumstances, can undoubtedly explain some of the improvement observed in many therapeutic situations and in uncontrolled studies in which the symptoms of individual patients "before" and "after" treatment are compared.[24-26]

Moreover, many people, lay or learned, and including physicians, seem to assume that events are evenly distributed in time. For those who happen to work in a marketing department and who are unaware of the uneven distribution of the time interval between relatively rare events in real life, the occurrence of series of cases of "miraculous cures" is the "reward" that makes up for sleepless nights over reports of clusters of severe adverse events and, consequently, gloomy sales perspectives. It is no wonder that any positive reports are uncritically accepted and used to reinforce marketing morale and as support for the promotion of drugs.

Pharmacopolitics

Medical traditions and drug policies differ among all major drug markets. These days, all large pharmaceutical companies have generously staffed influential departments of regulatory or medical affairs to coordinate their pharmacopolitical activities. Journalists, communication specialists, and even humanists are recruited in an attempt to improve the dialogue with certain sectors of society and with the general public.[3]

SOCIAL IMAGE OF DRUG MAKERS

For some reason or other, society appears to have a preference for drug problems over other health issues, some of which could certainly deserve a more thorough scrutiny in terms of medical justification and cost. A corollary to this observation is that "diagnostic abuses" or scandals because of uncritical overuse (which undoubtedly exist) are virtually unheard of, whereas drug companies often receive negative publicity for their promo-

tion and other activities. The explanation of this paradox may be the availability, in most developed countries, of good data on the use of medicines,
and that consumer advocates and the media therefore find it easier to find
information and focus on drug issues than on most other aspects of modern health care.

Pharmacopolitics involves the drug industry, the medical profession,
pharmacists, the general public, politicians, health authorities, and international organizations, to mention a few of the main players.[3] Consumer
advocates and the media also need special consideration, since pharmacoepidemiologists will sometimes be required to participate in public hear-
ings and debates on drug issues.

The Freedom of Information Act and the possibility of flawed use by
third parties (often "independent researchers") of data on drug safety are
of great concern to the pharmaceutical industry.[27] Almost any data taken out
of proper context and interpreted subjectively (read "unfriendly") could
cause major turmoil and adverse publicity, even to a company with the
highest ethical standards and the cleanest conscience. Credibility is essential when dealing with controversial safety issues, and pharmacoepidemiologists can achieve a good reputation in this respect only through open-
ness and by working at the highest ethical and scientific standards.

DRUG REGULATIONS

Pharmacoepidemiologic data of various types are frequently used to
put pressure on drug regulatory agencies to make new remedies available
more quickly. In particular, PMS studies are currently being offered as a
trade-off to obtain earlier approval of new drugs.

The first publication by Wardell[28] in 1973 of comparative data on the
introduction of new drugs in the UK and the US and the demonstration of
a "drug lag" in the latter market was the beginning of a campaign to speed
up the review of new drug applications. It was inferred that thousands of
lives per year might have been saved among American patients if beta-
adrenergic blockers had been introduced earlier in the US. The reluctance
of the Food and Drug Administration (FDA) to authorize the marketing of
some new drugs in the early 1970s was undoubtedly influenced by the
thalidomide disaster a decade earlier. Since then, the introduction of new
drugs in different countries has been carefully monitored. However, in
spite of a greater awareness of the problem, the overall FDA reviewing time
has not changed appreciably, except perhaps for important new drugs for
life-threatening illnesses.[29,30]

AIDS is currently a social issue in which epidemiologic data are used
to argue in favor of changes in drug regulations.[31,32] Lately, the drug industry and AIDS activists have joined forces to make "promising" new drugs

available to patients before formal registration. As a result of this pressure, an increasing number of drugs have been included in extended "compassionate use" schemes, like the treatment investigational new drug or the parallel track programs. It remains to be seen whether these changes represent a real benefit to patients and society or just turn out to be a dead end in the process of scientific drug evaluation. Nevertheless, this is another example of a field in which pharmacoepidemiologists find themselves involved in debates of public issues and where controversial decisions are often made.[1,33]

The spontaneous reporting system for unintended drug effects (UDEs) is an instrument that produces "signals," and other methods are required to assess the risks associated with the use of drugs in quantitative terms. Unfortunately, it is often not appreciated that novelty and commercial campaigns may introduce biases leading to relative overreporting of UDEs of recently marketed medicines.[14,16,19] It is perhaps more than a coincidence that several of the drugs withdrawn from the US and the UK markets during the 1970s and 1980s were heavily promoted products with rapid take-off of sales.[34] Obviously, in a system in which only a few percent of UDEs are reported under normal conditions, external factors such as increased attention, awareness, or publicity may easily produce a substantial increase in the frequency of notification.

Nevertheless, drugs in general appear to be remarkably well tolerated, and only 3–4% of drugs introduced under modern regulations are subsequently withdrawn in the light of a safety question.[35] This should be kept in mind to avoid the heated atmosphere that sometimes surrounds controversial drug withdrawals, where science gives way to emotional, political, or economic arguments with bizarre collateral uses of pharmacoepidemiologic data.

LEGAL ISSUES

Drug withdrawals for safety reasons often have important legal connotations. Although traditionally the situation in the US with regard to compensation for drug-induced injuries has been different from that in the rest of the world, this appears to be changing.[36,37] The European product liability directive of 1985 establishes strict liability for marketed pharmaceutical products. Some countries in different parts of the world (e.g., Sweden, New Zealand) have set up "no fault" schemes to provide compensation from a central body or fund without the need to prove negligence on the part of the manufacturers or other parties involved.

Sometimes healthy volunteers or patients are damaged as a result of their participation in clinical trials. Pharmacoepidemiologists will be required to give expert opinions on the "balance of probabilities" of the causal relationship between drug treatment and the injuries experienced.[38] They will then discover a new world of terms and interpretations radically different from the usual statistical and scientific concepts. For instance, to lawyers the word "probable" simply means "more than 50% likely"; they also have varying perceptions of risks and causal relationship.[39]

There is considerable potential for collateral interpretation of pharmacoepidemiologic data by the legal profession in other areas. Clinical trials showing efficacy in particular diseases are crucial for sustaining patent claims. Competition among companies is fierce, and pharmacoepidemiologists may get involved in legal battles over patent rights.

Summary

There is a delicate balance between pharmacoepidemiology as an academic discipline and a number of different nonscientific or collateral uses of data on drug effects and adverse reactions in society. The pharmaceutical industry is a melting pot of different personal attitudes and cultures, all of which are necessary, but frequently some are also contradictory.

The commercial use of pharmacoepidemiologic data is legitimate as long as good scientific standards are followed. However, this is often not the case and, in terms of the knowledge acquired, the results of industry-sponsored PMS studies have been rather disappointing. There is obviously room for improvement both in the methods of such studies and with regard to the use of resources.

Pharmacopolitics is another field in which drug data are used to influence the opinions and attitudes prevailing in society. Likewise, pharmacoepidemiologic data may sometimes be used by the legal profession, for example, for patent claims and to establish responsibilities in cases of drug-induced injuries.

Pharmacoepidemiologists should be aware of their roles as providers and interpreters of drug data in all these areas. There is a need for well-trained professionals who, without losing their scientific skills and integrity, learn and understand other attitudes and needs, and who are able to interact with different sectors of society.

References

1. Stolley PD. A public health perspective from academia. In: Strom BL, ed. Pharmacoepidemiology. New York: Churchill Livingstone, 1989:51-5.
2. Porta M, Carné X. Pharmacoepidemiology. In: Olsen J, Trichopoulos D, eds. Teaching epidemiology. What you should know and what you could do. New York: Oxford University Press, 1992:285-304.

3. Spilker B. Multinational drug companies. Principles and practices. 2nd ed. New York: Raven Press, Ltd., 1994.

4. Hlatky MA. Using databases to evaluate therapy. Stat Med 1991;10:647-52.

5. Byar DP. Problems with using observational databases to compare treatments. Stat Med 1991;10:663-6.

6. Do epidemiologists cause epidemics (editorial)? Lancet 1993;341:993-4.

7. Smith R. Hype from journalists and scientists. An unholy alliance (editorial). BMJ 1992;304: 730.

8. Freestone DS, Mitchell H. Inappropriate publication of trial results and potential for allegations of illegal share dealing. BMJ 1993;306:1112-4.

9. American College of Physicians ethical manual. Ann Intern Med 1992;117:947-60.

10. Hillman AL, Eisenberg JM, Pauly MV, Bloom BS, Glick H, Kinosian B, et al. Avoiding bias in the conduct and reporting of cost-effectiveness research sponsored by pharmaceutical companies. N Engl J Med 1991;324:1362-5.

11. Udvarshely S, Colditz GA, Rai A, Epstein AM. Cost–effectiveness and cost–benefit analysis in the medical literature. Are the methods being used correctly? Ann Intern Med 1992;116:238-44.

12. Waller PC, Wood SM, Langman MJS, Breckenridge A, Rawlins MD. Review of company postmarketing studies. BMJ 1992;304:1470-2.

13. Post-marketing surveillance—time to think again (editorial). Pharm Med 1992;6: 165-6.

14. Stephens MDB. Marketing aspects of company-sponsored postmarketing surveillance studies. Drug Saf 1993;8:1-8.

15. Strom BL. Study designs available for pharmacoepidemiology studies. In: Strom BL, ed. Pharmacoepidemiology. New York: Churchill Livingstone, 1989:13-26.

16. Faich GA, Guess HA, Kuritsky JN. Postmarketing surveillance for drug safety. In: Cato AE, ed. Clinical drug trials and tribulations. New York: Marcel Dekker, Inc., 1988:347-61.

17. Joint Committee of ABPI, BMA, CMS, and RCGP. Guidelines on postmarketing surveillance. Br Med J 1988;296:399-400.

18. Members of the ASPT Pharmacoepidemiology Section, Strom BL. Position paper on the use of purported postmarketing studies for promotional purposes. Clin Pharmacol Ther 1991;49:598-9.

19. Inman W. Prescriber profile and post-marketing surveillance. Lancet 1993;342:658-61.

20. Spilker B. Guide to clinical trials. New York: Raven Press, Ltd., 1991.

21. Boissel J-P, Alamercery Y, Sassano P. Are science and seeding "trials" compatible (abstract)? Control Clin Trials 1992;13:409.

22. Working Party of the MCA, RCGP, BMA, and ABPI. Guidelines for company-sponsored safety assessment of marketed drugs (SAMM guidelines). Br J Clin Pharmacol 1994;38:95-7.

23. Galton F. Regression towards mediocrity in hereditary stature. J Anthropol Inst 1886;15:246-63.

24. James KE. Regression toward the mean in uncontrolled clinical studies. Biometrics 1973;29:121-30.

25. Davis CE. The effect of regression to the mean in epidemiologic and clinical studies. Am J Epidemiol 1976;104:493-8.

26. Andersen B. Methodological errors in medical research. Oxford: Blackwell Scientific Publishers, 1990.

27. Stang P, Fox J. The Freedom of Information Act: the apple in Eden. J Clin Res Pharmacoepidemiol 1990;4:125-6.
28. Wardell WM. Introduction of new therapeutic drugs in the United States and Great Britain: an international comparison. Clin Pharmacol Ther 1973;14:773-90.
29. DiMasi JA, Seibring MA, Lasagna L. New drug development in the United States from 1963 to 1992. Clin Pharmacol Ther 1994;55:609-22.
30. Seo PS, Kaitin KI. FDA's review of new drug applications: recent trends. J Clin Res Pharmacoepidemiol 1992;6:159-68.
31. Schulman SR, Raiford DS. FDA regulations provide broader access to unapproved drugs. J Clin Pharmacol 1990;30:585-7.
32. Cawthorn RE. Interacting with activists: homework that pays off. Pharmaceut Exec 1992;September:58-62.
33. Stolley PD. Shortcuts in drug evaluation. Clin Pharmacol Ther 1992;52:1-3.
34. Bakke OM, Wardell WM, Lasagna L. Drug discontinuations in the United Kingdom and the United States, 1964–1983: issues of safety. Clin Pharmacol Ther 1984;35:559-67.
35. Bakke OM, Manocchia M, de Abajo F, Kaitin KI, Lasagna L. Drug safety discontinuations in the United Kingdom, the United States, and Spain from 1974 through 1993: a regulatory perspective. Clin Pharmacol Ther 1995;58:108-17.
36. Dodds-Smith I. Product liability issues arising out of the introduction of strict liability and procedures for dealing with multi-claimant cases. In: Goldberg A, Dodds-Smith I, eds. Pharmaceutical medicine and the law. London: Royal College of Physicians, 1991:47-62.
37. Brahams D. Introduction to the legal aspects of pharmaceutical medicine. In: Burley DM, Clarke JM, Lasagna L, eds. Pharmaceutical medicine. 2nd ed. London: Edward Arnold, 1993:320-52.
38. Hodges C. Harmonisation of European controls over research: ethics committees, consent, compensation, and indemnity. In: Goldberg A, Dodds-Smith I, eds. Pharmaceutical medicine and the law. London: Royal College of Physicians, 1991:63-90.
39. Bromberg MJ. Epidemiology in pharmaceutical liability litigation. Sword, shield, or booby trap? J Clin Res Drug Dev 1988;2:79-82.

19

Standards of Postmarketing Surveillance: Past, Present, and Future

Bert Spilker

Abstract

The standards (i.e., the scientific principles that underlie commonly accepted practice) of post-marketing surveillance (PMS) activities are discussed specifically in the context of relationships between regulatory authorities and pharmaceutical companies. The current state of PMS within most companies should be interpreted as representing important progress and not as an ideal state. The cardinal rule for using multipurpose databases is that patient diagnoses must be confirmed; the same validation principle applies to other types of studies. Standards for other innovative designs and the British guidelines for PMS are discussed. Developing new standards for pharmacoepidemiologic studies may contribute to the discipline's reaching maturity by the turn of the century.

Outline

T here are few fields of medicine that have evolved as rapidly over the last 15 years as postmarketing surveillance (PMS). Evolution is evident in the methods, standards, and results of this scientific discipline. It is informative to examine and compare the status of PMS as it existed at the dawn of the last decade, as it exists today, and as it will most likely appear at the dawn of the next century. The standards of PMS are defined briefly and discussed in terms of their development, after which the following selected issues are discussed.

1. Principles governing relationships between regulatory authorities and companies
2. Reporting unintended drug effect data to regulatory authorities
3. Organizing PMS activities within companies
4. Standards for establishing unintended drug effect causality
5. Standards of methodology for PMS studies
6. Establishment of standards and guidelines for conduct of PMS activities
7. Standards for regulatory agency conduct regarding PMS

Definition of Standards and How They Are Developed

Standards are defined operationally in this chapter as the scientific principles that underlie commonly accepted practice. Standards are not immutable; rather, they evolve over time, as scientific practices and professional behavior change. Pharmacoepidemiologic standards are established and influenced by a variety of groups involved in conducting studies reporting unintended drug effects, writing about this area, and developing the practice of the field in other ways.

Standards probably are influenced most strongly by regulatory authorities when they pass regulations or promote guidelines to influence current conduct and practice. Government task forces and committees outside the aegis of regulatory authorities also have played a role in this field, as described later in this chapter. Pharmaceutical companies influence the standards, particularly when they determine that obtaining the best data possible makes good business sense and this goal is encouraged. Academicians who are active in this field also influence standards.

Another group that affects the form standards take is professional societies. The International Society of Pharmacoepidemiology (ISPE) has members from academia, industry, regulatory authorities, and various other institutions and plays an important role in the development of PMS standards. Professional trade associations (e.g., Pharmaceutical Manufacturers Association) also have played a major role in influencing both the direction and growth in this field. Finally, there are many individuals associated with pharmacoepidemiology who influence standards through their writings, speeches, and peer pressure.

Principles Governing Relationships Between Regulatory Authorities and Companies

It is difficult to generalize about relationships in this area, but a few basic principles are evident, the most important being the positive value of cooperation between regulatory authorities and pharmaceutical companies. What changes over time is how well this principle is fulfilled through the standards of PMS practice and through the spirit of cooperation.

A marked degree of cooperation has existed between several of the larger regulatory authorities (e.g., in the US and France) and corporate sponsors. Although some disagreements previously existed, currently exist, and probably will continue to exist, both groups approach most issues with a positive attitude toward seeking agreement and improving standards.

Most regulatory authorities have begun to allow earlier marketing of important new medicines in exchange for sponsor guarantees to conduct adequate PMS studies. The most well-known example to date is zidovudine (Retrovir; Glaxo Wellcome). The early marketing of zidovudine is an important event for future breakthrough medicines. All companies would like to see this approach expanded to include most new medicines. Given current trends, I believe that this is likely to occur significantly by the year 2000. Some skeptics state that more rapid approval of breakthrough medicines has occurred at the expense of all other medicines. The data to prove or disprove this assertion are not yet available.

Reporting Unintended Drug Effect Data to Regulatory Authorities

Ten years ago, few regulatory authorities in industrialized countries had requirements about what types of unintended drug effects they wanted reported and at what frequency the reports should be made. Practice was governed by impressions and inferences of regulators and the regulated, but it was not widely codified in regulations outside the US and the UK. Practices such as whether labeled (i.e., included in the package insert) or only unlabeled unintended drug effects were reported within a short, specified period often differed within a country, as well as from country to country. The allowable time for reporting unintended drug effects after they occurred also differed among countries, but most large regulatory agencies primarily were concerned with unintended drug effects that occurred within their borders.

The situation today is quite different, and some regulatory authorities (e.g., Sweden, Germany) want to learn about all serious unintended drug effects of medicines marketed in their country, regardless of where these occur. This change has been relatively rapid and, even within the short span of 10 years, has gone through several phases. Ten or more years ago, each interested regulatory authority began to evolve its own rules for the types of unintended drug effects to report and how frequently to report them. Each authority designed its own forms and created its own definitions. This increasingly complex situation was becoming a nightmare for pharmaceutical companies. Some described PMS as building a Tower of Babel. It became rapidly apparent that cooperation between regulatory authorities and companies could resolve many unnecessary complexities and benefit both groups as well as physicians and, ultimately, patients.

The Council of International Organizations of Medical Sciences (CIOMS) is an informal coalition of medical associations (e.g., American Medical Association), trade associations (e.g., International Federation of Pharmaceutical Manufacturers Associations), and regulatory authorities. The CIOMS is a neutral forum where the form, format, and content of unintended drug effect reports are discussed. A working group of regulators and industry representatives initially convened in 1987 under the auspices of CIOMS and made several recommendations. A pilot test of these recommendations for alert reporting has been judged successful. This effort originally involved regulatory authorities from six countries and manufacturers from seven. Uniform forms in English were designed to promote rapid and efficient submission of relevant unintended drug effect data from manufacturers to regulators. The primary goal of this program is to facilitate postmarketing reporting using common definitions and uniform reporting forms, categories, and frequencies. A second phase focuses on the content, format, and timing of reports for important unintended drug effects that are labeled and not serious. This program is another example of the extraordinary cooperation in the PMS field that has benefited all groups.

Future needs for collaborative efforts include steps to minimize, if not eliminate, variances between the forms, format, frequency, and contents of all types of periodic unintended drug effect reports. This is part of the European Economic Community harmonization that hopefully will occur over the next decade and may be based, in part, on the CIOMS model. A more distant goal relates to the formalization and harmonization of epidemiologic studies on a worldwide basis.

Organizing PMS Activities Within Companies

To gather, assemble, and report on unintended drug effects, most research- and development-based companies have established PMS departments over the last decade. In 1980, there were extremely few departments in the industry, although many, if not most, companies had specific professionals to correspond with physicians who reported unintended drug effects. This early precursor of the modern PMS department is as different from the large computer-assisted PMS groups of today as are the accounting scribes sitting on high stools, carefully writing numbers in a ledger in a Dickensian novel, from computer-assisted financial departments today. The modern PMS group designs a specific PMS program for each investigational medicine during Phase III. This package of studies is designed to obtain important medical data as early during the postmarketing period as possible, which may be considered to begin during Phase IIIb (i.e., after the regulatory submission has been made but prior to the drug's initial approval). The current state of PMS organizations within companies should be interpreted as representing important progress and not as being an ideal state.

DATABASES WITHIN COMPANIES

Numerous problems remain to be resolved in the area of PMS. One of these is how to determine whether a pharmaceutical company with two (or more) unintended drug effect surveillance sites should use a single, worldwide database or whether it should have separate databases at each site and share information on an open and periodic basis. The pros and cons of each approach are not presented here.

It is predicted that, in 10 years, almost all pharmaceutical companies will have centralized their unintended drug effect data-reporting facilities for ease of operations. Most companies will use a single worldwide database, despite a number of important limitations and potential problems with this approach (e.g., combining unintended drug effect data of differing qualities). Subsetting the data within the database according to its quality and validity undoubtedly will occur. Data also may be partitioned, based on country of origin or according to any other factor that can be flagged as the data are entered into the computer.

Standards for Establishing Unintended Drug Effect Causality

Causality is the assessment of a cause-and-effect relationship between two associated events. The likelihood of the cause-and-effect relationship usually is expressed in such terms as definite, probably, possible, unlikely, and definitely not. Causality assessments may be viewed on several levels. For individual patients, it is often critical to determine whether a medicine is the cause of the patient's unintended drug effect. The specific causality assessment helps to determine whether the drug should be discontinued. For individual clinical trials, the causality assessment often determines whether the trial itself must be prematurely terminated. For individual companies, it usually is critical to be aware of causal relationships between medicines and serious unintended drug effects that are reported. This assessment often plays a major role in the company's decision to continue or terminate the drug's development.

For large PMS studies and unintended drug effect evaluations, the assessment of causality usually is not relevant for interpreting the data, because it usually is not possible to obtain sufficient information on reported unintended drug effects. The information obtained is often fragmentary, unverified, and of variable quality. It often is impossible to obtain sufficient additional data to answer questions. The interpretation of such data, even from many large, well-known databases, is subject to substantial error if the data are analyzed too finely (i.e., to assess causality). Although causality has been found to be an important, and even critical, tool for Phase I and other clinical trials, it is less valuable, and sometimes even counterproductive, to evaluate causality in PMS studies.

TOOLS USED TO ASSESS CAUSALITY

The tools available to assess causality have evolved over 30 years from an emphasis on global introspection (i.e., assessment by an expert using clinical judgment, experience, and data on the specific case), to the use of algorithms (i.e., simple or complex preestablished questions that lead to an answer), to formal Bayesian logic, and, finally, to the use of natural history registries to establish background rates.

Up to the mid-1970s, global introspection was the method most widely used to establish causality between a drug and an unintended drug effect. This approach was criticized by various professionals who were able to demonstrate lack of agreement among experts who used these methods. Global introspection approaches also have been criticized by proponents of algorithms as being a less scientific and less valid method for establishing causality.[1]

Ten to 20 years ago, we were at the height of the "algorithm phase" for establishing the causality of purported drug-induced adverse reactions. At least 15 separate algorithms, many of which had a highly logical approach, were developed and published. It is no accident that many algorithms were developed by individuals trained as scientists and not by practicing clinicians.

During the 1980s, a sense of frustration developed with algorithms, particularly when insufficient clinical data were available to utilize the algorithm as designed. This was particularly common with complex (i.e., elaborate) algorithms that posed many questions. Algorithms are utilized retrospectively, often when some important information either is unavailable or was never obtained. Algorithms are not patient specific and are not necessarily correlated with medical decision-making. The more simple algorithms proved easiest to use.

A group of professionals active in this area developed a Bayesian approach to the causality issue during the mid-1980s, using concepts of formal logic. This methodology is probably as capable as any other method of yielding a definitive answer to the cause-and-effect issue. The method is well suited for assessing causality for individual patients and, therefore, could assist clinical treatment. This approach is unsuitable, however, for medicines for which a great deal of data are unavailable, because the method requires a substantial amount of prior knowledge. Therefore, the method is useful only for medicines in Phases III and IV. This method is also extremely time consuming and is not appropriate except when the importance of the clinical question justifies the use of a relatively large amount of resources.

At present the need to assess causality during clinical trials differs from the need to assess it during PMS. Clinical trials must consider it. In the future as well as today, when serious unlabeled unintended drug effects arise in clinical trials, a sponsor might want to use both global introspections and a moderately simple algorithm. If results differ, I would place more reliance on the former method to establish the strength of the association of the event with the medicine.

There will be an increased demand for natural history epidemiology in PMS studies. This means that registries of the natural history of disease will be used more in the future to establish the background rate of unintended drug effects in patients with that disease. This information will be compared with medicine-induced rates. Comparing the rates for unintended drug effects with the rates obtained in natural history registries will be more important for PMS evaluations than focusing on the attribution of individual adverse events with the drug.

Several registries that gathered unintended drug effect data in selected therapeutic areas were founded prior to the 1980s. In the US, this includes the National Registry of Drug-Induced Ocular Side Effects, the Registry of Tissue Reactions to Drugs, and the Hepatic Events Registry. The Dermatological Adverse Drug Reaction Reporting System was begun in 1980.

Standards of Methodology for PMS Studies

Several large and costly PMS cohort studies (e.g., prazosin, cimetidine) had been mounted by 1980, with a goal of enrolling approximately 10 000 patients each. This number had a somewhat mystical connotation and often was described as representing a balance between the minimum size necessary to observe most rare unintended drug effects (i.e., those with an incidence of less than 1 in 3000) and the maximum size that could be managed practically by a single company. Standard methods of assembling large cohorts of patients (e.g., conducting multicenter studies) were used for these PMS studies. These methods usually were applied to all medicines for which prospective PMS was considered, rather than custom designing different approaches for particular drugs. PMS studies sometimes involved retrospective analyses of data already collected, to look for increased incidence rates of unintended drug effects in specific groups of patients.

The balance between conducting retrospective and prospective studies has changed over the last 2 decades from a preponderance of large, prospective, cohort studies to a preponderance of studies involving a retrospective or mixed examination of data in large, multipurpose, automated, linked databases. The pendulum also has swung from most information and signals of possible unintended drug effects coming from passive intelligence gathering to a greater proportion of signals coming from active searching of published literature and more active solicitation and evaluation of spontaneously generated reports.

The most important single change in PMS over the last 15 years has been the development and use of large, multipurpose databases to evaluate purported drug-induced unintended drug effects. The cardinal rule today for using these multipurpose databases for record linkage studies is that patient diagnoses must be confirmed. Without this essential step, erroneous interpretations and conclusions based on misclassifications of patients are possible.

The same principle of validation also applies to other types of studies, such as those of clusters of unintended drug effects. This situation is well known to public health investigators. For example, a report that 50 people who had emesis at a dinner party all ate the chicken salad, or that 50 people who lived in a polluted environment developed cancer, must be checked carefully. It may turn out in the former case that there was a contact psychological reaction that began when someone was overheated and felt nauseous; in the latter case, many of the people involved may have had unassociated types of cancers or may have only recently moved to the area.

The discipline of PMS is still in the midst of a substantial effort to develop additional and broader, large, automated, linked, multipurpose databases. Without sufficient linkages within each database and without a sufficient number of databases, it is impossible to adequately address relevant PMS questions and important issues. An important industry-wide group initiated by Ciba-Geigy, Risk Assessment of Drugs–Analysis and Response (RAD-AR), helps to build sufficient database capacity for pharmacoepidemiology and helps to clarify the relationship between the benefits and risks of medicine. This group has four major functions or goals:

1. to explore and support the appropriate role of epidemiology in the pharmaceutical industry,
2. to serve as a forum for exchanging epidemiology and related information,
3. to serve as a coordinating group for intercompany activities relating to epidemiology, and
4. to act as a liaison between the pharmaceutical industry and other organizations (e.g., regulatory agencies, universities) for epidemiology-related activities.

One of RAD-AR's first projects was to assemble and issue a four-volume series, *International Drug Benefit/Risk Assessment Data Resource Handbook*.[2] The four volumes cover North America, the UK, Japan, and Germany/the Netherlands/Switzerland. These volumes are the most complete list of sources of databases and available information. RAD-AR has achieved success at both the national and international levels. At the national level, numerous groups have evaluated the pharmacoepidemiologic methods, standards, and capacity within their own country. At the international level, RAD-AR has achieved a network of many national groups and has helped to foster the formation of the ISPE.

Major pharmaceutical industry resources are being used to evaluate current databases in terms of the validity of diagnoses and data, as well as the completeness and linkability. Numerous large, automated databases with record linkage currently exist, primarily in the US (see Chapter 14). By the year 2000, many more probably will have been established in most other countries where new medicines are developed. One of the keys to developing more large linked databases outside the US is their endorsement by large international health organizations (e.g., the World Health Organization), which would encourage some countries to overcome their current reluctance to build such databases. This reluctance often is based on the perceived need to protect the privacy of individuals.

These large databases will become more efficient in the future as they are used to address important PMS questions. Most of the existing databases are available to companies on a contractual basis. These include databases of health maintenance organizations, states' Medicaid, consortiums of hospitals, and selected registries. It should be noted that these databases were not designed with pharmacoepidemiology studies in mind; they differ significantly from each other in the data they collect and in their ability for linking different types of data. As a result, there are numerous pros and cons of using each database from a pharmacoepidemiologic viewpoint.

Current major experiments in PMS methodology include prescription event monitoring by the Drug Safety Research Unit in England. This technique involves systematic sampling of up to a million prescriptions per year, chosen (from 350 million written) because of the medicine prescribed. Each of the prescribing physicians of these million prescriptions is sent a green form requesting information on whether the prescription involved a new diagnosis, referral, unexpected improvement, change of treatment, and whether any unintended drug effects occurred. The goal of the Drug Safety Research Unit is to conduct prescription event monitoring on all new major chemical entity medicines used within the National Health Service. Eventually, prescription event monitoring may also be used to test specific hypotheses in England (Wales, Scotland, and Ireland are not included in this survey).

Data obtained through prescription event monitoring must be interpreted with a great deal of caution because (1) patient diagnoses are not confirmed and validated, (2) a causal relationship of a unintended drug effect cannot actually be established, and (3) a high reporting rate of unintended drug effects may falsely suggest that the medicine is less safe than others. For example, if a new drug is promoted as being less liable than others to cause a certain unintended drug effect, physicians will tend to place more of their high-risk patients (for developing that unintended drug effect) on the medicine. Thus, a higher rate of that adverse experience may be noted with the drug, but may not reflect a true incidence figure for unintended drug effects.

Results of prescription event monitoring and other population-based methods are expected to differ from data obtained in drug development studies sponsored by pharmaceutical companies. This is because the unintended drug effect profile of a relatively healthy or select group of patients receiving a medicine, in a study conducted in a limited patient population (e.g., in clinical trials), will differ from the unintended drug effect profile obtained in all patients in a large population who receive the medicine. However, many physicians do not return any data on their patients to the Drug Safety Research Unit, and the data returned may not represent a true cross-section of what is occurring. Even if physicians do return the data to the Drug Safety Research Unit, the validity is uncertain. Moreover, the background incidence of most unintended drug effects measured is unknown. Thus, without population controls, excesses in frequency are difficult to interpret. The type of patients who are prescribed new medicines is also unknown. One final drawback of prescription event monitoring is that it requires a minimum of several months to gather sufficient data, whereas a multipurpose automated database may take only 1 hour or less to obtain suggestive PMS results.

Epidemiologic intelligence from sentinel sources, such as observations from physicians in letters sent to pharmaceutical companies, regulatory agencies, and the literature, will remain an important source of information for identifying unintended drug effects that should be further evaluated. Allegations from the media of important medical risks from marketed medicines will also remain a mechanism to trigger responses in both companies and regulatory agencies.

Establishment of Standards and Guidelines for Conduct of PMS Studies

There were no guidelines or standards for PMS studies prior to the establishment of the Joint Commission on Prescription Drug Use. The US Congress established the Commission in 1976 "to describe a postmarketing surveillance system that could be used to detect, quantitate, and describe the anticipated and unanticipated effects of marketed drugs, and to recommend a means by which information on the epidemiology of prescription drug use in the U.S. could be distributed regularly to interested parties in the United States."[3] The Commission's final report was issued on January 23, 1980, and contained five major recommendations:

1. A systematic and comprehensive system of PMS should be developed in the US.
2. Such a system should be able to detect important unintended drug effects that occur more frequently than once per thousand uses of a drug, to develop methods to detect less frequent reactions, and to evaluate the beneficial effects of drugs as used in ordinary practice. New methods will have to be developed for the study of delayed drug effects, including both therapeutic and adverse effects.
3. An integral function of the PMS system should be to report the uses and effects of new and old prescription drugs.
4. Recognizing the progress that the Food and Drug Administration (FDA) has made in the area of PMS in the last 3 years, the Commission recommends that PMS should be a priority program of the FDA and that the FDA should continue to strengthen its program in this area.
5. A private, nonprofit Center for Drug Surveillance should be established to further the development of a PMS system in the US. This center should foster cooperation among existing PMS programs, develop new methods for carrying out surveillance, train scientists

in the disciplines needed for doing PMS, and educate both providers and recipients of prescription drugs about the effects of these drugs.

The first four recommendations have been initiated to a large extent by the FDA and the pharmaceutical industry in the US, working jointly as well as independently. The last recommendation has not been implemented, but the need for a national center certainly could be debated.

In the UK, a group analogous to the Joint Commission on Prescription Drug Use was the Graham–Smith Working Party. There are currently no formal requirements that serve as standards for PMS studies in either country.

Many regulatory agencies believe that there should be formal criteria or decisional standards to determine what medicines require tests, what types of studies are needed, and how PMS studies should be established, monitored, and reported. In other words, many groups believe that the postmarketing period of a drug's life should be evaluated as systematically and carefully as the premarketing period. There are generally well designed standards for the premarketing period of new chemical entities, and these are being reviewed in a search for appropriate PMS standards.

No guidelines existed for PMS in 1980. At that time, the data used and combined in PMS often contained contaminants (inaccurate or incomplete data), and data were not validated for accuracy. The few studies conducted were mainly designed by clinical groups without training in epidemiologic methods. There were no guidelines at regulatory agencies to decide which drugs should be subject to PMS studies.

A set of 19 guidelines for PMS was proposed by a joint committee of the Association of the British Pharmaceutical Industry (ABPI), the British Medical Association, the Committee on Safety of Medicines, and the Royal College of General Practitioners. These guidelines were developed particularly for observational cohort studies sponsored by pharmaceutical companies. These 19 points are primarily principles and managerial guidelines rather than scientific guidelines or standards useful for the design and conduct of PMS studies. The British guidelines include a definition of PMS and describe basic principles underlying most studies (e.g., there should be a valid medical reason for undertaking the study). The guidelines state that studies should not be designed solely for promotional purposes and that any breaches of this guideline are to be reported to the Code of Practice Committee of the ABPI. Another guideline is that appropriate fees may be paid to physicians for completing data forms, but no other financial inducements may be offered.[4] These guidelines might best be viewed as starting points for the development of scientific guidelines.

Revised investigational new drug and new drug applications, plus regulatory commentary and additional guidelines written by the FDA during the 1980s, indicate gradually increasing and clarified regulatory requirements on what unintended drug effect data to report. This pertains to unintended drug effects that occur in clinical trials as well as after the drug is marketed. The frequency and timing of these reports are also more precisely specified for both short-term serious, unexpected, and unlabeled unintended drug effects, and those included in quarterly or annual reports.

In the US, the Emerging Epidemiological Monitoring Techniques Committee of the Pharmaceutical Manufacturers Association is actively and aggressively exploring the development of standards for the field of PMS equivalent to good laboratory practices. Forty companies are participating in discussions on this topic. In sharing their problems and perspectives, they have followed the public health approach of encouraging multiple groups to work together to help protect the well-being of patients using pharmaceutical products. Many practices that were standard 10 years ago are no longer acceptable today.

The ISPE created a set of guidelines, "Guidelines for Good Epidemiology Practices for Drug, Device, and Vaccine Research in the United States." These guidelines, as revised March 27, 1996, are available on the Internet at (http://www.hsph.harvard.edu/Organizations/DDIL/gep.html).

The guidelines propose practices and procedures in the following six areas:

I. Protocol
II. Organization and personnel
III. Facilities, resource commitment, and contractors
IV. Study conduct
V. Communication
VI. Archiving

This is an excellent set of guidelines and is highly recommended. Although they were developed from a US perspective, most, if not all, principles transcend national boundaries and are applicable worldwide.

While the above guidelines represent a major advance in pharmacoepidemiology, another recent trend has had the opposite effect. A number of countries have either proposed or are considering legislation on data privacy that would severely hamper the ability of pharmacoepidemiologists to conduct some of their research. Relevant societies, as well as individuals, must make legislators aware of the impact on research that seemingly reasonable measures for protecting individuals' privacy would have. Any legislation should be crafted to allow valid and worthwhile pharmacoepidemiology research to continue and to prosper.

Most research- and development-based pharmaceutical companies are opposed to the establishment of regulatory guidelines for the postmarketing period. They do not believe that the FDA has the regulatory authority or mandate to put forth these guidelines. Thus, no guidelines currently determine which medicines require PMS studies in the US and what types of studies should be performed. These decisions are handled on a case-by-case basis between the sponsor and the regulatory agency. The European Economic Community seeks cooperation with the US, and it is hoped that a general consensus between these groups can be reached. As a general principle, any guidelines enacted should consider the ability of sponsors to conduct PMS studies with available methods and databases, and should not force sponsors to adopt standards and methods that are beyond current capabilities.

More formal PMS guidelines undoubtedly will exist in the future. It is hoped that these scientific guidelines will be put together as a consensus of all interested parties and that they will represent state-of-the-art scientific principles that are realistic to achieve. Setting standards that are unrealistic in terms of the methodologies or resources required to meet those standards will be counterproductive and not in the best interests of patients, the ultimate group for whom standards are created.

Standards for Regulatory Agency Conduct Regarding PMS Activities

An undesirable pseudoscientific practice of the past has been termed the "fishing expedition." In this method, someone at a regulatory agency or academic center with access to a large database would enter into his or her keyboard the name of a drug and a number of adverse medical events to determine whether any association existed. If an academician found, in the initial evaluation, a higher rate of unintended drug effects associated with a medicine than anticipated, then an academic paper or a letter to the editor often resulted. The report could be picked up by the media or a regulatory authority and pursued further. If regulatory people conducted this fishing expedition, they would ask the relevant company how it intended to respond to the associations found. This letter might require the company to conduct a survey or study but, at the minimum, would require that the company respond. Because of the ease of deriving possible associations by looking at one unintended drug effect across multiple drugs or by examining various patient populations and multiple unintended drug effects for a single medicine, a single individual could potentially keep the entire pharmaceutical industry busy investigating such associations. This could occur despite the fact that most, or almost all, of these associations were not meaningful and could not be confirmed.

Obviously, the actual situation never deteriorated to this extent, and it is currently scientifically unacceptable for causality assessments to be derived in this nonscientific manner. Associations that should (or must) be analyzed usually arise from case studies, in the literature, or from reports received by a company or regulatory authority from physicians, sales representatives, or other sources.

Both the FDA in the US and the Department of Health in the UK periodically publish reports of purported associations. For example, if either agency receives an increased frequency of blood dyscrasia reports occurring with a particular medicine, it often will include those data in the newsletter that all physicians receive. The agency's intention, to alert physicians about a potential problem and to seek additional data to better define the numerator and denominator of its incidence, is quite worthwhile. Unfortunately, this method may have the effect of eliciting many additional reports that complicate rather than simplify the assessment of a drug's benefits and risks.

In the future, perhaps all regulatory agencies will adopt a more logical and scientifically sound approach to increased frequencies of reports of known unintended drug effects or to reports of serious new unintended drug effects. The first step should be to contact the medicine's sponsor, manufacturer, or distributor and to notify it of the purported unintended drug effect. One company's response may be to dispatch trained monitors to visit the sites where the reported cases occurred and to evaluate all available data. At the same time, both the company and regulatory agency would review their existing databases to determine what cases were reported previously and the details of those cases. These assessments could better establish the importance of the signal, evaluate whether specific risk factors were involved in the cases, and describe any characteristics common to two or more of the cases. Benefit/risk assessments would be determined, and a meeting would be arranged (if necessary) to plan the next stage of follow-up.

Any one or more of the following additional steps could be taken. A group of experts from academia, the government, or both could be brought together to review the data and make recommendations. The regulatory authority or sponsor could issue a notification to all physicians in the country to seek further information (i.e., examples). At this point, it would have to be determined whether the name of the specific drug or only the chemical or therapeutic class should be identified. The latter approach would prevent biasing physicians against a single medicine and would also minimize the chance of a fishing expedition. This approach would determine more fairly whether the unintended drug effect was characteristic of an entire class of medicines. Large, automated, multipurpose databases could be used to evaluate the hypothesis. Other types of epidemiologic studies could be conducted also. Additional prospective epidemiologic studies could be undertaken to evaluate the unintended drug effect. Finally, if specific risk factors were identified and the benefit/risk consideration dictated that specific patients should not receive the medicine, then package labeling changes could be negotiated and the new data disseminated, using a variety of techniques.

Summary

This brief discussion illustrates some of the vast changes in PMS that have evolved over the last 25 years and indicates a number of potential future trends. The field has moved from its own Dark Ages of the 1970s, when little consensus and no standards existed, into the light of the 1990s. Pharmacoepidemiology needs to continue to move forward and develop further to refine the scientific standards and guiding principles that represent signs of a more mature discipline. Practitioners of pharmacoepidemiology should accept this challenge, whether individually or through appropriate organizations. Let us hope that the scientific growth of the field of PMS and the development of standards for its conduct continue, and that the once fledgling and fragmented field reaches maturity by the turn of the next century.

References

1. Kramer MS. Assessing causality of adverse drug reactions: global introspection and its limitations. Drug Inf J 1986;20:433-8.
2. Pharma Corporation and the Degge Group. International drug benefit/risk assessment data resource handbook. Basel, Switzerland: Ciba-Geigy, 1988.
3. Melmon K. Final report of the Joint Commission on Prescription Drug Use. US Senate Committee on Labor and Human Resources. Subcommittee on Health and Scientific Research. Washington, DC: US Government Printing Office, 1980.
4. Joint Committee of ABPI, BMA, CSM, and RCGP. Guidelines on post-marketing surveillance. Br Med J 1988;296:399-400.

20

Pharmacoepidemiology of Asthma Deaths

Neil Pearce
Richard Beasley
Julian Crane
Carl Burgess

Abstract

The pharmacoepidemiology of asthma deaths involves several distinctive features, including the rarity of asthma death, the problems of diagnosis, the occurrence of most deaths outside the hospital, and the self-administration and irregular use of asthma medications. The most striking features of asthma mortality during this century have been the epidemics of asthma deaths that occurred in six countries in the 1960s and again in New Zealand in the 1970s. These epidemics followed the introduction of isoprenaline forte (isoproterenol) and fenoterol, respectively; these are high-dose, poorly selective, full agonists, with relatively greater cardiac adverse effects than more selective beta$_2$-agonists. Case–control studies in New Zealand and Canada have found that patients prescribed fenoterol were at a higher risk of asthma death than were patients prescribed other beta-agonists. Attention is now shifting to the possible role of regular use of beta-agonists (as a class) in more gradual increases in asthma mortality in recent decades. However, this latter hypothesis is much more difficult to investigate since, in most industrialized countries, beta-agonists are used by virtually all asthmatic persons, and the problems of confounding by asthma severity are much greater. Thus, it is unlikely that these more general issues can be fully resolved by pharmacoepidemiologic studies, but epidemiology will clearly continue to have an important role to play, in combination with experimental and clinical studies, in investigating the effects of recent changes in the management of asthma.

Outline

A sthma treatment has been the subject of controversy for thousands of years. The word "asthma" comes from a Greek word meaning "panting,"[1] but reference to asthma can also be found in ancient Egyptian, Hebrew, and Indian medical writings.[2,3] One of the earliest documented examples of successful asthma treatment occurred in the 16th century, when Gerolamo Cardano was called from Italy to Edinburgh to treat John Hamilton, the Archbishop of St. Andrews. Hamilton's treatment included diet, purging, regular exercise, sleep, and substitution of unspun silk for feathers in the mattress; this kept him alive long enough to be hanged by the Scottish Reformers.[1]

In the following centuries, treatments for asthma have included foxes' lungs, Syrup of Garlick, Tincture of Lavender, Saffron Lozenges, and Smoked Amber with Tobacco (17th century); bloodletting and gentle vomits (18th century); whiffs of chloroform, lobelia, and morphine (19th century); and marijuana, petroleum, oil, and various "asthma powders" including extracts of daṯ...ḁ that were sold without restriction in shops and on street corners (early 20th century). Since the 1940s, asthma treatment has been transformed by the identification of beta-receptors and by the development of beta-agonist drugs with increasing activity for the beta$_2$-receptor; these have been the mainstay of asthma management since their introduction. The beta$_2$-agonists provide symptomatic relief by relieving bronchospasm; however, in the past decade, as inflammation has come to be viewed as the fundamental problem in asthma, there has been increasing emphasis on antiinflammatory drugs.[4,5]

Modern asthma management is presumably based on a more scientific understanding of the disease than earlier approaches. However, modern asthma drugs, such as the beta-agonists and corticosteroids, were primarily tested for short-term efficacy (when used as recommended), and their acute adverse effects (when overused in an acute attack) and chronic adverse effects (when used regularly) were not adequately tested either before or after their introduction. There is currently increasing concern about the safety and efficacy of beta-agonists and their possible role in asthma deaths.[6] Almost all studies to date of asthma deaths have concentrated on this issue, which is the focus of this chapter, but we also briefly discuss studies involving other asthma drugs.

Asthma Deaths

Osler[7] observed that "the asthmatic pants into old age," and asthma deaths were rare in the first half of this century.[8] Asthma death continues to be a rare event, and asthma is not usually regarded as life-threatening; thus, asthma deaths are usually considered to be avoidable, and any increase in the asthma death rate is viewed with concern. The most striking changes in asthma mortality during the past century were the epidemics of asthma deaths in six countries in the 1960s and again in New Zealand in the 1970s. These have been superimposed on a more gradual underlying increase in asthma mortality in many countries since the 1940s.[9]

There is a hierarchy of pharmacoepidemiologic study designs that can be used to investigate the causes of asthma deaths in general and of asthma mortality epidemics in particular. In terms of increasing the level of complexity and validity, these include the following: case series reports, analyses of time trends, and analytical studies (cohort and case–control studies). We will discuss these approaches when reviewing pharmacoepidemiologic studies of the 1960s' and 1970s' epidemics.

Several key features of the pharmacoepidemiology of asthma deaths should first be considered. First, one of the implications of asthma deaths being infrequent is that randomized controlled trials are usually not feasible for the assessment of the adverse effects of therapy, and cohort studies require large numbers of patients with relatively severe asthma.

Second, there are major problems of diagnosis of asthma death in infants and elderly persons; thus, almost all analyses of asthma mortality are confined to the 5- to 34-year age group because the diagnosis of asthma death is more firmly established.[10]

Third, most asthma deaths occur outside the hospital, without a physician's being in attendance[11]; thus, the mechanism of death is usually unknown, and information is often not available on the drugs used immediately prior to death. Thus, it is usually necessary to study the regular prescribed medication (which can be ascertained from routine records), even if an acute effect of medication is hypothesized.

Finally, asthma medication is self-administered, and use is often irregular. For example, beta-agonist use is related to (and confounded by) the frequency and severity of symptoms, and some patients may occasionally (or frequently) use very large quantities of beta-agonists in an acute attack,[12] but this may not be known if the attack is fatal. Thus, confounding by severity is a major concern in pharmacoepidemiologic studies of asthma deaths, particularly in studies that examine actual medication use.

The 1960s' Epidemics

CASE SERIES AND CASE REPORTS

Isoprenaline (isoproterenol) was the first pure beta-agonist to be synthesized, and its introduction in the 1940s was considered a great advance in asthma treatment, although concerns were soon expressed about the overuse of isoprenaline and the development of refractory asthma.[13] Beta-agonist sales increased markedly with the introduction of the pressurized aerosol (metered-dose inhaler) in the early 1960s; it was at this time that the first reports linking beta-agonists to asthma deaths appeared. For example, Greenberg and Pines[14] provided the following warning:

> *We suspect that patients with asthma may be killing themselves by the excessive use of sympathomimetic agents in the form of metered or pressurized aerosols containing isoprenaline, orciprenaline, or adrenaline.*

ANALYSES OF TIME TRENDS

These case reports led to analyses of time trends, which found that major asthma mortality epidemics were occurring in six developed countries: England and Wales, Scotland, Ireland, New Zealand, Australia, and Norway; other countries such as Germany and the US did not experience epidemics (Figure 1[8]). When investigating such an increase in mortality, researchers must first assess whether the increase in the death rates is real.[15] Speizer et al.[16] conducted a detailed examination of the mortality trends in the 5- to 34-year age group in England and Wales. They concluded that the epidemic was real and was not due to changes in death certification, disease classification, diagnostic practice, or asthma prevalence, but was because of an increase in case fatality due to new methods of treatment. In particular, they found that the sudden increase in asthma deaths followed the introduction of pressurized beta-agonist aerosols in 1961 and paralleled the subsequent increase in sales.

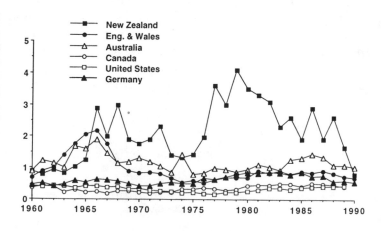

Figure 1
International Patterns of Asthma Mortality per 100 000 Persons Aged 5–34 Years Between 1960 and 1990. Eng. = England. Adapted from Reference 8.

MECHANISMS

Almost all of these deaths occurred outside the hospital,[11] and direct information on drug use was scanty. However, it was noted that the relief of symptoms by isoprenaline could enable a patient to tolerate worsening hypoxia and to unduly delay seeking medical help.[17] Animal studies suggested that direct toxicity of isoprenaline could be potentiated under conditions of hypoxemia; thus, whereas high doses of isoprenaline would be safe under normal conditions, such doses would not be safe when the patient was hypoxemic.[18,19] In this context, it was considered significant that most asthma deaths occur outside the hospital under conditions of hypoxemia, whereas asthma deaths rarely occur in the hospital when high doses of beta-agonists are administered with oxygen.[20] It may also be relevant that the cardiac effects of beta-agonists are greater in young persons,[21] that the increase in mortality was greatest in the 10- to 19-year age group, and that "at these ages children have begun to act independently and may be particularly prone to misuse a self-administered form of treatment."[16]

THE ISOPRENALINE FORTE HYPOTHESIS

Nevertheless, there was a major anomaly with the aerosol hypothesis: There had also been considerable sales of aerosols in the US and several other countries that did not experience mortality epidemics. This paradox was resolved by further analyses conducted by Stolley.[22] He found that a high-dose formulation of isoprenaline (isoprenaline forte) had been licensed in only eight countries. Six of these were the countries that had mortality epidemics, and these coincided with the introduction of the drug; in the other two countries (the Netherlands and Belgium), the preparation was introduced relatively late, and sales volumes were low; no mortality epidemics occurred in countries in which isoprenaline forte was unlicensed, such as Sweden, Canada, West Germany, and the US.[22] Some anomalies still remained in the time trend data, but these were generally minor. For example, in some countries the death rate declined before sales of isoprenaline forte began to decline, but the mortality decline followed widespread publicity about the mortality epidemic and the elimination of nonprescription availability of beta-agonist aerosols.

CASE–CONTROL STUDIES

Although the time trend data were compelling, the protagonists on both sides of the isoprenaline forte debate were agreed that the most definitive approach would have been to perform a cohort or case–control study.[22-24] In practice, a case–control study is the more feasible option since asthma deaths are rare.[25] However, formal case–control studies were never performed because the epidemic declined (following the issuing of warnings and the fall in sales) before there was time to conduct them.

The potential hazards of beta-agonist aerosols are now disputed in many texts and reviews.[26-28] In fact, little new evidence has appeared since 1972, with the exception of further analyses conducted by Stolley and Schinnar[29] that strengthened Stolley's original conclusions. The process of "reinterpretation" of the 1960s' epidemic was based on the minor anomalies in the time trend data, which were emphasized (and to some extent exaggerated) in subsequent reviews that contained no new data but merely referenced other reviews.[30] Other factors such as delays in seeking medical help also began to receive greater emphasis.[26-28] However, it is very difficult to envisage how (non-drug-induced) delays could have spontaneously occurred and then regressed in some countries (which "coincidentally" were the countries in which isoprenaline forte sales were high) but not in others (which "coincidentally" were countries in which isoprenaline forte sales were low or zero).

The Second New Zealand Epidemic

Given the reluctance of respiratory physicians to accept the epidemiologic evidence on the role of isoprenaline forte in the 1960s' epidemics, it is perhaps not surprising that history repeated itself. In 1976, a second asthma mortality epidemic began in New Zealand but not in other countries.

CASE SERIES AND CASE REPORTS

The epidemic was reported in 1981 by Wilson et al.,[31] who noted an apparent increase in the number of young people who were dying suddenly from acute asthma in Auckland and reviewed 22 fatal cases. Their findings were as follows:

> *In 16 patients death was seen to be sudden and unexpected. Although all were experiencing respiratory distress, most were not cyanosed and the precipitate nature of their death suggested a cardiac event, such as arrest, inappropriate to the severity of their respiratory problem. ... The only reasonable explanation is that the change must be a reflection of changes in the patterns of treatment of asthma in Auckland.*

Interestingly, an accompanying table showed that 10 of the 13 persons classified as sudden deaths for which the drug information was recorded had been prescribed fenoterol (at a time when the drug accounted for <30% of national sales), but this was not noted in the text that concentrated on a possible class effect of beta-agonists in combination with oral theophyllines.[31]

TIME TRENDS

Jackson et al.[32] subsequently investigated the international time trends and found that this new epidemic appeared to be confined to New Zealand. As for the 1960s' epidemic, they concluded that the new epidemic was real and could not be explained by changes in the classification of asthma deaths, inaccuracies in death certification, changes in diagnostic fashions, or changes in the incidence or prevalence of asthma. The most likely explanation, as for the 1960s' epidemics, was that the epidemic was due to an increased case fatality rate related to changes in the management of asthma in New Zealand.

The possibility of a role of a class effect of beta-agonists was investigated in time trend analyses by Keating et al.,[33] who found that the mortality epidemic had started in 1976, but that overall sales of inhaled beta-agonists had only begun to increase markedly in 1979. Thus, Sears and Beaglehole[34] subsequently concluded that "the temporal relationship between increased sales and deaths does not suggest a direct causal relationship."

THE NEW ZEALAND ASTHMA MORTALITY SURVEY

A national survey of asthma deaths in persons younger than 70 years during August 1981–July 1983 was subsequently conducted by the Asthma Task Force. Unfortunately, the study did not include a control group, and the findings are therefore difficult to interpret. Nevertheless, the authors[35] concluded that a number of factors contributed to asthma deaths, including inadequate functional assessment of the severity of asthma, inappropriate drug therapy with overreliance on beta-agonists and underuse of corticosteroids, delay in seeking and in some cases providing medical care, inadequate emergency care, and lack of follow-up after treatment of acute attacks. However, the authors produced no evidence that any of these factors had suddenly increased in 1976 in New Zealand (but not in other countries). The report did not specify any criteria for overuse, but concluded that "excessive use of bronchodilator drugs did not account for the high mortality rates."[35] However, a subsequent report by two members of the same group[36] noted the following:

> Most patients whose final episodes had lasted for several hours had repeatedly used their inhaled bronchodilator aerosol, and in some cases a domiciliary nebuliser, to administer large doses of beta-agonist, without seeking additional therapy with corticosteroids.

THE FENOTEROL HYPOTHESIS

Thus, there was no plausible explanation for the second New Zealand mortality epidemic until the fenoterol hypothesis was proposed by Crane et al.[37] in 1989. This hypothesis stemmed initially from published reports of the greater cardiovascular adverse effects of fenoterol and from incidental information that fenoterol was used by a relatively high proportion of asthmatic persons who died.[31,38] These observations prompted a reexamination of the time trend data.[37] This revealed that fenoterol was introduced to New Zealand in April 1976 and that the epidemic began in the same year (Figure 2). It was also observed that fenoterol represented less than 5% of the market in most other countries and was not available in the US. Although fenoterol had a 50% market share in West Germany, the per capita sales of fenoterol were only one-third as high as in New Zealand, and mortality had in fact nearly doubled in the 10 years following the introduction of fenoterol.[39] A further observation was that fenoterol was marketed as a 200-µg/puff preparation (compared with 100 µg/puff for salbutamol [albuterol]), whereas the drug was approximately twice as potent as salbutamol on a weight basis; thus, the marketed formulation was effectively a forte preparation at two to four times the strength of salbutamol.[40] Finally, a series of laboratory studies found that repeated inhalation of fenoterol resulted in increased cardiac adverse effects than associated with salbutamol or isoprenaline.[20]

Case–Control Studies of Asthma Deaths

In response to these observations, a series of case–control studies were conducted to investigate the possible role of fenoterol in the second New Zealand asthma mortality epidemic. We will first discuss the general study design issues involved in such studies, which include comparing the safety of one drug (e.g., fenoterol) with that of other drugs in the same class (e.g., salbutamol).

Figure 2
Fenoterol Market Share and New Zealand Asthma Deaths per 100 000 Persons Aged 5–34 Years Between 1974 and 1990.

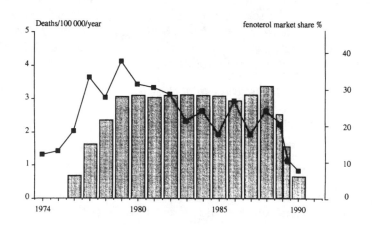

GENERAL PRINCIPLES

Although a randomized trial involving asthma deaths would be impractical and unethical, it is important to consider the principles that would be involved in such a trial as an aid to designing an appropriate case–control study.[25] There would be two major methodologic issues in a trial comparing fenoterol with salbutamol.

The first issue is the treatment regimen that would be randomized. This could involve randomization of the beta-agonist during acute attacks or randomization of the regular prescribed beta-agonist. There would be major practical problems with randomization at the time of acute attacks. However, asthma patients also tend to use their regular prescribed beta-agonist for relief in acute attacks. Thus, the most reasonable approach would be to randomize the regular prescribed beta-agonist therapy,[41] regardless of whether the hypothesis under study involved chronic or acute adverse effects. Patients who were experiencing acute attacks with an increasing frequency or severity might subsequently have changes to their medication, including changes to their beta-agonist, but it would be incorrect to take such changes into account, since these might result in serious bias. The correct approach would be to analyze the data according to the intention-to-treat principle.[25,41]

The second methodologic problem is that, although randomization should make the two groups similar with respect to their average chronic asthma severity, this cannot be guaranteed. Thus, it would be important to gather information on markers of chronic asthma severity at the time of randomization and to adjust for confounding by the baseline asthma severity. However, it would be incorrect to consider subsequent changes in acute or chronic severity and to control for subsequent asthma severity in the analysis, since this subsequent severity could be a result of treatment (i.e., it could be an intermediate step in the causal pathway leading from exposure to asthma death).[25] This consideration is not merely theoretical, since regular use of fenoterol increases chronic asthma severity,[42] and this could also occur with other beta-agonists.

These two major methodologic concerns of the hypothetical clinical trial would also apply to a case–control study. First, when determining whether there is a hazardous effect of treatment, researchers find that it is most appropriate to consider the regular prescribed medication of the cases and controls. It is inappropriate to consider changes in medication or the medication actually used during the final attack (if it is accepted that an effect exists, however, this latter information may be relevant in determining the mechanism).

Second, the treatment groups might differ according to their chronic asthma severity; it is therefore important to gather information on markers of chronic asthma severity. Once again, only the usual chronic severity would be relevant, not the severity of the final attack.

SEVERITY MARKERS

Four studies[43-46] have examined the association between markers of asthma severity and the risk of asthma death in adults. These have involved three markers of chronic asthma severity: (1) a hospital admission during the previous 12 months; (2) prescription of three or more categories of asthma drugs; and (3) prescription of oral corticosteroids. All three markers of chronic asthma severity were found to be associated with an increased risk of subsequent death, but the strongest association was found with the marker of "a hospital admission for asthma in the previous 12 months."[8]

MATCHING FOR SEVERITY

There is very little evidence of selective prescribing of fenoterol in the populations in which the New Zealand studies were conducted.[47] Nevertheless, confounding by severity is of general concern in studies of this type, and controlling for asthma severity may be difficult in case–control studies of asthma deaths, if (as is usual) the controls are chosen as a random sample of the study base.[48] For example, in the study by Rea et al.,[43] 39% (17/44) of patients dying of asthma had had a hospital admission for asthma in the previous year (the best marker of chronic asthma severity), compared with only 5% (2/44) of community asthma controls. Such an imbalance would make it impossible to control for chronic asthma severity in the analysis unless the controls have been matched (directly or indirectly) on chronic severity.

A direct match for severity ("pair matching") would involve taking each case and ensuring that the matched controls were identical to the case with respect to certain markers of chronic asthma severity. An indirect approach (analogous to frequency matching) might involve selecting controls from (nonfatal) hospital admissions for asthma, rather than from asthmatic persons in general. This latter approach is supported by the case–control study of Rea et al.[43] that used two control groups: a community control group chosen from asthmatic persons in general and an asthma hospital admission control group. The study found that (as noted above) there were major differences in asthma severity when the asthma deaths were compared with the community controls, but there were virtually no differences in asthma severity when the asthma deaths were compared with hospital admission controls.

THE NEW ZEALAND CASE–CONTROL STUDIES

The New Zealand case–control studies were designed in light of the above methodologic considerations. In the first study,[37] cases were obtained from the previous New Zealand asthma mortality survey and included all asthma deaths in the 5- to 45-year age group during 1981–1983 (Table 1);

Table 1
Studies of Fenoterol and Asthma Deaths

Studies	Study Period	Age Group (y)	Study Base	Cases (n)	Controls (n)	Matching for Severity
First New Zealand study	1981–1983	5–45	all asthmatics	117	468	yes (hospital admission controls)
Second New Zealand study	1977–1981	5–45	patients with a hospital admission for asthma in previous year	58	227	yes (hospital admission controls)
Third New Zealand study	1981–1987	5–45	patients with a hospital admission for asthma in previous year	112	427/448	yes (hospital admission controls)
Saskatchewan study	1980–1987	5–54	patients with 10 different asthma prescriptions in 1978–1987	44	233	partial (matching for previous admission)

Studies	Information Source		Main Exposure Information	Additional Information	Information on Use	Severity Markers
	Cases	Controls				
First New Zealand study	family doctor	hospital records	prescribed medication[a]	nil	no	hospital admissions, oral steroids, ≥3 categories of drugs
Second New Zealand study	hospital records	hospital records	prescribed medication[a]	nil	no	hospital admissions, oral steroids, ≥3 categories of drugs
Third New Zealand study	hospital records	hospital records	prescribed medication[a]	nil	no	hospital admissions, oral steroids, ≥3 categories of drugs, peak flows, pCO_2
Saskatchewan study	prescription records	hospital records	dispensed medication	number of units/mo	no	hospital admissions, oral steroids, ≥3 categories of drugs

[a]Prescribed medication is equivalent to dispensed medication because prescribed beta-agonists were free of charge during 1977–1987.

controls were chosen from (nonfatal) hospital admissions for asthma during the same period. The only asthma drug that was associated with a significantly increased risk of death was fenoterol (Table 2). Confounding by severity was assessed by examining subgroups defined by the three markers of severity (Table 3). In these subgroups the fenoterol relative risk was markedly increased, ranging from 2.2 to 13.3 in the most severe subgroup. These findings strongly indicate that the association between fenoterol and asthma deaths was not due to confounding by severity, since in this situation the fenoterol relative risk would have decreased as the analysis was increasingly restricted to the most severe subgroup[41,49]; instead, the opposite was observed.

A number of criticisms were made of this case–control study,[50-52] but the most valid criticism was one that was also noted in the original report,[37] namely, that the data for prescribed medicines were obtained from different sources for the cases and controls. This problem was addressed in a second New Zealand case–control study[53] of asthma deaths in 5- to 45-year-olds during 1977–1981. As in the first study, asthma deaths were compared with hospital admission controls, but the new study was restricted to deaths and hospital admission controls who had had a previous admission for asthma during the previous 12 months. This enabled the collection of prescribing information for cases and controls from hospital records for the prior admission, thereby overcoming the potential problem of information bias. The fenoterol relative risk was 2.0 (Table 2); as before, the relative risk increased markedly when the analysis was restricted to the most severe subgroups of asthmatics (Table 3).

A third national case–control study examined the same hypothesis in the same age group during 1981–1987.[54] Once again, the study was restricted to cases and controls who had had a previous admission for asthma in the previous 12 months. However, in this study, two control groups were used: control group A involved hospital admission controls (as before), whereas control group B comprised a random (unmatched) sample of the study base (comprising asthmatic persons with a prior admission for asthma in the previous 12 months). Whichever control group was used, fenoterol was associated with an increased risk of asthma death (Tables 2 and 3), but the alternative control group suggested by critics of the previous studies[52] yielded stronger relative risks than the approach used before (Table 3).

A final piece of evidence concerning the role of fenoterol in the second New Zealand epidemic is that, following the warnings about the use of fenoterol by persons with severe asthma issued in mid-1989, the mortality rate fell significantly.[55] During 1983–1988, the New Zealand mortality rate per 100 000 persons in the 5- to 34-year age group averaged 2.3 (Figure 2), and the death rate was 2.2 in the first half of 1989. In the second half of 1989 (after warnings were issued about the safety of fenoterol), the death rate fell

Table 2
Findings from Case-Control Studies of Fenoterol and Asthma Deaths[a]

Studies	Fenoterol Odds Ratio	Fenoterol 95% CI	Salbutamol Odds Ratio	Salbutamol 95% CI	Oral Beta-Agonists Odds Ratio	Oral Beta-Agonists 95% CI	Oral Theophyllines Odds Ratio	Oral Theophyllines 95% CI	Sodium Cromoglycate Odds Ratio	Sodium Cromoglycate 95% CI	Inhaled Corticosteroids Odds Ratio	Inhaled Corticosteroids 95% CI
First New Zealand study	1.6	1.0 to 2.3	0.7	0.5 to 1.1	1.1	0.7 to 1.7	1.4	1.0 to 2.2	1.2	0.7 to 2.0	1.3	0.9 to 2.0
Second New Zealand study	2.0	1.1 to 3.6	0.7	0.7 to 1.2	1.2	0.7 to 2.1	1.1	0.6 to 2.0	1.0	0.5 to 1.9	0.7	0.4 to 1.2
Third New Zealand study[b]	2.1	1.4 to 3.2	0.6	0.4 to 1.0	1.2	0.7 to 1.9	1.1	0.6 to 1.9	0.8	0.4 to 1.4	1.0	0.6 to 1.6
Saskatchewan study	5.3	2.5 to 11.5	1.0	0.5 to 2.0	1.8	0.9 to 3.5	3.7	1.6 to 8.4	1.8	0.9 to 3.6	1.6	0.8 to 3.3

Markers of Chronic Asthma Severity

	≥3 Categories of Asthma Drugs		Admission in Past Year		Prescribed Oral Corticosteroids	
	Odds Ratio	95% CI	Odds Ratio	95% CI	Odds Ratio	95% CI
First New Zealand study	1.8	1.2 to 2.7	1.5	1.0 to 2.3	1.4	0.9 to 2.2
Second New Zealand study	0.7	0.4 to 1.2	1.0	0.6 to 1.8	1.0	0.5 to 1.9
Third New Zealand study[b]	1.1	0.7 to 1.8	1.5	1.0 to 2.3	1.2	0.8 to 1.8
Saskatchewan study	4.4	1.9 to 10.5	1.0[c]		3.1	1.5 to 6.5

[a]In each instance, the odds ratio refers to the relative risk of asthma death in persons who were prescribed the drug compared with persons who were not prescribed the drug.
[b]Findings using control group A (see Table 3) as reference category.
[c]Controls were matched on this variable.

Table 3
Fenoterol Relative Risks in Subgroup Analyses[a]

			Subgroup						
	Overall		Admission in Past Year		Prescribed Oral Corticosteroids		Admission in Past Year and Prescribed Oral Corticosteroids		
Studies	Odds Ratio	95% CI	Odds Ratio	95% CI	Odds Ratio	95% CI	Odds Ratio	95% CI	
First New Zealand study	1.6	1.0 to 2.3	2.2	1.1 to 4.1	6.5	2.7 to 15.3	13.3	3.5 to 51.2	
Second New Zealand study	2.0	1.1 to 3.6	3.9	1.8 to 8.5	5.8	1.6 to 21.0	9.8	2.2 to 43.4	
Third New Zealand study[b]	2.1	1.4 to 3.2	2.5	1.4 to 4.2	3.2	1.5 to 6.8	2.8	1.1 to 6.9	
Third New Zealand study[c]	2.7	1.7 to 4.1	2.7	1.5 to 4.8	3.8	1.7 to 8.5	4.0	1.5 to 11.0	

[a]In each instance, the odds ratio refers to the relative risk of asthma death in persons in the subgroup who were prescribed fenoterol compared with persons who were not prescribed fenoterol.
[b]Control group A (matched for severity using hospital admission controls).
[c]Control group B (not matched for severity).

to 1.1; it fell further to 0.8 in 1990 (when availability of the drug was formally restricted) and remained at this level in 1991 and 1992. Although the link between the restrictions of fenoterol and the fall in mortality was subsequently questioned,[56] the data are nevertheless consistent with the fenoterol hypothesis and inconsistent with hypotheses relating to a possible class effect of beta-agonists[57] (see below).

THE SASKATCHEWAN STUDY

Support for the New Zealand findings has come from a Canadian study[58] funded by Boehringer Ingelheim, the manufacturer of fenoterol (Table 1). The study was based on a valuable pharmacoepidemiology database comprising the computerized files of the Saskatchewan Drug Plan; it examined 44 asthma deaths in the province of Saskatchewan during 1980–1987 and 233 controls. When the data were analyzed in an identical manner to that of the New Zealand analyses, the fenoterol relative risk in Saskatchewan was 5.3, with nearly one-half of the patients who died having been prescribed fenoterol compared with 16% of the controls (Table 2); the salbutamol relative risk was 1.0. Thus, the findings were even stronger than those in New Zealand when the studies were analyzed in an identical manner.

The authors interpreted some of their findings as reflecting a class effect of beta-agonists (discussed below), but they conceded that the study showed that fenoterol was more hazardous than other beta-agonists in the dosage in which it was marketed. The accompanying editorial in the *New England Journal of Medicine* concluded that there was enough doubt about the safety of fenoterol to avoid it altogether.[59] Hensley[60] subsequently noted that the Saskatchewan study supported the New Zealand findings on fenoterol and concluded that "the weight of evidence and availability of alternative medication should lead to a recommendation that fenoterol not be used to treat asthma." Although the authors of the Saskatchewan study[61] disputed these conclusions, Hensley[62] emphasized that the main hypothesis of the Saskatchewan study "concerned the association between death from asthma and long-term use of fenoterol in the form in which it was dispensed" and that this conclusion was supported by the description of the study that was published before the study findings.[63]

The Saskatchewan study was generally very well designed, but there were two features of the study design that are questionable. First, the study was based on patients who had received 10 or more prescriptions for one or more asthma drugs over a 10-year period, and their medication was then assessed for the previous 12 months (prior to death for the cases and prior to the corresponding date for the controls). The diagnosis of asthma was confirmed for the deaths (cases), but not for the controls. In fact, many of the asthma drugs considered are also used to treat other diseases, and some controls may therefore not have had asthma; in other instances, they may have had asthma earlier in the 10-year period, but may have no longer had the disease at the time that their drug therapy was assessed. This may partly explain why almost every asthma drug was prescribed more frequently in cases than in controls and why all of the cases had been prescribed beta-agonists during the previous 12 months while 18% of the controls had not.

A second problem with the Saskatchewan study design is the lack of adequate matching for asthma severity; the New Zealand studies matched for severity by using hospital admission controls, whereas only partial matching (for a previous hospital admission) was used in the Saskatchewan study. This may also partly explain why almost every asthma drug was prescribed more frequently in cases than in controls.

These methodologic problems are unlikely to be of major significance in overall analyses comparing two drugs within a class (such as fenoterol and salbutamol), but they are of greater concern when investigating a class effect and particularly in analyses involving small subgroups of patients. Further analyses controlling for markers of asthma severity did not markedly affect the findings for asthma deaths and near-deaths (considered as a group), but the specific findings for asthma deaths alone were not reported in these further analyses.[64]

The Saskatchewan case–control findings were subsequently confirmed by the publication of the full cohort analysis by Suissa et al.[65] This was based on the same patient population as the nested case–control study, but involved two further asthma deaths that were identified after the publication of the case–control study. As expected, the findings were similar to those of the case–control analysis, although the fenoterol findings are somewhat stronger in the full cohort analysis. The death rate in those prescribed fenoterol alone (in the dosage in which it was marketed) was about eight times that in those prescribed salbutamol alone; one-half of the patients who died had been prescribed fenoterol (compared with <10% of the total cohort). These findings are even stronger than those in New Zealand when the studies were analyzed in an identical manner.

OTHER ASTHMA DRUGS

The New Zealand and Saskatchewan studies also reported findings on other prescribed asthma medications (Table 2). As noted above, the Saskatchewan study tended to show increased risks for most asthma drugs because of the lack of adequate matching. By contrast, the New Zealand studies showed little evidence of increased risks for asthma drugs other than fenoterol. In light of previous speculation on a possible interaction between beta-agonists and oral theophyllines,[31] it is interesting that oral theophyllines showed an increased risk in the Saskatchewan study and in some subgroup analyses of the New Zealand studies, but this pattern was not particularly strong or consistent.

A further New Zealand study[66] examined deaths during 1969–1976 (i.e., prior to the introduction of fenoterol), but the number of cases identified was very small. The study found a relative risk of 0.9 for salbutamol (95% CI 0.3 to 2.6) during this period. Despite the small numbers, the study findings are interesting because they indicate that there was little or no tendency for patients with unstable or life-threatening asthma to be switched to salbutamol, which was the newer and more potent drug (this bias had been hypothesized with regard to the studies of fenoterol). The findings are also consistent with the observation that mortality remained stable or declined in Western countries during the period that salbutamol was introduced.

Studying a Class Effect of Beta-Agonists

Until recently, asthma pharmacoepidemiology studies had concentrated on the causes of the mortality epidemics. However, in recent years attention has also focused on the gradual increase in mortality that has occurred in a number of countries during the 1980s, including the possibility that the increase in mortality could be due to a class effect of beta-agonists. In particular, Sears et al.[42] found that regular use of fenoterol led to increased asthma severity, O'Connor et al.[67] found that regular use of terbutaline led to tolerance to the nonbronchodilator effects, and van Schayck et al.[68] found that continuous bronchodilator treatment (with salbutamol or ipratropium bromide) without antiinflammatory treatment accelerates decline in ventilatory function. More recently, Chapman et al.[69] studied 341 people with asthma in a 4-week randomized, crossover trial of regular salbutamol (2 puffs 4 times daily) for 2 weeks and as needed for 2 weeks. When control end points were compared between treatment periods for each individual by two blinded investigators, there was no difference in symptom control between periods in 70 asthmatics but, in the remainder, control was achieved more often by regular than by as-needed salbutamol (166 vs. 69; $p < 0.0001$). However, the authors noted that the improvement was small and was achieved at the cost of approximately six puffs per day; furthermore, they noted that a decrease in symptoms may itself be hazardous when exposed unwittingly to an asthma inducer.

Unfortunately, in most developed countries, it is very difficult to investigate a class effect of beta-agonists by using epidemiologic studies because virtually all asthmatic persons are using these drugs, and there is no appropriate comparison group. This situation is analogous to a clinical trial in which there is no placebo group. Thus, the New Zealand studies of fenoterol and asthma mortality[37,53,54] essentially involved a comparison of fenoterol with other drugs within the same class and have not addressed the more difficult issue of a class effect.

Only the Saskatchewan study[58] has attempted to address this issue. In the initial analyses of this study, there was no evidence of an increased risk with beta-agonists other than fenoterol in the primary analyses (Table 2), but the authors also conducted several additional analyses that suggested the possibility of a class effect.

First, they carried out a multivariate analysis in which fenoterol, salbutamol, and a number of other drugs and severity markers were entered into the model simultaneously; the fenoterol relative risk increased from 5.3 to 9.1, and the salbutamol relative risk increased from 1.0 to 2.8.

Second, they conducted a "dose–response" analysis according to the number of units prescribed per month. Once again, this analysis showed increased risks for both fenoterol and salbutamol, but the fenoterol relative risks were higher at each level of prescribing; for example, prescribing of 25 or more units per month (compared with no units per month) carried a relative risk of 113.2 for fenoterol and 29.4 for salbutamol.

Finally, they fitted an exponential dose–response curve to the fenoterol and salbutamol data and estimated that the fenoterol and salbutamol dose–response curves would have been similar if fenoterol had been marketed in 100-μg doses (i.e., one-half of the dose actually marketed).

There are several problems with these additional analyses, however.[70] The analyses that involved entering salbutamol and fenoterol simultaneously into a logistic regression model essentially involved the questionable independent comparisons of the fenoterol and salbutamol groups with the very small group of patients who were not prescribed either drug.[71] Since very few people were prescribed both drugs, virtually all of the statistical information comes from the comparisons of the "fenoterol only" and the "salbutamol only" groups with the group prescribed "neither drug." As noted above, this latter group included some persons who were not prescribed any beta-agonists (or in some cases were not prescribed any asthma drugs) during the previous 12 months; this group had a very low asthma death rate and probably included many persons with very mild asthma and some people who did not have asthma at all.

Concerning the dose–response analyses, the number of units prescribed per month is likely to be a very strong marker of chronic asthma severity; in fact, if the data are stratified on this severity marker, then the data show similar patterns to the New Zealand findings, with the fenoterol relative risk tending to increase as the analysis is restricted to the most severe subgroups. Thus, the "dose adjustment" involves comparing two dose–response curves, both of which are likely to be strongly confounded by asthma severity.

A further problem with the dose adjustment is that an exponential dose–response curve was assumed. This led to the conclusion that the fenoterol curve would have been similar to the salbutamol curve if fenoterol had been marketed in one-half of the actual dose (i.e., 100 μg/puff). However, assuming a linear dose–response relationship (which is the more orthodox approach) would have resulted in comparability of the curves at a level of about one-quarter of the dose in which fenoterol was marketed (i.e., 50 μg/puff), a dose concentration that is more compatible with the findings of experimental studies.[20]

Further doubt is cast on the dose–response findings by the observation that, if these were valid, there should have been mortality epidemics in many countries with the major increases in beta-agonist sales in recent years. These have not occurred, although, as noted above, there has been a gradual increase in the mortality rate in many countries. Similarly, the New Zealand time trend data are inconsistent with the hypothesis that the epidemic may have been due to a class effect of beta-agonists.[57]

Discussion

In summary, the most striking features of the epidemiology of asthma mortality during this century have been the epidemics of asthma deaths that occurred in six countries with the introduction of isoprenaline forte in the 1960s and again in New Zealand with the introduction of fenoterol in the 1970s. These epidemics have occurred only with isoprenaline forte and fenoterol, which have the distinction of being high-dose, poorly selective, full agonists, with relatively greater cardiac adverse effects. These epidemics waned after warnings were issued about the safety of isoprenaline forte and fenoterol.

Attention is now shifting to investigations of a possible role of regular use of beta-agonists and other aspects of modern medical management of asthma. However, there are considerably greater problems in studying a class effect of beta-agonists than in comparing individual drugs within this class. Thus, it is unlikely that these issues can be entirely resolved in pharmacoepidemiologic studies, but epidemiology will clearly continue to have an important role to play in collaboration with clinical and experimental studies.

Neil Pearce and Julian Crane are funded by Senior Research Fellowships, and the Wellington Asthma Research Group is supported by a Programme Grant from the Health Research Council of New Zealand. We thank Professor Michael Hensley and Dr. Paul Stang for their comments on the draft manuscript.

References

1. Keeney EL. The history of asthma from Hippocrates to Meltzer. J Allergy 1964;35:215-26.
2. Ellul-Micallef R. Asthma: a look at the past. Br J Dis Chest 1976;70:112-6.

3. Unger L, Harris MC. Stepping stones in allergy. Ann Allergy 1974;32:214-30.
4. Barnes P. A new approach to the treatment of asthma. N Engl J Med 1989;321:1517-27.
5. International consensus report on diagnosis and treatment of asthma. NIH Publication No. 92-3091. Washington, DC: US Department of Health and Human Services, 1992.
6. Breslin ABX. New developments in anti-asthma drugs. Med J Aust 1993;158:779-82.
7. Osler W. The principles and practice of medicine. 4th ed. Edinburgh: Pentland, 1901.
8. Pearce NE, Beasley R, Crane J, Burgess C. Epidemiology of asthma mortality. In: Holgate S, Busse W, eds. Asthma and rhinitis. Oxford: Blackwell Scientific, 1995:58-69.
9. Pearce NE, Crane J, Burgess C, Jackson R, Beasley R. Beta agonists and asthma mortality: déjà vu. Clin Exp Allergy 1991;21:401-10.
10. Sears MR, Rea HH, de Boer G, Beaglehole R, Gillies AJD, Holst PE, et al. Accuracy of certification of deaths due to asthma: a national study. Am J Epidemiol 1986; 124:1004-11.
11. Asthma deaths: a question answered (editorial). Br Med J 1972;2:443-4.
12. Windom HH, Burgess CD, Crane J, Pearce NE, Kwong T, Beasley R. The self-administration of inhaled beta agonist drugs during severe asthma. N Z Med J 1990;103: 205-7.
13. Lowell FC, Curry JJ, Schiller JW. A clinical and experimental study of isoprel in spontaneous and induced asthma. N Engl J Med 1949;240:45-51.
14. Greenberg MJ, Pines A. Pressurized aerosols in asthma (letter). Br Med J 1967;1:563.
15. Stolley P. Asthma mortality epidemics: the problem approached epidemiologically. In: Beasley R, Pearce NE, eds. The role of beta agonist therapy in asthma mortality. New York: CRC Press, 1993:49-63.
16. Speizer FE, Doll R, Heaf P. Observations on recent increase in mortality from asthma. Br Med J 1968;1:335-9.
17. Speizer FE, Doll R, Heaf P, Strang LB. Investigation into use of drugs preceding death from asthma. Br Med J 1968;1:339-43.
18. Collins JM, McDevitt DG, Shanks RG, Swanton JG. The cardiotoxicity of isoprenaline during hypoxia. Br J Pharmacol 1969;36:35-45.
19. Lockett MF. Dangerous effects of isoprenaline in myocardial failure. Lancet 1965;2: 104-6.
20. Beasley R, Pearce NE, Crane J, Windom H, Burgess C. Asthma mortality and inhaled beta agonist therapy. Aust N Z J Med 1991;21:753-63.
21. Kendall MJ, Woods KL, Wilkins MR, Worthington DJ. Responsiveness to beta adrenergic receptor stimulation: the effects of age are cardioselective. Br J Clin Pharmacol 1982;14:821-6.
22. Stolley PD. Why the United States was spared an epidemic of deaths due to asthma. Am Rev Respir Dis 1972;105:883-90.
23. Esdaile JM, Feinstein AR, Horwitz RI. A reappraisal of the United Kingdom epidemic of fatal asthma. Arch Intern Med 1987;147:543-9.
24. Lanes SF, Walker AM. Do pressurized bronchodilator aerosols cause death among asthmatics? Am J Epidemiol 1987;125:755-60.
25. Pearce NE, Crane J. Epidemiological methods for studying the role of beta agonist therapy in asthma mortality. In: Beasley R, Pearce NE, eds. The role of beta agonist therapy in asthma mortality. New York: CRC Press, 1993:67-83.
26. Fatal asthma (editorial). Lancet 1979;2:337-8.
27. Benatar SR. Fatal asthma. N Engl J Med 1986;314:423-9.
28. Paterson JW, Musk AW. Death in patients with asthma. Med J Aust 1987;147:53-5.

29. Stolley PD, Schinnar R. Association between asthma mortality and isoproterenol acrosols: a review. Prev Med 1978;7:319-38.

30. Stolley P. The bellman always rings thrice (letter). Ann Intern Med 1993;118:158.

31. Wilson JD, Sutherland DC, Thomas AC. Has the change to beta-agonists combined with oral theophylline increased cases of fatal asthma? Lancet 1981;1:1235-7.

32. Jackson RT, Beaglehole R, Rea HH, Sutherland DC. Mortality from asthma: a new epidemic in New Zealand. Br Med J 1982;285:771-4.

33. Keating G, Mitchell EA, Jackson R, Beaglehole R, Rea H. Trends in sales of drugs for asthma in New Zealand, Australia and the United Kingdom, 1975–81. Br Med J 1984;289:348-51.

34. Sears MR, Beaglehole R. Asthma mortality: a review of recent experience in New Zealand. J Allergy Clin Immunol 1987;80:319-25.

35. Sears MR, Rea HH, Beaglehole R, Gillies AJD, Holst PE, O'Donnell TV, et al. Asthma mortality in New Zealand: a two year national study. N Z Med J 1985;98:271-5.

36. Sears MR, Beaglehole R. Asthma morbidity and mortality: New Zealand. J Allergy Clin Immunol 1987;80:383-8.

37. Crane J, Pearce N, Flatt A, Burgess C, Jackson R, Kwong T, et al. Prescribed fenoterol and death from asthma in New Zealand, 1981–1983: a case–control study. Lancet 1989;1:917-22.

38. Sears MR, Rea HH, Fenwick J, Gillies AJD, Holst PE, O'Donnell TV, et al. 75 deaths in asthmatics prescribed home nebulisers. Br Med J 1987;294:477-80.

39. Beasley R, Crane J, Burgess C, Pearce NE, Jackson R. Fenoterol and severe asthma mortality (letter). N Z Med J 1989;102:294-5.

40. Grant IWB. Fenoterol and asthma deaths in New Zealand (letter). N Z Med J 1990;103:160-1.

41. Elwood JM. The New Zealand case–control studies on asthma deaths and fenoterol: interpretation and clinical and drug regulatory implications. In: Beasley R, Pearce NE, eds. The role of beta agonist therapy in asthma mortality. New York: CRC Press, 1993:85-123.

42. Sears MR, Taylor DR, Print CG, Lake DC, Qingqing L, Flannery EM, et al. Regular inhaled beta-agonist treatment in bronchial asthma. Lancet 1990;336:1391-6.

43. Rea HH, Scragg R, Jackson R, Beaglehole R, Fenwick J, Sutherland DC. A case–control study of deaths from asthma. Thorax 1986;41:833-9.

44. Crane J, Pearce NE, Burgess C, Woodman K, Robson B, Beasley R. Markers of risk of asthma death or readmission in the 12 months following a hospital admission for asthma. Int J Epidemiol 1992;21:737-44.

45. Ryan G, Musk AW, Perera DM, Stock H, Knight JL, Hobbs MST. Risk factors for death in patients admitted to hospital with asthma: a follow-up study. Aust N Z J Med 1991;21:681-5.

46. Strunk RC, Mrazek DA, Wolfson Fuhrmann GS, LaBrecque JF. Physiologic and psychological characteristics associated with deaths due to asthma in childhood. JAMA 1985;254:1193-8.

47. Beasley R, Burgess C, Pearce NE, Woodman K, Crane J. Confounding by severity does not explain the association between fenoterol and asthma death. Clin Exp Allergy 1994;24:660-8.

48. Pearce NE. What does the odds ratio estimate in a case–control study? Int J Epidemiol 1993;22:1189-92.

49. Sackett DL, Shannon HS, Browman GW. Fenoterol and fatal asthma (letter). Lancet 1990;1:46.

50. O'Donnell TV, Holst P, Rea HH, Sears MR. Fenoterol and fatal asthma (letter). Lancet 1989;1:1070-1.
51. Buist AS, Burney PGJ, Feinstein AR, Horwitz RI, Lanes SF, Rebuck AS, et al. Fenoterol and fatal asthma (letter). Lancet 1989;1:1071.
52. Poole C, Lanes SF, Walker AM. Fenoterol and fatal asthma (letter). Lancet 1990;1:920.
53. Pearce NE, Grainger J, Atkinson M, Crane J, Burgess C, Culling C, et al. Case–control study of prescribed fenoterol and death from asthma in New Zealand, 1977–1981. Thorax 1990;45:170-5.
54. Grainger J, Woodman K, Pearce NE, Crane J, Burgess A, Keane A, et al. Prescribed fenoterol and death from asthma in New Zealand 1981–7: a further case–control study. Thorax 1991;46:105-11.
55. Crane J, Pearce NE, Burgess C, Beasley R, Jackson R. Mortality from asthma in New Zealand (letter). BMJ 1992;304:1307.
56. Suissa S, Ernst P, Spitzer WO. Re: Asthma deaths in New Zealand (letter). BMJ 1992; 305:889.
57. Pearce N, Beasley R, Crane J, Burgess C, Jackson R. End of the New Zealand asthma mortality epidemic. Lancet 1995;345:41-4.
58. Spitzer WO, Suissa S, Ernst P, Horwitz RI, Habbick B, Cockcroft D, et al. The use of β-agonists and the risk of death and near death from asthma. N Engl J Med 1992; 326:501-6.
59. Burrows B, Lebowitz MD. The beta-agonist dilemma (editorial). N Engl J Med 1992; 326:560-1.
60. Hensley MJ. Fenoterol and death from asthma (letter). Med J Aust 1992;156:882.
61. Spitzer WO, Ernst P, Suissa S, Bolvin J-F, Horwitz RI, Habbick B, et al. Fenoterol and death from asthma (letter). Med J Aust 1992;157:568-9.
62. Hensley MJ. Fenoterol and death from asthma (letter). Med J Aust 1992;157:569.
63. Horwitz RI, Spitzer W, Buist S, Cockcroft D, Ernst P, Habbick B, et al. Clinical complexity and epidemiologic uncertainty in case–control research: fenoterol and asthma management. Chest 1991;100:1586-91.
64. Ernst P, Habbick B, Suissa S, Hemmelgarn B, Cockcroft D, Buist AS, et al. Is the association between inhaled beta-agonist use and life-threatening asthma because of confounding by severity? Am Rev Respir Dis 1993;148:75-9.
65. Suissa S, Ernst P, Boivin J-F, Horwitz RI, Habbick B, Cockroft D, et al. A cohort analysis of excess mortality in asthma and the use of inhaled β-agonists. Am J Respir Crit Care Med 1994;149:604-10.
66. Woodman K, Pearce NE, Beasley R, Burgess C, Crane J. Albuterol and deaths from asthma in New Zealand from 1969 to 1976: a case–control study. Clin Pharmacol Ther 1992;51:566-71.
67. O'Connor BJ, Aikman SL, Barnes PJ. Tolerance to the nonbronchodilator effects of inhaled beta-2 agonists in asthma. N Engl J Med 1992;327:1204-8.
68. van Schayck CP, Dompeling E, van Herwaarden CLA, Folgering H, Verbeek ALM, van der Hoogen HJM, et al. Bronchodilator treatment in moderate asthma or chronic bronchitis: continuous or on demand? A randomized controlled study. BMJ 1991; 303:1426-31.
69. Chapman KR, Kesten S, Szalai JP. Regular v as-needed inhaled salbutamol in asthma control. Lancet 1994;343:1379-82.
70. Crane J, Pearce N, Burgess C, Beasley R. Asthma and the β-agonist debate. Thorax 1995;50(suppl):S5-10.
71. Pearce NE, Crane J, Burgess C, Beasley R, Jackson R. Fenoterol, beta agonists and asthma deaths (letter). N Engl J Med 1992;327:355-6.

21

Pharmacoepidemiology of Psychiatric Disorders

Julie Magno Zito
Thomas J Craig

Abstract

The pharmacoepidemiology of neuropharmacologic drugs for psychiatric disorders is the subject of this chapter. The possibilities and limitations of the existing methods of determining neuropharmacologic drug efficacy and safety in psychiatric patients are discussed. Pharmacoepidemiologic methods can improve both the scientific evaluation and clinical use of these drugs by providing: (1) prevalence rates of drug use and unintended event rates from computerized information on large populations; (2) quantitative methods for risk/benefit assessments that incorporate multiple outcome measures, provide long-term effectiveness and safety data, and use statistical methods as well as epidemiologic reasoning to distinguish drug-induced from illness-based behaviors; and (3) systematic epidemiologic approaches to resolve dilemmas that involve the political, cultural, and social context in which drugs for psychiatric disorders are used. Collectively, these approaches seek an empirical basis for the development of clinical theory in psychiatric drug treatment.

Outline

harmacoepidemiology is defined in Chapter 1 as "the application of epidemiologic reasoning, methods, and knowledge to the study of the uses and effects (beneficial and adverse) of drugs in human populations." It was also defined by Rector[1] as "the study of the relationships of various factors to the frequency and distribution of pharmaceutical outcomes in a population." Pharmaceutical outcomes consist of three domains of measurable clinical phenomena, namely, the physiologic, psychological, and socioeconomic consequences of drug use. Because pharmacoepidemiologic methods can be used to address scientific questions on all three levels of the impact of drug use, they can add to the existing methods of determining drug efficacy[2] and safety.[3] These methods can be directed to the special needs of drug assessment in psychopharmacology, behavioral medicine, and behavioral pharmacology. This chapter reviews the pharmacoepidemiologic methods currently used to extend our knowledge of the relationship of neuropharmacologic drug use to human behavior and mental disorders. Recent work on drug use patterns in a mental health services model and treatment guidelines for mental disorders are included.

Neuropharmacologic Drugs and Behavioral Disorders

For the purpose of this discussion, neuropharmacologic drugs are defined as drugs that pass the blood–brain barrier and have intended or unintended behavioral effects. The major drug classes in this category consist of psychotropic drugs, but the term "neuroactive"[4] has been suggested to emphasize the role of additional pharmacologic classes of agents that exhibit behavioral effects, many of which are used in the treatment of psychiatric disorders. For example, anticholinergic agents and diphenhydramine are used to treat drug-induced parkinsonism in about 50% of antipsychotic inpatient exposures.[5] Antiepileptic drugs are also included in this category because of the relatively high prevalence of seizure disorder in psychiatric patients[6] as well as the prominent use of anticonvulsant drugs (e.g., carbamazepine, valproic acid) to treat patients with affective disorder who are resistant to standard drug treatment.[7] The most frequently used psychotropic drug classes are antipsychotic medications (pharmacologic class of neuroleptic drugs), antidepressant and anxiolytic-hypnotic medications, and mood stabilizers (e.g., lithium). Each class produces neuropharmacologic drug responses of both an intended (positive clinical response) and unintended (negative or adverse event) type. The term "behavioral toxicity" has been used to describe the adverse effects of drugs on behavioral or psychological functioning[8,9] and is receiving renewed interest in the psychiatric literature,[10,11] in part because the increased use of combinations of agents from various neuroactive classes increases the likelihood of behavioral toxicity.

In addition to the psychiatric indications mentioned above, there is a separate medical literature that describes the relationship between behavioral symptoms and drugs that produce neuropharmacologic effects secondary to the treatment of nonpsychiatric medical disorders. Consultation liaison psychiatrists are becoming aware of the frequency with which patients treated with digoxin at[12] and above[13] therapeutic serum concentrations often present as having a psychiatric disorder such as depression or dementia. Other examples include the report of depression associated with nifedipine,[14] ranitidine,[15] reserpine,[16] and beta-blockers.[17-19] In addition, physical disorders (e.g., peptic ulcer) are being treated with psychotropic drugs such as the antidepressant trimipramine[20] in patients who are not well controlled by changes in lifestyle and antacids or histamine$_2$-antagonists. "Psychobiology,"[21] "behavioral medicine," and "behavioral pharmacology"[22] are terms used to identify this area of specialization, although the latter term includes experimental psychological interventions such as operant conditioning, which uses drugs in a stimulus–response paradigm to alter behavior.

Interest in the psychobiologic aspects of drug use is growing as experts in areas such as cardiovascular medicine, oncology, rheumatology, and neurology are increasingly concerned with the role of personality, culture, and socioeconomic factors in the individual patient's response to long-term drug therapy. Both neuropharmacology and psychobiology could benefit from a greater coordination of terminology and methodology regarding drug use and human behavior. This would be a useful initial step in defining an area of specialization for the psychiatric pharmacoepidemiologist. The development of consultation liaison psychiatry as one of the newer specialties[23] suggests the importance of behavioral symptoms in medical patients, especially those receiving complex multidrug regimens. Curricula in this area should emphasize behavioral toxicity (drug-induced psychiatric symptoms) and loss of effectiveness of previously stabilized psychotropic drugs by the addition of neuroactive drugs.

The focus of this chapter is limited to the specific ways in which neuropharmacology can use quantitative epidemiologic methods. These methods will be described in four sections:

1. *population-based methods* from the longitudinal monitoring of large patient populations. Subsections address problems in optimal dosing of antipsychotic agents and the evaluation of clinical appropriateness;
2. *efficacy versus effectiveness* issues including limitations of the randomized, double-blind, controlled, clinical trial model and the gap between the outcome of research study populations and the clinical practice outcomes observed in large patient populations. Validity issues emerge from the discrepancies between some early study

inferences and more recent evidence of treatment failure. The discussion concludes with the case of clozapine as an illustration;

3. *drug safety* issues from postmarketing surveillance (PMS) programs to provide unintended event rates and to test hypotheses of possible drug-induced events; and
4. *specific drug decision-making methods* using statistical methods for optimizing psychotropic drug use in individual patients and patient subgroups.

Finally, several examples are given of policy questions in which epidemiologic methods can be used to aid the risk/benefit assessment of neuropharmacologic drug use for controversial indications.

Population-Based Methods

Developments in computer applications for psychiatry[24] include office records, diagnostic tools, and specialized treatment modalities such as psychotherapy and family therapy. More comprehensive applications related to inferences about the effectiveness and safety of medications are exceptional.

Feinstein[25] described the limitations of causal inferencing of drug effects from the standard clinical practice situation. To improve upon the logic of this process, therapeutic drug monitoring using a computerized longitudinal record of specific drug and response variables is suggested. For patients receiving neuropharmacologic drugs, this method involves the use of quantitative methods derived from pharmacokinetics, pharmacodynamics, and psychometric theory. Specifically, the drug serum concentration, pertinent laboratory or other test values, target response measures (e.g., structured scales for symptom reduction, occupational and social rehabilitation, hospitalized days), and unintended events are determined at regular intervals and longitudinally entered into a computerized database. Selected variables are then arranged in bivariate displays over time (the y-axis is the positive or negative response variable, and the x-axis is the clinic visit or assessment time). For example, the bivariate graphing of the phenytoin plasma concentration, daily dose, and seizure frequency versus time in the antiepileptic therapy of a pregnant seizure patient during the perinatal period illustrates the inferencing process related to drug clearance, bioavailability, and dosing of phenytoin in a patient-specific situation.[26] A psychopharmacologic example concerns the longitudinal monitoring of haloperidol and lithium.[27] An alternative system that uses ward-based microcomputer entry of clinical data was developed for public psychiatric hospitals in Texas.[28] The data collection system is intended to justify psychiatrists' choice of treatment and requires systemized drug evaluation at scheduled intervals.

Linkage of the longitudinally recorded drug variables with other computerized components of the medical record permits more elaborate epidemiologic evaluations of treatment and outcome. Where national systems, such as those of Sweden, have this capability, hypothesis-generating studies about such mental health issues as self-reported compliance among deinstitutionalized mentally ill persons are feasible.[29] In American hospitalized psychiatric populations, one example is the Mental Health Package of the Veterans Affairs (VA) that uses the MUMPS program language. It is being used in more than 170 hospitals to store variables on medication, demographics, and previous treatments, but, to our knowledge, large-scale drug epidemiology has been limited.[24]

Numerous epidemiologic studies were published on a pioneer system called the Multistate Information System (MSIS). When merged with computerized patient characteristics, MSIS linked diagnostic, selected clinical, and sociodemographic factors to medication use.[30] For more than a decade, the system has provided psychopharmacologic drug monitoring consisting of retrospective review of orders in exception to guidelines that were developed by a committee of experts.[31] The positive effect of computerized drug exception reporting on prescribing behavior was demonstrated empirically.[32] Based on users' suggestions, a revision was implemented using a readily available computer package (Pharmakon) so that review of both medical and psychotropic orders occurs prospectively (i.e., before the prescription is dispensed). In addition, the system data can be linked to computerized outcome measures such as discharge status and length of hospitalization, which serve as surrogate measures of global improvement. Retrieval and aggregation of these data and enhancement with specific ad hoc measures (e.g., symptom severity, research diagnosis) in random subsets of patients would enable large-scale epidemiologic evaluations of drug effectiveness and safety.

Using data retrieved from the MSIS database, the relationship between length of hospitalization and antipsychotic medication exposure was examined in newly admitted schizophrenic patients.[5] The univariate measure of outcome, length of hospitalization, was not related to the dose (low, moderate, high) of antipsychotic medication, suggesting that lower dosing will not impede discharge or, alternatively, that the multiplicity of factors related to discharge was not affected systematically by variation in dosing. Similarly, computerized data showed the pattern of psychotropic drug use in relation to the outcome of the schizophrenic episode for young adult males[33]; the study demonstrated that long-stay (>1 y) patients received more drug combinations and relatively higher doses of antipsychotic medications compared with short-stay (<180 d) patients. A study of psychotropic drug use in hospitalized children and adolescents revealed less specificity of drug class in relation to diagnosis than is typically seen in adults.[34] While these studies do not rule out bias due to severity of illness, they provide a rationale for additional prospective work so that illness factors (symptoms and functioning) can be incorporated into the model and for ongoing monitoring to assess appropriateness of the drug regimens as well as patient satisfaction.

Although not well appreciated in the past, ambulatory *medical* care visits are often the occasion in which psychiatric symptoms (e.g., depression) are assessed and treated. Data were derived from these settings by prospective monitoring of usual practice conditions during a 2-year period at three major US cities. The data were collected and analyzed, and the findings were widely disseminated as the Medical Outcomes Study.[35] Depression was found to be underdiagnosed[36] by medical clinicians (46–51%) compared with mental health specialists (78–87%) after adjusting for case-mix differences. Drug-specific prevalence for antidepressant medications was reported for 23%, while minor tranquilizer (anxiolytic) use was reported for 30% of the cohort of patients with current depressive disorder or depressive symptoms (n = 634) who visited general medical clinicians, psychiatrists, psychologists, or other therapists.[37] The appropriateness of anxiolytic drug use in this population deserves further study. The Medical Outcomes Study pioneered research in the general area of clinical health services and in mental health services, in particular.

Similarly, health maintenance organization (HMO) prescription data were used to estimate the prevalence of antidepressant prescriptions by practice specialty (primary vs. psychiatry).[38] Patients treated by psychiatrists were more likely to continue medications for more than 30 days and to achieve a dosage of 100 mg of imipramine or equivalents per day. In regard to children's use of psychotropic medications, a comparison of drug-specific prevalence[39] was made from samples of a state Medicaid program, a regional HMO, and a federal office-based survey, that is, the National Ambulatory Medical Care Survey (NAMCS), for children aged 5–14 years with orders (claims) for several frequently used psychotropic drugs. For example, methylphenidate prevalence was nearly twofold greater in the state Medicaid population (2.14%) than in the samples from an HMO (1.05%) or NAMCS encounters (1.38%). Subsequent research[40] among Medicaid enrollees in Maryland shows substantially lower (twofold) methylphenidate prescriptions for African-American youths compared with whites after accounting for geographic variation. Another drug variable, daily dose, is receiving attention in pharmacoepidemiologic studies. For example, methods for estimating daily dose from computerized prescription records have been reported for alprazolam in an HMO sample.[41]

Future studies in large database systems need to focus on treatment evaluation in specific patient populations using multiple outcome measures, such as symptom reduction, functional capacity, relapse rate, and patient satisfaction.[42] Multivariate analyses of treatment outcome might specify employment history and social functioning as covariates, since these variables have been identified as predictors of outcome from previous studies.[43,44] To the extent that the multivariate analytic approach accurately reflects the underlying nexus of patient and treatment variables, it should produce clinically meaningful as well as statistically significant results. Computerized and quantitative medical records will make these studies more feasible and less costly.

OPTIMAL DOSE DETERMINATION

This section explores the issue of how best to determine the usual dose range for a psychotropic agent; the case of antipsychotic medications is used as an example. Traditionally, the development of an acceptable dose range for a specific neuropharmacologic agent (e.g., an antipsychotic drug) is related to many factors in animal and human pharmacology. The mechanism of action of antipsychotic drugs involves blockade of dopaminergic receptors. Despite the well-accepted role of antipsychotic medications in managing psychosis, research leaders[45] now question whether antidopaminergic activity (pharmacologic effect) is a necessary and sufficient basis for antipsychotic efficacy (clinical effect) and whether antipsychotic efficacy is confounded by neurologic unintended effects in our studies of dose–response relationships. Moreover, the 1990s have occasioned the marketing of numerous antipsychotic agents with receptor activity profiles that are characterized as atypical. Among these are clozapine and olanzapine. Risperidone, sertindole, and quetiapine are other new agents competing with conventional neuroleptics. These developments highlight the current debate on antipsychotic dose–response effects[46] and, more broadly, on the balance of efficacy with safety for this widely used class of psychotropic drugs.

Since the dose–response relationship of antipsychotic drugs is so variable (because of large interpatient variability),[47,48] systematic methods to determine optimal dosing might involve empirically derived standards based on data from *population studies*. For example, in the study of antipsychotic therapy in newly admitted schizophrenic patients,[5] the average daily dose (expressed in chlorpromazine-equivalents) of high-potency agents was 2.7-fold greater than the dosage of low-potency agents. Since the excess exposure was not statistically associated with better treatment outcome, the dosing could be considered suboptimal because of the increased risk of tardive dyskinesia.[49] In addition, the excess drug exposure was translated into $1273, or 16.3% of the overall neuropharmacologic drug costs. This approach permits an empirically based clinical dosage and cost analysis. If the favorable outcome is the criterion, the optimal dosage could be defined as the dosage used in a cohort of patients with the best treatment outcome.

To be a valid approach, a large population with similar baseline characteristics must be assessed.

Population-based antipsychotic patterns are useful to illustrate the pronounced dosing patterns among countries. Average doses of antipsychotic medications were observed among 1141 patients treated during 1984 in seven regional mental health facilities in Italy.[50] The results were 471 ± 25.3 mg (SD) for high-potency agents versus 196 ± 8.9 mg for low-potency agents. As a comparison, two US studies showed 1034- versus 494-mg agents[51] or 1137- versus 419-mg agents,[5] for high- versus low-potency agents. Prescribing of antipsychotic medications in Italy results in less than *half* the average daily dose of US prescribing for severe mental disorders, while maintaining shorter hospitalizations.

In another illustration, a stepwise multiple regression model was applied by Hargreaves et al.[52] to analyze antipsychotic dosing trends from computerized drug data on 1490 admissions in California; the 50% decline in maximum and average daily dose over a 10-year period was not explained by fewer days in treatment and changing the choice of drug, leading the authors to conclude that the prescribing *behavior* had changed from earlier higher-dose to later lower-dose patterns. Surprisingly, this finding is not consistent with data from another region.[53] Sampling of discharge medical records from the inpatient unit of a community mental health center and a state hospital over a 10-year period showed *increased* antipsychotic dosing for schizophrenia. These regional differences may be valid, but such variation suggests the need for a national study in which a single method will be used across regions.

In the Texas system described earlier, a drug use model based on the epidemiologic concepts of sensitivity, specificity, and utility was used to determine clinical standards for antipsychotic drugs.[54] This example illustrates the potential for population-based data as an aid to validate dose ranges that had been established by early clinical trial data.

EVALUATION OF CLINICAL APPROPRIATENESS

National epidemiologic studies of psychiatric service needs and use are a relatively recent development. The most rigorous study of service use from a methodologic standpoint is based on a national probability sampling. The Epidemiologic Catchment Area (ECA) study found a 28.5% annual prevalence of mental and addictive disorders in the early 1980s with a 14.7% prevalence of services reported for these problems.[55] Earlier National Institute of Mental Health (NIMH)–funded household surveys exemplify this approach to document psychotropic drug patterns[56]; results showed that 15% of those reporting use of anxiolytic drugs reported more than 1 year of use. Although rigorous in sample selection, the considerable cost of household surveys, the low prevalence of psychotropic use among a community population, the limits of self-reported drug information, and the rapidity with which prescription drug survey data become obsolete make drug data from household surveys very scarce.

Smaller clinical surveys are a well-known approach to the evaluation of appropriate drug, dose, and combinations of drugs used in clinical practice, although they lack the generalizability of the national probability sample.[4,5,57] In public psychiatry, ad hoc surveys of prescribing have been a means of assessing a health service system that is generally regarded as underfunded and lacking in quality care. Polypharmacy continues to be a concern in recent reports[58] and is shown to persist even after the publication of proscribed practices.[59] Longitudinal data on the prescribing pattern of psychotropic drugs are rare.[60] A different approach to appropriateness is taken by the interdisciplinary team review of antipsychotic prescriptions after 6 months' use in severely and profoundly mentally retarded persons. This approach was reported to reduce medication (a presumed favorable outcome for this population) without a significant increase in major injuries.[61] Patient monitoring of the antipsychotic (neuroleptic) medications used to treat nursing home residents has been mandated by federal Omnibus Budget Reconciliation Act (OBRA) legislation since 1987. The law produced increased scrutiny of neuropharmacologic drug prescribing for individuals covered by Medicare and Medicaid reimbursement programs. The typical patient population in these studies consists of elderly nursing home residents.[62,63] An empirical study[64] of the use of antipsychotic drugs in nursing homes in Minnesota showed that annual rates of psychotropic drug use declined by one-third over the 4-year period from 3 years before enforcement to 1 year after. A hypothesized shift toward increased antianxiety agents (anxiolytic drugs) was not observed. OBRA regulations appear to be achieving their goals, but creative efforts should be used to avoid the equally unsatisfactory situation of underuse of antipsychotic medications or less-effective alternatives.

Efficacy Versus Effectiveness

In the 40 years since chlorpromazine was marketed for the treatment of acute and chronic psychosis, a large research and clinical literature has developed that supports the effectiveness of this antipsychotic agent, as well as the 20-odd congeners that have followed its introduction. Crane[65] estimated that more than 250 million patients had been exposed to these agents by the end of 1970. Such extensive somatic treatment has contributed to the growth of biologic psychiatry as an etiologic model for mental disorders. Along with this trend is a national research focus in the 1990s known as the "decade of the brain." Critics of this trend argue that, even if causation is biologic, treatment needs to be both somatic and psychosocial, as in the integrated biopsychosocial model. This topic is fertile ground for ongoing debate. Somatic treatment of mental disorders with antipsychotic medications followed from the substantial drug development work of the 1950s and 1960s. Antipsychotic drugs were marketed with the benefit of efficacy findings based on rigorous, short-term clinical trials, although, as time progressed, important questions about their long-term effectiveness and safety in clinical practice have arisen.

At present, antipsychotic drugs are widely used to treat the major psychotic disorders affecting children, adults, and elderly patients and less frequently used in the treatment of nonpsychotic and personality disorders. Nevertheless, the efficacy of the antipsychotic drugs continues to be the subject of reinterpretation.[44,66] The most recent challenge to the value of conventional antipsychotic drugs whose pharmacologic effect is based on "full" dopamine receptor occupancy comes from the availability of atypical agents (e.g., clozapine). Clozapine is an agent said to have "partial" dopamine receptor occupancy with a propensity for D-1 rather than D-2 receptors and substantial antiserotonergic, antihistaminic, and antimuscarinic blockade. However, the clinical effectiveness of atypical antipsychotic medications is the subject of controversy.[67] The controversy carries important implications for the next generation of antipsychotic agents. Similar issues are raised by reviewing three major psychotropic classes that were marketed after the antipsychotic drugs (i.e., antidepressants,[68,69] benzodiazepines,[70] and lithium[71]). Beyond the pharmacologic issues, these questions suggest a research–clinical practice gap between the inferences based on the original efficacy data from the randomized, double-blind, controlled, clinical trials (research) and the fact that there is a growing pool of treatment-refractory patients (clinical practice), up to one-third of treated schizophrenic patient populations.[72] To account for the apparent gap between research findings and real-world clinical practice patterns, it is necessary to review the research studies and to consider the following limitations of the clinical trial model in applying it to evaluate behavioral outcomes of neuropharmacologic drug use.

LIMITATIONS OF THE CLINICAL TRIAL MODEL IN PSYCHIATRY

Limitation 1. Clinical trials include *selected patients* and evaluate them on limited response measures in controlled settings. By comparison, population-based psychotropic drug use (prevalence) is evaluated by epidemiologic survey methods (e.g., for outpatient data such as those available from the NAMCS, an annual National Center for Health Statistics–sponsored survey of health resource use in the US).[73] The cross-sectional surveys provide estimates of outpatient drug use, albeit without dose exposure information, and show how psychotropic prescribing varies among primary care, psychiatry, and all other specialties.[74] In 1992, a companion survey called the National Hospital Ambulatory Medical Care Survey (NHAMCS) was inaugurated[75] so that data from hospital emergency department and outpatient department care would be available. Studies based on NAMCS and NHAMCS data can illustrate the usefulness of large database methods for generating hypotheses that can then be examined by more rigorous experimental methods. To illustrate, an NAMCS study used a sophisticated analysis to demonstrate gender bias in psychotropic drug prescribing by primary care clinicians when, after controlling for statistically significant symptoms, physician diagnoses, sociodemographic factors, and health service factors, researchers found that women were more likely to receive a prescription for anxiolytic and antidepressant medications.[76]

NAMCS limitations include failure to capture the full spectrum of psychiatric drug usage, which includes the more severely ill patient who requires greater dosage during the inpatient phase of a psychotic episode and then typically receives follow-up care from mental health outpatient services. In addition, psychotropic drug use occurs with institutionalized psychiatric or medically ill persons in nursing homes, as well as with deinstitutionalized psychiatric, elderly, and developmentally disabled persons living in various domiciliary care settings.[77] Among these patient populations there are distinct differences in the following: (1) diagnosis; (2) baseline level of intellectual, emotional, and behavioral functioning; (3) severity of illness in terms of acute target psychiatric symptoms; and (4) chronic need for supervised living arrangements as well as social and occupational rehabilitation. Given the range of clinical and social factors needed to characterize the patient receiving psychiatric drug treatment and the likelihood that treatment will be ongoing for many patients, the distinction between long-term treatment outcome and the more limited response measures of the typical clinical trial is understandable. Nevertheless, the problem calls for revision of our data collection systems.

Limitation 2. Clinical trials in patients with acute psychiatric disorders have reported *univariate outcomes* in short-term studies that do not generalize to all patients or to functional improvements. Of the hundreds of studies reporting the remission of acute psychosis with antipsychotic drugs, the most compelling evidence was provided in two rigorously conducted studies. In an NIMH collaborative study,[78] the response measure was acute symptom reduction; 75% of the patients who received chlorpromazine at a mean dosage of 700 mg per day showed moderate or greater improvement compared with 25% of placebo-treated patients. The Veterans Administration Collaborative Study evaluated patients who were readmitted with chronic schizophrenia and found a statistically significant greater improvement at 12 weeks in patients treated with fixed doses of chlorpromazine 400 mg/d compared with placebo-treated patients.[79] Despite early optimism and repeated replication of such positive findings, the short-term findings led to a number of unanticipated problems, such as lack of *persistence* of treatment response.

Current research is directed at finding efficacious treatments for the 25% of drug-treated nonresponders (often referred to as treatment refractory or treatment resistant) and the 25% of placebo responders. Studies that evaluate drug therapy in nonresponders include the schizophrenic patient with negative symptoms[80] and evaluations of targeted symptoms,[81,82] low-dose regimens[72] and the intermittent use of benzodiazepines (e.g., lorazepam)[83,84] to control agitated and aggressive behaviors in chronic schizophrenic or bipolar patients whose conditions have not been controlled by an antipsychotic drug or antipsychotic drug plus lithium. The individual treatment needs of specific patient subgroups will emerge from these studies to the extent that the studies reflect good design. For example, the study should incorporate the target behaviors of the patient population in question; provide detailed drug regimen data, particularly regarding recent past and baseline adjunctive drugs and their doses; use appropriate multidimensional outcome measures; and provide sufficient statistical power to detect the expected differences in outcome. The lack of complete drug regimen data in empirical investigations of mentally retarded persons has been cited as a major failing in that literature.[85] Failure to establish relative potency in comparative drug studies confounds outcome measures, and their findings produce confusing and sometimes erroneous conclusions.[86]

Limitation 3. Clinical trials of maintenance medication for chronic psychosis sometimes fail to take into account important, potentially *confounding factors*. The evaluation of drug therapy for the maintenance phase of treatment of the chronically psychotic patient relies on aggregating findings across the approximately 30 maintenance or withdrawal studies.[87] In an update of this meta-analysis, 35 controlled studies (n = 3500) were summarized and revealed a 16% relapse rate for drug-treated patients compared with a 58% rate for placebo-treated patients.[46] However, numerous arguments have been raised questioning the validity of this meta-analysis.[88]

A major confounding problem in withdrawal studies concerns a clinical syndrome associated with drug withdrawal.[89] During the first 4–6 weeks of antipsychotic drug withdrawal, dyskinesias may emerge that previously have been masked by the drug. Sometimes they are accompanied by cholinergic rebound effects manifested as nervousness, tremor, and gastrointestinal and flu-like symptoms and may present a clinical picture indistinguishable from clinical decompensation.[90] As a result, short-term withdrawal effects could have been reported as relapse (clinical decompensation). The extent to which short-term withdrawal effects of the patients withdrawn from an active antipsychotic drug are mistaken for relapse is unknown. Moreover, the drug withdrawal study design is limited by the fact that the experimental variable manipulated is discontinuation of drug and not dopaminergic function.[91] To minimize this problem, a drug withdrawal protocol may be used to allow gradual decrements over sufficient time periods for physiologic and behavioral readjustment. Alternatively, the study could add an inclusion criterion that specifies a study antipsychotic daily dose (expressed as a relative potency scale as chlorpromazine-equivalents [CPZ-EQs mg]) roughly equivalent for the current dose to prevent the confounding of treatment outcome by withdrawal effects.

There are particular studies or critiques that create doubts or provide alternative explanations about drug responsiveness.[92-98] For example, subgroups of schizophrenic patients with high premorbid functioning were demonstrated to benefit from drug therapy in one study[99] but not in another.[100] The limitations of studies using small sample sizes have been known for many years.[101] Newer studies of chronic schizophrenia have combined two or more interventions, such as maintenance drug therapy and a psychosocial intervention based on the stress-diathesis model. A review of this major research area is available.[102] Studies by Hogarty et al.[103] exemplify the combined intervention studies in which treatment outcome measurement is usually more comprehensive than in the older, single-intervention studies.

Maintenance treatment studies of both types of prospective parallel group studies (trials and drug-withdrawal relapse studies) have design limitations. The need, identified more than a decade ago, for an integrated conceptual approach[104] to drug and psychosocial treatment is quite evident from a current review of the drug therapy of psychiatric disorders. This approach would ensure that new pharmacologic agents would be evaluated in combined biologic and psychosocial treatment interventions in rigorously designed dosing studies with a goal of demonstrating the relationship of drug dosage to treatment outcome in chronic psychiatric disorders. If Food and Drug Administration (FDA) requirements for Phase III clinical trials included multifactor treatment outcomes for drugs indicated for the treatment of severe and persistent disorders, it is likely that the gap between early trial findings and the outcome for the ever-growing treatment-resistant population could be shortened.

Clozapine: Bridging the Gap? Clozapine, an atypical antipsychotic medication for treatment-resistant schizophrenia introduced to the US market in 1988, was evaluated in an essentially classic randomized, double-blind 6-week study of more than 200 patients, comparing the drug with standard treatment consisting of chlorpromazine.[105] A novel aspect of the study was a pretrial phase to rule out patients responsive to haloperidol, a standard antipsychotic treatment, to avoid the risk of exposing a treatment-responsive patient to clozapine because of its greater risk of agranulocytosis. To address the issue of effectiveness in the usual treatment setting, a statewide evaluation of clozapine[106] among 202 patients who met criteria similar to those of the Sandoz Collaborative Study[105] was undertaken. The study showed that a similar proportion of patients (one-third) improved as in the clinical trial, although the time to improvement was at least 12 weeks for this cohort of longer-stay hospitalized patients. The resistance to improvement was disappointing and may explain the less than 10% discharge rate at 1 year of treatment. Clinical trials for new agents such as clozapine illustrate that premarketing clinical trial data continue to be derived from studies that are focused on short-term symptom improvement. Despite this fact, the medication is indicated for the chronic, "treatment-resistant" individual for whom long-term effectiveness is needed. A more precise understanding of the role of antipsychotic drugs in long-term, functional improvement is most critically needed, and short-term clinical trials have generally failed to provide it. Efforts to lengthen trials should be undertaken, particularly since many chronically psychotic patients are in monitored treatment programs where study participation may be more feasible than in a general medical population. Methodologic issues related to clozapine's cost–effectiveness have been reviewed in terms of trial data compared with pharmacoepidemiologic outcome data.[107]

Safety Methods

Current concerns regarding the safety of marketed neuropharmacologic agents are reflected in the increasing number of case reports of neuroleptic malignant syndrome,[108,109] sudden deaths associated with antipsychotic and antidepressant use,[110,111] debate about whether particular cases of intoxication involving antipsychotic medications and lithium are recognized,[112,113] and the increased risk associated with rapid neuroleptization.[114] As previously discussed (see page 502), Baldessarini et al.[51] have documented and we have replicated[5] the relatively greater daily doses (CPZ-EQs) that are associated with the use of high-potency (low-dose) antipsychotic agents such as haloperidol and fluphenazine. This change in prescribing pattern has implications for the prevalence of chronic unintended events (e.g., tardive dyskinesia).

Efforts to revise antipsychotic dosing protocols are needed especially to minimize the following cycle: excess dose leads to unrecognized behavioral toxicity that is misidentified as symptom worsening and leads to increased dose.[115,116] Hopefully, studies currently under way (e.g., Patient Outcome Research Teams for Schizophrenia) will achieve their goals of developing and evaluating empirically based treatment recommendations. Other organizations (e.g., the American Psychiatric Association) are establishing practice guidelines based on a need to demonstrate quality clinical decision-making for their members and for external reimbursement organizations.[117] As part of this effort, a database called the Practice Research Network will collect the clinical assessment and treatment data of 1000 office-based psychiatrists who will volunteer data and conduct clinical research. In addition, studies are needed to establish accurate dosing conversions from one antipsychotic medication to another and to incorporate these dosing rules into clinical practice.[46,118] A large-scale, controlled, prospective study in the public sector (e.g., among VA or community mental health patients) would address this need. Safety issues are also related to the appropriate downward dosage titration to avoid acute drug withdrawal effects.[27,119,120]

POSTMARKETING SURVEILLANCE OF PSYCHOTROPIC MEDICATIONS

The need for denominator-based unintended event rates for marketed medications is a major thrust of pharmacoepidemiology, as noted in Chapter 5. Inman[3] has summarized the existing approaches to drug safety monitoring that focus on spontaneous reporting mechanisms (numerator-based) and described the need for routine denominator-based methods. Research leaders in psychiatry have discussed the need for PMS of psychotropic medications,[121] but have found that a feasible procedure for maintaining a constant level of vigilance in reporting events is still lacking. The need for funding or reliable carrot-stick methods to prod compliance with reporting programs was emphasized. A general introduction to PMS of psychotropic agents[122] describes how it might be used as a means of detecting new unintended reactions or beneficial effects (e.g., new therapeutic indications) and computing the actual population incidence. An example of PMS in Britain is described[123] as prescription-event monitoring; it captures drug data from National Health Service prescription records related to approximately 70% of the nation's general practitioners. Results of the monitoring for alprazolam, a benzodiazepine indicated for anxiety, anxiety-associated depression, and panic disorder, have been reported. The study relied on a "green form" survey of 8727 practitioners, with a response rate of 57%, to record unintended events. However, none of the dramatic effects (e.g., mania, hostility) that received widespread media coverage and raised concerns about its safety were observed. The authors acknowledge the likelihood of underreporting in this system. Another factor is the possibility that these behavioral toxicity symptoms were never recognized as such (and not reported) but were treated as part of the underlying or incipient illness.

OBSERVATIONAL STUDY METHODS FOR DRUG SAFETY

Observational studies have been used to evaluate mental and behavioral symptoms suspected of being drug induced. For example, the prevalence of drug-induced psychiatric symptoms was estimated to occur in 0.6% of general hospital admissions according to the Boston Collaborative Drug Surveillance Program.[124] Computerized outpatient drug records of HMO enrollees were used as the source of a cohort study of anticonvulsant use secondary to tricyclic antidepressant therapy in order to link seizures to antidepressant use. The findings do not generalize to the more severely ill patients who usually receive larger daily doses. Therefore, replication of this finding of low prevalence (<1 in 1000 exposures) in more severely ill patients and in patients with greater dose exposures would be useful.[125]

In smaller traditional prospective clinical studies, medication-related admissions of psychiatric patients in Israel were more prevalent (7.5%) than in studies of medical admissions.[126] Using a broader operational definition, Stewart et al.[127] found that one-third of all psychiatric admissions in the US were drug related. Replicating these findings in a VA hospital setting, one-third of the admissions were attributed to prescribed drug intoxication, adverse effects, or compliance, and total drug-related admissions had significantly longer hospitalizations than those with non-drug-related admissions.[128] A more recent German study[129] analyzed all drug-related admissions to two university psychiatric hospitals. For the 6-year period examined, 0.7% of 15 800 consecutive psychiatric admissions were associated with unintended reactions to medications. Older age, multiple-drug therapy, and high-dose, parenterally administered antipsychotics were important risk factors leading to psychiatric hospitalization. The 10-fold lower rate in Germany than in the previously described studies may reflect differences in prescribing patterns or patient populations or the long-term effect of an intensive unintended reaction monitoring program in Germany. None of these traditional approaches addresses the problem of the unrecognized drug-induced event (i.e., when drug-induced symptoms are attributed to a worsening of the underlying illness).

More recent computerized database approaches to drug adverse effect questions have taken advantage of the availability of Medicaid drug billing information. For example, the association of beta-blockers with depression was evaluated by observing the significantly greater frequency (23% vs. 10%) of tricyclic antidepressant medications among hypertensive patients taking beta-blockers compared with those taking methyldopa or reserpine. The finding was interpreted as supportive evidence of beta-blocker-induced depression based on a method free of most of the limitations of previous studies.[130]

In a cogent case–control study analysis, the risk of hip fracture in elderly patients was determined to be significantly increased for Medicaid enrollees receiving long half-life hypnotic-anxiolytic, tricyclic antidepressant, and antipsychotic medications. The risk increased in proportion to the dosage, and the effect persisted after stratifying for dementia.[131]

A sophisticated program to develop patient self-monitoring as a method for the PMS of unintended drug reactions[132] has been operating for more than 8 years, and has been validated. The validation study[133] indicated that patient-identified unintended clinical events associated with antibiotic or tricyclic antidepressant use closely matched those elicited by interview of the patients by the study staff. The ability of ambulatory patients to accurately discriminate probable unintended drug reactions from other unintended clinical events was dependent on the surveillance method and on the method for obtaining unintended clinical event reports.[134] Comparable reporting by psychiatric outpatients taking antidepressant medications and by patients receiving antibiotic therapies suggested that psychiatric patients can participate as reliably as others in the reporting of unintended drug reactions. The lack of an anticipated association between age and incidence of unintended drug reactions led the authors to conclude that a method of elicitation that minimizes the risk of recall bias is most desirable.[135]

The unrecognized drug-induced event is a problem of particular concern in neuropharmacology and pharmacoepidemiology. One attempt to overcome this dilemma is the intensive drug monitoring program that has been operating since 1979 in three psychiatric hospitals in Germany.[136] Randomly selected inpatients are observed by a psychiatrist drug monitor who classifies events according to a specific severity grading system. Severity is implicitly determined by rating the impact of therapy as follows: grade I, no change in medication; grade II, dosage reduction; and grade III, discontinuation of medication. After 32 months of monitoring, the grade III adverse (unintended) event was observed in 15% of patients compared with a rate of 9% in an organized spontaneous reporting system. The greater incidence reported in the denominator-based system supports the notion that systematic surveillance of unintended events helps to correct for the underreporting bias that is believed to occur in spontaneous reporting systems.

Phase III drug trials include routine monitoring of patients for unintended events. One of the most sophisticated psychopharmacologic drug assessment tools developed for this purpose is called Systematic Assessment for Treatment of Emergent Events (SAFTEE)[137] and involves a generalized review of body systems. In this approach, a regular quantitative assessment is made of the frequency and severity of all symptoms without regard to the origin of the symptom as illness based or drug related. Statistical analysis of the relationship among variables (e.g., symptom, severity, pattern, time of onset, drug and dose) makes it possible to identify an unintended event by statistical means, rather than by an a priori rule of clinical judgment.

A simplified version of SAFTEE was developed for routine clinical practice by using drug or dosage changes as a trigger. The feasibility of this approach was established in a pilot test that was based on acute admissions units and psychogeriatric units of a state hospital population.[138] The epidemiologic analysis that uses a statistical measure of the relationship among symptoms (putative unintended events) and drug or dose may be particularly useful in distinguishing drug-induced from illness-based behaviors. In addition, inverse statistical relationships may suggest new indications; for example, a protective effect may be hypothesized when the baseline incidence of a behavioral symptom such as depression is reduced in the presence of a drug that is not recognized as having an antidepressant effect.

DRUG-INDUCED VERSUS ILLNESS-BASED SYMPTOMS

This review highlights issues that suggest that a major task of the neuropharmacologist as the millennium approaches continues to be the need to distinguish drug-induced from illness-based symptoms. Behavioral toxicity symptoms[10] such as akathisia[139] and akinesia[140] were the subject of considerable debate before they were accepted as drug-induced phenomena. In the past, several marketed neuropharmacologic agents gained media and professional attention because of anecdotal reports of behavioral toxicity. For example, triazolam-associated confusion, amnesia, hallucinations, and agitation featured prominently in the clinical literature, in part because the individuals experiencing the effects were neurologists.[141] The effects were confirmed by analysis from the Spontaneous Reporting System of the FDA.[142] Earlier reports led to partial or complete withdrawal of triazolam or certain of its dosage forms from world markets including the Netherlands, France, Spain, Italy, and Germany.[143] These examples highlight the potential uses for pharmacoepidemiologic methods that permit the testing of hypotheses regarding the relationship between neuropharmacologic drug, dose, or drug combinations and behavioral effects such as selected psychological and behavioral unintended events (e.g., anxiety, agitation) in the usual practice setting rather than the research setting and with medication prescribed in a customary use fashion.

The history of triazolam use suggests a major target area where the aims of neuropharmacology and pharmacoepidemiology converge (i.e., to identify pronounced behavioral effects and their relationship to dosage as early as possible). To accomplish this aim, large prospective cohorts at specialized teaching and research centers could be formed for PMS of new agents as a condition of participation in Phase III clinical trials. Such projects would need public funding for their support. In addition, existing trial methods may benefit from a reevaluation of how complex domains such as memory loss are measured. Finally, an ethical dimension of the triazolam experience concerns whether effects that are intolerable in busy professionals are rated as tolerable by observers of clinical trial patients.

Specific Drug Decision-Making Methods

Sackett[144] listed five biases that may be operating when the clinician infers a causal association between a change in the patient's behavior and the introduction of a medication. These biases are spontaneous remission, regression effect, placebo effect, expectancy effect, and the obsequiousness bias. Some of these problems can be minimized by following the "N of 1" study method. This study design permits an evaluation of the effect of a medication in a single subject (on active drug/on placebo in a random assignment, double-blind design) in the customary clinical setting.[145,146] This approach can be a low-cost yet rigorous evaluation preliminary to the clinical trial for the assessment of marketed drugs for unlabeled indications (i.e., uses not approved by the FDA). For example, the method could be useful in determining the effectiveness of carbamazepine in treatment-resistant affective disorder patients and propranolol in treatment-resistant violent patients.

The effectiveness of a neuropharmacologic agent in specific subpopulations such as pregnant women, the elderly, and those with comorbid conditions can be determined by epidemiologic drug assessments. Recent interest in gender and ethnicity by the NIMH, for example, by its funding of research on mental disorders, is also apparent in the clinical literature[147,148] and in the FDA's creation of a women's health program. Aggregate data from the longitudinal monitoring of specific subpopulations can be used to make treatment decisions for these subgroups. For example, for the depressed patient with evidence of delayed cardiac conduction time, the risk/benefit ratio may favor the use of electroconvulsive therapy over tricyclic antidepressant drug therapy. The decision criteria would require a longitudinal record of quantitatively recorded symptom severity and a history of past medication exposure to determine whether there were adequate trials of nontricyclic alternatives. Compelling questions about the safety of psychotropic drugs in women can be found. For example, a case–control study[149] found a 17-fold increase in risk of total myocardial infarction associated with current use of psychotropic drugs among young women. These tentative findings occurred in a study whose primary aim was to study cardiovascular mortality among 16- to 39-year-old women and should be replicated. In addition, teratogenicity studies of fluoxetine[150] and lithium[151] are based on selected reporting by pregnant women and showed no increased risk of fetal malformation. In the case of fluoxetine and tricyclic antidepressants, there was an increased risk of miscarriage.

Despite intensive efforts of the past decade to improve diagnostic classification with the *Diagnostic and Statistical Manual of Mental Disorders: DSM-IV (Fourth Edition)*, therapeutic choice and outcome are still poorly predicted by symptomatology, except for homogeneous diagnostic categories. As an alternative to denominator-based classification, Thomsen[152] developed an inferential classification using Bayes' formula with correction for redundancy. For example, he calculated correlations of 0.57 between two symptom patterns and low-dose antipsychotic therapy. Refining his approach would involve the addition of other clinical variables such as chronicity (prior days hospitalized), employment history, and social functioning history that previous studies have demonstrated to predict outcome.[44]

POLICY QUESTIONS

There are a number of current controversies that involve the use of marketed medications for treating psychiatric patients. Since the early 1970s, the right of the hospitalized psychotic patient with an involuntary commitment status to refuse nonemergency drug treatment has been developing through judicial or regulatory decisions or by legislation.[72,153-155] The potential impact of these decisions on institutional psychiatric practice, where antipsychotic medication is the mainstay of treatment in more than 140 000 state hospitalized patients, is great. However, the implementation of review procedures may not be producing patient outcomes dramatically different from the prereview era.[156]

Reimbursement policies for psychiatric illness are currently being debated, and numerous prospective payment schemes are under investigation. Treatments and procedures have been proposed and disputed as alternatives to the use of diagnostic categories to predict length of stay.[157] Each of these schemes has implications that extend to drug treatment variables such as drug and dosage. Drug regimens that rapidly resolve symptoms and permit clinical management in the least costly environment are consistent with this model. However, this approach would have a negative impact on specific subgroups such as the low-functioning, treatment-resistant, persistently ill patient.

Efforts to resolve clinical dilemmas include the consensus development conference, a strategy that acknowledges the underlying social and political dimensions of science and technology. The conference aims to bring together all parties with vested interests as a means of resolving clinical practice dilemmas. To the extent that each interest group can evaluate the meaningfulness of the scientific literature on the efficacy and safety of somatic and psychotherapeutic interventions as well as the short- and long-term consequences of alternative approaches, the consensus development conference can be useful in framing the individual clinical decision within the larger societal context. In psychiatry, electroconvulsive therapy[158] and drug treatment of mood disorders[159] have been subjected to the consensus process.

Along with managed care trends and cost containment, the development and promulgation of clinical practice guidelines[160] for the treatment of mental disorders (e.g., depression) augur well for pharmacoepidemiology. This trend offers pharmacoepidemiology a great opportunity to examine the relationship between practice variation and therapy. Comparisons of psychotropic drug prevalence among staff model HMOs, preferred provider organizations, and independent practice associations, as well as Medicaid systems in both traditional fee-for-service and managed care settings, would be reasonably easy places to start.

There are two controversial drug-related topics that might benefit from public health-focused reviews of treatment and outcome: first, antipsychotic drug effectiveness in the nonemergency treatment of the drug-refusing involuntarily committed patient; and second, the management of the long-term patient with psychotic disorder by treatment adjuncts or alternatives to antipsychotic medications that are aimed at minimizing the risk of tardive dyskinesia.

Conclusion

In this chapter we have attempted to apply the organizing and analyzing principles of epidemiology to current knowledge of neuropsychiatric drug use for the treatment of mental disorders. It is a first step toward defining the realm for pharmacoepidemiologists to pursue in psychiatry. Hopefully, this approach will be more broadly adopted and lead to a refinement of the model. Recent pharmacoepidemiologic efforts in child psychiatry are fueled by the recognition of inadequate drug information from clinical trials for children.[161] In general, future benefits of pharmacoepidemiology include a greater integration of study findings, not only for short-term drug evaluation, but, most critically, for long-term effectiveness. As a long-term objective, psychiatric pharmacoepidemiology should increase the validity and appropriate application of information in the clinical science of neuropharmacology.

References

1. Rector TS. Pharmacoepidemiology: emerging roles for pharmacists (letter). Am J Hosp Pharm 1985;42:778, 783.
2. Lawson DH. Pharmacoepidemiology: a new discipline (editorial). Br Med J 1984; 289:940-1.
3. Inman W. Monitoring for drug safety. Philadelphia: JP Lippincott, 1980.
4. Ingman SR, Lawson IR, Pierpaoli PG, Blake P. A survey of the prescribing and administration of drugs in a long-term care institution for the elderly. J Am Geriatr Soc 1975;23:309-16.

5. Zito JM, Craig TJ, Wanderling J, Siegel C. Pharmaco-epidemiology in 136 hospital-ized schizophrenic patients. Am J Psychiatry 1987;144:778-82.

6. McKenna PJ, Kane JM, Parrish K. Psychotic syndromes in epilepsy. Am J Psychiatry 1985;142:895-904.

7. Post RM, Uhde TW, Roy-Byrne PP, Joffe RT. Antidepressant effects of carbamaze-pine. Am J Psychiatry 1986;143:29-34.

8. DiMascio A, Shader RI. Clinical handbook of psychopharmacology. New York: Science House, 1970.

9. Cole JO. Behavioral toxicity. In: Uhr L, Miller JG, eds. Drugs and behavior. New York: John Wiley, 1960.

10. Van Putten T, Marder SR. Behavioral toxicity of antipsychotic drugs. J Clin Psychiatry 1987;48(suppl):13-9.

11. Davis JM. Antipsychotic drugs. In: Kaplan HI, Sadock BJ, eds. Comprehensive text-book of psychiatry/V. Baltimore: Williams & Wilkins, 1989:1620.

12. Eisendrath SJ, Sweeney MA. Toxic neuropsychiatric effects of digoxin at therapeu-tic serum concentrations. Am J Psychiatry 1987;144:506-7.

13. Wamboldt FS, Jefferson JW, Wamboldt MZ. Digitalis intoxication misdiagnosed as depression by primary care physicians. Am J Psychiatry 1986;143:219-21.

14. Hullett FJ, Potkin SG, Levy AB, Ciasca R. Depression associated with nifedipine-induced calcium channel blockade. Am J Psychiatry 1988;145:1277-9.

15. Billings RF, Stein MB. Depression associated with ranitidine. Am J Psychiatry 1986; 143:915-6.

16. Goodwin FK, Bunney WE Jr. Depressions following reserpine: a reevaluation. Semin Psychiatry 1971;3:435-48.

17. Waal-Manning HJ. Hypertension: which beta-blocker? Drugs 1976;12:412-4.

18. Parker WA. Propranolol-induced depression and psychosis. Clin Pharm 1985;4:214-8.

19. Pollack MH, Rosenbaum JF, Cassem NH. Propranolol and depression revisited: three cases and a review. J Nerv Ment Dis 1985;173:118-9.

20. Nitter L Jr, Haraldsson A, Holck P, Hoy C, Munthe-Kass J, Myrhol K, et al. The effect of trimipramine on the healing of peptic ulcer. A double-blind study. Multicentre investigation—G.P. Scand J Gastroenterol Suppl 1977;43:39-41.

21. Weiner H. Psychobiology and human disease. New York: Elsevier, 1977.

22. Contemporary research in behavioral pharmacology. New York: Plenum Press, 1978.

23. Strain JJ, Taintor Z. Consultation-liaison psychiatry. In: Kaplan HI, Sadock BJ, eds. Comprehensive textbook of psychiatry/V. Baltimore: Williams & Wilkins, 1989: 1272-9.

24. Lieff J. Computer applications in psychiatry. Washington, DC: American Psychiatric Association Press, 1987:135.

25. Feinstein AR. Quality of data in the medical record. Comput Biomed Res 1970;3: 426-35.

26. Freed CR, Gal J, Manchester DK. Dosage of phenytoin during pregnancy (letter). JAMA 1985;253:2833-4.

27. Zito JM. Psychotherapeutic drug manual. New York: John Wiley, 1994:287-8.

28. Overall JE, Faillace LA, Rhoades HM, Johnson SR, Volkow N, Stone MA, et al. Computer-based monitoring of clinical care in a public psychiatric hospital unit. Hosp Community Psychiatry 1987;38:381-6.

29. Allgulander C. Psychoactive drug use in a general population sample, Sweden: cor-relates with perceived health, psychiatric diagnoses, and mortality in an automated record-linkage study. Am J Public Health 1989;79:1006-10.

30. Laska E, Siegel C, Simpson G. Automated review system for orders of psychotropic drugs. Arch Gen Psychiatry 1980;37:824-7.
31. Siegel C, Alexander MJ, Dlugacz YD, Fischer S. Evaluation of a computerized drug review system: impact, attitudes, and interactions. Comput Biomed Res 1984;17:419-35.
32. Craig TJ, Mehta RM. Clinician–computer interaction: automated review of psychotropic drugs. Am J Psychiatry 1984;141:267-70.
33. Zito JM, Craig TJ, Wanderling J, Siegel C, Green M. Pharmacotherapy of the hospitalized young adult schizophrenic patient. Compr Psychiatry 1988;29:379-86.
34. Zito JM, Craig TJ, Wanderling J. Pharmacoepidemiology of 330 child and adolescent psychiatric patients. J Pharmacoepidemiol 1994;3:47-62.
35. Wells KB, Stewart A, Hays RD, Burnam MA, Rogers W, Daniels M, et al. The functioning and well-being of depressed patients. Results from the Medical Outcomes Study. JAMA 1989;262:914-9.
36. Wells KB, Hays RD, Burnam MA, Rogers W, Greenfield S, Ware JE Jr. Detection of depressive disorder for patients receiving prepaid or fee-for-service care. Results from the Medical Outcomes Study. JAMA 1989;262:3298-302.
37. Wells KB, Katon W, Rogers B, Camp P. Use of minor tranquilizers and antidepressant medications by depressed outpatients: results from the Medical Outcomes Study. Am J Psychiatry 1994;151:694-700.
38. Simon GE, Von Korff M, Wagner EH, Barlow W. Patterns of antidepressant use in community practice. Gen Hosp Psychiatry 1993;15:399-408.
39. Zito JM, Riddle MA, Safer D, Johnson R, Fox M, Speedie S, et al. Pharmacoepidemiology of youth with treatments for mental disorders (abstract). Presented at the New Clinical Drug Evaluation Unit 35th Annual Meeting, Orlando, FL, June 2, 1995.
40. Zito JH, Safer DJ, dos Reis S, Magder LS, Riddle MA. Methylphenidate patterns among Medicaid youth. Psychopharmacol Bull 1997;33:143-7.
41. Johnson RE, McFarland BM, Corelle CA, Woodson GT. Estimating daily dose for pharmacoepidemiologic studies: alprazolam as an example. Pharmacoepidemiol Drug Saf 1994;3:139-45.
42. Schwartz CC, Myers JK, Astrachan BM. The outcome study in psychiatric evaluation research. Issues and methods. Arch Gen Psychiatry 1973;29:98-102.
43. Strauss JS, Carpenter WT Jr. The prediction of outcome in schizophrenia. II. Relationships between predictor and outcome variables: a report from the WHO international pilot study of schizophrenia. Arch Gen Psychiatry 1974;31:37-42.
44. Strauss JS, Carpenter WT Jr. Prediction of outcome in schizophrenia. III. Five-year outcome and its predictors. Arch Gen Psychiatry 1977;34:159-63.
45. Baldessarini RJ, Cohen BM, Teicher MH. Significance of neuroleptic dose and plasma level in the pharmacological treatment of psychoses. Arch Gen Psychiatry 1988;45:79-91.
46. Davis JM, Andriukaitis S. The natural course of schizophrenia and effective maintenance drug treatment. J Clin Psychopharmacol 1986;6(suppl):2S-10S.
47. Baldessarini RJ. Drugs and the treatment of psychiatric disorders. In: Gilman AG, Rall TW, Nies AS, Taylor P, eds. Goodman and Gilman's the pharmacological basis of therapeutics. 8th ed. New York: Pergamon, 1990.
48. Cohen BM. Neuroleptic drugs in the treatment of acute psychosis: how much do we really know? Psychopharmacol Ser 1988;5:47-61.
49. Tardive dyskinesia: a task force report of the American Psychiatric Association (APA) Press. Washington, DC: American Psychiatric Association Press, 1992:1.

50. Muscettola G, Bollini P, Pampallona S. Pattern of neuroleptic drug use in Italian mental health services. DICP Ann Pharmacother 1991;25:296-301.
51. Baldessarini RJ, Katz B, Cotton P. Dissimilar dosing with high-potency and low-potency neuroleptics. Am J Psychiatry 1984;141:748-52.
52. Hargreaves WA, Zachary R, LeGoullon M, Binder R, Reus V. Neuroleptic dose: a statistical model for analyzing historical trends. J Psychiatr Res 1987;21:199-214.
53. Reardon GT, Rifkin A, Schwartz A, Myerson A, Siris SG. Changing patterns of neuroleptic dosage over a decade. Am J Psychiatry 1989;146:726-9.
54. Overall JE, Garza-Trevino E, Rhoades HM, Volkow ND, Cecil S. Justifying neuroleptic drug treatment. Hosp Community Psychiatry 1989;40:749-51.
55. Regier DA, Narrow WE, Rae DS, Manderscheid RW, Locke BZ, Goodwin FK. The de facto US mental and addictive disorders service system. Epidemiologic catchment area prospective 1-year prevalence rates of disorders and services. Arch Gen Psychiatry 1993;50:85-94.
56. Mellinger GD, Balter MB, Uhlenhuth EH. Prevalence and correlates of the long-term regular use of anxiolytics. JAMA 1984;251:375-9.
57. Johnson RE, McFarland BH. Antipsychotic drug exposure in a health maintenance organization. Med Care 1993;31:432-44.
58. Muijen M, Silverstone T. A comparative hospital survey of psychotropic drug prescribing. Br J Psychiatry 1987;150:501-4.
59. Clark AF, Holden NL. The persistence of prescribing habits: a survey and follow-up of prescribing to chronic hospital in-patients. Br J Psychiatry 1987;150:88-91.
60. Williams P, Murray J, Clare A. A longitudinal study of psychotropic drug prescription. Psychol Med 1982;12:201-6.
61. Glaser BA, Morreau LE. Effects of interdisciplinary team review on the use of antipsychotic agents with severely and profoundly mentally retarded persons. Am J Ment Deficiency 1986;90:371-9.
62. Beardsley RS, Gardocki GJ, Larson DB, Hidalgo J. Prescribing of psychotropic medication by primary care physicians and psychiatrists. Arch Gen Psychiatry 1988;45:1117-9.
63. Garrard J, Makris L, Dunham T, Heston LL, Cooper S, Ratner ER, et al. Evaluation of neuroleptic drug use by nursing home elderly under proposed Medicare and Medicaid regulations. JAMA 1991;265:463-7.
64. Garrard J, Chen V, Dowd B. The impact of the 1987 federal regulations on the use of psychotropic drugs in Minnesota nursing homes. Am J Public Health 1995;85:771-6.
65. Crane GE. Clinical psychopharmacology in its 20th year. Late, unanticipated effects of neuroleptics may limit their use in psychiatry. Science 1973;181:124-8.
66. Carpenter WT Jr, Heinrichs DW, Hanlon TE. Methodologic standards for treatment outcome research in schizophrenia. Am J Psychiatry 1981;138:465-71.
67. Carpenter WT Jr, Conley RR, Buchanan RW, Breier A, Tamminga CA. Patient response and resource management: another view of clozapine treatment of schizophrenia. Am J Psychiatry 1995;152:827-32.
68. Barreira PJ, Vogel W. The clinical vs. research paradox in psychopharmacological research. Psychiatry Res 1988;25:109-10.
69. Woggon B. Unsolved problems in the pharmacotherapy of depression. Psychopharmacol Ser 1988;5:159-65.
70. Kales A, Kales JD. Shortcomings in the evaluation and promotion of hypnotic drugs (editorial). N Engl J Med 1975;293:826-7.
71. Schou M. Lithium prophylaxis: myths and realities. Am J Psychiatry 1989;146:573-6.

72. Kane JM. Dosage reduction strategies in the long-term treatment of schizophrenia. In: Kane JM, ed. Drug maintenance strategies in schizophrenia. Washington, DC: American Psychiatric Association Press, 1987:1-12.
73. Nelson C, McLemore T. The National Ambulatory Medical Care Survey: 1975–81 and 1985. DHHS Publication No. (PHS) 88-1754. Vital Health Stat [13] 1988;93:1-50.
74. Hohmann AA, Larson DB, Thompson JW, Beardsley RS. Psychotropic medication prescription in U.S. ambulatory medical care. DICP Ann Pharmacother 1991;25:85-9.
75. Rivera-Calimlim L, Hershey L. Neuroleptic concentrations and clinical response. Ann Rev Pharmacol Toxicol 1984;24:361-86.
76. Hohmann AA. Gender bias in psychotropic drug prescribing in primary care. Med Care 1989;27:478-90.
77. Avorn J, Dreyer P, Connelly K, Soumerai SB. Use of psychoactive medication and the quality of care in rest homes. Findings and policy implications of a statewide study. N Engl J Med 1989;320:227-32.
78. Cole J. Phenothiazine treatment in acute schizophrenia. Arch Gen Psychiatry 1964; 10:246-61.
79. Casey J, Bennett I, Lindley C. Drug therapy of schizophrenia. Arch Gen Psychiatry 1960;2:210-9.
80. Carpenter WT Jr, Heinrichs DW, Alphs LD. Treatment of negative symptoms. Schizophr Bull 1985;11:440-52.
81. Carpenter WT Jr, Heinrichs DW, Hanlon TE. A comparative trial of pharmacologic strategies in schizophrenia. Am J Psychiatry 1987;144:1466-70.
82. Carpenter WT Jr, Heinrichs DW. Early intervention, time-limited, targeted pharmacotherapy of schizophrenia. Schizophr Bull 1983;9:533-42.
83. Arana GW, Ornsteen ML, Kanter F, Friedman HL, Greenblatt DJ, Shader RI. The use of benzodiazepines for psychotic disorders: a literature review and preliminary clinical findings. Psychopharmacol Bull 1986;22:77-87.
84. Wolkowitz OM, Pickar D, Doran AR, Breier A, Tarell J, Paul SM. Combination alprazolam-neuroleptic treatment of the positive and negative symptoms of schizophrenia. Am J Psychiatry 1986;143:85-7.
85. Agran M, Moore S, Martin JE. Research in mental retardation: underreporting of medication information. Res Dev Disabil 1988;9:351-7.
86. McKane JP, Robinson AD, Wiles DH, McCreadie RG, Stirling GS. Haloperidol decanoate v. fluphenazine decanoate as maintenance therapy in chronic schizophrenic in-patients. Br J Psychiatry 1987;151:333-6.
87. Davis JM. Overview: maintenance therapy in psychiatry: I. Schizophrenia. Am J Psychiatry 1975;132:1237-45.
88. Tobias LL, MacDonald ML. Withdrawal of maintenance drugs with long-term hospitalized mental patients: a critical review. Psychol Bull 1974;81:107-25.
89. Gardos G, Cole JO, Tarsy D. Withdrawal syndromes associated with antipsychotic drugs. Am J Psychiatry 1978;135:1321-4.
90. Lieberman J. Cholinergic rebound in neuroleptic withdrawal syndromes. Psychosomatics 1981;22:253-4.
91. Levine J, Schooler N, Severe J. Discontinuation of oral and depot fluphenazine in schizophrenic patients after one year of continuous medication: a controlled study. In: Cattabeni F, Racagni G, Spano P, Costa E, eds. Long-term effects of neuroleptics. New York: Raven Press, 1980:483-94.
92. Leff JP, Wing JK. Trial of maintenance therapy in schizophrenia. Br Med J 1971;3: 599-604.

93. Rappaport M, Hopkins HK, Hall K, Belleza T, Silverman J. Are there schizophrenics for whom drugs may be unnecessary or contraindicated? Int Pharmacopsychiatry 1978;13:100-11.
94. Rosen B, Engelhardt DM, Freedman N, Margolis R. The hospitalization proneness scale as a predictor of response to phenothiazine treatment. J Nerv Ment Dis 1968; 146:476-80.
95. Saenger G. Patterns of change among "treated" and "untreated" patients seen in psychiatric community mental health clinics. J Nerv Ment Dis 1970;150:37-50.
96. Paul G, Lentz R. Psychosocial treatment of chronic mental patients: milieu vs. social-learning programs. Cambridge: Harvard University Press, 1977.
97. Mosher LR, Menn AZ. Community residential treatment for schizophrenia: two-year follow-up. Hosp Community Psychiatry 1978;29:715-23.
98. Esterson A, Cooper DG, Laing RD. Results of family-orientated therapy with hospitalized schizophrenics. Br Med J 1965;5476:1462-5.
99. Klein DF, Rosen B. Premorbid asocial adjustment and response to phenothiazine treatment among schizophrenic inpatients. Arch Gen Psychiatry 1973;29:480-5.
100. Goldstein MJ, Rodnick EH, Evans JR, May PR, Steinberg MR. Drug and family therapy in the aftercare of acute schizophrenics. Arch Gen Psychiatry 1978;35:1169-77.
101. Peto R, Pike MC, Armitage P, Breslow NE, Cox DR, Howard SV, et al. Design and analysis of randomised clinical trials requiring prolonged observation of each patient. I. Introduction and design. Br J Cancer 1976;34:585-612.
102. Schooler NR, Hogarty GE. Medication and psychosocial strategies in the treatment of schizophrenia. In: Meltzer H, ed. Psychopharmacology: the third generation of progress. New York: Raven Press, 1987:1111-9.
103. Hogarty GE, Schooler N, Ulrich RF, Mussare F, Ferro P, Herron E. Fluphenazine and social therapy in the aftercare of schizophrenic patients. Relapse analyses of a two-year controlled study of fluphenazine decanoate and fluphenazine hydrochloride. Arch Gen Psychiatry 1979;36:1283-94.
104. Karasu TB. Psychotherapy and pharmacotherapy: toward an integrative model. Am J Psychiatry 1982;139:1102-13.
105. Kane J, Honigfeld G, Singer J, Meltzer H, Clozaril Collaborative Study Group. Clozapine for the treatment-resistant schizophrenic. Arch Gen Psychiatry 1988;45: 789-96.
106. Zito JM, Volavka J, Craig TJ, Czobor P, Banks S, Vitrai J. Pharmacoepidemiology of clozapine in 202 inpatients with schizophrenia. Ann Pharmacother 1993;27:1262-9.
107. Zito JM, Provenzano G. Pharmaceutical decisionmaking: pharmacoepidemiology or pharmacoeconomics—who's in the driver's seat? Psychopharmacol Bull 1995; 31:735-44.
108. Levenson JL. Neuroleptic malignant syndrome. Am J Psychiatry 1985;142:1137-45.
109. Sternberg DE. Neuroleptic malignant syndrome: the pendulum swings (editorial). Am J Psychiatry 1986;143:1273-5.
110. Craig TJ. Medication use and deaths attributed to asphyxia among psychiatric patients. Am J Psychiatry 1980;137:1366-73.
111. Zugibe FT. Sudden death related to the use of psychotropic drugs. Philadelphia: WB Saunders, 1980:75-90.
112. Goldney RD, Spence ND. Safety of the combination of lithium and neuroleptic drugs. Am J Psychiatry 1986;143:882-4.
113. Miller F, Menninger J. Correlation of neuroleptic dose and neurotoxicity in patients given lithium and a neuroleptic. Hosp Community Psychiatry 1987;38:1219-21.

114. Bollini P, Andreani A, Colombo F, Bellantuono C, Beretta P, Arduini A, et al. High-dose neuroleptics: uncontrolled clinical practice confirms controlled clinical trials. Br J Psychiatry 1984;144:25-7.

115. Osser DN. Use of antidepressants in schizophrenia: diagnostic problems (letter). Arch Gen Psychiatry 1990;47:979-80.

116. Weiden P. Clinical nonrecognition of neuroleptic-induced movement disorders: a cautionary study. Am J Psychiatry 1987;144:1148-53.

117. Zarin D, Pincus HA, McIntyre JS. Practice guidelines (editorial). Am J Psychiatry 1993;150:175-7.

118. Kane JM, Woerner M, Sarantakos S. Depot neuroleptics: a comparative review of standard, intermediate, and low-dose regimens. J Clin Psychiatry 1986;47(suppl): 30-3.

119. McMahon T. Anti-depressant and antipsychotic withdrawal syndromes (abstract). Neurobehav Toxicol Teratol 1985;7:2.

120. Noyes R Jr, Clancy J, Coryell WH, Crowe RR, Chaudhry DR, Domingo DV. A withdrawal syndrome after abrupt discontinuation of alprazolam. Am J Psychiatry 1985;142:114-6.

121. Hollister LE, Overall JE. Experience with a failed postmarketing drug surveillance program. J Clin Pharmacol 1984;24:3-5.

122. Fisher S. Postmarketing surveillance of adverse drug reactions. In: Meltzer H, ed. Psychopharmacology: the third generation of progress. New York: Raven Press, 1987:1667-73.

123. Edwards JG, Inman WH, Pearce GL, Rawson NS. Prescription-event monitoring of 10,895 patients treated with alprazolam. Br J Psychiatry 1991;158:387-92.

124. Danielson DA, Porter JB, Lawson DH, Soubrie C, Jick H. Drug-associated psychiatric disturbances in medical inpatients. Psychopharmacology 1981;74:105-8.

125. Jick H, Dinan BJ, Hunter JR, Stergachis A, Ronning A, Perera DR, et al. Tricyclic antidepressants and convulsions. J Clin Psychopharmacol 1983;3:182-5.

126. Hermesh H, Shalev A, Munitz H. Contribution of adverse drug reaction to admission rates in an acute psychiatric ward. Acta Psychiatr Scand 1985;72:104-10.

127. Stewart RB, Springer PK, Adams JE. Drug-related admissions to an inpatient psychiatric unit. Am J Psychiatry 1980;137:1093-5.

128. Salem RB, Keane TM, Williams JG. Drug-related admissions to a Veterans' Administration psychiatric unit. Drug Intell Clin Pharm 1984;18:74-6.

129. Wolf B, Grohmann R, Schmidt LG, Ruther E. Psychiatric admissions due to adverse drug reactions. Compr Psychiatry 1989;30:534-45.

130. Avorn J, Everitt DE, Weiss S. Increased antidepressant use in patients prescribed beta-blockers. JAMA 1986;255:357-60.

131. Ray WA, Griffin MR, Schaffner W, Baugh DK, Melton LJ. Psychotropic drug use and the risk of hip fracture. N Engl J Med 1987;316:363-9.

132. Fisher S, Bryant SG. Postmarketing surveillance of adverse drug reactions: patient self-monitoring. J Am Board Fam Pract 1992;5:17-25.

133. Fisher S, Bryant SG, Solovitz BL, Kluge RM. Patient-initiated postmarketing surveillance: a validation study. J Clin Pharmacol 1987;27:843-54.

134. Fisher S, Bryant SG. Postmarketing surveillance: accuracy of patient drug attribution judgments. Clin Pharmacol Ther 1990;48:102-7.

135. Bryant SG, Fisher S, Prinsley DM, Olins NJ, Larson DB. Effects of age on reporting of adverse clinical events: results from two postmarketing surveillance methods. Pharmacotherapy 1991;11:249-55.

136. Schmidt LG, Grohmann R, Helmchen H, Langscheid-Schmidt K, Muller-Oerling-hausen B, Poser W, et al. Adverse drug reactions. An epidemiological study at psychiatric hospitals. Acta Psychiatr Scand 1984;70:77-89.

137. Levine J, Schooler N. SAFTEE: a technique for the systematic assessment of side effects in clinical trials. Psychopharmacol Bull 1986;22:343-6.

138. Zito J, Craig TJ, Wanderling JA, Siegel C. SAFTEE-EPI: pilot study of a computerized adverse drug reaction monitoring system. Pharmacoepidemiol Newsl 1987;2:6.

139. Van Putten T. The many faces of akathisia. Compr Psychiatry 1975;16:43-7.

140. Rifkin A, Quitkin F, Klein DF. Akinesia. Arch Gen Psychiatry 1975;32:672-4.

141. Morris HH, Estes ML. Traveler's amnesia. Transient global amnesia secondary to triazolam. JAMA 1987;258:945-6.

142. Wysowski DK, Barash D. Adverse behavioral reactions attributed to triazolam in the Food and Drug Administration's Spontaneous Reporting System. Arch Intern Med 1991;151:2003-8.

143. Bixler EO, Kales A, Manfredi RL, Vgontzas AN, Tyson KL, Kales JD. Triazolam (letter). Lancet 1991;337:1612.

144. Sackett DL. Bias in analytic research. J Chronic Dis 1979;32:51-63.

145. Porta MS. The search for more clinically meaningful research designs: single-patient randomized clinical trials (editorial). J Gen Intern Med 1986;1:418-9.

146. Guyatt G, Sackett D, Taylor DW, Chong J, Roberts R, Pugsley S. Determining optimal therapy—randomized trials in individual patients. N Engl J Med 1986;314: 889-92.

147. Yonkers KA, Kando JC, Cole JO, Blumenthal S. Gender differences in pharmacokinetics and pharmacodynamics of psychotropic medication. Am J Psychiatry 1992; 149:587-95.

148. Gurwitz JH, Col NF, Avorn J. The exclusion of the elderly and women from clinical trials in acute myocardial infarction. JAMA 1992;268:1417-22.

149. Thorogood M, Cowen P, Mann J, Murphy M, Vessey M. Fatal myocardial infarction and use of psychotropic drugs in young women. Lancet 1992;340:1067-8.

150. Pastuszak A, Schick-Boschetto B, Zuber C, Feldkamp M, Pinelli M, Sihn S, et al. Pregnancy outcome following first-trimester exposure to fluoxetine (Prozac). JAMA 1993;269:2246-8.

151. Jacobson SJ, Jones K, Johnson K, Ceolin L, Kaur P, Sahn D, et al. Prospective multicenter study of pregnancy outcome after lithium exposure during first trimester. Lancet 1992;339:530-3.

152. Thomsen IS. Analysis of syndromes using Bayes's formula. Acta Psychiatr Scand 1984;69:143-50.

153. Tancredi L. The rights of mental patients: weighing the interests. J Health Polit Policy Law 1980;5:199-204.

154. Brooks A. The right to refuse antipsychotic medications: law and policy. Rutgers Law Rev 1987;39:339-76.

155. Appelbaum PS. The right to refuse treatment with antipsychotic medications: retrospect and prospect. Am J Psychiatry 1988;145:413-9.

156. Zito JM. Final report of NIMH study RO1MH44688: drug treatment refusal in severe mental illness, June 30, 1993. Unpublished report. Bethesda, MD: National Institute of Mental Health Services Branch, 1993.

157. Siegel C, Alexander MJ, Lin S, Laska E. An alternative to DRGs. A clinically meaningful and cost-reducing approach. Med Care 1986;24:407-17.

158. Consensus conference. Electroconvulsive therapy. JAMA 1985;254:2103-8.

159. NIMH/NIH Consensus Development Conference statement. Mood disorders: pharmacologic prevention of recurrences. Consensus Development Panel. Am J Psychiatry 1985;142:469-76.
160. Rush AJ. Clinical practice guidelines. Good news, bad news, or no news? Arch Gen Psychiatry 1993;50:483-90.
161. Zito JM, Riddle MA. Psychiatric pharmacoepidemiology for children. Child Adolesc Psychiatr Clin North Am 1995;4:77-95.

22

Pharmacoepidemiology and Coronary Heart Disease
Michael A Lewis

Abstract

Coronary heart disease (CHD) is one of the most prevalent conditions in industrialized nations. Consequently, the use of medications directed at the prevention and treatment of this condition is, particularly in the elderly, extremely high. Observational studies have established independent and treatable risk factors for CHD, such as hypertension and hypercholesterolemia. However, primary prevention trials have not shown the reductions in CHD that would be expected from the risk reductions achieved with drug treatment of risk factors. Clinical trials of acute myocardial infarction and secondary prevention trials, on the other hand, have shown the benefits of specific medications and have changed the conventions for acute and secondary treatments of this condition. This chapter begins with the risk factors for CHD and the pros and cons of their treatment with specific agents, and highlights the agents currently thought to be beneficial for the treatment of advanced stages of CHD. The chapter concludes with an appraisal of changes in therapeutic strategies due to the results of epidemiologic studies, and addresses the cost/benefit relationships of modern treatments.

The three arteries on which the heart depends for its blood supply have become the focus of immense healthcare efforts. The patency of these arteries and thus the ventricular function of the heart itself are threatened by the development of atherosclerotic plaques on the arterial wall. These plaques narrow the lumen of the coronary arteries and lead to coronary heart disease (CHD) or ischemic heart disease, which is characterized by reduced cardiac function and eventually by chest pain, also known as angina pectoris. The progression of atherogenesis, a process related to both aging and the presence of specific predisposing factors, might lead to the formation of a thrombus at the site of an atherosclerotic plaque.[1] This sudden obstruction is the most frequent cause of acute myocardial infarction (AMI), an event that is often fatal. The ensuing lack of oxygen and nutrients results in tissue death within the affected area if the obstruction is not removed.

Survival and future prognosis depend on the quantity and the location of heart tissue destroyed. AMI is frequently associated with a reduced function of the heart as a whole, either for reasons of sheer tissue destruction and cardiac muscle insufficiency, or because important transmission pathways are interrupted, causing arrhythmias. The prevention, treatment, and prognosis of AMI, either with or without medications, have been major focuses of cardiovascular epidemiology. A discussion pertaining to the factors influencing CHD development and the drug treatment available for the prevention and treatment of AMI follows.

Epidemiology of Coronary Heart Disease

CHD is the leading cause of death worldwide, but mortality rates vary widely by country.[2-4] In the US, approximately 30% of deaths, or 600 000 per year, are due to CHD. Although at younger ages this condition primarily afflicts men, CHD seems to be increasing in women.[5] Because the percentage of persons over age 65—especially over 85—is increasing in most industrialized countries more rapidly than other age groups,[6] and because CHD is closely related to aging, this condition will become even more prevalent in the future. Consequently, CHD will require large investments in medical care and drug treatments.

Specifically in the US, CHD mortality as measured by official mortality statistics had escalated to epidemic proportions from the beginning of the century, peaking in the mid-1960s. It has since declined by 42% (age adjusted) from 1963 to 1985.[7] The reasons for the increase and for the decline are not precisely known. The deficiencies perceived with official statistics, which might be influenced by revisions of the *International Classification of Diseases*, changes or differences in diagnostic customs, coding customs, and the single-cause coding procedure,[2,3] have led to the development of methodologies designed to improve the understanding of factors that might influence the course of CHD.

Observational studies, such as the Framingham Heart Study,[8] were the first to address the role of risk factors in the development of CHD. Large primary intervention trials, for example, the Multiple Risk Factor Intervention Trial (MRFIT), have sought to assess the influence of risk factor reduction.[9] Population-based studies, such as the Minnesota Heart Study,[10] and studies based on hospital discharge records in Worcester,[11] have led to an understanding of trends in AMI and general medical care. Large monitoring and cohort studies have been established to investigate the long-term influences of risk factors and treatments. The ongoing multinational Monitoring of Trends and Determinants in Cardiovascular Disease (MONICA) Project[5,12] is planned for 10 years in 26 countries and combines survey and AMI register studies to determine the association between population risk factor levels and attack or incidence rates of AMI. It also includes a medical care component to assess the impact of treatment changes on trends in AMI case fatality. The comprehensive, US-based Atherosclerotic Risk in Communities (ARIC) Study focuses on the development of atherosclerosis[13] and investigates the atherosclerotic status and risk of a cohort of 16 000 probands in four US communities.

Population monitoring and drug utilization cohorts with follow-up studies might, in the long run, be able to address questions of the effectiveness of cardiovascular drug use on a cumulative scale. These observational studies may not be adequate to establish small benefits of preventive, acute, and secondary treatments because they are prone to uncontrolled confounding and are unable to establish treatment effects. The current focus of research efforts lies on drug efficacy, which is best established by an experimental approach: the randomized, controlled trial.[14]

Since the effects to be observed are small and because, as a rule in epidemiology, a single study is not conclusive, two new approaches have been developed. Particularly for AMI treatments, large, simple clinical trials that provide data on a large number of patients are conducted on a multicentric basis.[15] Examples are the International Study of Infarct Survival (ISIS)[16] and the Gruppo Italiano per lo Studio della Streptochinasi nell'Infarto Miocardico (GISSI) trial series.[17] This approach assumes that specific characteristics of patients can be neglected in favor of large numbers. The difficulty might be the introduction of an unknown variation in the study population that is not reflected in the association between exposure and outcome. The advantages are that they make clinical trials more feasible, more comparable, and possibly more realistic because they provide a better reflection of clinical practice.

The second approach is the meta-analysis of the results of several smaller studies that have investigated the same exposures with the same outcomes.[18] The summary results of these meta-analyses provide an odds ratio with much tighter confidence intervals than any of the individual studies, so that a clear direction of treatment effect—if one is present—is obtained. This technique has received much criticism, but it has established a firm position as a valuable objective descriptive method.[18] The difficulties of comparing studies with different design details are obvious. Another serious limitation is the potential for publication bias, which may begin with an author's unwillingness to write up a study yielding a "null" or contradictory result and end with journals declining to publish information they deem unimportant. The introduction of large, multicenter simple clinical trials offsets this disadvantage, because the results of these expensive studies will be published. When the specific circumstances and caveats are kept in mind, both methods supply a basis for medical decision-making that would otherwise be left to the intuition of the individual practitioner. A future direction is the development of methodologies and databases to facilitate cumulative meta-analyses that can provide timely and scientifically supported treatment advice to clinicians.[19]

Risk Factors for Coronary Heart Disease

Primary prevention has been directed at the control of the major risk factors: hypertension, hypercholesterolemia, and smoking. Although other influences and lifestyle factors have been identified, these three still constitute the main factors that might be treated medically.

HYPERTENSION

Arterial hypertension is common in all industrialized countries, and its prevalence approaches or exceeds 50% in the elderly.[20] The benefits of medical treatment of malignant hypertension in uncontrolled studies were so pronounced that randomized trials appeared neither necessary nor desirable.[21] Treatment of severe hypertension with diastolic blood pressures over 115 mm Hg also appears beneficial, particularly for stroke prevention.[22] Although most studies have demonstrated that diastolic blood pressure above 90 mm Hg is positively and independently associated with the primary incidence of stroke and CHD,[23] the benefits of treatment of mild-to-moderate hypertension with a diastolic blood pressure between 90 and 114 mm Hg are still not clearly established.[24] Apart from its role as a risk factor for CHD, mild hypertension causes no discomfort, and its treatment is in fact associated with such adverse effects as hypotension and impotence, which tend to reduce the overall quality of life. However, current recommendations advocate the treatment of mild hypertension in acknowledgment of its etiologic association with CHD.[25]

Angiotensin-converting enzyme (ACE) inhibitors, beta-blockers, calcium-channel blockers, peripheral alpha$_1$-adrenergic receptor blockers, and thiazide diuretics are used in hypertension treatment.[26,27] Of these, ACE inhibitors, beta-blockers, and calcium-channel blockers have additional cardiovascular treatment indications. The ACE inhibitor captopril is primarily a vasodilating agent indicated initially for congestive heart failure and hypertension,[28] particularly in the elderly.[29] Beta-blockers comprise two groups of structurally similar drugs: those that inhibit all beta-receptors (beta$_1$- and beta$_2$-; noncardioselective) and those that block only beta$_1$-receptors (cardioselective).[30] The cardioselective beta-blockers are particularly useful for the treatment of CHD, hypertension, and arrhythmias. The major calcium-channel blockers nifedipine, verapamil, and diltiazem rank among the 10 best-selling drugs in the US and are used for treatment of hypertension and angina pectoris.[31] Observational studies have found an increase in mortality related to calcium-channel blocker use among patients with CHD, so this drug group may not be appropriate for that indication.[32,33]

A "stepped-care" approach has been recommended widely as an empiric method for the treatment of hypertension.[25] This approach encourages the use of diuretics or beta-blockers as initial monotherapy for hypertension and has become largely accepted in clinical practice, as evidenced by drug utilization studies showing diuretics and beta-blockers to be the most frequently prescribed drugs for hypertension.[34,35] However, the worldwide trend toward an increase in the use of ACE inhibitors indicates the rapid acceptance of new treatment venues.[36-40] Because of their efficacy as monotherapy, ACE inhibitors are currently considered one of the first-line drugs for hypertension treatment. Despite the stepped-care guidelines, treatment patterns show wide international variations. Thus, hypertension is more likely to be treated with drugs in Northern Ireland than in Norway or Sweden.[41] Beta-blockers are preferred in Sweden as first choice, whereas thiazides are preferred in Northern Ireland and Norway. In Germany, physicians begin treatment at higher levels of diastolic blood pressure than in the US, and clearly prefer beta-blockers as step-one therapy for young patients, while prescribing diuretics for the majority of older patients.[42]

In the US, the preference for hypertension treatment in the elderly has shifted from beta-blockers to calcium-channel blockers.[43] Beta-blocking drugs can reduce the risk of coronary and cerebrovascular disease in the older patient with hypertension, but should probably be used in smaller doses than those prescribed in younger patients.[27] The net effect on the prevention of hypertensive complications, including CHD, appears to be independent of the agent used.[44]

Although drug therapy slows progression in the severity of hypertension, it does not seem to have had the expected impact on coronary outcomes.[45] The results of observational studies suggest that a lowering of diastolic blood pressure by 5–6 mm Hg in the general population should reduce CHD by 25–40%.[23] However, primary prevention trials showed only a statistically nonsignificant 10% reduction in CHD morbidity and mortality.[45] The Oslo Study[46] found that the CHD mortality rate at 10 years was significantly greater in the drug-treated group than in the untreated control group. Even a meta-analysis of 14 unconfounded randomized trials of antihypertensive drugs (chiefly diuretics or beta-blockers) with a 5–6 mm Hg reduction in diastolic blood pressure showed that fatal and nonfatal CHD was reduced by only 14% (p < 0.01), with a nonsignificant reduction of 11% for fatal CHD.[47] This corresponds to only half the epidemiologically expected CHD reduction. The clearest indication for antihypertensive treatment seems to be a sufficiently high risk of stroke.[27,47] The cause for the unexpectedly slight effect of hypertension treatment is not entirely clear. It may be explained partly by the adverse effect of diuretics and beta-adrenergic blockers, for example, on both lipid and carbohydrate metabolism.[48,49] Although beta-blockers were shown to reduce platelet activity[50] and endothelial permeability for lipoproteins, and to reduce the influx of calcium into the plaque,[51] their role in primary prevention is not clear.[52] The adverse lipid effects observed with thiazide diuretics are theoretically large enough to reduce the CHD preventive effect by almost 50%. In recognition of their lack of adverse lipid effects and their tolerability, first-line therapy with alpha$_1$-adrenoreceptor inhibitors,[53,54] ACE inhibitors, and calcium-channel blockers has become increasingly common,[6] although the use of the latter in patients with CHD is being reassessed because of a suspicion of increased mortality.[32,33]

Awareness of the need to treat hypertension, because of its association with CHD, has increased the prevalence of hypertension treatment. This treatment and the availability of more expensive drugs have substantially increased the drug costs associated with treating hypertension.[55] In Germany, about two-thirds of the increased cost of treating hypertension is caused by changing prescription patterns.[56] A cost-effectiveness analysis of treating mild hypertension showed that the net healthcare benefits, measured in quality-adjusted life years, ranged from –2 days (a net negative effect of treatment) to 64 days in men and from –18 days to 35 days in women.[57] Diuretic monotherapy was still found to be the most cost-effective, followed by beta-blockers and then ACE inhibitors. Depending on the mode of payment, the increased cost of treatment with these newer drugs will have an impact on the patient, on her or his willingness to be treated, and on compliance.[55] On the other hand, a relatively inexpensive drug such as reserpine, which might be as effective as the new drugs, has remained largely unresearched, in part because of a spurious and since-refuted association with breast cancer.[58-60] The newest recommendations for the treatment of hypertension[25] have been criticized because they do not include new drugs, such as ACE inhibitors,[39] and because they neglect the use of old drugs.[58]

HYPERCHOLESTEROLEMIA

Abnormalities in plasma lipoprotein metabolism play a central role in the pathogenesis of atherosclerosis. These conditions are genetically determined and range from patients with a retarded clearance of plasma low-density lipoprotein (LDL) cholesterol to the most severe form of homozygous familial hypercholesterolemia. The primary indicators for an increased cardiovascular risk are an elevated total cholesterol with an increased plasma concentration of LDL and a reduced concentration of high-density lipoprotein (HDL) cholesterol. The most prevalent condition is primary moderate hypercholesterolemia characterized by a plasma total cholesterol concentration above 6.2 mmol/L (240 mg/dL) and an LDL-cholesterol concentration above 4.14 mmol/L (160 mg/dL).[61] It is estimated that about 25% of the American population aged 20–74 years have serum cholesterol concentrations of 6.21 mmol/L or greater.[62] Despite some inconsistencies in the results of trials and observational studies, it has become widely accepted that lowering cholesterol also reduces the risk of CHD.[63] Because of the association found between raised serum cholesterol concentrations and an increased risk of CHD in epidemiologic studies and animal experiments, various working groups have advocated a reduced intake of saturated fat and cholesterol for the general population.[64,65]

The most commonly used hypolipidemic agents are the fibric acids, which include clofibrate, gemfibrocil, fenofibrate, and bezafibrate. They lower total cholesterol concentrations only moderately (~10–20%), but they are generally well tolerated.[66] The bile acid sequestrants cholestyramine and colestipol lower plasma cholesterol concentrations by 15–30%. Niacin, in turn, suppresses the hepatic synthesis of lipoprotein and may also have an effect on reducing cardiovascular mortality.[67] However, many patients do not tolerate bile acid sequestrants or niacin very well, so that their usefulness as cholesterol-lowering agents is limited. Hydroxymethylglutaryl-coenzyme A (HMG-CoA) reductase inhibitors, such as lovastatin, simvastatin, and pravastatin, markedly reduce the concentrations of LDL cholesterol in patients with primary moderate or severe hypercholesterolemia and also appear to raise HDL.[61,68] Although no important short-term adverse effects have been reported, lovastatin may predispose to myopathy if given in combination with cyclosporin, gemfibrozil, or niacin,[61] and it is recommended for the severe familial or nonfamilial forms of hypercholesterolemia. Unless total cholesterol concentrations are high, attempts to raise low concentrations of HDL cholesterol should be restricted to lifestyle changes, such as smoking cessation, exercise, and weight loss.[69] The first-line drugs are bile acid sequestrants or niacin.[62] The treatment goal is an LDL cholesterol concentration below 3.36 mmol/L (130 mg/dL); treatment failures by other means constitute a fair indication for HMG-CoA reductase inhibitors. The rapidly increasing use of lovastatin suggests that in practice the indication of HMG-CoA reductase inhibitors is not restricted to these recommendations.

Several primary prevention trials have been undertaken to establish the effect of treatment in comparison with an untreated group, beginning with early dietary interventions[70] and including lipid-lowering agents such as clofibrate,[71] colestipol,[72] cholestyramine,[73] and gemfibrozil.[66] The majority of these trials were conducted on middle-aged white men. The Helsinki Heart Study,[66] the major study using the fibric acid gemfibrozil, showed a 34% lower risk of definite CHD among men who were assigned active treatment, compared with the placebo group. The major study to investigate the effects of the bile acid sequestrant cholestyramine is the Lipid Research Clinics Coronary Primary Prevention Trial,[73] a randomized, double-blind study that showed a significant difference in myocardial infarction rates in the treatment group. The degree of cholesterol reduction was proportional to the dosage, and the best results were achieved for patients who fully complied with the study regimen. A randomized, controlled trial of three treatments in high-risk men with increased LDL and a family history of heart disease showed that (1) conservative dietary treatment was less effective than medication and (2) a combination of either niacin or lovastatin with colestipol slows the progression of coronary artery lesions by more than 30%.[74]

Although the large primary prevention trials have shown that the incidence of CHD events was reduced, only one found a reduction in mortality from heart disease. Several studies have shown excess deaths from accidents and suicides in the treatment groups. Despite nearly 120 000 patient-years under treatment and control conditions and a reduction of CHD mortality ($p = 0.04$), meta-analysis of primary intervention trials fails to show improvement of overall mortality.[75] Another meta-analysis suggests that cholesterol lowering in itself is beneficial and attributes adverse effects to fibrinates and hormones.[76] However, the significant association between cholesterol reduction and deaths from such causes as suicide, accidents, and other forms of violence shown in both medical and dietary control studies remains a puzzle. Since data exist on the association between a low serum cholesterol concentration and violent social behavior in animals and humans, this aspect would require further attention. The lack of effect on total mortality and the increases in noncardiovascular mortality in some treatment groups have caused serious concern about the use of cholesterol-lowering drugs.[77] Nonetheless, drug treatment of hypercholesterolemia has risen dramatically in the US from 1978 to 1988.[78] Estimates from 13 million prescription sales indicate a minimum of 1 million Americans under drug treatment in 1988, with the leading drug being lovastatin, closely followed by gemfibrozil. Similar developments have taken place in the UK.[77] In the

US, 25% of the population could thus become subject to treatment.[62] Although lipid lowering might reduce the number of incident events and thus the costs associated with their treatment, the growing consensus is that lipid-lowering drugs should be reserved for individuals with severe hypercholesterolemia who are at high risk of CHD.[79,80]

CIGARETTE SMOKING

Nicotine abuse is one of the modifiable CHD risk factors, and part of the recent decline of CHD mortality in the US is attributed to the reduction of smokers in the population. Nicotine stimulates the sympathetic nervous system, increases vascular tone, increases platelet aggregation and plasma fibrinogen concentrations, and has an unfavorable effect on the lipid profile.[81] Smoking 20 cigarettes a day approximately doubles the risk of CHD.[82] Besides being independent risk factors, nicotine and high cholesterol tend to interact. Thus, cigarette-smoking adults experience a fall in HDL of more than 6 mg/dL, which is not explained by other factors, whereas the HDL fraction rises in individuals who quit smoking.[83] Other lipoprotein fractions do not seem to be affected. Intervention strategies are directed at quitting the smoking habit. Medications developed to aid in smoking cessation include nicotine gum and sustained-release nicotine transdermal patches. These medications, however, do not provide treatment of the addiction to nicotine. During their administration, they have the same cardiovascular disadvantages as cigarette smoking, and they might themselves provoke a coronary event.

CONTRACEPTION/HORMONE SUBSTITUTION

The use of any oral contraceptive agent increases the risk of venous thromboembolism by about a factor of four, from 1 in 10 000 women-years to 4 in 10 000 women-years, and an increased risk of AMI and stroke has also been suspected. Although ethinyl estradiol is thought to be the responsible agent, the results of major case–control studies comparing progestagens indicate that the more recently introduced progestagens are associated with a slightly higher risk of venous thromboembolism compared with progestagens that have been on the market for a longer length of time.[84,85] Because of possible influences of diagnostic and prescribing habits and attrition of susceptible persons in treatment cohorts, these studies also address potential biases affecting observational research. On the other hand, the more recently introduced progestagens appear to be associated with a lower risk of AMI.[86]

Most studies on postmenopausal women indicate that their risk of AMI increases compared with the premenopausal status. One study states that this is only true for surgically induced menopause, where the increased risk may be removed by use of replacement estrogens.[87] In its 10-year follow-up, the Nurses' Health Study[88] concludes that women with postmeno-pausal estrogen use have 44% less risk of major CHD than a comparable group of untreated women. The ARIC Study has shown that the combined use of progestin and estrogen is associated with an even more favorable lipid profile than estrogen use alone and additionally influences hemostatic factors favorably.[89] Based on the improved lipid profile and fibrinogen reduction, the estimate of CHD risk reduction from this study is 42%, with an additional benefit potentially derived from a decrease in the factor VII concentrations found for estrogen–progestin users. Postmenopausal hormone replacement therapy therefore has the potential of significantly reducing the risk of CHD in older women.

ALCOHOL

There has been a suspicion that moderate alcohol consumption may be protective against ischemic heart disease.[90] This effect was noted in the Nurses' Health Study, showing a 70% risk reduction for CHD, with a slight increase in subarachnoid hemorrhage among 34- to 59-year-old nurses.[91] On the other hand, a cohort study of 7735 men aged 40–59 years in England attributed the reduced risk of ischemic heart disease among light drinkers to the lower prevalence of concomitant risk factors, such as smoking and hypertension, in this group.[92] Other studies have consistently shown alcohol use to be associated with elevated blood pressure in what appears to be a causal relationship.[93] However, even after adjustment for known cardiac risk factors, a very large study of 51 529 health professionals aged 40–75 years showed an inverse relationship between alcohol consumption and the risk of CHD.[94] This 10-year retrospective study with a 2-year prospective follow-up showed a clear dose relationship with a multivariate risk of 0.57 (95% CI 0.35 to 0.79) for individuals who consumed more than 50 g of alcohol a day, and the study still showed significant reduction in CHD risk at 10–15 g, the equivalent of one glass of wine. The action of alcohol is thought to be due to the associated rise in HDL cholesterol. Although it was argued that alcohol raises only HDL-3 subfractions, both subfractions 2 and 3 were found to be protective.[95] An overall protective effect can, of course, be assumed only for moderate alcohol consumption. The hazards of alcoholism are well known and would offset any cardioprotective effect.

Preventing the Acute Event in High-Risk Patients

The medications used in treatment of AMI are directed at symptomatic relief, but they have increasingly been studied with a view toward preventing AMI. The drugs used primarily in the treatment of angina pectoris include nitrates,[19] calcium-channel blockers,[34,96] beta-blockers,[97] and ACE inhibitors.[98] Platelet aggregation inhibitors, particularly aspirin, play a special role in the prevention of thrombi that cause AMI.

Calcium-channel blockers reduce vasospasm that might lead to AMI, and they significantly reduce myocardial oxygen demand, render cells more resistant to ischemia, inhibit epinephrine-induced platelet aggregation, and might reduce atherogenesis.[99] On the whole, however, the anti-ischemic effects of calcium-channel blockers are controversial, and safety issues have been raised for this group in observational studies.[32,33] For beta-blockers, studies have shown a 13% reduction of AMI in patients with unstable angina but no reduction of cardiac mortality.[97] On the other hand, one study has shown a positive effect on survival for hospitalized AMI patients who had regularly received beta-blockers before the event,[100] so that the role of beta-blockers in the prevention of and death from AMI still needs further research. While the ACE inhibitor enalapril was shown to reduce overall deaths and hospitalizations for heart failure significantly in comparison with both placebo[101] and nitrate,[102] there is also some evidence that use of enalapril may be associated with a reduction in deaths due to AMI[101] and particularly of sudden death.[102] A variation found in the gene encoding ACE may be associated with CHD, so that circulating ACE can serve as an indicator for AMI risk independently of the presence of classical risk factors.[103]

The role of the platelet aggregation inhibitor aspirin (acetylsalicylic acid) in reducing the risk of AMI has been recognized, and its role has become increasingly certain.[104,105] Unintended drug effects (UDE) associated with aspirin use are gastrointestinal bleeding[106] and, very rarely, the induction of Reye's syndrome in children and even adults during viral illness.[107] Clinically, dosages of 80–325 mg daily or every other day have been proven to be effective, preceded by a loading dose of 160 mg for maximum platelet inhibition.[105,108,109] Other platelet aggregation inhibitors do not appear to have significant advantages for the prevention of AMI. Thus, neither dipyridamole nor sulfinpyrazone has been conclusively shown to prevent stroke or AMI when used singly. Ticlopidine is a more potent platelet inhibitor than aspirin, but it is considerably more expensive and might produce severe, reversible neutropenia (<1%), diarrhea (20%), skin rash (14%), and increases in total cholesterol in 9% of those treated.[110]

The reduction of AMI risk was so pronounced in the treatment group (RR 0.56; 95% CI 0.45 to 0.70) that the aspirin component of the Physicians' Health Study[111] was prematurely terminated. Several smaller studies have also documented the effectiveness of low-dose aspirin.[112] In addition, aspirin has been implicated in reducing the risk of fatal colon cancer.[113] On the other hand, a large British trial similar to the Physicians' Health Study showed no reduction of AMI risk in the aspirin-treated group.[114] Alternate-day aspirin therapy has been shown to prevent myocardial infarction (MI) in patients with chronic stable angina and is associated with an 87% reduction in the risk for MI.[104] These studies indicate that aspirin is effective in the primary prevention of heart attacks.[105,115]

The onset of AMI exhibits a daytime distribution pattern, with a peak occurrence during the morning hours.[116] It may also have a weekly variation.[117] Several studies have shown peaks of MI incidence around 9 am. This is attributed to such factors as early morning blood pressure increases, enhanced platelet aggregability, and decreased fibrinolytic activity.[81] The circadian phenomenon has led to the development of the concept of "triggering" events, acute risks that contribute to AMI and that might be eliminated with the appropriate medication on a 24-hour basis.[118] In particular, patients treated with beta-blockers did not exhibit the early morning peak incidence.[119,120] Studies on alterations of circadian patterns through medications are directed at determining the appropriate timing and form of medication intake to reduce the incidence of AMI during the high-risk early morning period.[121] However, the majority of studies on circadian AMI patterns are conducted on hospitalized patients and do not include the sizable group of out-of-hospital fatal events.

To summarize primary prevention, the impact of drug therapy on the natural history of CHD has been disappointing. Although excesses of such risk factors as hypertension and hypercholesterolemia are detected in some cases, a reduction of risk factors is not paralleled by a reduction of events, so that the optimistic view on risk factor intervention is being replaced by a more critical perspective.[122] Full risk factor prevention would turn a large percentage of the healthy population into patients, at substantial cost to health service systems.[77] The long-term use of drugs as preventive measures should be reserved for those high-risk groups in whom at least a short-term balance of benefit has been shown by controlled trials.[79,123] In addition, the single-factor approach toward risk treatment needs to be replaced by one that considers both the desired effect and the potential adverse effects induced by the drug on other risk factors.

Treatment of Acute Myocardial Infarction

The major end point of coronary heart disease is AMI, which is associated with a high case fatality. Approximately 55% of patients aged 25–74 years do not survive this event.[124,125] It is found that 30% of all AMI patients never reach the hospital and that the majority of deaths occur within the first hour after the infarct. This emphasizes the need for primary prevention, the need for research on triggering mechanisms of AMI, and the need for research on treatments that could be provided on site by care providers to support the patient before he or she reaches the hospital. Besides support of general function and rhythm control, the treatment of AMI is directed at the immediate limitation of infarct size.[126] This implies that the patient must arrive at a treatment site as soon as possible after coronary artery occlusion has occurred, making timing an important treatment factor to consider. The time of application has been shown to be important for beta-blockers, for which the ISIS-1 trial showed benefit only if given within the first 48 hours,[16] and particularly for thrombolysis, where administration is generally restricted to the period within the first 6 hours after onset of AMI. The major acute treatments are beta-blocking agents[16,127]; thrombolysis[17]; and intravenous nitrates, aspirin, and anticoagulants.[128] Treatment with intravenous magnesium has gained attention.[129]

BETA-BLOCKERS

The benefit of early intravenous treatment with beta-blockers is fairly well established. It is estimated that 200 patients need to be treated with a beta-blocker to avoid one early death, one early reinfarction, and one early cardiac arrest.[16] Thus, hospital patients treated for AMI with a beta-blocker (atenolol) showed a 15% lower case fatality than did the placebo group, and most of the benefit was found within the first day of treatment. Compared with most preventive strategies, the cost/benefit relationship of acute treatment with beta-blockers is very good.

THROMBOLYTIC THERAPY

The most common agents used to recanalize a thrombotic artery are streptokinase, urokinase, alteplase, and anistreplase.[130-132] All these agents activate the fibrinolytic system of the blood, acting as plasminogen activators that in turn break up the blood clot in the occluded artery. Controlled clinical trials in patients with AMI have demonstrated that intravenously administered thrombolytic agents, such as streptokinase,[17] anisoylated plasminogen streptokinase activator complex (anistreplase), and recombinant tissue plasminogen activator (alteplase),[133] recanalize occluded arteries, reduce the size of the infarct, improve ventricular function, and reduce early mortality if given within the first 6 hours after the event. Whereas streptokinase is not a new drug and is fairly inexpensive, alteplase is new and expensive. The advantages of alteplase, which affect only a very small proportion of patients, are probably too small to offset its cost, which in 1988 was 10 times that of streptokinase (and was 7 times higher in 1993[134]) and could not be incorporated in the fee charged for uncomplicated MI in the US under normal, nontrial conditions.[135] Major adverse effects are hemorrhages into the necrotic area of the heart, which convert ischemic into hemorrhagic infarcts and may result in myocardial rupture. This does not seem to occur more frequently in patients treated with alteplase compared with an untreated group.[133] Studies on adverse effects comparing different agents vary. Whereas in one study the incidence rates of adverse-specific bleeding 24 hours or 96 hours after administration of streptokinase versus alteplase appear to be similar,[136] other studies show significantly higher rates of cerebral bleeding with alteplase (0.7%) than with streptokinase (0.3%; $p < 0.0001$).[137] A further complication that might occur is the primary resistance to recanalization (in 15–50% of patients) or the reocclusion of the coronary artery after successful thrombolysis in 5–15% of patients. Because the infusion of the thrombolytic agents itself has a procoagulant effect and the traumatized segment of the vessel wall is particularly sensitive to reocclusion, a single therapeutic approach is probably not optimal.[138] A comparison of adjunctive therapy of thrombolysis, specifically alteplase with heparin and with low-dose aspirin, has shown that 82% of the heparin-treated group maintained arterial patency compared with only 52% of the aspirin-treated group,[139] so that adjunctive heparin seems recommendable. The recent Global Utilization of Streptokinase and Tissue Plasminogen Activator for Occluded Coronary Arteries (GUSTO) trial, which included 41 000 patients in four treatment groups, has confirmed this approach and has shown a slight advantage of recombinant alteplase over streptokinase, with an estimated saving of six lives in 1000 treatments.[134] Only borderline effects of thrombolysis on long-term survival were shown in one population-based register study of patients after AMI.[140]

ASPIRIN

In the acute treatment of AMI, aspirin alone was found to reduce cardiovascular mortality by 23% compared with a placebo group.[141] When aspirin is given in addition to the thrombolytic agent streptokinase, mortality in the treated group was reduced by 42%. In the aspirin-treated group, the risk of reinfarction and nonfatal stroke is significantly reduced by 50% without association with any significant increase in cerebral hemorrhage. Thus, aspirin and streptokinase appear to have an additive effect.

NITRATES

Nitrates are vasodilators that improve myocardial perfusion and usually provide prompt symptomatic relief of angina pectoris.[142] Although no single study on the administration of intravenous nitrates—either nitroprusside or nitroglycerin—has been very persuasive, a meta-analysis of these studies showed a reduction of mortality of about 35% compared with the untreated groups.[143] This is considerably greater than the benefit achieved with other drug groups. The basis of action is again the limitation of infarct size by reduction of myocardial oxygen demand.

CALCIUM-CHANNEL BLOCKERS

The results of studies on the treatment of AMI with calcium-channel blockers have been largely disappointing. None of the randomized trials on nifedipine has shown a benefit from use of nifedipine in terms of mortality reduction or reduction of creatinine kinase MB band, a cardiac enzyme the concentration of which is associated with infarct size.[144,145] The Trial of Early Nifedipine Treatment (TRENT) Study was terminated prematurely because the mortality was 10.2% for nifedipine and 9.2% for the placebo group.[145] There is mounting evidence from observational studies that calcium-channel blockers are not appropriate for acute or chronic treatment of patients with CHD or AMI.[32,33,140]

Compared with the effects found in primary prevention, the effects established for acute treatment of AMI have been more positive. The results of clinical trials have been instrumental in shaping currently accepted treatments that seem to be rapidly integrated into clinical practice. This is shown best by the increased use of antiplatelet drugs, beta-blockers, and fibrinolytic drugs over time, but it is also shown by the reduced use of calcium-channel blockers.[146-148] These developments also show that trials and clinical pharmacoepidemiology have achieved a firm position within the practice of medicine. Because of the severity of the condition, UDEs in medications used for the acute treatment of AMI are only a secondary consideration, unless they are included as an outcome. This is the case, for example, in the studies on streptokinase or aspirin, in which hemorrhage is an expected pharmacologic problem.[141] However, even large, simple clinical trials could not include the numbers of patients required to detect and attribute completely unexpected, rare type B events.

Secondary Prevention

The long-term survival of patients with AMI following discharge from the hospital is poorer than that of a comparable sample of the general population.[149] This survival disadvantage is most pronounced within the first year after the event. As in acute-phase treatments, the majority of studies examining the effect of medications on long-term survival and reinfarction are randomized, controlled trials in which a treatment group is compared with a nontreatment or placebo group. Compared with the hospital-based trials, these follow-up trials are much more prone to bias because of compliance, concomitant drug treatments, and additional morbidity, so that actual drug effects might be difficult to ascertain. On the other hand, "clean" follow-up trials might ascertain a drug effect, but this might be applicable only to a very restricted population, not to post-AMI patients as a whole.

BETA-BLOCKERS

An overview of follow-up studies including about 20 000 post-AMI patients shows a 20% reduction of mortality within the first 2–3 years under beta-blockade, and a similar reduction was found for the rate of reinfarction.[97] The beta-blockers successfully used in secondary prevention trials were timolol, propranolol, and metoprolol. Metoprolol is the most commonly used beta-blocker in secondary prevention, as found in population-based studies,[150] and beta-blockade is associated with a significant improvement in long-term survival.[140]

ANGIOTENSIN-CONVERTING ENZYME INHIBITORS

Recent studies have shown this drug group to be useful in post-AMI treatment for the prevention of ventricular dilatation in response to myocardial damage (remodeling), where its influence on the ejection fraction was better than that of diuretic treatment alone.[151] Both captopril and enalapril also reduce ventricular arrhythmias by reducing plasma norepinephrine and increasing serum and total body potassium.[152] There are as yet too few studies to adequately assess the role of ACE inhibitors in either primary or secondary prophylaxis of AMI; nonetheless, current developments in clinical use show that their indication is being expanded to encompass postinfarction treatment even in the absence of conclusive evidence.[153] Furthermore, captopril given after AMI was found to reduce both total and cardiovascular mortality significantly in a randomized trial on a selected group of 2231 patients.[154] A similar but nonsignificant trend was found for enalapril.[155,156]

ASPIRIN

It is estimated that the administration of low doses of aspirin for 1 month prevents 2.5 deaths and 1–2 nonfatal reinfarctions or strokes for every 100 patients with suspected MI.[141] Individual studies have shown benefits with regard to reinfarction and total mortality ranging from 5% to 50%.[140] The advantage of aspirin over anticoagulation therapy is the lower cost, ease of administration, and less need for monitoring.[115]

CALCIUM-CHANNEL BLOCKERS

The most prevalent calcium-channel blocker, nifedipine, had no significant effect on survival or reinfarction rates within 10 months after the onset of the event in two placebo-controlled trials.[157,158] In fact, an overview showed that the relative risk of death for patients treated with calcium-channel blockers is about 6% higher than that for the untreated groups.[97] No influence was seen for diltiazem on overall mortality,[159] but a reduced reinfarction rate was found in the subgroup of patients with non-Q-wave AMI (5.2% in the treated vs. 9.3% in the untreated group).[160] A reduced rate of reinfarction was also found for verapamil, but total mortality was not significantly reduced.[161] The results of observational studies have suggested that nifedipine in particular may be associated with an increased risk of death when used in treating patients after AMI.[33,140] Although a long-term effect of calcium antagonists on atherosclerosis might be perceived only for longer study periods, the current results are not in favor of calcium antagonists.

ANTIARRHYTHMIC AGENTS

Especially in patients after MI, asymptomatic ventricular ectopic depolarizations are associated with an increased probability of cardiac arrest.[162] One of the most startling results of standard treatment in past years was published by the Cardiac Arrhythmia Suppression Trial (CAST) investigators[163] on the Class I antiarrhythmic agents encainide and flecainide after MI. Contrary to the general assumption, users of these drugs were found to be at an increased risk of death, so that it now appears inappropriate to treat any patient with asymptomatic ventricular arrhythmia, as was the rule before the CAST. This is a clear example of a single, important study's influence on policy (the Food and Drug Administration restricted the use of these agents) and treatment conventions almost immediately. It also illustrates clearly the importance of outcome-oriented surveillance of treatments for specific conditions and for accepted treatment conventions. The CAST investigators were unable to explain the mechanism underlying the excess mortality with flecainide and encainide. Design faults based on disregard of elimination, intoxication, or lack of active drug were largely discounted by the investigators.[163-165] The major adverse effects of antiarrhythmic agents are proarrhythmias (the drugs themselves increase the risk of arryhthmias) and sleep disturbances. Although numerous antiarrhythmic agents are available, the likelihood of a good response is approximately 50% for the most effective (flecainide), and tolerance tends to be poor.[166] Smaller prospective trials have shown that amiodarone for asymptomatic complex arrhythmias decreases mortality in the first year after MI.[167] Post-AMI magnesium treatment was associated with a 55% higher 1-year incidence of cardiac events than was a placebo group, so this form of treatment is not recommended at present.[168]

NITRATES

The vast majority of post-AMI patients are treated with nitrates,[150,169] but data on the effect of nitrates in secondary prophylaxis are sparse. One study found that survival of cardiac patients treated with nitrates is improved compared with that of untreated patients.[170] However, studies showing a definite advantage of long-term, post-AMI nitrate therapy still need to be performed.

Secondary prevention is directed at a high-risk population of postinfarct patients, and has become a focus of large trials. Trials involving follow-up are subject to response and compliance problems. The compliance problem has resulted in two evaluation approaches, that is, the "intention-to-treat" and the "fastidious" or "per protocol" approaches.[14] The intention-to-treat approach implies that all patients take their medications as directed, regardless of compliance. This would come closest to reflecting the effect of a drug within a general population (effectiveness), but obscures a potential treatment effect. Most studies publish the intention-to-treat analyses. The fastidious approach best reflects drug action if the drug is taken as indicated (efficacy), but it is prone to selection bias due to potential differences between patients who choose to adhere to a regimen and those who do not. These methodologic problems were addressed when the Coronary Drug Project published results showing improved survival in a subgroup analysis of adherers versus nonadherers of a clofibrate cholesterol-lowering regimen,[171] but no difference was found in the overall analysis of treated versus placebo groups. A similar compliance-associated effect on postinfarction mortality was found in a secondary prevention trial of propranolol.[172] In this placebo-controlled study on 2175 post-MI patients, the effect of compliance was adjusted for severity and psychosocial factors. Compliance was strongly associated with 1-year mortality in both the placebo group (odds ratio of poor compliers = 2.7) and the propranolol group (odds ratio = 2.8). These strong associations between the level of adherence and long-term mortality, which imply that noncompliers may be a special group of patients at higher risk of death, deserve further research. Both intention-to-treat and fastidious analyses are therefore valuable approaches for an accurate assessment of the public health impact of a treatment. The question remains whether trials of secondary prevention tell the full story. The majority of patients who have had an AMI have multiple medical conditions treated with multiple agents. The effects of multimedication on patients after AMI are not well researched. In Germany, patients are, on average, discharged from the hospital with four or five cardiovascular drugs, and complications arising from drug–drug interactions alone could affect as many as 65% of the patients.[150,169] Because of the complexity of treatments and response in the post-AMI phase, a more comprehensive form of postmarketing surveillance in natural populations is required to enhance the results of trials. This is particularly true for highly prevalent drug uses, such as calcium-channel blockers, the effectiveness of which is contestable.[32,33,140]

Summary

The high prevalence of CHD has made its medical treatment an intensive area of research, furthering results that have changed clinical practice and that have moved treatment modes from an intuitive to a scientific approach, particularly in the area of acute care. The new era in the management of CHD is marked by comprehensive treatment guidance through epidemiologic methods from observational studies to clinical trials. Drug risks, although present, play a minor role in CHD treatment. This is because the high case fatality of the acute event offsets the concentration on risk in favor of the search for an effective treatment. For the areas of primary and secondary prevention, prospective, controlled trials are needed to ascertain whether the increased costs of newly developed drugs are justified by potential benefits.[36] In a highly contested market, however, this places the bias in favor of newer medications, which receive much more research attention. In part, this research is forced by the market penetration of medications, such as ACE inhibitors, which are increasingly used after AMI, and the HMG-CoA reductase inhibitors, which have achieved a dominant position among lipid-lowering drugs.[78] In view of its cost and given the availability of a less expensive alternative, the enthusiastic reception of alteplase remains a puzzle.[133] The importance of research on traditional treatments has been underlined by the results of the CAST, which showed the treated group to be at higher risk of death,[163] but also by the results on the positive effects of aspirin.[104,105] Despite the many advantages of trials, however, they cannot address questions concerning adverse effects, interactions, use, and effects of these agents within the heterogeneous population for which cardiovascular drugs are targeted. Only intensified observational research will provide evidence of the effectiveness of cardiovascular drugs within the general population and will show whether medications such as beta-blockers or calcium-channel blockers actually do live up to their promise. Effective health care is supplied only when trial results are enhanced by postmarketing surveillance studies that establish cost/benefit and risk/benefit relationships on a population basis.

The author thanks W. Foerg, PharmD, Pharmacy of the Augsburg Central Hospital, and U. Hazijenko, MONICA Augsburg Coronary Event Register, for their help in preparing the literature searches.

References

1. Davies MJ, Thomas AC. Plaque fissuring—the cause of acute myocardial infarction, sudden ischaemic death and crescendo angina. Br Heart J 1985;53:363-73.
2. La Veccia C, Levi F, Lucchini F, Negri E. Trends in mortality from cardiovascular and cerebrovascular disease (in German). Soz Präventivmed 1993;(suppl 1):S3-71.

3. Uemura K, Pisa Z. Trends in cardiovascular disease mortality in industrialized countries since 1950. World Health Stat Q 1988;41:155-78.
4. Beaglehole R. International trends in coronary heart disease mortality, morbidity, and risk factors. Epidemiol Rev 1990;121:1-15.
5. Keil U, Filipiak B, Döring A, Hense HW, Lewis M, Löwel H, et al. Monitoring trends and determinants in cardiovascular disease in Germany: results of the MONICA Project, Augsburg, 1985–1990. MMWR Morb Mortal Wkly Rep 1992;41(suppl):171-9.
6. Schoenberger JA. Epidemiology and evaluation: steps toward hypertension treatment in the 1990s. Am J Med 1991;90:3S-7S.
7. Thom TJ, Maurer J. Time trends for coronary heart disease mortality and morbidity. In: Higgins MW, Luepker RV, eds. Trends in coronary heart disease mortality. The influence of medical care. New York: Oxford University Press, 1988.
8. Dawber TR, Meadors GF, Moore FE Jr. Epidemiologic approaches to heart disease: the Framingham Heart Study. Am J Public Health 1951;41:279-86.
9. Kannel WB, Neaton JD, Wentworth D, Thomas HE, Stamler J, Hulley SB, et al., for the MRFIT Research Group. Overall and coronary heart disease mortality rates in relation to major risk factors in 325,348 men screened for MRFIT. Am Heart J 1986; 112:825-36.
10. McGovern PG, Folsom AR, Sprafka JM, Burke GL, Doliszny KM, Demirovic J, et al. Trends in survival of hospitalized myocardial infarction in patients between 1970 and 1985. Circulation 1992;85:172-9.
11. Goldberg RJ, Gore JM, Gurwitz JH, Alpert JS, Brady P, Strohsnitter W, et al. The impact of age on the incidence and prognosis of initial acute myocardial infarction: the Worcester Heart Attack Study. Am Heart J 1989;117:543-9.
12. World Health Organization MONICA Project (Monitoring of Trends and Determinants in Cardiovascular Disease): a major international collaboration. WHO MONICA Project Principal Investigators. J Clin Epidemiol 1988;41:105-14.
13. The Atherosclerosis Risk in Communities (ARIC) Study: design and objectives. The ARIC Investigators. Am J Epidemiol 1989;129:687-702.
14. Feinstein A. Clinical epidemiology. The architecture of clinical research. Philadelphia: WB Saunders, 1985.
15. Yusuf S, Collins R, Peto R. Why do we need some large, simple randomized trials? Stat Med 1984;3:409-20.
16. Randomised trial of intravenous atenolol among 16027 cases of suspected acute myocardial infarction: ISIS-1. First International Study of Infarct Survival Collaborative Group. Lancet 1986;2:57-66.
17. Effectiveness of intravenous thrombolytic treatment in acute myocardial infarction. Gruppo Italiano per lo Studio della Streptochinasi nell'Infarto Miocardico (GISSI). Lancet 1986;1:397-401.
18. Spitzer WO, ed. The challenge of meta-analysis. Potsdam international consultation on meta-analysis. J Clin Epidemiol 1995;48:1-172.
19. Antman EM, Lau J, Kupelnick B, Mosteller F, Chalmers TC. A comparison of results of meta-analyses of randomized control trials and recommendations of clinical experts. Treatments for myocardial infarction. JAMA 1992;268:240-8.
20. Dahlöf B, Lindholm LH, Hansson L, Schersten B, Ekbom T, Wester PO. Morbidity and mortality in the Swedish Trial in Old Patients with Hypertension (STOP-Hypertension). Lancet 1991;338:1282-5.
21. Harrington M, Kincaid-Smith P, McMichael J. Results of treatment of malignant hypertension. Br Med J 1959;2:969-89.

22. Effects of treatment on morbidity in hypertension. Results in patients with diastolic blood pressures averaging 115 through 129 mm Hg. JAMA 1967;202:1028-34.
23. MacMahon S, Peto R, Cutler J, Collins R, Sorlie P, Neaton J, et al. Blood pressure, stroke, and coronary heart disease. Part 1. Prolonged differences in blood pressure: prospective observational studies corrected for the regression dilution bias. Lancet 1990;335:765-74.
24. Treating mild hypertension. Report of the British Hypertension Society working party. BMJ 1989;298:694-8.
25. The fifth report of the Joint National Committee on Detection, Evaluation, and Treatment of High Blood Pressure (JNC V). Arch Intern Med 1993;153:154-83.
26. Black HR. Choosing initial therapy for hypertension. A personal view. Hypertension 1989;13(suppl):I149-53.
27. Dall JL. Hypertension in the elderly. Am J Med 1989;87:38S-40S.
28. Deedwania PC. Angiotensin-converting enzyme inhibitors in congestive heart failure. Arch Intern Med 1990;150:1798-805.
29. Barabino A, Galbariggi G, Pizzorni C, Lotti G. Comparative effects of long-term therapy with captopril and ibopamine in chronic congestive heart failure in old patients. Cardiology 1991;78:243-56.
30. Borchard U. Clinical pharmacology of beta-receptor blockers (in German). Basel: Aesopus Verlag, 1989.
31. Pearle DL. Calcium antagonists in acute myocardial infarction. Am J Cardiol 1988; 61:22B-5B.
32. Furberg CD, Psaty BM, Myers JF. Nifedipine: dose-related increase in mortality in patients with coronary heart disease. Circulation 1995;92:1326-31.
33. Psaty BM, Heckbert SR, Koepsell TD. The risk of myocardial infarction associated with antihypertensive drug therapies. JAMA 1995;274:620-5.
34. Davidson RA, Meuleman JR. Initial treatment of hypertension: a questionnaire survey. J Clin Hypertens 1986;2:339-45.
35. Manolino TA, Cutler JA, Furberg CD, Psaty BM, Whelton PK, Applegate WB. Trends in pharmacologic management of hypertension in the United States. Arch Intern Med 1995;155:829-37.
36. Ray WA, Schaffner W, Oates JA. Therapeutic choice in the treatment of hypertension. Initial treatment of newly diagnosed hypertension and secular trends in the prescribing of antihypertensive medications for Medicaid patients. Am J Med 1986; 81:9-16.
37. Sinclair B, Jackson R, Beaglehole R. Patterns in the drug treatment of hypertension in Auckland, 1982–7. N Z Med J 1989;102:491-3.
38. Hense HW, Tennis P. Changing patterns of antihypertensive drug use in a German population between 1984 and 1987. Results of a population based cohort study in the Federal Republic of Germany. Eur J Clin Pharmacol 1990;39:1-7.
39. Weber MA, Laragh JH. Hypertension: steps forward and steps backward. The Joint National Committee fifth report. Arch Intern Med 1993;153:149-52.
40. Houston MC. Hypertension strategies for therapeutic intervention and prevention of end-organ damage. Prim Care 1991;18:713-53.
41. Griffiths K, McDevitt DG, Andrew M, Baksaas I, Helgeland A, Jervell J, et al. Therapeutic traditions in Northern Ireland, Norway and Sweden. II. Hypertension. WHO Drug Utilization Research Group (DURG). Eur J Clin Pharmacol 1986;30:521-5.
42. Weiland SK, Keil U, Spelsberg A, Hense HW, Haertel U, Gefeller O, et al. Diagnosis and management of hypertension by physicians in the Federal Republic of Germany. J Hypertens 1991;9:131-4.

43. Byyny RL. Epidemiologic aspects of elderly hypertensive patients and the results of treatment with nitrendipine. J Cardiovasc Pharmacol 1989;10(suppl):S27-32.
44. Wilhelmsen L, Berglund G, Elmfeldt D, Fitzsimons T, Holzgreve H, Hosie J, et al. Beta-blockers versus diuretics in hypertensive men: main results from the HAPPHY trial. J Hypertens 1985;5:561-72.
45. Kannel WB. Implications of the primary prevention trials against coronary heart disease. J Hypertens 1990;8(suppl):S245-50.
46. Leren P, Helgeland A. Coronary heart disease and treatment of hypertension. Some Oslo Study data. Am J Med 1986;80:3-6.
47. Collins R, Peto R, MacMahon S, Hebert P, Fiebach NH, Eberlein KA, et al. Blood pressure, stroke, and coronary heart disease. Part 2. Short-term reductions in blood pressure: overview of randomised drug trials in their epidemiological context. Lancet 1990;335:827-38.
48. Nakamura H. Effects of antihypertensive drugs on plasma lipids. Am J Cardiol 1987;60:24E-8E.
49. Grimm RH. Antihypertensive therapy: taking lipids into consideration. Am Heart J 1991;122:910-8.
50. Winther K, Hansen K, Klysner RI, Geisler A, Knudsen B, Glazer S, et al. Platelet aggregation and beta blockers. Lancet 1985;1:224-5.
51. Cruickshank JM. Beta-blockers, plasma lipids, and coronary heart disease. Circulation 1990;82(suppl):II60-5.
52. Wikstrand J, Berglund G, Tuomilehto J. Beta-blockade in the primary prevention of coronary heart disease in hypertensive patients. Review of present evidence. Circulation 1991;84(suppl):VI93-100.
53. de Planque BA. A double-blind comparative study of doxazosin and prazosin when administered with beta-blockers or diuretics. Am Heart J 1991;121:304-11.
54. Wessels F. Double-blind comparison of doxazosin and enalapril in patients with mild or moderate essential hypertension. Am Heart J 1991;121:299-303.
55. Hurley SF, Williams SL, McNeil JJ. Trends in prescribing of antihypertensive drugs in Australia, 1977–1987. Med J Aust 1990;152:259-66.
56. Bock KD. Changing prescription patterns: impact on costs. J Hypertens 1987;5 (suppl):S83-5.
57. Kawachi I, Malcolm LA. The cost–effectiveness of treating mild-to-moderate hypertension: a reappraisal. J Hypertens 1991;9:199-208.
58. Lederle FA, Applegate WB, Grimm RH. Reserpine and the medical marketplace. Arch Intern Med 1993;153:705-6.
59. Reserpine and breast cancer. Report from the Boston Collaborative Drug Surveillance Program, Boston University Medical Center. Lancet 1974;2:669-71.
60. Shapiro S, Parsells JL, Kaufmann WD, Stolley PD, Schottenfeld D. Risk of breast cancer in relation to the use of Rauwolfia alkaloids. Eur J Clin Pharmacol 1984; 26:143-6.
61. Grundy SM. HMG-CoA reductase inhibitors for treatment of hypercholesterolemia. N Engl J Med 1988;319:24-33.
62. Report of the National Cholesterol Education Program Expert Panel on Detection, Evaluation, and Treatment of High Blood Cholesterol in Adults. The Expert Panel. Arch Intern Med 1988;148:36-69.
63. Tyroler HA. Review of lipid-lowering clinical trials in relation to observational epidemiologic studies. Circulation 1987;76:515-22.
64. Strategies for the prevention of coronary heart disease: a policy statement of the European Atherosclerosis Society. Eur Heart J 1987;8:77-88.

65. Consensus conference. Lowering blood cholesterol to prevent heart disease. JAMA 1985;253:2080-6.
66. Frick MH, Elo O, Haapa K, Heinonen OP, Heinsalmi P, Helo P, et al. Helsinki Heart Study: primary prevention trial with gemfibrozil in middle-aged men with dyslipidemia. Safety of treatment, changes in risk factors, and incidence of coronary heart disease. N Engl J Med 1987;317:1237-45.
67. Canner PL, Berge KG, Wenger NK, Stamler J, Friedman L, Prineas RJ, et al. Fifteen years' mortality in Coronary Drug Project patients: long-term benefit with niacin. J Am Coll Cardiol 1986;8:1245-55.
68. Therapeutic response to lovastatin (mevinolin) in nonfamilial hypercholesterolemia. A multicenter study. The Lovastatin Study Group II. JAMA 1986;256:2829-34.
69. Grundy SM, Goodman DS, Rifking BM, Cleeman JI. The place of HDL in cholesterol management. Arch Intern Med 1989;149:505-9.
70. Dayton S, Pearce ML, Hashomoto S, Dixon WJ, Tomiyasu U. A controlled clinical trial of a diet high in unsaturated fat in preventing complications of atherosclerosis. Circulation 1969;39-40(suppl 2):1-63.
71. A co-operative trial in the primary prevention of ischaemic heart disease using clofibrate. Report from the Committee of Principal Investigators. Br Heart J 1978;40:1069-118.
72. Dorr AE, Gunderson K, Schneider JC, Spencer TW, Martin WB. Colestipol hydrochloride in hypercholesterolemic patients—effect on serum cholesterol and mortality. J Chronic Dis 1978;31:5-14.
73. The Lipid Research Clinics Coronary Primary Prevention Trial results. I. Reduction in incidence of coronary heart disease. JAMA 1984;251:351-64. II. The relationship of reduction in incidence of coronary heart disease to cholesterol lowering. JAMA 1984;251:365-74.
74. Brown G, Albers JJ, Fisher LD, Schaefer SM, Lin JT, Kaplan C, et al. Regression of coronary artery disease as a result of intensive lipid-lowering therapy in men with high levels of apolipoprotein B. N Engl J Med 1990;323:1289-97.
75. Muldoon MF, Manuck SB, Matthews KA. Lowering cholesterol concentration and mortality: a quantitative review of primary prevention trials. BMJ 1990;301:309-14.
76. Gould AL, Rossouw JE, Santanello NC, Heyse JF, Furberg CD. Cholesterol reduction yields clinical benefit. A new look at old data. Circulation 1995;91:2274-82.
77. Davey Smith G, Pekkanen J. Should there be a moratorium on the use of cholesterol lowering drugs? BMJ 1992;304:431-4.
78. Wysowski DK, Kennedy DL, Gross TP. Prescribed use of cholesterol-lowering drugs in the United States, 1978 through 1988. JAMA 1990;263:2185-8.
79. Davey Smith G, Song F, Sheldon TA. Cholesterol lowering and mortality: the importance of considering initial level of risk. BMJ 1993;306:1367-73.
80. Oliver MF. National cholesterol policies. Eur Heart J 1993;14:581-3.
81. Willich SN. Acute myocardial infarction: circadian variation, triggers, and prevention (in German). Darmstadt: Steinkopff, 1992.
82. Castelli WP, Dawber TR, Feinleib M, Garrison RJ, McNamara PM, Kannel WB. The filter cigarette and coronary heart disease: the Framingham Heart Study. Lancet 1981;1:109-13.
83. Fortmann SP, Haskell WL, Williams PT. Changes in plasma high density lipoprotein cholesterol after changes in cigarette use. Am J Epidemiol 1986;124:706-10.
84. Farley TMM, Meirik O, Chang CL, Marmot MG, Poulter NR. World Health Organization Collaborative Study of Cardiovascular Disease and Steroid Hormone Contraception. Effect of different progestagens in low oestrogen oral contraceptives on venous thromboembolic disease. Lancet 1995;346:1582-8.

85. Spitzer WO, Lewis MA, Heinemann LAJ, Thorogood M, MacRae KD, Transnational Research Group on Oral Contraceptives and Health in Young Women. Third generation oral contraceptives and risk of venous thromboembolic disorders: an international case–control study. BMJ 1996;312:83-8.

86. Lewis MA, Spitzer WO, Heinemann LAJ, MacRae KD, Bruppacher R, Thorogood M, Transnational Research Group on Oral Contraceptives and Health in Young Women. Third generation oral contraceptives and risk of myocardial infarction: an international case–control study. BMJ 1996;312:88-90.

87. Colditz GA, Willet WC, Stampfer MJ, Rosner B, Speizer FE, Hennekens CH. Menopause and the risk of coronary heart disease in women. N Engl J Med 1987;316:1105-10.

88. Stampfer MJ, Colditz GA, Willet WC, Manson JE, Rosner B, Speizer FE, et al. Postmenopausal estrogen therapy and cardiovascular disease. Ten-year follow-up from the Nurses' Health Study. N Engl J Med 1991;325:756-62.

89. Nabulsi AA, Folsom AR, White A, Patsch W, Heiss G, Wu KK, et al. Association of hormone-replacement therapy with various cardiovascular risk factors in postmenopausal women. N Engl J Med 1993;328:1069-75.

90. Marmot MG. Alcohol and coronary heart disease. Int J Epidemiol 1984;13:160-7.

91. Stampfer MJ, Colditz GA, Willet WC, Speizer FE, Hennekens CH. A prospective study of moderate alcohol consumption and the risk of coronary disease and stroke in women. N Engl J Med 1988;319:267-73.

92. Shaper AG, Phillips AN, Pocock SJ, Walker M. Alcohol and ischaemic heart disease in middle-aged British men. Br Med J 1987;294:733-7.

93. Klatsky AL, Friedman GD, Armstrong MA. The relationship between alcoholic beverage use and other traits to blood pressure: a new Kaiser Permanente study. Circulation 1986;73:628-36.

94. Rimm EB, Giovannucci EL, Willet WC, Colditz GA, Ascherio A, Rosner B, et al. Prospective study of alcohol consumption and risk of coronary artery disease in men. Lancet 1991;338:464-8.

95. Stampfer MJ, Sacks FM, Salvini S, Willett WC, Hennekens CH. A prospective study of cholesterol, apolipoproteins, and the risk of myocardial infarction. N Engl J Med 1991;325:373-81

96. Nayler WG. Calcium antagonists. San Diego: Academic Press, 1988.

97. Yusuf S, Wittes J, Friedman L. Overview of results of randomized clinical trials in heart disease. I. Treatments following myocardial infarction. II. Unstable angina, heart failure, primary prevention with aspirin, and risk factor modification. JAMA 1988;260:2088-93,2259-63.

98. Akhras F, Jackson G. The role of captopril as single therapy in hypertension and angina pectoris. Int J Cardiol 1991;33:259-66.

99. Loaldi A, Polese A, Montorsi P, De Cesare N, Fabbiocchi F, Ravagnani P, et al. Comparison of nifedipine, propranolol and isosorbide dinitrate on angiographic progression and regression of coronary arterial narrowings in angina pectoris. Am J Cardiol 1989;64:433-9.

100. Nidorf SM, Parsons RW, Thompson PL, Jamrozik KD, Hobs MST. Reduced risk of death at 28 days in patients taking a beta-blocker before admission to hospital with myocardial infarction. BMJ 1990;300:71-4.

101. Effect of enalapril on survival in patients with reduced left ventricular ejection fractions and congestive heart failure. The SOLVD Investigators. N Engl J Med 1991;325:293-302.

102. Cohn JN, Johnson G, Ziesche S, Cobb F, Francis G, Tristani F, et al. A comparison of enalapril with hydralazine–isosorbide dinitrate in the treatment of chronic congestive heart failure. N Engl J Med 1991;325:303-10.

103. Cambien F, Poirier O, Lecerf L, Evans A, Cambou JP, Arveiler D, et al. Deletion polymorphism in the gene for angiotensin-converting enzyme is a potent risk factor for myocardial infarction. Nature 1992;359:641-4.

104. Ridker PM, Manson JE, Gaziano JM, Burin JE, Hennekens CH. Low-dose aspirin therapy for chronic stable angina: a randomized, placebo-controlled clinical trial. Ann Intern Med 1991;114:835-9.

105. Collaborative overview of randomized trials of antiplatelet therapy—I: Prevention of death, myocardial infarction, and stroke by prolonged antiplatelet therapy in various categories of patients. Antiplatelet Trialists' Collaboration. BMJ 1994;308: 81-106.

106. Levy M, Miller DR, Kaufman DW, Siskind V, Schwingl P, Rosenberg L, et al. Major upper gastrointestinal bleeding. Relation to the use of aspirin and other nonnarcotic analgesics. Arch Intern Med 1988;148:281-5.

107. Peters LJ, Wiener GJ, Gillam J, Van Noord G, Geisinger KR, Roach S. Reye's syndrome in adults. Arch Intern Med 1986;146:2401-3.

108. A comparison of two doses of aspirin (30 mg vs. 283 mg a day) in patients after a transient ischemic attack or minor ischemic stroke. The Dutch TIA Trial Study Group. N Engl J Med 1991;325:1261-6.

109. Kearon C, Hirsh J. Optimal dose for starting and maintaining low-dose aspirin. Arch Intern Med 1993;153:700-2.

110. Hass WK, Easton JD, Adams HP Jr, Pryse-Phillips W, Molony BA, Anderson S, et al. A randomized trial comparing ticlopidine hydrochloride with aspirin for the prevention of stroke in high-risk patients. N Engl J Med 1989;321:501-7.

111. Final report on the aspirin component of the ongoing Physicians' Health Study. Steering Committee of the Physicians' Health Study Research Group. N Engl J Med 1989;321:129-35.

112. Nyman I, Larsson H, Wallentin L, the Research Group on Instability in Coronary Artery Disease in Southern Sweden. Prevention of serious cardiac events by low-dose aspirin in patients with silent myocardial ischaemia. Lancet 1992;340:497-501.

113. Thun MJ, Nomboodiri MM, Heath CW. Aspirin use and reduced risk of fatal colon cancer. N Engl J Med 1991;325:1593-6.

114. Peto R, Gray R, Collins R, Wheatley K, Hennekens C, Jamrozik K, et al. A randomised trial of the effects of prophylactic daily aspirin among male British doctors. Br Med J 1988;296:320-31.

115. Fuster V, Dyken ML, Vokonas PS, Hennekens C. Aspirin as a therapeutic agent in cardiovascular disease. Circulation 1993;2:659-75.

116. Willich SN, Löwel H, Lewis M, Arntz R, Baur R, Winther K, et al. Association of wake time and the onset of myocardial infarction. Circulation 1991;84(suppl):VI62-7.

117. Willich SN, Löwel H, Lewis M, Hörmann A, Arntz H-R, Keil U. Weekly variation of acute myocardial infarction. Increased Monday risk in the working population. Circulation 1994;90:87-93.

118. Muller JE, Tofler GH. Circadian variation in cardiovascular disease. N Engl J Med 1991;325:1038-9.

119. Muller JE, Stone PH, Turi ZG, Rutherford JD, Czeisler CA, Parker C, et al. Circadian variation in the frequency of onset of acute myocardial infarction. N Engl J Med 1985;313:1315-22.

120. Willich SN, Linderer T, Wegscheider K, Leizorovicz A, Alamercery I, Schröder R, et al. Increased morning incidence of myocardial infarction in the ISAM study: absence with prior beta blockade. Circulation 1989;80:853-8.
121. Lewis M, Willich SN, Löwel H, Schubert F, Arntz H, TRIMM Study Group. Does cardiovascular drug use influence circadian variation of acute myocardial infarction (abstract)? J Clin Res Pharmacoepidemiol 1991;5:164.
122. Oliver MF. Doubts about preventing coronary heart disease. Multiple interventions in middle aged men may do more harm than good. BMJ 1992;304:393-4.
123. Rose G. Preventive medicine: aims and ethics. Pharm Med 1987;2:103-7.
124. Löwel H, Herman B, Lewis M, Holtz H, Quietzsch D, Hörmann A, et al. Registration methods and estimates of morbidity and mortality of acute myocardial infarction. Results from East and West Germany. Ann Epidemiol 1993;3(suppl):S69-78.
125. Löwel H, Lewis M, Hörmann A, Keil U. Case finding, data quality aspects and comparability of myocardial infarction registers: results of a south German register study. J Clin Epidemiol 1991;44:249-60.
126. Yusuf S, Sleight P. Limitation of myocardial infarct size. Present status. Drugs 1983; 25:441-50.
127. Yusuf S, Peto R, Lewis J, Collins R, Sleight P. Beta-blockade during and after myocardial infarction: an overview of the randomized trials. Prog Cardiovasc Dis 1985; 27:335-71.
128. Lau J, Antman EM, Jiminez-Silva J, Kupelnick B, Mosteller F, Chalmers TC. Cumulative meta-analysis of therapeutic trials for myocardial infarction. N Engl J Med 1992;327:248-54.
129. Teo KK, Yusuf S, Collins R, Held PH, Peto R. Effects of intravenous magnesium in suspected myocardial infarction: overview of randomised trials. BMJ 1991;303: 1499-503.
130. Collen D. Biological properties of plasminogen activators. In: Sobel BE, Collen D, Grossbard EB, eds. Tissue plasminogen activator in thrombolytic therapy. Basel: Marcel Dekker, 1987.
131. A prospective trial of intravenous streptokinase in acute myocardial infarction (I.S.A.M.). Mortality, morbidity, and infarct size at 21 days. The I.S.A.M. Study. N Engl J Med 1986;314:1465-71.
132. Anderson HV, Willerson JT. Thrombolysis in acute myocardial infarction. N Engl J Med 1993;329:703-9.
133. Gertz SD, Kragel AH, Kalan JM, Braunwald E, Roberts WC, TIMI Investigators. Comparison of coronary and myocardial morphologic findings in patients with and without thrombolytic therapy during fatal first acute myocardial infarction. Am J Cardiol 1990;66:904-9.
134. An international randomized trial comparing four thrombolytic strategies for acute myocardial infarction. The GUSTO Investigators. N Engl J Med 1993;329:673-82.
135. Vogel JH, Setty RK, Coughlin BJ, Avolio RM, McFadden RB. Intravenous streptokinase in acute myocardial infarction at the community hospital: a six-year experience. Am J Cardiol 1988;62:25K-7K.
136. McLeod DC, Coln WG, Thayer CF, Perfetto EM, Hartzema AG. Pharmacoepidemiology of bleeding events after use of r-alteplase or streptokinase in acute myocardial infarction. Ann Pharmacother 1993;27:956-62.
137. O'Donnel M. Battle of the clotbusters. BMJ 1991;302:1259-61.
138. Gold HK. Conjunctive antithrombotic and thrombolytic therapy for coronary artery occlusion. N Engl J Med 1990;323:1483-5.

139. Hsia J, Hamilton WP, Kleiman N, Roberts R, Chaitman BR, Ross AM, Heparin–Aspirin Reperfusion Trial (HART) Investigators. A comparison between heparin and low-dose aspirin as adjunctive therapy with tissue plasminogen activator for acute myocardial infarction. N Engl J Med 1990;323:1433-7.
140. Koenig W, Löwel H, Lewis M, Hörmann A. Long-term survival after myocardial infarction: relationship with thrombolysis and discharge medication. Results of the Augsburg Myocardial Infarction Follow-up Study, 1985 to 1993. Eur Heart J 1996;17:1199-206.
141. Randomised trial of intravenous streptokinase, oral aspirin, both, or neither among 17,187 cases of suspected acute myocardial infarction: ISIS-2. ISIS-2 (Second International Study of Infarct Survival) Collaborative Group. Lancet 1988;2:349-60.
142. De Caterina R, Gianessi D, Mazzone A, Bernini W. Mechanisms for the in vivo antiplatelet effects of isosorbide dinitrate. Eur Heart J 1988;9(suppl A):45-9.
143. Yusuf S, Collins R, MacMahon S, Peto R. Effect of intravenous nitrates on mortality in acute myocardial infarction: an overview of the randomised trials. Lancet 1988;1:1088-92.
144. Sirnes PA, Overskeid K, Pedersen TR, Bathen J, Drivenes A, Froland GS, et al. Evolution of infarct size during the early use of nifedipine in patients with acute myocardial infarction: the Norwegian Nifedipine Multicenter Trial. Circulation 1984;70:628-44.
145. Wilcox RG, Hampton JR, Banks DC, Birkhead JS, Brooksby JA, Burns-Cox CJ, et al. Trial of early nifedipine in acute myocardial infarction: the TRENT Study. Br Med J 1986;293:1204-8.
146. Collins R, Julian D. British Heart Foundation surveys (1987 and 1989) of United Kingdom treatment policies for acute myocardial infarction. Br Heart J 1991;66:250-5.
147. Lamas GA, Pfeffer MA, Hamm P, Wertheimer J, Eouleau JL, Braunwald E. Do the results of randomized clinical trials of cardiovascular drugs influence medical practice? N Engl J Med 1992;327:241-7.
148. Lewis M, Löwel H, Hörmann A. The usefulness of population-based coronary event registers for the evaluation of drug use. Cardiovasc Dis Epidemiol Newsl 1992;48:88-9.
149. Hennig H, Gilpin EA, Covell JW, Swan EA, O'Rourke RA, Ross J. Prognosis after acute myocardial infarction: a multivariate analysis of mortality and survival. Circulation 1979;59:1124-36.
150. Lewis M, Löwel H, Hörmann A. Medical treatment of patients with acute myocardial infarction before and after the acute event. Results of the Augsburg Coronary event register (in German). Soz Präventivmed 1994;39:75-85.
151. Sharpe N, Murphy J, Smith H, Hannon S. Treatment of patients with symptomless left ventricular dysfunction after myocardial infarction. Lancet 1988;1:255-9.
152. Dargie HJ, Cleland JG. Arrhythmias in heart failure—the role of amiodarone. Clin Cardiol 1988;11(suppl):II26-30.
153. Lamas GA, Pfeffer MA. Left ventricular remodeling after acute myocardial infarction: clinical course and beneficial effects of angiotensin-converting enzyme inhibition. Am Heart J 1991;121:1194-202.
154. Pfeffer MA, Braunwald E, Moyé LA, Basta L, Brown JE, Cuddy TE, et al. Effect of captopril on mortality and morbidity in patients with left ventricular dysfunction after myocardial infarction. N Engl J Med 1992;327:669-77.
155. Effect of enalapril on mortality and the development of heart failure in asymptomatic patients with reduced left ventricular ejection fractions. SOLVD Investigators. N Engl J Med 1992;327:685-91.

156. Swedberg K, Held P, Kjekshus J, Rasmussen K, Ryden L, Wedel H, Consensus II Study Group. Effects of early administration of enalapril on mortality in patients with acute myocardial infarction. N Engl J Med 1992;327:678-84.
157. Secondary Prevention Reinfarction Israeli Nifedipine Trial (SPRINT). A randomized intervention trial of nifedipine in patients with acute myocardial infarction. The Israeli SPRINT Study Group. Eur Heart J 1988;9:354-64.
158. Goldbourt U, Behar S, Reicher-Reiss H, Zion M, Mandelzweig L, Kaplinsky E, SPRINT Study Group. Early administration of nifedipine in suspected acute myocardial infarction. The Secondary Prevention Reinfarction Israel Nifedipine Trial 2 Study. Arch Intern Med 1993;153:345-53.
159. The effect of diltiazem and reinfarction after myocardial infarction. The Multicenter Diltiazem Postinfarction Trial Research Group. N Engl J Med 1988;319:385-92.
160. Gibson RS, Boden WE, Théraux P, Strauss HD, Pratt CM, Gheorghiade M, et al. Diltiazem and reinfarction in patients with non-Q-wave myocardial infarction. Results of a double-blind, randomized, multicenter trial. N Engl J Med 1986;315:423-9.
161. Effect of verapamil on mortality and major events after acute myocardial infarction (the Danish Verapamil Infarction Trial II—DAVIT II). Am J Cardiol 1990;66:779-85.
162. Ruberman W, Weinblatt E, Goldberg JD, Frank CW, Shapiro S. Ventricular premature beats and mortality after myocardial infarction. N Engl J Med 1977;297:750-7.
163. Preliminary report: effect of encainide and flecainide on mortality in a randomized trial of arrhythmia suppression after myocardial infarction. The Cardiac Arrhythmia Suppression Trial (CAST) Investigators. N Engl J Med 1989;321:406-12.
164. Galloe AM, Graudal N. Cardiac Arrhythmia Suppression Trial (letter). N Engl J Med 1991;325:584-5.
165. Echt DS. Cardiac Arrhythmia Suppression Trial (reply to letter). N Engl J Med 1991;325:585.
166. Salerno DM, Gillingham KJ, Berry DA, Hodges M. A comparison of antiarrhythmic drugs for the suppression of ventricular ectopic depolarizations: a meta-analysis. Am Heart J 1990;120:340-53.
167. Burkart F, Pfisterer M, Kiowski W, Follath F, Burckhardt D. Effect of antiarrhythmic therapy on mortality in survivors of myocardial infarction with asymptomatic ventricular arrhythmias: Basel Antiarrhythmic Study of Infarct Survival (BASIS). J Am Coll Cardiol 1990;16:1711-8.
168. Galloe AM, Rasmussen HS, Jorgensen LN, Aurup P, Balslov S, Cintin C, et al. Influence of oral magnesium supplementation of cardiac events among survivors of an acute myocardial infarction. BMJ 1993;307:585-7.
169. Lewis M, Löwel H, Stieber J, Engelbrecht R, Hörmann A, John J. Drug–drug interactions in the prescriptions of patients before and after acute myocardial infarction: results from the MONICA Augsburg coronary event register (in German). Soz Präventivmed 1991;36:9-17.
170. Rapaport E. Influence of long-acting nitrate therapy on the risk of reinfarction, sudden death, and total mortality on survivors of acute myocardial infarction. Am Heart J 1985;110:276-80.
171. Influence of adherence to treatment and response of cholesterol on mortality in the coronary drug project. Coronary Drug Project Group. N Engl J Med 1980;303:1038-41.
172. Horwitz RI, Viscoli CM, Berkman L, Donaldson RM, Horwitz SM, Murray CJ, et al. Treatment adherence and risk of death after a myocardial infarction. Lancet 1990;336:542-5.

23

An Annotated Bibliography of Pharmacoepidemiologic Studies

Abraham G Hartzema
Donald C McLeod

This bibliography of pharmacoepidemiologic studies was compiled after an extensive survey of the literature through 1997. A structured approach was taken in compiling a master list of pharmacoepidemiologic studies published in the scientific literature. The two major databases, MEDLINE of the National Library of Medicine and *International Pharmaceutical Abstracts* of the American Society of Health-System Pharmacists, were explored.

For searching, the terms *epidemiologic methods, cross-sectional studies, longitudinal studies, cohort studies,* and *case–control studies* were used in combination with the search terms *drug* and *medication;* the term *pharmacoepidemiology* was searched also. We did not search the literature on the term *clinical trial* because clinical trials are used mainly to study the effectiveness of the drug for its primary indication. Some clinical trials appeared in search results, but were omitted from this bibliography.

The references obtained were downloaded in a master file and sorted by date of reference and author's name; duplicate entries were omitted. In the next step, a second database was created that contained selected references from the first database. The selection criteria included the following: authors' names or study needed to be included and articles as indicated by the title that had no relationship to pharmacoepidemiology were omitted, as were case studies, clinical trials examining the efficacy of a drug product or the comparative efficacy of two compounds, pharmacokinetic studies, and animal or human toxicology studies.

Studies using pharmacoepidemiologic methods, primarily case–control and cohort, were abstracted, and the following characteristics were included in the annotation: drug name, drug category, drug dosing criteria, treatment duration, validation of exposure, study methodology, total number of patients enrolled, population selection criteria, sample frame limitations, number of cases, number of controls, comparability of controls, drug event, validation of outcome, elimination of alternative explanations, and findings.

In addition, an index of the studies was compiled using the annotations. The number following the index term refers to the reference number of the article. These are indexed by year of publication and the number of the study and are sorted by alphabetical order of the first author's name. Because of methodologic refinements over the last few years, we have broadened the methodologic index categories with those for nested case–control studies, population-based studies, and so on. Older studies that may have appeared in these more refined categories are still indexed by the original index categories.

The bibliography was compiled with the primary intention to demonstrate the research efforts in the area of pharmacoepidemiology and to stimulate such efforts. References were selected to reflect the spectrum in types of pharmacoepidemiologic studies as well as the different study methods used in these studies. In an effort to illustrate the strengths and limitations of existing studies, we cited some references despite their methodologic weaknesses. Other studies may have been unintentionally omitted, but because of their merit should have been included.

Although we provide a comprehensive overview of the pharmacoepidemiology literature, it is not complete. The citations included are listed chronologically by year and alphabetically by first author's name within the year of publication. The bibliography is accompanied by a structured annotation system. In the annotation and indexing of the study methodology, drug exposure, and categorization of unintended effects, the terminology of the authors was adhered to whenever logical.

In addition, some articles of pertinence known to the authors, but not identified by the above computer search, were included in the bibliography. Over the past several years, an enormous increase in the number of pharmacoepidemiologic case–control and cohort studies published in the literature can be observed.

The authors thank Xingyue Huang and Maarit Korhonen, our graduate research assistants, for their considerable assistance in database searching and compiling and editing the bibliography.

INDEX OF DRUG NAMES

Drug Names—Reference Numbers

YY:NN   YY = Year of publication
          NN = Sequence number of
          article sorted by
          author's name within
          year of publication

See also Index of Drug Categories

INDEX OF DRUG CATEGORIES

Drug Categories—Reference Numbers

YY:NN   YY = Year of publication
         NN = Sequence number of
              article sorted by
              author's name within
              year of publication

See also Drug Names

96:4; 96:12; 96:16; 96:21; 96:27; 96:32; 96:33;
96:38; 96:39; 96:41; 96:45; 96:46; 96:50;
96:54; 96:55; 96:56; 96:58; 96:63; 97:1; 97:2;
97:4; 97:6; 97:9; 97:10; 97:11; 97:13
estrogens 90:25; 91:27; 91:30; 91:32; 92:7; 93:4;
93:9; 93:30; 93:37; 93:39; 94:6; 94:13; 95:6;
95:11; 95:12; 95:28; 95:36; 95:55; 95:62; 95:67;
96:16; 96:21; 96:27; 96:32; 96:38; 96:39;
96:41; 96:46; 97:2; 97:6; 97:9; 97:10; 97:11
fluoride supplements 90:24; 95:33
fungicides 96:40
glaucoma agents 94:10
glucocorticoids 91:3; 91:6; 91:23; 92:1; 92:6;
93:17; 93:22; 94:9; 95:22; 96:15; 96:48; 97:5
gold compounds 95:4
gold salts 93:2; 96:35
growth hormone 91:10; 93:11
histamine₂-receptor antagonists 90:16; 96:18;
96:37
histamine₂-receptor blockers 94:3
hypnotics 95:35; 95:43; 95:64
immunomodulators 94:16
immunosuppressants 93:12
lipid-lowering agents (see cholesterol-lipid-
lowering agents)
luteinizing hormone–releasing hormone
agonist 97:12
methylxanthines 95:63
multivitamins 96:6
narcotics (see opioid analgesics)
neuroleptics 93:13; 93:23; 94:4
nitrosatable agents 95:10
nonsteroidal antiinflammatory drugs (see
NSAIDs)
NSAIDs 91:2; 91:4; 91:13; 91:15; 91:18; 91:19;
91:23; 91:25; 91:26; 92:17; 92:19; 92:23;
92:24; 92:25; 93:2; 93:3; 93:15; 93:20; 93:24;
93:29; 93:31; 93:34; 94:2; 94:8; 94:12; 95:15;
95:16; 95:21; 95:23; 95:26; 95:32; 95:34;
95:38; 95:42; 95:47; 95:54; 95:60; 95:68;
95:70; 95:71; 96:10; 96:14; 96:17; 96:22;
96:23; 96:30; 96:31; 96:35; 96:36; 96:44;
96:49; 96:60; 97:3
nutritional supplements 90:31
opioid analgesics 92:22; 95:18
oral contraceptives (see estrogen–progestins)
ovulation inducers 90:18; 94:15; 95:5; 96:7
penicillins 91:28; 92:21; 93:6; 93:34; 94:23
phenothiazines 91:16; 92:18
plasmodicides 94:7
progestins 91:8; 91:30; 91:32; 92:20; 95:65
proton pump inhibitors 94:3; 96:18; 96:37
quinolones 96:53

radiographic contrast media 93:18
sedatives 90:15; 95:18; 95:43; 95:53
spermicides 95:72
sulfonamides 92:15; 92:21; 94:5; 94:11
teratogens 90:4
thiazide diuretics (see diuretics)
thrombolytics 90:9; 91:7; 92:4; 92:14; 93:21
thyroid hormones 92:8; 95:73
tocolytics 94:8
tricyclic antidepressants 91:5; 92:22
vaccines 93:10; 95:3
vasodilators 91:17; 95:18
vitamins 90:29; 90:32; 93:5; 93:16; 93:32; 93:36;
95:9; 95:17; 95:20; 95:40; 95:57; 95:58; 95:59;
96:13; 96:24; 96:47
xanthines (see methylxanthines)

INDEX OF DRUG EVENTS

Drug Events—Reference Numbers

YY:NN   YY = Year of publication
NN = Sequence number of
article sorted by
author's name within
year of publication

abdominal discomfort 96:40
adrenal hypoplasia 96:62
adverse drug reactions: see general drug
events
agranulocytosis 92:15
AIDS survival 92:9; 93:8
akathisia 93:13
Alzheimer disease 95:54; 96:41
anaphylaxis 93:18; 93:34
aplastic anemia 96:35
asthma (see deaths, asthma) 90:21; 95:22; 96:29
birth 96:9
birth defects (see congenital malformations)
birth weight 96:15
bleeding (see hemorrhage)
blood cell abnormalities
agranulocytosis 91:17; 92:15
anemia 91:22
aplastic anemia 91:17; 93:2; 96:35
leukopenia 93:38
neutropenia 93:15

INDEX OF STUDY METHODOLOGIES

Study Methodologies—Reference Numbers

YY:NN   YY = Year of publication
         NN = Sequence number of
               article sorted by
               author's name within
               year of publication

case–control study 96:3; 96:4; 96:6; 96:7; 96:10; 96:14; 96:16; 96:23; 96:24; 96:25; 96:26; 96:28; 96:31; 96:33; 96:35; 96:36; 96:37; 96:44; 96:45; 96:46; 96:49; 96:50; 96:51; 96:52; 96:54; 96:56; 96:60; 96:61; 96:62; 97:3; 97:5; 97:6; 97:11

case–control study, nested 90:3; 91:13; 91:23; 92:6; 92:13; 93:16; 93:25; 94:1; 94:3; 94:11; 94:13; 94:20; 96:11; 96:13; 96:20; 96:29; 96:39; 96:41; 96:43; 96:63; 97:13

case–control study, population-based 97:1

case–control study, prospective 90:29; 91:1; 91:4; 91:8; 92:2; 92:21; 93:5; 95:9; 96:1

case–control study, retrospective 90:2; 90:4; 90:10; 90:11; 90:12; 90:13; 90:15; 90:16; 90:17; 90:18; 90:19; 90:21; 90:28; 90:31; 90:32; 90:33; 91:2; 91:3; 91:4; 91:9; 91:14; 91:15; 91:16; 91:18; 91:19; 91:22; 91:25; 92:3; 92:10; 92:12; 92:14; 92:17; 92:18; 92:19; 92:20; 92:23; 92:26; 93:1; 93:2; 93:3; 93:5; 93:17; 93:18; 93:19; 93:29; 93:34; 93:35; 93:36; 94:10; 94:15; 94:19; 94:20; 94:21; 94:22; 95:10; 95:11; 95:15; 95:18; 95:27; 95:30; 95:32; 95:39; 95:40; 95:41; 95:45; 95:46; 95:50; 95:56; 95:61; 95:66; 95:67; 95:70; 95:71; 95:73; 96:1; 96:22; 97:10

case–control study, retrospective, hospital-based 95:26; 95:36; 95:37; 95:48; 95:65; 95:75

case–control study, retrospective, population-based 90:22; 90:23; 90:25; 91:17; 91:30; 92:11; 93:20; 94:14; 94:17; 95:2; 95:5; 95:8; 95:13; 95:25; 95:42; 95:51; 95:57; 95:58; 95:59; 95:62; 95:68; 96:6; 96:44; 96:45; 96:47; 96:49; 96:54; 96:61; 97:4

case review, retrospective 94:4; 97:10

clinical trial 90:9; 91:26; 93:10; 93:22

cohort study 96:8; 96:17; 97:8

cohort study, cross-sectional 96:27

cohort study, population-based 96:57

cohort study, prospective 90:7; 90:8; 90:14; 90:19; 90:24; 90:27; 91:10; 91:20; 91:21; 91:22; 91:31; 92:4; 92:5; 92:7; 92:8; 92:16; 93:12; 93:13; 93:21; 93:23; 93:24; 93:27; 93:30; 93:32; 93:38; 94:6; 94:9; 94:23; 95:1; 95:3; 95:4; 95:6; 95:7; 95:12; 95:16; 95:17; 95:19; 95:20; 95:21; 95:23; 95:24; 95:29; 95:34; 95:35; 95:38; 95:43; 95:47; 95:49; 95:52; 95:54; 95:63; 95:64; 95:69; 95:72; 96:9; 96:12; 96:21; 96:34; 96:42; 96:58; 97:7

cohort study, retrospective 90:1; 90:6; 90:20; 90:26; 90:29; 91:5; 91:6; 91:7; 91:8; 91:11; 91:16; 91:24; 91:27; 91:28; 91:29; 91:32; 92:1; 92:7; 92:9; 92:13; 92:22; 92:24; 92:25; 93:4; 93:6; 93:7; 93:8; 93:9; 93:11; 93:14; 93:15; 93:26; 93:28; 93:31; 93:33; 93:37; 94:2; 94:5; 94:8; 94:12; 94:13; 94:16; 94:18; 94:22; 95:14; 95:28; 95:31; 95:32; 95:44; 95:53; 95:55; 95:60; 95:74; 96:5; 96:15; 96:18; 96:19; 96:32; 96:48; 97:9

computer simulation 93:39

crossover trial, randomized, double-blind, placebo-controlled 95:22

cross-sectional study 91:13; 93:29; 95:7; 95:38; 95:54; 96:38

patient fellowship study 96:2

patient follow-up study 94:7

Poisson regression 96:59

postmarketing surveillance study 92:19

prescription sequencing study 90:30; 92:2; 92:12; 97:8

prospective 93:10

prospective patient follow-up study 96:40; 96:53

prospective, randomized 90:5; 93:22

prospective recruitment 96:55

randomized 91:26; 96:30

reported 92:15

retrospective 91:12; 97:12

Legend: OR = odds ratio; CI = confidence interval; RR = relative risk

90:1   Andersson M, et al. High risk of therapy-related leukemia and preleukemia after therapy with prednimustine, methotrexate, 5-fluorouracil, mitoxantrone, and tamoxifen for advanced breast cancer. Cancer 1990;65:2460-4

Drug Name: prednimustine, methotrexate, fluorouracil, mitoxantrone, tamoxifen   *Drug Category:* antineoplastic agents   *Drug Treatment Duration:* varies: until disease progression, refusal of therapy, or death   *Validation of Drug Exposure:* recorded during chemotherapy session   *Study Methodology:* cohort study, retrospective   *Population Selection Criteria:* women treated for advanced breast cancer, having had a mastectomy or tumorectomy   *Total Number of Subjects:* 71   *Case Subjects:* 5 treated   *Drug Event:* cancer (leukemia)   *Validation of Outcome:* physical examination; measurement of hemoglobin, platelet, and leukocyte counts; bone marrow examination   *Rule Out Alternative Explanation:* high dosages   *Results:* RR for overt leukemia = 339 (95% CI 41 to 1223); 2 cases observed versus 0.0059 cases expected; intensive combination chemotherapy with alkylating agents may be harmful for treating advanced breast cancer

90:2   Belongia EA, et al. An investigation of the cause of the eosinophilia–myalgia syndrome associated with tryptophan use. N Engl J Med 1990;323:357-65

Drug Name: tryptophan   *Drug Category:* amino acid supplement   *Validation of Drug Exposure:* telephone questionnaire, interview   *Study Methodology:* case–control study, retrospective   *Population Selection Criteria:* controls are users of tryptophan with and without eosinophilia–myalgia syndrome   *Total Number of Subjects:* 120   *Case Subjects:* 63 (with symptoms), 33 (without symptoms)   *Drug Event:* eosinophilia–myalgia syndrome   *Validation of Outcome:* self-referral, correspondence with physicians   *Results:* 97% of cases; 60% of controls' drugs were from the same manufacturer (OR = 19.3, 95% CI 2.5 to 844.9; p < 0.001); the outbreak resulted from the ingestion of a chemical constituent associated with tryptophan-manufacturing conditions

90:3   Curtis RE, et al. Leukemia following chemotherapy for breast cancer. Cancer Res 1990;50:2741-6

Drug Category: antineoplastic agents   *Validation of Drug Exposure:* cancer registries   *Study Methodology:* nested case–control and a follow-up of a previous cohort study   *Population Selection Criteria:* women treated with adjuvant chemotherapy for breast cancer   *Total Number of Subjects:* 13 734   *Case Subjects:* 24 developed leukemia   *Drug Event:* cancer (leukemia)   *Validation of Outcome:* tumor registries   *Results:* cases had an 11.9-fold risk of leukemia (95% CI 2.6 to 55); women treated with adjuvant chemotherapy for breast cancer are at an increased risk of leukemia

90:4   Cziezel A, Rácz J. Evaluation of drug intake during pregnancy in the Hungarian case–control surveillance of congenital anomalies. Teratology 1990;42:505-12

Drug Category: teratogens   *Drug Treatment Duration:* during pregnancy   *Validation of Drug Exposure:* questionnaire   *Study Methodology:* case–control study, retrospective   *Population Selection Criteria:* newborns   *Total Number of Subjects:* 21 546 healthy newborns, 10 698 with malformations, 828 with Down's syndrome   *Drug Event:* congenital malformations   *Validation of Outcome:* physician diagnoses, autopsies   *Rule Out Alternative Explanation:* mother's comorbidities   *Results:* 26.8% of women used no drugs during pregnancy, 2.0 = the mean number of drugs; the use of true human teratogenic drugs is rare, and the risk of morphologic effects is low

90:5   DeWood MA, Wolbach RA. Randomized double-blind comparison of side effects of nicardipine and nifedipine in angina pectoris. The Nicardipine Investigation Group. Am Heart J 1990;119:468-78

Drug Name: nicardipine, nifedipine   *Drug Category:* calcium-channel blockers   *Drug Dosing Criteria:* nicardipine 30 mg tid, nifedipine 20 mg tid   *Drug Treatment Duration:* 8 weeks   *Study Methodology:* prospective randomized trial, two parallel groups: (I) with nifedipine unintended effects; (II) without nifedipine unintended effects   *Population Selection Criteria:* patients 21 years or older with a primary diagnosis of angina pectoris   *Total Number of Subjects:* cohort I: n = 140; cohort II: n = 110   *Control Subjects:* in both cohorts, groups randomly assigned to nicardipine or nifedipine therapy   *Drug Event:* dizziness, flushing, headache   *Results:* dizziness: nifedipine 18%, nicardipine 6%; p = 0.02; patients experiencing adverse effects of dizziness, flushing, and headache while using nifedipine are likely to develop them again if reexposed

90:6   Ginsberg JS, et al. Heparin effect on bone density. Thromb Haemost 1990;64:286-9

Drug Name: heparin   *Drug Category:* anticoagulants   *Drug Treatment Duration:* ≥ 1 month   *Validation of Drug Exposure:* medical records   *Study Methodology:* cohort study, retrospective   *Population Selection Criteria:* premenopausal women   *Total Number of Subjects:* 122   *Case Subjects:* 61 previously treated with heparin   *Drug Event:* osteoporosis, fracture   *Validation of Outcome:* patient interview, absorptiometry of the spine and wrist   *Rule Out Alternative Explanations:* relations between density and osteoporosis   *Results:* heparin causes a reduction in bone density

90:7   Golding J, et al. Factors associated with childhood cancer in a national cohort study. Br J Cancer 1990;62:304-8

Drug Category: various: analgesics   *Drug Treatment Duration:* during pregnancy   *Study Methodology:* cohort study, prospective   *Population Selection Criteria:* infants delivered during one specified week   *Total Number of Subjects:* 132   *Case Subjects:* 33 developed cancer by age 10 years   *Drug Event:* cancer (childhood)   *Validation of Outcome:* death certification, cancer registry, and follow-up interviews at age 5 and 10 years   *Rule Out Alternative Explanation:* differential recall bias   *Results:* statistically significant associations between antenatal X-rays (OR = 2.75), antenatal smoking (OR = 2.69), use of analgesics during labor (OR = 4.11), and drugs administered to neonate (≥ 1 wk) (OR = 2.6) and cancer

90:8   Green DM, et al. Severe hepatic toxicity after treatment with vincristine and dactinomycin using single- or divided-dose schedules: a report from the National Wilms' Tumor Study. J Clin Oncol 1990;8:1525-30

Drug Name: actinomycin D, vincristine   *Drug Category:* antineoplastic agents   *Drug Dosing Criteria:* 15, 56, or 60 µg/kg   *Drug Treatment Duration:* one dose of actinomycin, 10 weeks of vincristine   *Validation of Drug Exposure:* flow sheets from tumor study   *Study Methodology:* cohort study, prospective   *Population Selection Criteria:* children in tumor study, had nephrectomy   *Total Number of Subjects:* 319 treated with either drug   *Case Subjects:* 38 severe hepatic toxicity after treatment   *Drug Event:* gastrointestinal abnormalities (hepatic disease)   *Validation of Outcome:* flow sheets from tumor study   *Results:* frequency of severe hepatic toxicity: 14.3% (60 µg/kg), 3.7% (45 µg/kg), 2.8% (15 µg/kg) (p = 0.025); suggests an increased frequency of severe hepatic toxicity with the higher, single-dose schedule

90:9   Gruppo Italiano per lo Studio della Sopravvivenza nell'Infarto Miocardico (GISSI). GISSI-2: a factorial randomised trial of alteplase versus streptokinase and heparin versus no heparin among 12 490 patients with acute myocardial infarction. Lancet 1990;336:65-71

Drug Name: streptokinase, r-alteplase, heparin   *Drug Category:* thrombolytics; anticoagulants   *Drug Dosing Criteria:* streptokinase 1.5 MU for 30–60 minutes; alteplase 100 mg for 3 hours; heparin 12 500 U sc bid   *Drug Treatment Duration:* until discharge from hospital   *Validation of Drug Exposure:* medical, hospital records   *Study Methodology:* multicenter open clinical trial   *Population Selection Criteria:* admitted to coronary care units within 6 hours of onset of acute myocardial infarction, no contraindications to heparin   *Total Number of Subjects:* 12 490   *Case Subjects:* 3122 patients per group, 4 groups total: streptokinase, alteplase, heparin, and no heparin   *Drug Event:* stroke, hemorrhage   *Validation of Outcome:* clinical records   *Results:* incidences for total adverse events: streptokinase 22.5%; alteplase 23.1% (RR = 1.04, 95% CI 0.95 to 1.13); heparin 22.7%; no heparin 22.9% (RR = 0.99, 95% CI 0.91 to 1.08); streptokinase and alteplase appear equally effective for infarction patients

90:10   Jick H, et al. A comparison of the risk of hypoglycemia between users of human and animal insulin. 1. Experience in the UK. Pharmacotherapy 1990;10:395-7

Drug Name: insulin   *Drug Category:* antidiabetic agents   *Validation of Drug Exposure:* medical, hospital, and clinical records   *Study Methodology:* case–control study, retrospective   *Population Selection Criteria:* insulin-dependent diabetics 10–49 years   *Total Number of Subjects:* 490   *Case Subjects:* 121 with hypoglycemia: 97 using human, 17 using animal, 7 using both insulin types   *Control Subjects:* 3699 without hypoglycemia: 306 using human, 51 using animal, 12 using both insulin types   *Drug Event:* hypoglycemia   *Validation of Outcome:* discharge summaries, verbal reports   *Rule Out Alternative Explanation:* not identifying all cases/episodes   *Results:* human versus animal insulin for hypoglycemia RR = 0.8 (95% CI 0.4 to 1.6); there is no difference in risk between users of human versus animal insulin

90:11   Kaldor JM, et al. Leukemia following chemotherapy for ovarian cancer. N Engl J Med 1990;322:1-6

Drug Name: busulfan, chlorambucil, cyclophosphamide, melphalan, thiotepa   *Drug Category:* antineoplastic agents   *Drug Dosing Criteria:* low versus high dose defined with respect to median dose   *Validation of Drug Exposure:* medical records   *Study Methodology:* case–control study, retrospective   *Population Selection Criteria:* 114 cases of leukemia following ovarian cancer identified in cancer registries and international hospitals   *Total Number of Subjects:* 456   *Control Subjects:* 342   *Cases:* 114   *Drug Event:* cancer (leukemia)   *Validation of Outcome:* leukemia histologically confirmed   *Results:* overall chemotherapy RR = 12 (95% CI 4.4 to 32)

	Relative Risk	
Drug	Low Dose	High Dose
busulfan	3.6	33.0 (p < 0.01)
chlorambucil	14.0 (p < 0.05)	23.0 (p < 0.01)
cyclophosphamide	2.2	4.1
melphalan	12.0 (p < 0.05)	23.0 (p < 0.01)
thiotepa	8.3 (p < 0.05)	9.7

90:12   Kaldor JM, et al. Leukemia following Hodgkin's disease. N Engl J Med 1990;322:7-13

Drug Name: procarbazine, mechlorethamine   *Drug Category:* antineoplastic agents   *Validation of Drug Exposure:* medical records   *Study Methodology:* case–control study, retrospective   *Population Selection Criteria:* treated for Hodgkin's disease, experiencing no relapse   *Total Number of Subjects:* 618   *Case Subjects:* 168 developed leukemia following treatment for Hodgkin's ≥1 year later   *Drug Event:* cancer (leukemia)   *Validation of Outcome:* medical records   *Rule Out Alternative Explanation:* confounding factors/variables, only following up one type of treatment, unequal therapy treatment, cases under reported   *Results:* chemotherapy alone associated with leukemia RR = 9.0 (95% CI 4.1 to 20); chemo- and radiotherapy RR = 7.7 (95% CI 3.9 to 15); chemotherapy for Hodgkin's disease greatly increases leukemia risk

90:13 Kaufman DW, et al. Diazepam use in relation to breast cancer: results from two case–control studies. Am J Epidemiol 1990;131:483-90

Drug Name: diazepam   *Drug Category:* anticonvulsants, antianxiety agents   *Validation of Drug Exposure:* interview   *Study Methodology:* two case–control studies, retrospective   *Total Number of Subjects:* study 1, 5009; study 2, 1821   *Case Subjects:* study 1—3078 breast cancer, 1259 other cancer, 672 no cancer; study 2—607 breast cancer, 1214 no cancer   *Drug Event:* cancer (breast)   *Validation of Outcome:* interview   *Rule Out Alternative Explanation:* selection bias, association between drug's use and the tendency for diagnosis   *Results:* for regular diazepam use before breast cancer diagnosis RR = 1.0 (95% CI 0.6 to 1.7) for cancer controls and RR = 0.8 (95% CI 0.4 to 1.8) for noncancer controls; data suggest that regular diazepam use does not increase the risk of breast cancer

90:14 LaCroix AZ, et al. Thiazide diuretic agents and the incidence of hip fracture. N Engl J Med 1990;322:286-90

Drug Category: diuretics   *Validation of Drug Exposure:* interviews, household surveys   *Study Methodology:* cohort study, prospective   *Population Selection Criteria:* ≥65 years   *Total Number of Subjects:* 9518   *Case Subjects:* 242 (with hip fractures)   *Drug Event:* fracture (hip)   *Validation of Outcome:* annual interviews, proxy and hospital reports   *Rule Out Alternative Explanation:* duration on medication treatment unknown   *Results:* RR for hip fracture = 0.63 (95% CI 0.46 to 0.86) adjusted for community and age and RR = 0.68 (95% CI 0.49 to 0.94) multivariate; in older subjects, the use of thiazide diuretic agents is associated with about a one-third decreased risk of hip fracture

90:15 Laegreid L, et al. Congenital malformations and maternal consumption of benzodiazepines: a case–control study. Dev Med Child Neurol 1990;32:432-41

Drug Category: sedatives, antianxiety agents, benzodiazepines   *Drug Treatment Duration:* during pregnancy   *Validation of Drug Exposure:* serum benzodiazepine concentrations   *Study Methodology:* case–control study, retrospective   *Population Selection Criteria:* children born 1985–1986   *Total Number of Subjects:* 134   *Case Subjects:* 25   *Control Subjects:* 109—paired sampling, chosen by the next neonatally surviving sibling of a child with cerebral irritation or depression   *Drug Event:* congenital malformations   *Validation of Outcome:* diagnostic hospital register, autopsies   *Results:* OR = 23 (p = 0.00006 Fisher's exact test)

90:16 La Vecchia C, et al. Histamine-2-receptor and gastric cancer risk. Lancet 1990;336:355-7

Drug Name: cimetidine, ranitidine   *Drug Category:* histamine$_2$-receptor antagonists   *Validation of Drug Exposure:* interview, questionnaire   *Study Methodology:* case–control study, retrospective   *Population Selection Criteria:* admitted into hospitals   *Total Number of Subjects:* 2064   *Case Subjects:* 563 newly diagnosed stomach cancer   *Control Subjects:* 1501 acute illnesses, not neoplastic or gastrointestinally related   *Drug Event:* cancer (gastric)   *Validation of Outcome:* hospital diagnoses   *Rule Out Alternative Explanation:* recall bias, not a population-based study, limited histamine$_2$-receptor antagonist treatment   *Results:* RR for ever use = 1.8 (95% CI 1.2 to 2.7), for 5–9 years of use RR = 3.1 (95% CI 1.8

to 5.3), for >10 years of use RR = 0.2 (95% CI 0.03 to 0.8); there is an increased risk of gastric cancer with the first few years of histamine₂-receptor antagonist treatment

90:17 McKinney PA, et al. Chronic myeloid leukemia in Yorkshire: a case–control study. Acta Haematol 1990;83:35-8

Drug Name: digoxin, methyldopa, nifedipine   *Drug Category:* digitalis agents, antihypertensive agents, calcium-channel blockers   *Validation of Drug Exposure:* patient interview by trained interviewers with medical confirmation if available   *Study Methodology:* case–control study, retrospective   *Population Selection Criteria:* cases included with hematologic finding of chronic myeloid leukemia in people aged 15 years and older and residents of the Yorkshire Health Region between January 10, 1979, and September 27, 1986   *Total Number of Subjects:* 363   *Control Subjects:* 241   *Cases:* 122   *Comparability of Controls:* age (±3 y)- and gender-matched hospital controls   *Drug Event:* cancer (leukemia)   *Validation of Outcome:* hospital and physician records   *Results:* ORs: diuretics OR = 4.0 (95% CI 1.9 to 8.8; p < 0.001); methyldopa OR = 9.8 (95% CI 0.9 to 483.0; p < 0.06); digoxin OR = 2.4 (95% CI 0.6 to 10.9; p < 0.28); beta-blockers OR = 2.2 (95% CI 1.1 to 4.5; p < 0.02); nifedipine OR = 7.3 (95% CI 1.3 to 75.1; p < 0.02; excess risks were associated with heart disease and related drugs; weak associations were revealed with occupational and/or hobby exposure to irradiation

90:18 Mills JL, et al. Risk of neural tube defects in relation to maternal fertility and fertility drug use. Lancet 1990;336:103-4

Drug Category: ovulation inducers   *Validation of Drug Exposure:* telephone interview   *Study Methodology:* case–control study, retrospective   *Population Selection Criteria:* women who have had a child   *Total Number of Subjects:* 1690   *Case Subjects:* 571 children with neural tube defects, 546 children with other nonrelated abnormalities, 573 children with no apparent malformations   *Drug Event:* neural tube defects, congenital malformations   *Validation of Outcome:* prenatal diagnoses, delivery, ultrasound examination   *Rule Out Alternative Explanation:* recall and information biases   *Results:* fertility drug use rate for neural tube defects OR = 1.28 (95% CI 0.39 to 4.51), no abnormalities OR = 0.80 (95% CI 0.27 to 2.27); fertility drug use was not significantly more frequent for neural tube defects than for other or no abnormalities

90:19 O'Riordan T, et al. Adjuvant antibiotic therapy in duodenal ulcers treated with colloidal bismuth subcitrate. Gut 1990;31:999-1002

Drug Name: bismuth subcitrate, metronidazole, amoxicillin   *Drug Category:* antibacterials   *Drug Dosing Criteria:* colloidal bismuth subcitrate (CBS) 120 mg qid, metronidazole 200 and 400 mg tid, amoxicillin 500 mg tid   *Drug Treatment Duration:* 4 weeks   *Validation of Drug Exposure:* tablet counts   *Study Methodology:* cohort study, prospective   *Population Selection Criteria:* have duodenal ulcer   *Total Number of Subjects:* 141   *Case Subjects:* CBS alone 43, CBS with amoxicillin 18, CBS with metronidazole 200 mg 23, CBS with metronidazole 400 mg 26, CBS with adjuvant metronidazole and amoxicillin 31   *Drug Event:* gastrointestinal abnormalities (gastritis, *H. pylori* infection, duodenal ulcer)   *Validation of Outcome:* endoscopy, antral biopsy   *Rule Out Alternative Explanation:* development of antibiotic resistance   *Results:* 93% sensitive before and 86% resistant after treatment; CBS with adjuvant metronidazole significantly improves the eradication of *H. pylori* compared with CBS alone

90:20 Palmer AJ, et al. Mortality associated with captopril and enalapril: a report from the DHSS Hypertension Care Computing Project. J Hypertens 1990;8:521-4

Drug Name: captopril, enalapril   *Drug Category:* angiotensin-converting coenzyme inhibitor   *Validation of Drug Exposure:* hypertension electronic records   *Study Methodology:* cohort study, retrospective   *Population Selection Criteria:* with hypertension   *Total Number of Subjects:* 739   *Case Subjects:* 368 captopril, 371 enalapril   *Drug Event:* death   *Validation of Outcome:* blood, urine measurements, bilateral renal artery stenosis   *Rule Out Alternative Explanation:* congestive heart failure   *Results:* mortality for captopril versus enalapril RR = 1.37 (95% CI 0.63 to 2.98); mortality with enalapril is probably similar to that of captopril, and their crude mortality rate was comparable with those of other hypertensive agents

90:21   Pearce N, et al. Case–control study of prescribed fenoterol and death from asthma in New Zealand, 1977–81. Thorax 1990;45:170-5

Drug Name: fenoterol   *Drug Category:* bronchodilators, beta-adrenoreceptor agonists   *Validation of Drug Exposure:* hospital records, prescriptions, general practitioners' letters   *Study Methodology:* case–control study, retrospective   *Population Selection Criteria:* prescribed fenoterol; in hospital during 1977–1981; 5–45 years old   *Total Number of Subjects:* 285   *Case Subjects:* 58 died of asthma   *Control Subjects:* 227 age matched   *Drug Event:* death, asthma   *Validation of Outcome:* discharge records, national mortality records, statistics records   *Rule Out Alternative Explanation:* bias of drugs used versus event   *Results:* asthma death in patients taking fenoterol OR = 1.99 (95% CI 1.12 to 3.55; p = 0.02), inhaled fenoterol for ≥3 asthma drugs OR = 2.98 (95% CI 1.15 to 7.70; p = 0.02), previous admission within the past 12 months OR = 3.91 (95% CI 1.79 to 8.54; p < 0.01), oral corticosteroids OR = 5.83 (95% CI 1.62 to 21.0; p = 0.01); inhaled fenoterol increases the risk of mortality in patients with severe asthma

90:22   Psaty BM, et al. Beta blockers and the primary prevention of nonfatal myocardial infarction in patients with high blood pressure. Am J Cardiol 1990;66:12G-4G

Drug Category: beta-adrenoreceptor antagonists   *Drug Treatment Duration:* average duration = 7.5 years   *Validation of Drug Exposure:* inpatient medical records, physician diagnoses, hospital records, death records   *Study Methodology:* population-based case–control study, retrospective   *Population Selection Criteria:* health maintenance organization enrollees with pharmacologically treated hypertension, 30–79 years old   *Total Number of Subjects:* 863   *Case Subjects:* 126 with nonfatal myocardial infarction   *Drug Event:* myocardial infarction   *Validation of Outcome:* measurement of blood pressure, time of death   *Rule Out Alternative Explanation:* other known risk factors for coronary artery disease   *Results:* RR for nonfatal myocardial infarction = 0.62 (95% CI 0.38 to 0.99); beta-blockers may prevent first events of nonfatal myocardial infarction in hypertensive people

90:23   Psaty BM, et al. The relative risk of incident coronary heart disease associated with recently stopping the use of β-blockers. JAMA 1990;263:1653-7

Drug Category: beta-adrenoreceptor antagonists   *Validation of Drug Exposure:* pharmacy database, prescriptions, discharge abstracts, information systems, death registry   *Study Methodology:* population-based case–control study, retrospective   *Population Selection Criteria:* receiving medication for hypertension, 30–79 years old, no history of coronary heart disease   *Total Number of Subjects:* 985   *Case Subjects:* 248 hospitalized/died from first event of coronary heart disease, 1982–1984   *Drug Event:* coronary heart disease   *Validation of Outcome:* discharge abstracts, death registry, information systems   *Rule Out Alternative Explanation:* noncompliance to medication, misclassification of death/illness   *Results:* coronary heart disease RR = 4.5 (95% CI 1.1 to 18.5) for recently stopping beta-blockers; recently stopping receiving beta-blockers is a risk factor for an incident event of coronary heart disease in patients with high blood pressure

90:24   Riggs BL, et al. Effect of fluoride treatment on the fracture rate in post-menopausal women with osteoporosis. N Engl J Med 1990;322:802-9

Drug Name: fluoride   *Drug Category:* fluoride supplements   *Drug Dosing Criteria:* 75 mg per day   *Drug Treatment Duration:* 4 years   *Validation of Drug Exposure:* counting pills   *Study Methodology:* cohort study, prospective   *Population Selection Criteria:* postmenopausal white women 50–75 years old with osteoporosis   *Total Number of Subjects:* 135   *Case Subjects:* 66   *Drug Event:* osteoporosis, fracture (bone)   *Validation of Outcome:* bone roentgenography, radiologic examinations, measures of bone mineral density   *Rule Out Alternative Explanation:* bias from dropouts, sources of unintended effects questionable   *Results:* new vertebral fractures: placebo—136, fluoride—163 (insignificant); nonvertebral fractures: placebo—24, fluoride—72 (p < 0.01); severe unintended effects: placebo—24, fluoride—54; fluoride therapy increases cancellous but decreases bone mineral density and increases skeletal fragility; conclusion: treatment for postmenopausal osteoporosis is noneffective

90:25   Rubin GL, et al. Estrogen replacement therapy and the risk of endometrial cancer: remaining controversies. Am J Obstet Gynecol 1990;162:148-54

Drug Name: estrogen replacement therapy   *Drug Category:* estrogens   *Drug Treatment Duration:* ≥3 consecutive months   *Validation of Drug Exposure:* self-reports, telephone interview   *Study Methodology:* population-based case–control study, retrospective   *Population Selection Criteria:* women with ≥3 consecutive months of estrogen replacement at >40 years of age   *Total Number of Subjects:* 1182   *Case Subjects:* 196   *Drug Event:* cancer (endometrial)   *Validation of Outcome:* histology reports and slides, National Cancer Institute data collection   *Rule Out Alternative Explanation:* selection, informational and detection biases   *Results:* ≥2 years of estrogen, localized cancer RR = 2.8 (95% CI 1.6 to 4.6), extrauterine cancer RR = 2.9 (95% CI 0.9 to 9.4), endometrial cancer RR = 2.1 (2–5 y of therapy) and RR = 3.5 (≥6 y of therapy); use of estrogen replacement therapy without concurrent progestin therapy, especially ≥2 years, increases the risk of endometrial adenocarcinoma

90:26   Senturia YD, Peckham CS. Children fathered by men treated with chemotherapy for testicular cancer. Eur J Cancer 1990;26:429-32

Drug Category: antineoplastic agents   *Validation of Drug Exposure:* standardized data collection forms   *Study Methodology:* cohort study, retrospective   *Population Selection Criteria:* child of a man with testicular cancer, community controls   *Total Number of Subjects:* 131   *Case Subjects:* 96 fathered child while on chemotherapy   *Control Subjects:* 96 matched, fathered child while not on chemotherapy, other matched community controls   *Drug Event:* congenital malformations   *Validation of Outcome:* general practitioner's records   *Results:* RR for malformations = 1.0 (95% CI 0.41 to 2.40); no evidence found that children fathered by chemotherapy patients have an increased risk of congenital malformations

90:27   Sibai BM, et al. A comparison of no medication versus methyldopa or labetalol in chronic hypertension during pregnancy. Am J Obstet Gynecol 1990;162:960-7

Drug Name: methyldopa, labetalol   *Drug Category:* antihypertensive agents, beta-adrenoreceptor antagonists   *Drug Dosing Criteria:* methyldopa 750 mg/day, 4-g/day maximum; labetalol 300 mg/day, 2.4-g/day maximum   *Drug Treatment Duration:* ≥8 months (27.5-wk average)   *Study Methodology:* cohort study, prospective   *Population Selection Criteria:* pregnant women   *Total Number of Subjects:* 263   *Case Subjects:* 86 labetalol, 87 methyldopa   *Drug Event:* hypertension   *Validation of Outcome:* blood pressure measurement, birth records   *Rule Out Alternative Explanation:* confounding factors   *Results:* no differences with regard to preeclampsia, abruptio placentae, preterm delivery, gestational age at delivery, birth weight, growth retardation, or neonatal head circumference were observed; treatment of maternal blood pressure during pregnancy did not improve perinatal outcome

90:28 Slutsker L, et al. Eosinophilia–myalgia syndrome associated with exposure to tryptophan from a single manufacturer. JAMA 1990;264:213-7

Drug Name: tryptophan *Drug Category:* amino acid supplement *Validation of Drug Exposure:* self-report, telephone surveys *Study Methodology:* case–control study, retrospective *Population Selection Criteria:* tryptophan consumption *Total Number of Subjects:* 151 *Case Subjects:* 58 with syndrome *Drug Event:* eosinophilia–myalgia syndrome (EMS) *Validation of Outcome:* physician reports, self-referral, phone-conducted questionnaires *Rule Out Alternative Explanation:* cases have another common denominator; tryptophan itself, along with individual factors, causes EMS *Results:* 98% of cases, 30% of survey controls, and 48% of volunteer controls used from the same manufacturer; EMS is related to a contaminant/alteration in a subset of tryptophan

90:29 Stryker WS, et al. Diet, plasma levels of beta-carotene and alpha-tocopherol, and risk of malignant melanoma. Am J Epidemiol 1990;131:597-611

Drug Name: vitamin E, vitamin A *Drug Category:* vitamins *Validation of Drug Exposure:* food frequency questionnaire, blood sample *Study Methodology:* case–control study, prospective *Population Selection Criteria:* ≥18 years old, first visit to dermatology clinic *Total Number of Subjects:* 452 *Case Subjects:* 204 *Drug Event:* cancer (malignant melanoma) *Results:* OR (highest vs. lowest quintile) = 0.9 (95% CI 0.5 to 1.5) for plasma beta-carotene; OR = 0.7 (95% CI 0.5 to 1.3) for plasma alpha tocopherol; OR = 0.7 (95% CI 0.4 to 1.2) for carotene intake; OR = 0.7 (95% CI 0.4 to 1.3) for total vitamin E intake; alcohol consumption association with risk of melanoma = 2.1 (p = 0.03); little protective effect from increased plasma concentrations of retinol, alpha tocopherol, or carotenoids was found

90:30 Thiessen BQ, et al. Increased prescribing of antidepressants subsequent to β-blocker therapy. Arch Intern Med 1990;150:2286-90

Drug Name: propranolol *Drug Category:* beta-adrenoreceptor antagonists, antidepressants *Validation of Drug Exposure:* records of a prescription drug plan checked against both drug rules and the health insurance registry file *Study Methodology:* prescription sequencing study *Population Selection Criteria:* ≥20 years old, receiving/having received beta-blocker treatment for chronic illness *Total Number of Subjects:* of 672 863 eligible, 3218 new beta-blocker users were studied *Case Subjects:* 237 received antidepressants by 12 months after treatment *Drug Event:* depression *Validation of Outcome:* antidepressive prescriptions *Rule Out Alternative Explanation:* selection bias, comparability of drug use in previous studies in other databases *Results:* propranolol, overall risk for antidepressant use RR = 4.8 (95% CI 4.1 to 5.5) and RR = 2.1 for other study drug users; for propranolol, RR of antidepressant use varied with age, was longest in 20- to 39-year-old group, and changed with age

90:31 Van't Veer P, et al. Selenium in diet, blood, and toenails in relation to breast cancer: a case–control study. Am J Epidemiol 1990;131:987-94

Drug Name: selenium *Drug Category:* nutritional supplements *Validation of Drug Exposure:* interview, biologic specimens *Study Methodology:* case–control study, retrospective *Population Selection Criteria:* women 25–44 or 55–64 years old *Total Number of Subjects:* 371 *Case Subjects:* 133 *Drug Event:* cancer (breast) *Validation of Outcome:* cancer registries *Rule Out Alternative Explanation:* breast cancer associated with gastrointestinal cancer *Results:* multivariate adjusted OR for breast cancer = 1.6 (95% CI 0.8 to 3.4) for dietary amount, 2.0 (95% CI 0.9 to 4.4) for plasma concentration, 0.9 (95% CI 0.4 to 1.9) for erythrocyte concentration, and 1.1 (95% CI 0.6 to 2.1) for toenail concentrations of selenium; no association was found between selenium and breast cancer

90:32   Werler MM, et al. Maternal vitamin A supplementation in relation to selected birth defects. Teratology 1990;42:497-503

Drug Name: vitamin A   *Drug Category:* vitamins   *Drug Treatment Duration:* during pregnancy   *Validation of Drug Exposure:* interview of mothers, logbooks, and contact with nurseries   *Study Methodology:* case–control study, retrospective   *Population Selection Criteria:* infants with malformations   *Total Number of Subjects:* 5267   *Case Subjects:* 2658 defects involving structures developed from cranial neural crest cells   *Control Subjects:* 2609 having other malformations   *Drug Event:* congenital malformations   *Validation of Outcome:* records of study on birth defects   *Rule Out Alternative Explanation:* unknown doses of vitamin A, disease misclassification, chromosomal abnormalities, and Mendelian disorders   *Results:* RR for lunar month 1 = 2.5 (95% CI 1.0 to 6.2), for lunar month 2 RR = 2.3 (95% CI 0.9 to 5.8), for lunar month 3 RR = 1.6 (95% CI 0.6 to 4.5); maternal vitamin A supplements increase the risk of defects arising from cranial neural crest–derived cells

90:33   Zalzstein E, et al. A case–control study on the association between first trimester exposure to lithium and Ebstein's anomaly. Am J Cardiol 1990;65:817-8

Drug Name: lithium carbonate   *Drug Category:* antimanics   *Drug Treatment Duration:* first trimester of pregnancy   *Validation of Drug Exposure:* medical history records for both parents   *Study Methodology:* case–control study, retrospective   *Population Selection Criteria:* infants having either Ebstein's anomaly or neuroblastoma   *Total Number of Subjects:* 227   *Case Subjects:* 59 born 1971–1988 with Ebstein's anomaly   *Control Subjects:* 168 with neuroblastoma   *Drug Event:* Ebstein's anomaly   *Validation of Outcome:* displacement of septal cusp >8 mm/m², medical charts, cineangiography <1970, M-mode or two-dimensional echocardiography ≥1970   *Rule Out Alternative Explanation:* recall bias for drug use, mothers with adverse outcome recall drug use incorrectly, teratogenic drugs are more likely to be recalled than nonteratogenic drugs   *Results:* the 59 cases of Ebstein's anomaly rule out with 80% power and an alpha of 0.05, and an increased risk of greater than 28-fold. The likelihood of spontaneous occurrence of Ebstein's anomaly in a woman taking lithium is 1 in 2 million; there is an association between prenatal exposure to lithium and Ebstein's anomaly

91:1   Albers MM, et al. Chronic use of the calcium-channel blocker nifedipine has no significant effect on bone metabolism in men. Bone 1991;12:39-42

Drug Name: nifedipine   *Drug Category:* calcium-channel blockers   *Drug Dosing Criteria:* average of 40 mg/day   *Drug Treatment Duration:* average of 3 years   *Validation of Drug Exposure:* self-report   *Study Methodology:* case–control study, prospective   *Population Selection Criteria:* white men with a history of significant coronary artery disease and treatment with nifedipine for more than 2 years' duration   *Total Number of Subjects:* 22   *Case Subjects:* 11   *Control Subjects:* 11   *Drug Event:* osteoporosis   *Validation of Outcome:* photon absorptiometer   *Rule Out Alternative Explanation:* nifedipine has a longer-lasting effect not seen in the short time span of the cases' drug exposure; men have a lower bone turnover, small sample size   *Results:* no significant differences were noted in bone mineral density at the lumbar spine, proximal femur, and proximal and distal radius; no significant differences in the parameters of bone turnover or hormones affecting calcium metabolism and bone were found

91:2   Bashein G, et al. Preoperative aspirin therapy and reoperation for bleeding after coronary artery bypass surgery. Arch Intern Med 1991;151:89-93

Drug Name: aspirin   *Drug Category:* nonsteroidal antiinflammatory drugs   *Treatment Duration:* week prior to coronary artery bypass grafts (CABG)   *Validation of Exposure:* medical record review   *Study Methodology:* case–control study, retrospective

Population Selection Criteria: CABG patients reoperated on for bleeding   *Total Number of Subjects:* 270 patients 1984–1987   *Number of Cases:* 90   *Number of Controls:* 180   *Drug Event:* hemorrhage, CABG   *Validation of Outcome:* hospital records   *Results:* aspirin increased reoperation, transfusions, intensive care, and hospital stays; bleeding not predictable by preoperative coagulation tests

91:3   Butler CR, et al. Bone mineral content in patients with rheumatoid arthritis: relationship to low-dose steroid therapy. Br J Rheumatol 1991;30:86-90

Drug Category: glucocorticoids   *Drug Dosing Criteria:* low dose: <10 mg/day   *Study Methodology:* case–control study, prospective   *Population Selection Criteria:* with rheumatoid arthritis   *Total Number of Subjects:* 142   *Case Subjects:* 71   *Control Subjects:* 71   *Drug Event:* osteoporosis, fracture   *Validation of Outcome:* single-photon absorptiometry and radioimmunoassay   *Rule Out Alternative Explanation:* confounding factors (i.e., age, disease duration, gender, Larsen index, and use of second-line drugs)   *Results:* steroid therapy was associated with a reduced bone mineral content in men (1.16 ± 0.29 vs. 1.32 ± 0.23; $p < 0.05$) and postmenopausal (0.76 ± 0.24 vs. 0.91 ± 0.25; $p < 0.02$) but not premenopausal women (1.1 ± 0.28 vs. 1.1 ± 0.17); symptomatic fractures were more common in steroid-treated patients than in those who had not received steroids (10/71 vs. 2/71; $p < 0.05$)

91:4   Campbell K, Steele RJC. Drugs and complicated diverticular disease: a case–control study. Br J Surg 1991;78:190-1

Drug Category: nonsteroidal antiinflammatory drugs (NSAIDs)   *Validation of Drug Exposure:* medical records   *Study Methodology:* case–control study, retrospective   *Population Selection Criteria:* admitted to hospital with complete medication profile   *Total Number of Subjects:* 150   *Case Subjects:* 50   *Control Subjects:* 100 total: 50 randomly selected from all emergency hospital admissions and 50 with uncomplicated diverticular disease   *Drug Event:* gastrointestinal (diverticulosis)   *Validation of Outcome:* hospital admission and clinical assessment (i.e., barium enema, colonoscopy)   *Results:* 48% of the cases were taking NSAIDs at the time of admission, compared with 18% and 20% of the control groups, respectively, indicating a strong association between the ingestion of NSAIDs and the development of severe complications of diverticular disease; the estimated OR for this association was 4.0 (95% CI 1.37 to 13.03; $p < 0.01$)

91:5   Caravati EM, Bossart PJ. Demographic and electrocardiographic factors associated with severe tricyclic antidepressant toxicity. J Toxicol Clin Toxicol 1991;29:31-43

Drug Name: various   *Drug Category:* tricyclic antidepressants, antidepressants   *Validation of Drug Exposure:* hospital records of serum tricyclic antidepressant concentrations   *Study Methodology:* cohort study, retrospective   *Population Selection Criteria:* admitted to emergency care at hospital, serum screen positive for tricyclic antidepressants   *Total Number of Subjects:* 106   *Case Subjects:* major toxicity 65 (seizures, endotracheal intubation, coma, arrhythmias, hypertension, or death occurred)   *Drug Event:* cardiac arrhythmia, seizures   *Validation of Outcome:* electrocardiograms, heart rate, serum concentration measurements   *Results:* the presence of the parameters for major toxicity (listed above) was positively associated with an increased chance of severe toxicity

91:6   Carson JL, et al. The low risk of upper gastrointestinal bleeding in patients dispensed corticosteroids. Am J Med 1991;91:223-8

Drug Category: glucocorticoids   *Validation of Drug Exposure:* Michigan Medicaid billing database   *Study Methodology:* cohort study, retrospective   *Population Selection Criteria:* dermatitis or asthma treated with corticosteroids   *Total Number of Subjects:* 19 880   *Case Subjects:* upper gastrointestinal (UGI) bleeding 45   *Drug Event:* hemorrhage (gastrointestinal)   *Validation of Outcome:* medical records   *Results:* incidence = 2.8, 23.0, and 15.9 cases per 10 000 person-months for no UGI history, receiving anticoagulants, and a UGI history, respectively; therapy preventing UGI bleeding should be restricted to high-risk patients, if used at all, because the incidence of UGI bleeding in patients treated with corticosteroids is so low

91:7   Christensen JH, et al. The effect of streptokinase on chest pain in acute myocardial infarction. Pain 1991;46:31-4

Drug Name: streptokinase   *Drug Category:* thrombolytics   *Validation of Drug Exposure:* hospital records   *Study Methodology:* cohort study, retrospective   *Population Selection Criteria:* acute myocardial infarction and consequent chest pain   *Total Number of Subjects:* 152   *Case Subjects:* 76   *Drug Event:* chest pain   *Validation of Outcome:* analgesic administration   *Rule Out Alternative Explanation:* selection, information biases *Results:* the median duration of pain was reduced significantly in cases (3.5 h) compared with controls (24 h); streptokinase given in the acute phase of myocardial infarction effectively reduces the duration of cardiac chest pain

91:8   Faundes A, et al. Ovulatory dysfunction during continuous administration of low-dose levonorgestrel by subdermal implants. Fertil Steril 1991;56:27-31

Drug Name: levonorgestrel (Norplant)   *Drug Category:* progestins   *Study Methodology:* case–control study, prospective   *Population Selection Criteria:* women without contraindications to Norplant   *Total Number of Subjects:* 43   *Case Subjects:* 31   *Drug Event:* ovulatory dysfunction   *Validation of Outcome:* clinical evaluation   *Results:* 55% experienced some form of dysfunction, which possibly contributes to the high contraceptive effectiveness of Norplant

91:9   Felson DT, et al. Thiazide diuretics and the risk of hip fracture: results from the Framingham study. JAMA 1991;265:370-3

Drug Category: diuretics   *Study Methodology:* case–control study, retrospective   *Population Selection Criteria:* thiazide diuretic user, postmenopausal woman   *Total Number of Subjects:* 848   *Case Subjects:* 176 (had a first hip fracture)   *Control Subjects:* 672   *Drug Event:* fracture (bone)   *Validation of Outcome:* personal interviews, hospitalization records, telephone calls to subjects not examined, death reviews, and a fracture list specific to this study   *Rule Out Alternative Explanation:* small numbers of former users, potentially confounding factors, not accounting for calcium intake, not recording the specific drug used or the dosage prescribed, others   *Results:* there is a nonsignificant, modest protective effect of any recent thiazide use; recent thiazide-only users experienced significant protection against fracture (adjusted OR = 0.31, 95% CI 0.11 to 0.88), and recent users of combination drugs containing thiazides experienced no protection (adjusted OR = 1.16, 95% CI 0.44 to 3.05)

91:10   Fradkin JE, et al. Creutzfeldt–Jakob disease in pituitary growth hormone recipients in the United States. JAMA 1991;265:880-4

Drug Name: growth hormone, human   *Drug Category:* growth hormone   *Drug Treatment Duration:* variable, median duration of 100 months   *Validation of Drug Exposure:* identified through National Hormone and Pituitary Program records   *Study Methodology:* follow-up study, cohort study, prospective   *Population Selection Criteria:* recipients of human growth hormone   *Total Number of Subjects:* 6284   *Drug Event:* Creutzfeldt–Jakob disease   *Validation of Outcome:* telephone interview   *Rule Out Alternative Explanation:* relatively small numbers of cases   *Results:* seven cases have occurred to date, all among the nearly 700 drug recipients who started therapy before 1970; the median duration of therapy of 100 months in the cases was significantly longer than 41 months for all patients starting treatment before 1970

91:11 Gerstman BB, et al. Oral contraceptive estrogen dose and the risk of deep venous thromboembolic disease. Am J Epidemiol 1991;133:32-7

Drug Name: oral contraceptives *Drug Category:* estrogen–progestins *Drug Dosing Criteria:* <50 µg, 50 µg, >50 µg *Validation of Drug Exposure:* prescription information recorded in Medicaid Informational System *Study Methodology:* cohort study, retrospective *Population Selection Criteria:* females in Michigan Medicaid program, 15–44 years old, with at least one oral contraceptive prescription in 1980–1986 *Total Number of Subjects:* 234 218 *Drug Event:* thromboembolism (venous) *Validation of Outcome:* hospital medical records *Rule Out Alternative Explanation:* false diagnoses, biased information *Results:* intermediate dose: thromboembolism RR = 1.5 (95% CI 1.0 to 2.1; p = 0.04), high dose RR = 1.7 (95% CI 0.9 to 3.0; p = 0.06); the lower doses of estrogen reduce the risk of deep venous thromboembolic disease compared with the higher doses

91:12 Grainger J, et al. Prescribed fenoterol and death from asthma in New Zealand, 1981–7: a further case–control study. Thorax 1991;46:105-11

Drug Name: fenoterol *Drug Category:* bronchodilators, beta-adrenoreceptor agonists *Treatment Duration:* long-term inhaler use *Validation of Exposure:* medical records *Study Methodology:* retrospective analysis of national asthma mortality survey *Population Selection Criteria:* recorded asthma deaths in New Zealand 1981–1987 *Total Number of Subjects:* 112 *Number of Controls:* group A: 427 asthma patients admitted to hospital same year and with previous admission; group B: 448 patients admitted same year as death case *Drug Event:* death (asthma) *Validation of Outcome:* medical record review *Rule Out Alternative Explanation:* other drugs, illnesses *Results:* fenoterol OR group A = 2.11 (95% CI 1.37 to 3.23; p < 0.01); group B = 2.66 (95% CI 1.74 to 4.06; p < 0.01)

91:13 Griffin MR, et al. Nonsteroidal antiinflammatory drug use and increased risk for peptic ulcer disease in elderly persons. Ann Intern Med 1991;114:257-63

Drug Name: fenoprofen, piroxicam, tolmetin, meclofenamate, ibuprofen, indomethacin, sulindac, naproxen *Drug Category:* nonsteroidal antiinflammatory drugs (NSAIDs) *Drug Treatment Duration:* none, indeterminant, ≥30 days, 31–90 days, or ≥90 days *Validation of Drug Exposure:* computerized records and prescriptions *Study Methodology:* case–control study, nested *Population Selection Criteria:* Tennessee Medicaid enrollee ≥65 years old *Total Number of Subjects:* 8478 *Case Subjects:* 1415 hospitalized for peptic ulcer or upper gastrointestinal disease *Drug Event:* gastrointestinal abnormalities (peptic ulcer) *Validation of Outcome:* hospital records, death certificates, surgery, endoscopy, roentgenograms, autopsy *Rule Out Alternative Explanation:* selection bias, result bias, other confounding factors *Results:* RRs for peptic ulcer among NSAID current users versus nonusers: overall = 4.1 (95% CI 3.5 to 4.7), lowest dose = 2.8 (95% CI 1.8 to 4.3), highest dose = 8.0 (95% CI 4.4 to 14.8); RR among first-month NSAID use = 7.2 (95% CI 4.9 to 10.5); the use of nonaspirin NSAIDs is associated with increased risk of serious ulcer disease and may be responsible for a large fraction of peptic ulcer disease in elderly persons

91:14 Heidrich FE, et al. Diuretic drug use and the risk for hip fracture. Ann Intern Med 1991;115:1-6

Drug Category: diuretics *Validation of Drug Exposure:* inpatient, enrollment, and pharmacy databases *Study Methodology:* case–control study, retrospective *Population Selection Criteria:* Group Health Cooperative of Puget Sound elderly patients hospitalized due to a hip fracture between 1977 and 1983 and age- and gender-matched, population-based control patients *Total Number of Subjects:* 924 *Case Subjects:* 462 *Control Subjects:* 462 *Drug Event:* fracture (hip) *Validation of Outcome:* databases used to obtain drug exposure validation *Rule Out Alternative Explanation:* potential confounders were noted, limitation by lack of direct patient contact to verify data abstraction and other reasons *Results:* the adjusted risk for hip fracture for current furosemide use was 3.9 (95% CI 1.5 to 10.4); according to this study, use of thiazide diuretics did not protect against hip fracture and cannot be recommended for fracture prevention; current furosemide use was also associated with hip fracture

91:15   Holvoet J, et al. Relation of upper gastrointestinal bleeding to nonsteroidal antiinflammatory drugs and aspirin: a case–control study. Gut 1991;32:730-4

Drug Name: aspirin   *Drug Category:* nonsteroidal antiinflammatory drugs (NSAIDs)   *Validation of Drug Exposure:* questionnaire   *Study Methodology:* case–control study, retrospective   *Population Selection Criteria:* cases—patients admitted to hospital for hematemesis or melena; controls—matched admitted patients   *Total Number of Subjects:* 322   *Case Subjects:* 161   *Drug Event:* hemorrhage (gastrointestinal)   *Validation of Outcome:* gastroenterologists' records   *Rule Out Alternative Explanation:* preexisting ulcers   *Results:* highly significant difference between cases and controls in NSAID use (OR = 7.4; p < 0.001; 95% CI 3.7 to 14.7) and aspirin use (OR = 2.2; p= 0.025; 95% CI 1.3 to 4.0); highly significant difference with the presence of antecedents of peptic ulcer disease (OR = 5.5; p < 0.001; 95% CI 3.2 to 9.6); the attributable risk for NSAID use was 0.30 (95% CI 0.23 to 0.37) and for aspirin use was 0.14 (95% CI 0.08 to 0.20)

91:16   Isaac NE, et al. Exposure to phenothiazine and risk of cataract. Arch Ophthalmol 1991;109:256-60

Drug Category: antipsychotic agents, phenothiazines   *Drug Treatment Duration:* none, recent, long-term, 2–5 years, or 1-year length   *Validation of Drug Exposure:* hospital pharmacy database   *Study Methodology:* matched cohort study, retrospective   *Population Selection Criteria:* born before 1932 (≥60 y)   *Total Number of Subjects:* 45 301   *Case Subjects:* 4674 developed cataracts   *Control Subjects:* 40 627   *Drug Event:* cataracts   *Validation of Outcome:* hospital records' database   *Rule Out Alternative Explanation:* use of drugs indicates more disease states and therefore a greater contact with medical services, phenothiazine causes anticholinergic adverse effects, and manner of use of antipsychotic drugs leads to a lack of an association   *Results:* the use of antipsychotic or other phenothiazine drugs increased the risk of cataract extraction by roughly 3.5 times in individuals with use in the prior 2–5 years; risk was also increased in individuals with prior use of antidiabetic agents, systemic steroids, and benzodiazepines; there was no elevated risk associated with the use of antihypertensives, and there was no protective effect for aspirin, acetaminophen, or ibuprofen

91:17   Kelly JP, et al. Risks of agranulocytosis and aplastic anemia in relation to the use of cardiovascular drugs: the International Agranulocytosis and Aplastic Anemia Study. Clin Pharmacol Ther 1991;49:330-41

Drug Name: furosemide, propranolol, dipyridamole, digoxin, acetyldigoxin   *Drug Category:* vasodilators, calcium-channel blockers, digitalis agents, beta-adrenoreceptor antagonists, antihypertensive agents, diuretics   *Drug Treatment Duration:* drug use (any) in past 6 months   *Validation of Drug Exposure:* patient interview   *Study Methodology:* population-based case–control study, retrospective   *Population Selection Criteria:* hospital patients   *Total Number of Subjects:* 2140   *Case Subjects:* 270 (hospitalized with agranulocytosis)   *Drug Event:* blood cell abnormalities (agranulocytosis, aplastic anemia)   *Validation of Outcome:* clinical diagnosis, blood tests   *Rule Out Alternative Explanation:* limited use of some test drugs, other drugs causing agranulocytosis   *Results:* RRs for agranulocytosis for propranolol = 2.5, dipyridamole = 3.8, digoxin = 2.5, acetyldigoxin = 9.9 (all significantly associated with event, as well as procainimide and aprindine); furosemide was the only significantly associated drug for aplastic anemia (RR = 3.1)

91:18   Laporte JR, et al. Upper gastrointestinal bleeding in relation to previous use of analgesics and non-steroidal anti-inflammatory drugs. Lancet 1991;337:85-9

Drug Category: analgesics, nonsteroidal antiinflammatory drugs   *Validation of Drug Exposure:* questionnaire   *Study Methodology:* case–control study, retrospective   *Population Selection Criteria:* patients admitted to hospital—cases with hematemesis or melena and a primary diagnosis of acute upper gastrointestinal (UGI) bleeding, matched controls   *Total Number of Subjects:* 2440   *Case Subjects:* 630   *Drug Event:* hemorrhage (gastrointestinal)   *Validation of Outcome:* admission to hospital/hospital records   *Rule Out Alternative Explanation:* selection bias, age bias   *Results:* OR for aspirin = 7.2 (95% CI 5.4 to 9.6), indomethacin = 4.9 (95% CI 2.0 to 12.2), naproxen = 6.5 (95% CI 2.2 to 19.6), piroxicam = 19.1 (95% CI 8.2 to 44.3); paracetamol, propyphenazone, and dipyrone did not increase the risk; there was a higher incidence of UGI bleeding among the elderly; previous ulcer and UGI history did not affect ORs

91:19   Manson JE, et al. A prospective study of aspirin use and primary prevention of cardiovascular disease in women. JAMA 1991;266:521-7

Drug Name: aspirin   *Drug Category:* analgesics, nonsteroidal antiinflammatory drugs   *Drug Dosing Criteria:* 1–3, 4–6, 7–14, or ≥15 per week, each assumed to be 325 mg   *Validation of Drug Exposure:* questionnaires for 1980, 1982, and 1984   *Study Methodology:* cohort study, prospective, including 6 years of follow-up   *Population Selection Criteria:* US registered female nurses 34–65 years, free of diagnosed coronary heart disease, stroke, and cancer at baseline   *Total Number of Subjects:* 87 687   *Drug Event:* myocardial infarction   *Validation of Outcome:* medical record examinations, follow-up questionnaire   *Rule Out Alternative Explanation:* recall bias possible, confounders, reasons for using aspirin may be associated with a reduced risk, others   *Results:* there were 516 important vascular events; the RR for a first myocardial infarction was 0.68 (95% CI 0.52 to 0.89; p = 0.005) of those taking 1–6 aspirin tablets per week compared with no aspirin; after simultaneous adjustment for risk factors for coronary disease, the RR was 0.75 (95% CI 0.58 to 0.99; p = 0.94)

91:20   McCarthy GM, Skillings JR. A prospective cohort study of the orofacial effects of vincristine neurotoxicity. J Oral Pathol Med 1991;20:345-9

Drug Name: vincristine   *Drug Category:* antineoplastic agents   *Drug Dosing Criteria:* 1–2 mg   *Drug Treatment Duration:* one dose weekly for ≥4 weeks   *Validation of Drug Exposure:* clinic records   *Study Methodology:* cohort study, prospective   *Population Selection Criteria:* cancer patients receiving vincristine   *Total Number of Subjects:* 40   *Case Subjects:* 26 (developed neurotoxicity)   *Drug Event:* neurotoxicity   *Validation of Outcome:* telephone interview, baseline interviews, oral examinations   *Rule Out Alternative Explanation:* recall bias   *Results:* 65% developed symptoms of neurotoxicity in orofacial area significantly associated with younger age and single marital status

91:21   Moore RD, et al. Long-term safety and efficacy of zidovudine in patients with advanced human immunodeficiency virus disease. Arch Intern Med 1991;151:981-6

Drug Name: zidovudine   *Drug Category:* antiretrovirals   *Study Methodology:* cohort study, prospective   *Population Selection Criteria:* prescribing zidovudine to treat HIV infection   *Total Number of Subjects:* 866 eligible of 2876 screened   *Case Subjects:* 500 (AIDS), 366 (AIDS-related complex)   *Drug Event:* drug events, general   *Validation of Outcome:* medical, hospital records   *Rule Out Alternative Explanation:* dose or concurrent use of other medications not controlled   *Results:* pretreatment factors and treatment for a high proportion of time significantly associated with increased survival time; serious leukopenia occurred in 37% and serious anemia occurred in 32% of patients

91:22 Pedersen-Bjergaard J, et al. Increased risk of myelodysplasia and leukemia after etoposide, cisplatin, and bleomycin for germ-cell tumors. Lancet 1991;338:359-63

Drug Name: etoposide, cisplatin, bleomycin *Drug Category:* antineoplastic agents *Drug Dosing Criteria:* standard (2000 mg/m²) or high dose (3000 mg/m²), cumulative doses *Validation of Drug Exposure:* administration *Study Methodology:* case–control study, retrospective *Population Selection Criteria:* with germ-cell tumors treated with chemotherapy *Total Number of Subjects:* 212 *Case Subjects:* 5 *Drug Event:* cancer (leukemia) *Validation of Outcome:* physical examination, radiographs, and laboratory tests *Results:* the mean cumulative risk of leukemic complications was 4.7% (standard error = 2.3) 5.7 years after start of therapy; compared with the general population, the risk of overt leukemia was 336 (95% CI 92 to 861)

91:23 Piper JM, et al. Corticosteroid use and peptic ulcer disease: role of nonsteroidal anti-inflammatory drugs. Ann Intern Med 1991;114:735-40

Drug Category: glucocorticoids, nonsteroidal antiinflammatory drugs (NSAIDs) *Validation of Drug Exposure:* pharmacy file, nursing home file *Study Methodology:* case–control study, nested *Population Selection Criteria:* in Tennessee Medicaid program, ≥65 years old *Total Number of Subjects:* 8478 *Case Subjects:* 1415 (hospitalized with a confirmed peptic ulcer or episode of upper gastrointestinal bleeding 1984–1986) *Drug Event:* peptic ulcer, hemorrhage (gastrointestinal) *Validation of Outcome:* surgery, endoscopy, roentgenogram, autopsy, hospital discharge records, death certificates *Rule Out Alternative Explanation:* use of drugs from other sources, noncompliance, only elderly population studied, making results not applicable to non-Medicaid or younger populations, other risk factors *Results:* RR for patients receiving corticosteroids but not NSAIDs = 1.1 (95% CI 0.5 to 2.1); RR for those receiving both drugs = 4.4 (95% CI 2.0 to 9.7)

91:24 Rosa FW. Spina bifida in infants of women treated with carbamazepine during pregnancy. N Engl J Med 1991;324:674-7

Drug Name: carbamazepine *Drug Category:* anticonvulsants *Drug Treatment Duration:* during pregnancy *Validation of Drug Exposure:* Medicaid database records *Study Methodology:* cohort study, retrospective *Population Selection Criteria:* Medicaid-registered pregnant women who delivered between 1980 and 1988 and took anticonvulsant agents during pregnancy *Total Number of Subjects:* 1490 *Case Subjects:* 4 *Drug Event:* spina bifida *Validation of Outcome:* Medicaid database records *Rule Out Alternative Explanation:* confounding by maternal exposure to other drugs not indicated, selection bias and others unlikely *Results:* there were 4 cases found—3 exposed maternally to carbamazepine, and 1 exposed to other anticonvulsants

91:25 Sandler DP, et al. Nonsteroidal anti-inflammatory drugs and the risk for chronic renal disease. Ann Intern Med 1991;115:165-72

Drug Category: nonsteroidal antiinflammatory drugs (NSAIDs) *Drug Treatment Duration:* <2 years, 2–4 years, and >4 years *Validation of Drug Exposure:* telephone interviews *Study Methodology:* multicenter case–control study, retrospective *Population Selection Criteria:* cases were hospitalized between 1980 and 1982 with discharge diagnosis of newly diagnosed chronic renal dysfunction and a serum creatinine concentration consistently at or above 130 mmol/L (1.5 mg/dL); controls were randomly chosen by telephone screening *Total Number of Subjects:* 1060 *Case Subjects:* 544 *Control Subjects:* 516 *Drug Event:* renal failure *Validation of Outcome:* hospital discharge diagnoses *Rule Out Alternative Explanation:* difference between men and women, misclassification of exposure, NSAIDs used to treat symptoms of undiagnosed renal disease, detection bias, misclassification of controls, and other possible confounding factors *Results:* a twofold risk for chronic renal disease was associated with previous daily use of NSAIDs (adjusted OR = 2.1, 95% CI 1.1 to 4.1), limited predominantly to men >65 years with daily use (OR = 10.0, 95% CI 1.2 to 82.7)

91:26   Seddon JM, et al. Low-dose aspirin and risks of cataract in a randomized trial of U.S. physicians. Arch Ophthalmol 1991;109:252-5

Drug Name: aspirin   *Drug Category:* nonsteroidal antiinflammatory drugs   *Drug Dosing Criteria:* 325 mg on alternate days *Drug Treatment Duration:* varies—average of 60.2 months   *Validation of Drug Exposure:* self-acclamation, questionnaires   *Study Methodology:* randomized trial   *Population Selection Criteria:* healthy male US physicians 40–84 years old   *Total Number of Subjects:* 22 071   *Case Subjects:* 10 654   *Drug Event:* cataracts   *Validation of Outcome:* written consent forms, ophthalmologists' diagnoses, questionnaires sent to ophthalmologists   *Rule Out Alternative Explanation:* random misclassification, confounding factors, delayed effect   *Results:* RR for cataract abstraction (aspirin vs. placebo) = 0.80 (95% CI 0.56 to 1.15); RR for cataracts (aspirin vs. placebo) = 0.95 (95% CI 0.74 to 1.22)

91:27   Spector TD, et al. Does estrogen replacement therapy protect against rheumatoid arthritis? J Rheumatol 1991;18:1473-6

Drug Name: estrogen replacement therapy   *Drug Category:* estrogens   *Drug Treatment Duration:* ≥3 months   *Validation of Drug Exposure:* clinical records   *Study Methodology:* cohort study, retrospective   *Population Selection Criteria:* women 35–64 years old   *Total Number of Subjects:* 4326   *Case Subjects:* 1075   *Control Subjects:* 3251   *Drug Event:* rheumatoid arthritis   *Validation of Outcome:* questionnaire   *Rule Out Alternative Explanation:* clinical observers not blinded, data were from 1987 rather than the 1958 American Rheumatology Association criteria, selection bias   *Results:* 8 cases occurred in the postmenopausal control cohort and 6 in the case cohort; the incidence rates were 19.7/10 000 for estrogen replacement users and 12.3/10 000 for controls; the RRs for the estrogen users were 1.62 (95% CI 0.56 to 4.74); the data do not support the previous observation of a fourfold reduction in the drug event among estrogen replacement users

91:28   Strom BL, et al. A population-based study of Stevens–Johnson syndrome: incidence and antecedent drug exposures. Arch Dermatol 1991;127:831-8

Drug Category: penicillins   *Validation of Outcome:* Computerized Online Medicaid Pharmaceutical Analysis and Surveillance System (COMPASS)   *Study Methodology:* population-based cohort study, retrospective   *Population Selection Criteria:* patient in COMPASS Medicaid records from 1980 to 1983 for Michigan and Minnesota, and in 1983 for Florida who had been with Medicaid before hospitalization for the event   *Total Number of Subjects:* 21   *Case Subjects:* 19 with documented Stevens–Johnson syndrome and 2 with toxic epidermal necrolysis   *Drug Event:* Stevens–Johnson syndrome   *Validation of Outcome:* COMPASS   *Rule Out Alternative Explanation:* possible differences between patient reports obtained for the study and those unobtainable for the study, underdiagnosis of the disease, turnover rate and other variations within the Medicaid program, and random variation   *Results:* the incidence rates of the disease were 7.1 (95% CI 6.1 to 8.2) in Michigan, 2.6 in Minnesota (95% CI 1.6 to 4.0), and 6.8 in Florida (95% CI 4.3 to 10.3) per million per year; penicillins, especially aminopenicillins, were frequently used in the 19 cases

91:29   Strom BL, et al. No causal relationship between transdermal scopolamine and seizures: methodologic lessons for pharmacoepidemiology. Clin Pharmacol Ther 1991;50:107-13

Drug Name: transdermal copolamine, diphenhydramine, meclizine, prochlorperazine, promethazine   *Drug Category:* antiemetics   *Validation of Drug Exposure:* Computerized

Online Medicaid Pharmaceutical Analysis and Surveillance System (COMPASS) and primary medical records   *Study Methodology:* cohort study, retrospective   *Population Selection Criteria:* taking one of the five drugs listed above and recorded in COMPASS in Michigan for January 1980–1986 and in Florida for January 1982–1986   *Total Number of Subjects:* 197 348   *Case Subjects:* 1013 exposed to transdermal scopolamine, 15 experiencing seizures after taking transdermal scopolamine   *Control Subjects:* all the rest, exposed to the other drugs   *Drug Event:* seizures   *Validation of Outcome:* COMPASS   *Rule Out Alternative Explanation:* random error; confounding variables; information, selection, and misclassification biases; and misclassification of patient and control subjects   *Results:* a fourfold-increased risk of seizures after transdermal scopolamine use was observed in the claims data; on examination of the primary medical records, all patients experiencing seizures after use of the drug either had seizures before receiving the drug or did not really have seizures; the data do not confirm the existence of an association between seizures and the use of transdermal scopolamine

91:30   Voigt LF, et al. Progestagen supplementation of exogenous oestrogens and risk of endometrial cancer. Lancet 1991;338:274-7

Drug Category: progestins, estrogens, estrogen–progestins   *Drug Treatment Duration:* <10 days/month, >10 days/month, ≥6 months of total progestagen therapy   *Validation of Drug Exposure:* patient or telephone interview   *Study Methodology:* population-based case–control study, retrospective   *Population Selection Criteria:* women aged 40–65 years   *Total Number of Subjects:* 340   *Case Subjects:* 158   *Control Subjects:* 182   *Drug Event:* cancer (breast, endometrial)   *Validation of Outcome:* cancer surveillance system   *Results:* the risk of endometrial cancer among women using unopposed estrogen for over 3 years was more than five times that of women using no hormones (RR = 5.7, 95% CI 2.5 to 12.8), those who had also used a progestagen for at least 6 months of that time had an RR of 1.6 (95% CI 0.6 to 3.9)

91:31   Warram JH, et al. Excess mortality associated with diuretic therapy in diabetes mellitus. Arch Intern Med 1991;151:1350-6

Drug Category: diuretics   *Study Methodology:* cohort study, prospective   *Population Selection Criteria:* white, normal creatinine concentrations at baseline, outpatients enrolled in study of ophthalmologic laser treatment study with diabetes and severe retinopathy   *Total Number of Subjects:* 759   *Case Subjects:* 139 died   *Drug Event:* death   *Validation of Outcome:* death certificate and medical records reviewed by a mortality committee   *Results:* cardiovascular mortality was higher in patients treated for hypertension than in patients with untreated hypertension; after adjusting for differences in risk factors, cardiovascular mortality was 3.8 times higher in patients treated with diuretics alone than in patients with untreated hypertension (p < 0.001)

91:32   Wolf PH, et al. Reduction of cardiovascular disease-related mortality among postmenopausal women who use hormones: evidence from a national cohort. Am J Obstet Gynecol 1991;164:489-94

Drug Name: estrogen replacement therapy   *Drug Category:* progestins, estrogens, estrogen–progestins   *Drug Treatment Duration:* ≤16.3 years   *Validation of Drug Exposure:* treatment/therapy   *Study Methodology:* cohort study, retrospective   *Population Selection Criteria:* white, postmenopausal women ≥55 years old   *Total Number of Subjects:* 1944   *Case Subjects:* 631 died (of these, 347 died from cardiovascular disease)   *Drug Event:* death   *Validation of Outcome:* death certificate with cause coded by the rules of the International Classification of Diseases   *Rule Out Alternative Explanation:* other cardiovascular risk factors, other biases   *Results:* RRs for:

history of diabetes	= 2.38 (95% CI 1.73 to 3.26)
previous myocardial infarction	= 2.12 (95% CI 1.56 to 2.86)
smoking	= 2.18 (95% CI 1.69 to 2.81)
high blood pressure	= 1.49 (95% CI 1.14 to 1.94)
death from cardiovascular disease	= 0.66 (95% CI 0.48 to 0.90)
(among those experiencing natural menopause)	= 0.69 (95% CI 0.45 to 1.06)

Postmenopausal hormone therapy reduces the risk of death from cardiovascular disease

92:1 Anaissie E, et al. Listeriosis in patients with chronic lymphocytic leukemia who were treated with fludarabine and prednisone. Ann Intern Med 1992;117:466-9

Drug Name: fludarabine, prednisone *Drug Category:* antineoplastic agents, glucocorticoids *Study Methodology:* cohort study, retrospective *Population Selection Criteria:* patients with chronic lymphocytic leukemia receiving care between 1980 and 1990 *Total Number of Subjects:* 795: 248 treated with both drugs, 160 treated with fludarabine alone, 387 receiving conventional chemotherapy *Drug Event:* listeriosis *Validation of Outcome:* cancer center's records *Rule Out Alternative Explanation:* confounding effect from corticosteroid administration, small number of cases, others *Results:* 7 of the cases developed drug event (1.7%, 95% CI 0.2% to 6%) compared with none of the controls (95% CI 0% to 0.9%; p = 0.015); the 7 were treated with both drugs; none of 160 patients treated with fludarabine only (p = 0.045 by Fisher's exact test)

92:2 Bright RA, Everitt DE. Beta-blockers and depression. Evidence against an association. JAMA 1992;267:1783-7

Drug Category: beta-adrenoreceptor antagonists, antidepressants *Validation of Drug Exposure:* prescription claims for the drugs *Study Methodology:* prescription sequencing study (case–control) *Population Selection Criteria:* enrollee of Medicaid and having a depression marker (antidepressant drugs, in-hospital depression diagnosis, or electroconvulsive therapy) *Total Number of Subjects:* 4302 *Drug Event:* depression *Validation of Outcome:* Medicaid claims for depression markers *Rule Out Alternative Explanation:* case definition, sensitivity of depression markers, assessment of drug exposure, others *Results:* case patients overall were more likely to have taken drug (OR = 1.45, 95% CI 1.29 to 1.62); controlling for confounders resulted in a null effect (OR = 0.98, 95% CI 0.87 to 1.12); the OR was consistently lower for case patients with a depression diagnosis or electroconvulsive therapy than for cases with only antidepressant use as a marker

92:3 Curtis RE, et al. Risk of leukemia after chemotherapy and radiation treatment for breast cancer. N Engl J Med 1992;326:1745-51

Drug Names: melphalan, cyclophosphamide *Drug Category:* antineoplastic agents *Validation of Drug Exposure:* cancer registry records, hospital charts, oncology clinic records *Study Methodology:* case–control study, retrospective *Population Selection Criteria:* women with invasive breast cancer, 1973–1985 *Total Number of Subjects:* 82 700 population cohort study, 354 in study *Number of Cases:* 90 *Number of Controls:* 264 *Drug Event:* cancer (leukemia) *Validation of Outcome:* registry files *Results:* dose-dependent risks were observed after radiotherapy and treatment with melphalan and cyclophosphamide; melphalan was 10 times more leukemogenic than cyclophosphamide (RR = 31.4 vs. 3.1); there was little increase in the risk associated with total cyclophosphamide doses of <20 000 mg

92:4 De Jaegere PP, et al. Intracranial hemorrhage in association with thrombolytic therapy: incidence and clinical predictive factors. J Am Coll Cardiol 1992;19:289-94

Drug Name: streptokinase   *Drug Category:* thrombolytics   *Treatment Duration:* single dose   *Validation of Drug Exposure:* hospital records in the Netherlands   *Study Methodology:* cohort study, prospective   *Population Selection Criteria:* mycocardial infarction treated with streptokinase   *Total Number of Subjects:* 2469 (75% streptokinase)   *Number of Cases:* 24 (1%)   *Number of Controls:* 48 (matched 2/case)   *Drug Event:* hemorrhage (intracranial)   *Validation of Outcome:* hospital records   *Results:* RRs: oral anticoagulants <therapy, weight <70 kg, and age >65 y

92:5   Dravet C, et al. Epilepsy, antiepileptic drugs, and malformations in children of women with epilepsy: a French prospective cohort study. Neurology 1992;42(suppl 5):75-82

Drug Name: valproic acid, phenytoin, phenobarbital   *Drug Category:* anticonvulsants   *Validation of Drug Exposure:* questionnaires sent to healthcare workers and professionals, plasma concentrations measured by physicians each trimester of patients' pregnancies   *Study Methodology:* cohort study, prospective   *Population Selection Criteria:* pregnant women   *Total Number of Subjects:* 117 183 births in the study period   *Case Subjects:* 227 outcomes of pregnancy bearing 229 infants   *Drug Event:* congenital malformations, microcephaly   *Validation of Outcome:* birth defects registry, mail or telephone to the physicians   *Results:* 7% of the cases and 1.36% of the general population had malformations; no significant relationship was found between type and severity of epilepsy and occurrence of malformations of isolated microcephaly; valproic acid and phenytoin were the most teratogenic; the malformations observed in cases whose mothers received valproic acid, phenytoin, or phenobarbital were not seen in cases whose mothers were not exposed to those drugs; phenytoin plus phenobarbital was more teratogenic than phenobarbital alone; benzodiazepines in combinations had a borderline, nonspecific effect on microcephaly

92:6   Ernst P, et al. Risk of fatal and near-fatal asthma in relation to inhaled corticosteroid use. JAMA 1992;268:3462-4

Drug Name: various   *Drug Category:* glucocorticoids   *Drug Dosing Criteria:* inhaled   *Validation of Drug Exposure:* Saskatchewan database   *Study Methodology:* nested case–control analysis of a historical cohort; a further analysis   *Population Selection Criteria:* 5–54 years old, dispensed 10 or more asthma drugs from 1978–1987, having at least one hospitalization for asthma in prior 2 years, having received social assistance   *Total Number of Subjects:* 784   *Case Subjects:* 129: 44 deaths and 85 near-deaths   *Control Subjects:* 655   *Drug Event:* death (asthma)   *Validation of Outcome:* death or occurrence of hypercarbia, intubation, and mechanical ventilation during an acute attack of asthma found in death certificates, coroner's reports, autopsy reports, and hospital discharge summaries   *Results:* subjects dispensed one or more metered-dose inhaler of beclomethasone per month on average over a 1-year period had significantly lower risk of fatal and near-fatal asthma (OR = 0.1, 95% CI 0.02 to 0.6), after accounting for the risk associated with use of other medications and adjusting for the markers of risk of adverse events related to asthma

92:7   Falkeborn M, et al. The risk of acute myocardial infarction after oestrogen and oestrogen–progestagen replacement. Br J Obstet Gynaecol 1992;99:821-8

Drug Category: estrogens, estrogen–progestins   *Validation of Drug Exposure:* pharmacy records   *Study Methodology:* population-based cohort study, prospective   *Population Selection Criteria:* women ≥35 years, prescribed noncontraceptive estrogens during 1977–1980   *Total Number of Subjects:* 23 174   *Case Subjects:* 227   *Drug Event:* myocardial infarction   *Validation of Outcome:* hospital admission inpatient registry   *Rule Out Alternative Explanation:* possible selection bias, loss of follow-up due to migration out of the region, misclassification of drug exposure, others *Results:* 227 actual cases occurred versus 281.1 cases expected (RR = 0.81, 95% CI 0.71 to 0.92); women who were younger than 60 years at entry into the study and prescribed estradiol compounds (1–2 mg) or conjugated estrogens (0.625–1.25 mg) showed a significant 30% reduction of the RR = 0.69 (95% CI 0.54 to 0.86); those prescribed a combined estradiol–levonorgestrel brand also demonstrated a significantly lowered RR = 0.53 (95% CI 0.30 to 0.87); the risk estimates were near unity during the first year of follow-up but decreased during subsequent years; exposure to the weak estrogen estriol did not alter the risk

92:8   Franklyn JA, et al. Long-term thyroxine treatment and bone mineral density. Lancet 1992;340:9-13

Drug Name: thyroxine, levothyroxine   *Drug Category:* thyroid hormones   *Drug Dosing Criteria:* various—mean, 191 µg/d; SD ± 50 µg/d   *Drug Treatment Duration:* long-term; mean, 7.9 years; range, 1–19 years   *Study Methodology:* cohort study, prospective *Population Selection Criteria:* no present or previous therapy with estrogens, thiazide diuretics, calcium, vitamin D, or tamoxifen   *Total Number of Subjects:* 98   *Case Subjects:* 49   *Control Subjects:* 49   *Drug Event:* osteoporosis   *Validation of Outcome:* dual-energy X-ray absorptiometry   *Results:* the patients showed no evidence of lower bone mineral density than the controls nor was bone mineral density correlated with dose, duration of therapy, or cumulative intake or with tests of thyroid function; there was a decrease in bone density with age in both groups

92:9   Graham NM, et al. The effects on survival of early treatment of human immunodeficiency virus infection. N Engl J Med 1992;326:1037-42

Drug Name: zidovudine   *Drug Category:* antiretrovirals   *Drug Treatment Duration:* ≤3 years   *Validation of Drug Exposure:* hospital and clinic records   *Study Methodology:* cohort study, retrospective   *Population Selection Criteria:* high-risk men seropositive for HIV-1 *Total Number of Subjects:* 2568   *Number of Cases:* 304 deaths   *Number of Controls:* historical data   *Drug Event:* AIDS survival   *Validation of Outcome:* hospital and clinic records   *Rule Out Alternative Explanation:* CD4 count, cell count, *Pneumocystis carinii* pneumonia prophylaxis   *Results:* zidovudine alone RR death = 0.45 at 6 months, 0.59 at 12 months, 0.70 at 18 months (all significant), and 0.81 at 24 months (not significant)

92:10   Grainger J, et al. Prescribed fenoterol and death from asthma in New Zealand, 1981–7: a further case–control study. Thorax 1991;46:105-11

Drug Name: fenoterol   *Drug Category:* bronchodilators, beta-adrenoreceptor agonists *Validation of Drug Exposure:* data extracted from the case notes, the accident and emergency department notes, and the general practitioner's letter   *Study Methodology:* case–control study, retrospective   *Population Selection Criteria:* 5–45 years old, admitted to hospital for asthma between 1981 and 1987   *Total Number of Subjects:* 897   *Case Subjects:* 112   *Control Subjects:* 875: Group A—427 admissions of asthma in the previous 12 months, Group B—448 just one hospital admission within the 12 months   *Drug Event:* death (asthma)   *Validation of Outcome:* National Health Statistics Center records *Rule Out Alternative Explanation:* potential for confounding by asthma severity, others *Results:* the inhaled fenoterol OR was 2.11 (95% CI 1.37 to 3.23; p < 0.01) for Group A and 2.66 (95% CI 1.74 to 4.06; p < 0.01) for Group B; markers of chronic asthma severity were associated with asthma death with Group B but not Group A

92:11   Gross TP, et al. The risk of epithelial ovarian cancer in short-term users of oral contraceptives. Am J Epidemiol 1992;136:46-53

Drug Name: oral contraceptives   *Drug Category:* estrogen–progestins   *Drug Treatment Duration:* short term (3–11 mo use)   *Validation of Drug Exposure:* patient interview conducted by trained female staff using questionnaires   *Study Methodology:* population-based case–control study, retrospective   *Population Selection Criteria:* US women 20–54 years old   *Total Number of Subjects:* 2212   *Case Subjects:* 283 with cancer: 41 oral contraceptive users, 242 never users   *Control Subjects:* 1929 without cancer: 412 users, 1517 never users   *Drug Event:* cancer (ovarian)   *Validation of Outcome:* patient interviews   *Results:* the age- and parity-adjusted RR of cancer for the cases versus controls was 0.6 (95% CI 0.4 to 0.9); important factors in risk of cancer were family history of ovarian cancer, reasons for stopping use of oral contraceptives, and latency (the time between first taking the pill and disease diagnosis)

92:12   Gurwitz JH, et al. Antihypertensive drug therapy and the initiation of treatment for diabetes mellitus. Ann Intern Med 1992;118:273-8

Drug Category: antihypertensive agents, thiazides, antidiabetic agents   *Validation of Drug Exposure:* Medicaid records   *Study Methodology:* prescription sequencing study (case–control)   *Population Selection Criteria:* New Jersey Medicaid enrollees ≥35 years old   *Total Number of Subjects:* 23 710   *Case Subjects:* 11 855 newly started on a hypoglycemic agent (oral agent or insulin) between 1981 and 1990   *Control Subjects:* 11 855   *Drug Event:* hyperglycemia   *Validation of Outcome:* Medicaid hospitalization records indicating first initiation of hypoglycemic therapy   *Rule Out Alternative Explanation:* surveillance bias, selection factors   *Results:* after adjusting for risk factors, initiation of hypoglycemics was increased for users of virtually all antihypertensive agents relative to nonusers; the estimated RR for cases versus controls was 1.40 (95% CI 1.26 to 1.58) for patients taking thiazide diuretics and ranged from 1.56 to 1.77 for patients receiving other antihypertensives; a higher risk was associated with multiple-agent regimens OR = 1.93 (95% CI 1.75 to 2.13), including thiazide diuretics; OR = 1.76 (95% CI 1.49 to 2.07), when thiazides were excluded

92:13   Kamb ML, et al. Eosinophilia–myalgia syndrome in L-tryptophan-exposed patients. JAMA 1992;267:77-82

Drug Name: tryptophan   *Drug Category:* amino acid supplement   *Validation of Drug Exposure:* psychiatrist office records   *Study Methodology:* cohort study, retrospective, nested case–control studies   *Population Selection Criteria:* patients of one psychiatrist in South Carolina   *Total Number of Subjects:* 418   *Drug Event:* eosinophilia–myalgia syndrome   *Validation of Outcome:* chart reviews and telephone and in-person interviews   *Rule Out Alternative Explanation:* patient-related confounding factors   *Results:* risk for definite event was associated with a certain brand's dose and age of patient; 47 cases (11%) were definite and 68 (16%) were possible cases, most of which involved patients using the particular brand; among the brand users, 45 definite cases (29%) and 36 possible cases (23%) were found

92:14   Kase CS, et al. Intracranial hemorrhage after coronary thrombolysis with tissue plasminogen activator. Am J Med 1992;92:384-90

Drug Name: r-alteplase, heparin   *Drug Category:* thrombolytics, anticoagulants   *Drug Dosing Criteria:* 4000–5000 units heparin iv, various doses of alteplase   *Validation of Drug Exposure:* hospital records   *Study Methodology:* case–control study, retrospective   *Population Selection Criteria:* entered into 1 of 16 clinical trials within 6 hours of onset of chest pain   *Total Number of Subjects:* 1700   *Case Subjects:* 9   *Drug Event:* hemorrhage (intracranial)   *Validation of Outcome:* clinical diagnosis   *Rule Out Alternative Explanation:* small number of people with the event, local cerebrovascular factors, and others   *Results:* 9 of 1700 (0.53%) of those administered the experimental drug developed the hemorrhage

92:15   Keisu M, Ekman E. Sulfasalazine-associated agranulocytosis in Sweden, 1972–1989: clinical features and estimation of its incidence. Eur J Clin Pharmacol 1992;43:215-8

Drug Name: sulfasalazine *Drug Category:* sulfonamides, antibacterials *Treatment Duration:* any *Validation of Drug Exposure:* report submitted to Swedish drug-monitoring system (fatal cases' medical record requested) *Study Methodology:* reported cases compared with national usage *Population Selection Criteria:* sulfasalazine *Total Number of Subjects:* estimated 345 *Number of Cases:* 117 *Drug Event:* agranulocytosis *Validation of Outcome:* medical records *Rule Out Alternative Explanation:* other drugs analyzed *Results:* incidence during first 30 days of prescription = 1/2400, days 31–90 = 1/700, and days 91–365 = 1/11 200 (serious estimate was 1/1750 patient-years of exposure)

92:16 Lishner M, et al. Maternal and fetal outcome following Hodgkin's disease in pregnancy. Br J Cancer 1992;65:114-7

Drug Category: antineoplastic agents *Treatment Duration:* any during pregnancy *Validation of Exposure:* clinic, hospital records *Study Methodology:* retrospective chart review versus matched control group, cohort study, prospective *Population Selection Criteria:* concomitant Hodgkin's disease and pregnancy *Total Number of Subjects:* 50 *Number of Cases:* 48 *Number of Controls:* 67 *Drug Event:* congenital malformations *Validation of Outcome:* hospital, clinic records *Rule Out Alternative Explanation:* matched controls *Results:* 20-year survival of mothers the same in cases as controls; no increased fetal malformations (only patients receiving chemotherapy in the first trimester gave birth to a child with hydrocephaly who subsequently died)

92:17 Mellemgaard A, et al. Risk of kidney cancer in analgesics users. J Clin Epidemiol 1992;45:1021-4

Drug Category: nonsteroidal antiinflammatory drugs *Drug Treatment Duration:* presumed regular use *Validation of Drug Exposure:* information gathered from discharge register *Study Methodology:* case–control study, retrospective *Population Selection Criteria:* discharged from hospital since 1977 with a diagnosis of rheumatoid arthritis, osteoarthritis, or back pain *Total Number of Subjects:* 155 554 *Case Subjects:* 9572 cancers *Drug Event:* cancer (renal) *Validation of Outcome:* cancer register *Rule Out Alternative Explanation:* surveillance bias, conservative estimates due to misclassification, positive selection bias present, others *Results:* the risk of cancer of the urinary tract was slightly increased (RR = 1.31) because of an increased risk of renal cell carcinoma (RR = 1.40); the RR was higher in individuals with rheumatoid arthritis than among individuals with osteoarthritis or back pain, and higher among women than men

92:18 Mortensen PB. Neuroleptic medication and reduced risk of prostate cancer in schizophrenic patients. Acta Psychiatr Scand 1992;85:390-3

Drug Category: antipsychotic agents, phenothiazines *Validation of Drug Exposure:* case records *Study Methodology:* case–control study, retrospective *Population Selection Criteria:* chronic schizophrenic inpatients *Total Number of Subjects:* 6168 in the whole cohort study, 114 in the study *Case Subjects:* 38 *Control Subjects:* 76 *Drug Event:* cancer (prostate) *Validation of Outcome:* cancer registry *Rule Out Alternative Explanation:* potential risk factors such as marital status, duration of hospitalization, and age at first psychiatric hospitalization; an association between cancer and the circumstances leading up to neuroleptic treatment *Results:* there was a reduction in the risk for prostate cancer among those treated with high-dose phenothiazines, primarily chlorpromazine of 15 g or more, cumulatively

92:19 Nobili A, et al. Non-steroidal anti-inflammatory drugs and upper gastrointestinal bleeding, a post-marketing surveillance case–control study. Pharmacoepidemiol Drug Saf 1992;1:65-72

Drug Category: nonsteroidal antiinflammatory drugs *Drug Treatment Duration:* either exposed or not *Validation of Drug Exposure:* questionnaire during patient interview

Study Methodology: case–control study, retrospective; postmarketing surveillance study *Population Selection Criteria:* admitted to hospital between January 1987 and December 1988   *Total Number of Subjects:* 1764   *Case Subjects:* 441   *Control Subjects:* 1323   *Drug Event:* hemorrhage (gastrointestinal)   *Validation of Outcome:* admission to hospital with hematemesis and/or melena   *Results:* there was a strong association for aspirin intake, in the week (OR = 11.2, 95% CI 7.8 to 16.9) and the month (OR = 6.9, 95% CI 4.6 to 10.2) preceding hospitalization

92:20   Pardthaisong T, et al. The long-term growth and development of children exposed to Depo-Provera during pregnancy or lactation. Contraception 1992;45:313-24

Drug Name: medroxyprogesterone   *Drug Category:* progestins   *Validation of Drug Exposure:* family planning clinic records and interview   *Study Methodology:* case–control study, retrospective   *Population Selection Criteria:* women identified in a family planning clinic who gave birth to children still alive at the time of the follow-up   *Total Number of Subjects:* 3579   *Case Subjects:* 1207 exposed during pregnancy, 1215 exposed during breastfeeding   *Control Subjects:* 1167   *Drug Event:* growth suppression   *Validation of Outcome:* weights, heights, signs of onset of puberty   *Rule Out Alternative Explanation:* bias due to the self-reporting of pubic hair growth   *Results:* with the exception of the delay in onset of reported pubic hair growth among exposed girls, there were no significant effects on attainment of puberty (RR = 1.1, 95% CI 0.8 to 1.6) after adjusting for socioeconomic factors

92:21   Petri M, Allbritton J. Antibiotic allergy in systemic lupus erythematosus: a case–control study. J Rheumatol 1992;19:265-9

Drug Name: tetracycline, erythromycin   *Drug Category:* sulfonamides, penicillins, cephalosporins, antibacterials   *Validation of Drug Exposure:* in-person or telephone questionnaire   *Study Methodology:* case–control study, prospective   *Total Number of Subjects:* 585   *Case Subjects:* 221 with systemic lupus erythematosus   *Control Subjects:* 364 relatives and best friends   *Drug Event:* hypersensitivity   *Validation of Outcome:* in-person or telephone questionnaire   *Rule Out Alternative Explanation:* recall bias possible, balancing error between cases and controls, interview bias   *Results:* antibiotic allergy was common in patients with lupus exposed to the drug: 27% penicillin/cephalosporin, 31% sulfonamide, 7% tetracycline, and 13% erythromycin; allergy to penicillin/cephalosporin (OR = 2.3, 95% CI 1.5 to 3.6), sulfonamides (OR = 2.4, 95% CI 1.2 to 4.7), and erythromycin (OR = 4.8, 95% CI 1.5 to 14.9) was significantly more common in cases than in controls

92:22   Ray WA, et al. Psychoactive drugs and the risk of injurious motor vehicle crashes in elderly drivers. Am J Epidemiol 1992;136:873-83

Drug Category: benzodiazepines, tricyclic antidepressants, opioid analgesics, antihistamines   *Drug Treatment Duration:* current, former, nonknown, unknown   *Validation of Drug Exposure:* Medicaid program files   *Study Methodology:* cohort study, retrospective   *Population Selection Criteria:* 65–84 years old with valid driver's license during 1984–1988   *Total Number of Subjects:* 16 262   *Case Subjects:* 6600 former users, 4993 unknown, and 5530 current users   *Control Subjects:* 21 578   *Drug Event:* motor vehicle crashes   *Validation of Outcome:* driver's license files and police reports   *Rule Out Alternative Explanation:* alcohol use, driving frequency, underreporting, misclassification   *Results:* the RR of injurious crash involvement for current users of any psychoactive drug was 1.5 (95% CI 1.2 to 1.9), for benzodiazepines 1.5 (95% CI 1.2 to 1.9), and for tricyclic antidepressants 2.2 (95% CI 1.3 to 3.5); the RR increased with dose: 2.4 (95% CI 1.3 to 4.4) for at least 20 mg of diazepam and 5.5 (95% CI 2.6 to 11.6) for at least 125 mg of amitriptyline

92:23   Riddel RH, et al. Non-steroidal antiinflammatory drugs as possible cause of collagenous colitis: a case–control study. Gut 1992;33:683-6

Drug Category: nonsteroidal antiinflammatory drugs (NSAIDs)   *Drug Treatment Duration:* variable, ≥6 months   *Validation of Drug Exposure:* clinical records, written replies from physicians, cases, and/or controls   *Study Methodology:* case–control study, retrospective   *Population Selection Criteria:* having had large bowel biopsy specimens taken   *Total Number of Subjects:* 62   *Case Subjects:* 31   *Control Subjects:* 31   *Drug Event:* gastrointestinal (colitis)   *Validation of Outcome:* surgical pathology files, records of weekly gastrointestinal biopsy   *Rule Out Alternative Explanation:* known relationship between arthritis and collagenous colitis   *Results:* the long-term use (>6 mo) was significantly more common in the cases (n = 19) than the controls (n = 4) (p < 0.02); patients using NSAIDs had diarrhea after the use of the drugs, average of 5.5 years; SD 4.4; range 0.5 to 15 years; in three patients with collagenous colitis, diarrhea improved after withdrawing drugs; dechallenge in one was followed by a recurrence of diarrhea that improved after rechallenge

92:24   Rodríguez LAG, et al. The role of non-steroidal anti-inflammatory drugs in acute liver injury. BMJ 1992;305:865-8

Drug Category: nonsteroidal antiinflammatory drugs (NSAIDs)   *Validation of Drug Exposure:* database health records   *Study Methodology:* cohort study, retrospective   *Population Selection Criteria:* either currently using or had used NSAIDs   *Total Number of Subjects:* 228 392 total, 34 hospital admissions   *Case Subjects:* 16 current users   *Control Subjects:* 18 past users   *Drug Event:* hepatic disease   *Validation of Outcome:* hospital admission for the drug event   *Rule Out Alternative Explanation:* number and type of other medications, only assessing hospital admission cases (no self-limiting injuries were assessed), lack of clinical tests to show severe liver damage   *Results:* the incidence rate among current users was 9 per 100 000 person-years (95% CI 6 to 15 per 100 000 person-years); subjects currently using NSAIDs had twice the risk of newly diagnosed liver injury as past users (rate ratio = 2.3, 95% CI 1.1 to 4.9) and an excess risk of 5 per 100 000 person-years; age- and gender-adjusted risk ratio was 1.7 (95% CI 0.8 to 3.7); there was no increased risk with long-term duration of treatment (rate ratio = 1.0, 95% CI 0.3 to 3.5)

92:25   Rodríguez LAG, et al. Nonsteroidal antiinflammatory drugs and gastrointestinal hospitalizations in Saskatchewans: a cohort study. Epidemiology 1992;3:337-42

Drug Names: diclofenac, indomethacin, naproxen, piroxicam, sulindac   *Drug Category:* nonsteroidal antiinflammatory drugs (NSAIDs)   *Validation of Drug Exposure:* Saskatchewan Department of Health database files   *Study Methodology:* cohort study, retrospective   *Population Selection Criteria:* first receipt of a prescription for diclofenac, indomethacin, naproxen, piroxicam, or sulindac between January 1982 and December 1986   *Total Number of Subjects:* 228 392   *Case Subjects:* 2302   *Drug Event:* gastrointestinal abnormalities (toxicity)   *Validation of Outcome:* hospitalization with gastric, duodenal, gastrojejunal, or peptic ulcer with bleeding and/or perforation, hemorrhage of the gastrointestinal tract, other gastrointestinal diagnoses   *Rule Out Alternative Explanation:* age showed a strong association with the risk of gastrointestinal hospitalization   *Results:* current users of NSAIDs had an increased risk of gastrointestinal hospitalization (RR = 3.9, 95% CI 3.5 to 4.4); RR decreased as time since the last prescription increased; 2.2 (95% CI 1.9 to 2.6) for recent past users and 1.3 (95% CI 1.1 to 1.5) for less-recent past users; indomethacin users had the highest RR and sulindac users had the lowest

92:26   Woodman K, et al. Albuterol and deaths from asthma in New Zealand from 1969 to 1976: a case–control study. Clin Pharmacol Ther 1992;51:566-71

Drug Name: albuterol *Drug Category:* bronchodilators, beta-adrenoreceptor agonists *Validation of Drug Exposure:* hospital records *Study Methodology:* case–control study, retrospective *Population Selection Criteria:* ages 5–45 years, hospitalized with asthma *Total Number of Subjects:* 139 *Case Subjects:* 17 asthma deaths *Control Subjects:* 57 (group A) and 65 (group B) *Drug Event:* death (asthma) *Validation of Outcome:* hospital records *Rule Out Alternative Explanation:* small number of cases, few records of actual cases retrieved *Results:* the inhaled albuterol OR was 0.88 (95% CI 0.29 to 2.26) with control group A and 1.40 (95% CI 0.48 to 4.09) with control group B; the findings indicate that albuterol was not associated with deaths from asthma after its introduction

93:1 Back EE, et al. Risk factors for developing eosinophilia–myalgia syndrome among L-tryptophan users in New York. J Rheumatol 1993;20:666-72

Drug Name: tryptophan *Drug Category:* amino acid supplement *Treatment Duration:* ≥2 weeks *Validation of Exposure:* case reports and medical records (use of nonprescription drugs) *Study Methodology:* case–control study, retrospective *Population Selection Criteria:* patients with eosinophilia–myalgia syndrome (EMS) in New York *Number of Cases:* 113 *Number of Controls:* 95 (also users of drug) *Drug Event:* EMS *Validation of Outcome:* medical records tracing of drug to manufacturer by lot *Results:* risk of EMS greater after December 1, 1988 (OR = 25.8); risk increased with dose, age, and use of drug as sedative

93:2 Baumelou E, et al. Epidemiologic study of aplastic anemia in France: a case–control study. Blood 1993;81:1471-8

Drug Name: gold sodium thiomylate, penicillamine, colchicine, acetaminophen *Drug Category:* antigout agents, gold salts, nonsteroidal antiinflammatory drugs *Treatment Duration:* retrospective 5 years, 1 year *Validation of Exposure:* interviews (personally, proxy) using standardized questionnaires *Study Methodology:* case–control study, retrospective *Population Selection Criteria:* French national registry; aplastic anemia cases with depressed hemoglobin (≤10 g/100 mL) and reticulocyte (≤50 × 10^9/L) or granolycyte (≤1.5 × 10^9/L) and platelet (≤100 × 10^9/L) counts *Number of Cases:* 147 *Number of Controls:* 287 hospitalized and 108 neighbors; matched for age (± 5 y), gender, and interviewer *Drug Event:* blood cell abnormalities (aplastic anemia) *Validation of Outcome:* bone marrow biopsy *Rule Out Alternative Explanation:* occupational/nonoccupational toxic environmental factors, genetic disease, consanguinity *Results:* 5 previous years: gold salts, D-penicillamine (OR = 4.9); colchicine (OR = 4.1); allo/thiopurinol (OR = 3.6); acetaminophen, salicylate (OR = 1.8 to 2.0); frequent salicylate use during previous year (OR = 5.0)

93:3 Carson JL, et al. Safety of nonsteroidal antiinflammatory drugs with respect to acute liver disease. Arch Intern Med 1993;153:1331-6

Drug Category: nonsteroidal antiinflammatory drugs (NSAIDs) *Treatment Duration:* any *Validation of Exposure:* computerized Medicaid data (COMPASS) in Michigan and Florida *Study Methodology:* case–control study, retrospective *Population Selection Criteria:* acute hepatitis without identifiable cause 1980–1987 *Total Number of Subjects:* 107 *Number of Cases:* 107 (incidence, 2.2/100 000/y) *Number of Controls:* 4/case matched for age, gender, and state *Drug Event:* gastrointestinal abnormalities (hepatic disease) *Validation of Outcome:* review of abstracted hospital records *Rule Out Alternative Explanation:* hepatitis with other causes excluded *Results:* adjusted OR for prescription NSAID use = 1.2 (95% CI 0.5 to 2.8) (not significant); nonprescription NSAID use not determined

93:4 Colton T, et al. Breast cancer in mothers prescribed diethylstilbestrol in pregnancy. Further follow-up. JAMA 1993;269:2096-100

Drug Name: diethylstilbestrol (DES)   *Drug Category:* estrogens   *Treatment Duration:* at birth   *Validation of Exposure:* hospital records   *Study Methodology:* cohort study, retrospective   *Population Selection Criteria:* use of DES at birth of child from 1940 to 1960   *Total Number of Subjects:* 3029   *Number of Controls:* 3029   *Drug Event:* cancer (breast)   *Validation of Outcome:* hospital and medical records   *Results:* RR = 1.35 (95% CI 1.05 to 1.74) earlier and has remained essentially the same; risk does not appear to increase greatly over time

93:5   Cornelissen M, et al. Increased incidence of neonatal vitamin K deficiency resulting from maternal anticonvulsant therapy. Am J Obstet Gynecol 1993;168:923-8

Drug Name: vitamin K   *Drug Category:* anticonvulsants, vitamins   *Drug Treatment Duration:* average, 11 years; range, 1–23 years   *Study Methodology:* case–control study, prospective   *Population Selection Criteria:* pregnant women   *Total Number of Subjects:* 50   *Case Subjects:* 25   *Control Subjects:* 25   *Drug Event:* vitamin K deficiency   *Validation of Outcome:* vitamin K concentration in the fetal cord blood sample   *Rule Out Alternative Explanation:* lower maternal concentration of vitamin K due to fasting before giving birth, others   *Results:* protein induced by vitamin K absence of factor II (PIVKA-II) was detectable in 54% of the case cord samples and in 20% of the controls (p = 0.01); in both groups, the vitamin K_1 cord blood concentration was predominantly below the detection limit; the maternal vitamin K_1 concentrations were lower in cases than controls (Wilcoxon's rank sum test; p < 0.05), but PIVKA-II was rarely present

93:6   Derby LE, et al. Cholestatic hepatitis associated with flucloxacillin. Med J Aust 1993:158:596-600

Drug Name: flucloxacillin   *Drug Category:* penicillins, antibacterials   *Treatment Duration:* one or more prescriptions   *Validation of Exposure:* medical office computer data from 600 general practitioners in the UK (VAMP)   *Study Methodology:* cohort study, retrospective   *Population Selection Criteria:* prescription for flucloxacillin   *Total Number of Subjects:* 132 087   *Number of Cases:* 11 (additional 3 in control group)   *Number of Controls:* 145; 844 patients with prescription for oxytetracycline   *Drug Event:* gastrointestinal abnormalities (hepatic disease)   *Validation of Outcome:* medical record review of potential cases   *Rule Out Alternative Explanation:* other causes of hepatitis   *Results:* flucloxacillin is a likely cause of cholestatic hepatitis; risk of 7.6/100 000 users (95% CI 3.6 to 13.9)

93:7   Derby LE, et al. Erythromycin-associated cholestatic hepatitis. Med J Aust 1993;158:600-2

Drug Name: erythromycin   *Drug Category:* antibacterials   *Treatment Duration:* one or more prescriptions   *Validation of Exposure:* medical office computer data from 600 general practitioners in the UK (VAMP)   *Study Methodology:* cohort study, retrospective   *Population Selection Criteria:* prescription for any erythromycin product   *Total Number of Subjects:* 366 064   *Number of Cases:* 13   *Number of Controls:* none   *Drug Event:* gastrointestinal abnormalities (hepatic disease)   *Validation of Outcome:* medical record review of potential cases   *Rule Out Alternative Explanation:* other known causes of hepatitis   *Results:* erythromycin is a risk factor, 3.6 cases per 100 000 (95% CI 1.9 to 6.1)

93:8   Easterbrook PJ, et al. Rate of CD4 cell decline and prediction of survival in zidovudine-treated patients. AIDS 1993;7:959-67

Drug Name: zidovudine   *Drug Category:* antiretrovirals   *Treatment Duration:* 12 months   *Validation of Exposure:* hospital records   *Study Methodology:* cohort study, retrospective   *Population Selection Criteria:* HIV-1 seropositive   *Total Number of Subjects:* 1415 (various stages of AIDS)   *Number of Cases:* 1415   *Drug Event:* AIDS survival   *Validation of Out-*

come: hospital records   *Results:* rate of CD4 decline during first year predictive of survival; occurrence of CD4 rise after start of zidovudine not predictive

93:9 Finucane FF, et al. Decreased risk of stroke among postmenopausal hormone users. Arch Intern Med 1993;153:73-9

Drug Name: estrogen replacement therapy   *Drug Category:* estrogens   *Treatment Duration:* long term   *Validation of Exposure:* interviews, physical examinations   *Study Methodology:* national cohort (US) study, retrospective   *Population Selection Criteria:* white, postmenopausal patients on estrogen   *Total Number of Subjects:* 1910   *Number of Cases:* 250 (64 deaths)   *Number of Controls:* 1513 in an earlier study   *Drug Event:* stroke   *Validation of Outcome:* discharge data from hospitals and nursing homes and death certificates   *Results:* stroke RR of estrogen users = 0.69 (95% CI 0.47 to 1.00) and of death = 0.37 (95% CI 0.14 to 0.92)

93:10 Fishbein DB, et al. Risk factors for systemic hypersensitivity reactions after booster vaccinations with human diploid cell rabies vaccine: a nationwide prospective study. Vaccine 1993;11:1390-5

Drug Name: rabies vaccine (human diploid cell)   *Drug Category:* vaccines   *Treatment Duration:* booster injection   *Validation of Exposure:* clinical trial records   *Study Methodology:* prospective enrollment, not blinded clinical trial   *Population Selection Criteria:* three previous doses of HDCV and rabies neutralizing titer ≤1:5; patients identified from sera submitted to testing laboratory   *Total Number of Subjects:* 98   *Number of Cases:* 6   *Drug Event:* hypersensitivity   *Validation of Outcome:* medical records, interviews   *Results:* intramuscular primary vaccination and intradermal boosters may increase chance of hypersensitivity

93:11 Fradkin JE, et al. Risk of leukemia after treatment with pituitary growth hormone. JAMA 1993;270:2829-32

Drug Name: growth hormone, human   *Drug Category:* growth hormone   *Treatment Duration:* mean, 9–10 years   *Validation of Exposure:* records of National Hormone and Pituitary Program (NHPP)   *Study Methodology:* cohort study, retrospective   *Population Selection Criteria:* growth failure patients treated in NHPP during 1963–1985   *Total Number of Subjects:* 6284   *Number of Cases:* 6   *Number of Controls:* 2.26 cases expected in general population   *Drug Event:* cancer (leukemia, lymphoma)   *Validation of Outcome:* Medicaid   *Results:* no excess of lymphoma; RR of leukemia = 2.6 (90% CI 1.2 to 5.2) in extended follow-up

93:12 Fuhrer JA, et al. Impact of time-interval after transplantation and therapy with fibrates on serum cholesterol levels in renal transplant patients. Clin Nephrol 1993;39:265-71

Drug Name: prednisone, azathioprine, cyclosporine   *Drug Category:* immunosuppressants, cholesterol-lipid-lowering agents   *Treatment Duration:* 3 and 5 years   *Validation of Exposure:* clinic records   *Study Methodology:* cohort study, prospective   *Population Selection Criteria:* renal transplants, Mammern, Switzerland   *Total Number of Subjects:* 210   *Number of Cases:* 103 at 3 years; 66 at 5 years   *Number of Controls:* patients stratified based on drug regimens   *Drug Event:* hypercholesterolemia   *Validation of Outcome:* clinic records   *Rule Out Alternative Explanation:* patients with confounding diseases excluded   *Results:* patients treated with cyclosporine alone or cyclosporine/prednisone have higher cholesterol concentrations than do patients taking prednisone/azathioprine; fibrates can be used as therapy

93:13 Green BH, et al. Prospective data on the prevalence of abnormal involuntary movement among elderly people living in the community. Acta Psychiatr Scand 1993;87:418-21

Drug Category: antipsychotic agents, neuroleptics *Treatment Duration:* any *Validation of Exposure:* personnel interviews 3 years apart *Study Methodology:* cohort study, prospective *Population Selection Criteria:* persons >65 years in Liverpool, England *Total Number of Subjects:* 701 *Drug Event:* tardive dyskinesia, akathisia *Validation of Outcome:* personal interviews by psychiatrists *Rule Out Alternative Explanation:* other causes sought *Results:* tardive dyskinesia incidence of 0.72%, akathisia incidence of 1.57%; usually associated with organic mental disorder, not neuroleptic use

93:14   Greenberg S, et al. Trimethoprim–sulfamethoxazole induces reversible hyperkalemia. Ann Intern Med 1993;119:291-5

Drug Name: trimethoprim/sulfamethoxazole (TMP/SMX) *Drug Category:* antibacterials *Treatment Duration:* ≥6 days *Validation of Exposure:* hospital records *Study Methodology:* cohort study, retrospective *Population Selection Criteria:* HIV-1 patient with symptomatic infection *Total Number of Subjects:* 51 *Number of Cases:* 25 *Number of Controls:* 26 *Drug Event:* hyperkalemia *Validation of Outcome:* hospital record *Rule Out Alternative Explanation:* patients receiving potassium supplements or interacting drugs excluded *Results:* TMP/SMX increased potassium by 1.1 mmol/L 10 days after starting high-dose therapy (p < 0.0001)

93:15   Jick H, et al. Nonsteroidal antiinflammatory drugs and certain rare, serious adverse events: a cohort study. Pharmacotherapy 1993;13:212-7

Drug Name: diclofenac, naproxen, piroxicam *Drug Category:* nonsteroidal antiinflammatory drugs (NSAIDs) *Treatment Duration:* one or more prescriptions *Validation of Exposure:* computerized data in general practitioners' offices in the UK (VAMP) *Study Methodology:* cohort study, retrospective *Population Selection Criteria:* prescription for NSAIDs *Total Number of Subjects:* 42 361 (diclofenac), 50 676 (naproxen), and 17 676 (piroxicam) (102 644 total) *Drug Event:* blood cell abnormalities (hemolytic anemia, neutropenia); gastrointestinal abnormalities (pancreatitis) *Validation of Outcome:* medical record review *Results:* one reaction of each probably occurred with the drugs (1 reaction to each drug)—very low risk

93:16   Klebanoff MA, et al. The risk of childhood cancer after neonatal exposure to vitamin K. N Engl J Med 1993;329:905-8

Drug Name: vitamin K *Drug Category:* vitamins *Treatment Duration:* at birth *Validation of Exposure:* medical records collaborative perinatal project *Study Methodology:* nested case–control study *Population Selection Criteria:* children born in 1959–1966 *Total Number of Subjects:* 54 795 *Number of Cases:* 48 by eighth birthday *Number of Controls:* 5/case *Drug Event:* cancer (childhood) *Validation of Outcome:* clinic, hospital records *Results:* vitamin K given to 68% of cases and 71% of controls; OR = 0.47 (95% CI 0.41 to 1.71) for leukemia and 1.08 for other cancers; no association was found

93:17   Kotaniemi A, et al. Estimation of central osteopenia in children with chronic polyarthritis treated with glucocorticoids. Pediatrics 1993;91:1127-30

Drug Category: glucocorticoids *Treatment Duration:* long term *Validation of Exposure:* clinic and hospital records *Study Methodology:* case–control study, retrospective *Population Selection Criteria:* girls aged 7–19 years with juvenile chronic polyarthritis treated with glucocorticoids *Number of Cases:* 43 *Number of Controls:* 44 *Drug Event:* osteoporosis *Validation of Outcome:* hospital records *Results:* reduced bone mineral density, bone size, and volumetric density at lumbar spine and femoral neck (p ≤ 0.02)

93:18   Lang DM, et al. Elevated risk of anaphylactoid reaction from radiographic contrast media is associated with both β-blocker exposure and cardiovascular disorder. Arch Intern Med 1993;153:2033-40

Drug Category: radiographic contrast media, beta-adrenoreceptor antagonists *Treatment Duration:* any *Validation of Exposure:* hospital records *Study Methodology:* case–control study, retrospective *Population Selection Criteria:* patients receiving intravenous contrast media *Total Number of Subjects:* 34 371 *Number of Cases:* 122 *Number of Controls:* one or two per case *Drug Event:* anaphylaxis *Validation of Outcome:* hospital records *Results:* major life-threatening anaphylactoid reaction (AR) associated with cardiovascular disorder, OR = 7.71 (95% CI 1.04 to 57.23); severe AR associated with beta-blockers (OR = 7.67, 95% CI 1.79 to 32.85)

93:19 Lidegaard Ø. Oral contraception and risk of a cerebral thromboembolic attack: results of a case–control study. BMJ 1993;306:956-63

Drug Name: oral contraceptives *Drug Category:* estrogen–progestins *Validation of Exposure:* mail questionnaire *Study Methodology:* case–control study, retrospective *Population Selection Criteria:* women admitted with a cerebral thromboembolism to all Danish medical, neurologic, neurosurgical, and gynecologic departments for 1985–1989 *Number of Cases:* 320 *Number of Controls:* 1197 *Matched for:* age, same day and month of birth, same age as age at attack *Drug Event:* thromboembolism (cerebral), stroke *Confounder Control:* age, smoking, years of schooling, use of different types of oral contraceptives *Results:* 50 µg estrogen (OR = 2.9, 95% CI 1.6 to 5.4); 30–40 µg estrogen (OR = 1.8, 95% CI 1.1 to 2.9); progestogen (OR = 0.9, 95% CI 0.4 to 2.4); a 50% increase of cerebral thromboembolic attacks among cigarette smokers occurred

93:20 McCredie M, et al. Different roles for phenacetin and paracetamol in cancer of the kidney and renal pelvis. Int J Cancer 1993;53:245-9

Drug Name: phenacetin, acetaminophen *Drug Category:* nonsteroidal antiinflammatory drugs *Validation of Drug Exposure:* questionnaire *Study Methodology:* population-based case–control study, retrospective *Population Selection Criteria:* 20–79 years old, New South Wales *Total Number of Subjects:* 1159 *Case Subjects:* 636: 489 with renal-cell cancer; 147 with renal pelvic cancer *Control Subjects:* 523 *Drug Event:* cancer (renal) *Validation of Outcome:* cancer registry *Rule Out Alternative Explanation:* interview bias not likely, recall bias possible, others *Results:* the risk of renal pelvic cancer was increased by phenacetin/aspirin compound analgesics (RR = 12.2, 95% CI 6.8 to 22.2) more than by paracetamol (RR = 1.3, 95% CI 0.7 to 2.4); the risk for the highest tertile of paracetamol users was doubled (RR = 2.0, 95% CI 0.9 to 4.4) compared with nonusers of any analgesics; the risk of renal-cell cancer was 1.4 (95% CI 0.9 to 2.3) for phenacetin/aspirin compounds and 1.5 (95% CI 1.0 to 2.3) for paracetamol taken in any form

93:21 McLeod DC, et al. Pharmacoepidemiology of bleeding events after use of r-alteplase or streptokinase in acute myocardial infarction. Ann Pharmacother 1993;27:956-62

Drug Name: streptokinase, r-alteplase *Drug Category:* thrombolytics *Treatment Duration:* single-dose bolus infusion (96-h observation) *Validation of Exposure:* medical record *Study Methodology:* prospective dynamic cohort patients with acute myocardial infarction *Population Selection Criteria:* 36 US hospitals *Total Number of Subjects:* 626 *Number of Cases:* 419 (r-alteplase) *Number of Controls:* 207 (streptokinase) *Drug Event:* hemorrhage (general, intracranial) *Validation of Outcome:* retrospective medical record review *Rule Out Alternative Explanation:* comorbidity and concomitant exposure to aspirin, heparin, warfarin *Control:* demographic and therapeutic variables *Results:* in the first 24 hours, 21.5% of r-alteplase and 15.9% of streptokinase patients experienced bleeding events; in the 96-hour period, incidence was 30.5% versus 31.9%; bleeding events: 18.4% perivascular access site; 6.4% gastrointestinal, 5.0% skin/soft tissue/muscle, 3.4% urinary, 2.2% pulmonary, 1.9% systemic, and 1.4% oral; intracranial bleeding occurred in 4 r-alteplase and 2 streptokinase patients; 4 of these patients died; bleeding type and incidence were similar with each drug

93:22 Merkus PJ, et al. Long-term effect of inhaled corticosteroids on growth rate in adolescents with asthma. Pediatrics 1993;91:1121-6

Drug Name: albuterol, budesonide *Drug Category:* bronchodilators, beta-adrenoreceptor agonists, glucocorticoids *Treatment Duration:* median, 22 months *Validation of Exposure:* clinical trial and medical records *Study Methodology:* prospective, randomized, double-blind trial *Population Selection Criteria:* asthmatic teenagers (mean age, 12.8 y) in Leiden, Netherlands *Number of Cases:* 40 *Number of Controls:* 80 *Drug Event:* growth suppression *Validation of Outcome:* trial records *Results:* growth rate in males less than in females, who were similar to controls; albuterol plus budesonide patients grew more than albuterol plus placebo patients, but less than controls; budesonide was not responsible for delayed growth (delayed puberty may be the reason)

93:23 Morgenstern H, Glazer WM. Identifying risk factors for tardive dyskinesia among long-term outpatients maintained with neuroleptic medications. Arch Gen Psychiatry 1993;50:723-33

Drug Category: neuroleptics, antipsychotic agents *Treatment Duration:* 3 months to 33 years *Validation of Exposure:* outpatient mental health clinic records *Study Methodology:* cohort study, prospective *Population Selection Criteria:* maintenance neuroleptic therapy *Total Number of Subjects:* 398 *Number of Cases:* 62 new tardive dyskinesia cases *Drug Event:* tardive dyskinesia *Validation of Outcome:* clinic records *Results:* 5-year risk of 20%; tardive dyskinesia rate positively affected by age, being nonwhite, and neuroleptic dose

93:24 Mulberg AE, et al. Identification of nonsteroidal antiinflammatory drug–induced gastroduodenal injury in children with juvenile rheumatoid arthritis. J Pediatr 1993;122:647-9

Drug Category: nonsteroidal antiinflammatory drugs (NSAIDs) *Treatment Duration:* long term *Validation of Exposure:* clinic records *Study Methodology:* cohort study, prospective *Population Selection Criteria:* children with juvenile rheumatoid arthritis managed with NSAIDs *Number of Cases:* 17 (abdominal complaints) *Drug Event:* hemorrhage (gastrointestinal) *Validation of Outcome:* clinic records *Results:* 69% had anemia, epigastric pain and anemia present in 47%, endoscopic diagnoses made in 76%, NSAIDs associated with significant gastrointestinal abnormalities in children

93:25 Olsen JH, et al. Phenobarbital, drug metabolism, and human cancer. Cancer Epidemiol Biomarkers Prev 1993;2:449-52

Drug Name: phenobarbital *Drug Category:* anticonvulsants *Treatment Duration:* long term *Validation of Exposure:* clinic records, Danish cancer registry *Study Methodology:* nested case–control study *Population Selection Criteria:* epileptic patients with lung and bladder cancers *Total Number of Subjects:* 8004 *Number of Cases:* 104 lung, 18 bladder *Number of Controls:* 322 *Drug Event:* cancer (lung, bladder) *Validation of Outcome:* clinic records *Rule Out Alternative Explanation:* smoking *Results:* bladder cancer inversely related to phenobarbital use; drug may induce hepatic drug-metabolizing enzymes that deactivate bladder carcinogens found in cigarette smoking

93:26 Pallares R, et al. Cephalosporins as risk factors for nosocomial *Enterococcus faecalis* bacteremia. Arch Intern Med 1993;153:1581-6

Drug Category: cephalosporins, antibacterials *Treatment Duration:* short-term hospital therapy *Validation of Exposure:* hospital medical records *Study Methodology:* cohort with matched control study, retrospective *Population Selection Criteria:* all cases with culture-positive *E. faecalis* bacteremia   *Total Number of Subjects:* 312   *Number of Cases:* 156   *Number of Controls:* 156   *Drug Event: E. faecalis* infection   *Validation of Outcome:* hospital medical records   *Rule Out Alternative Explanation:* other variables, that is, catheters, studied   *Results:* OR cephalosporin use = 5.1 (adjusted OR = 4.8, 95% CI 2.3 to 9.8)

93:27   Pedersen-Bjergaard J, et al. Therapy-related myelodysplasia and acute myeloid leukemia: cytogenetic characteristic of 115 consecutive cases and risk in seven cohorts of patients treated intensively for malignant diseases in the Copenhagen series. Leukemia 1993;7:1975-86

Drug Category: antineoplastic agents   *Treatment Duration:* any   *Validation of Exposure:* clinic records   *Study Methodology:* cohort (cohorts of different cancer types) study, prospective   *Population Selection Criteria:* patients with therapy-related myelodysplasia or acute myeloid leukemia   *Number of Cases:* 115   *Drug Event:* cancer (leukemia)   *Validation of Outcome:* clinic records, cytogenetic studies   *Results:* akylating agents and drugs targeting DNA-topoisomerase II are leukemogenic, combination more so than either class alone; alkylating agents alone increase risk 1% per year from years 2–8

93:28   Piper JM, et al. Prenatal use of metronidazole and birth defects: no association. Obstet Gynecol 1993;82:348-52

Drug Name: metronidazole   *Drug Category:* antibacterials   *Validation of Exposure:* computerized Tennessee Medicaid data   *Study Methodology:* cohort study, retrospective   *Population Selection Criteria:* prescription for metronidazole 30 days before to 120 days after last normal menstrual period   *Total Number of Subjects:* 1387   *Number of Cases:* 96   *Number of Controls:* 1387 (80 cases of birth defects)   *Drug Event:* congenital malformations   *Validation of Outcome:* nurse review of hospital records   *Rule Out Alternative Explanation:* race, age, parity, education   *Results:* drug RR = 1.2 (95% CI 0.8 to 1.6), not significant

93:29   Savage RL, et al. Variation in the risk of peptic ulcer complications with non-steroidal antiinflammatory drug therapy. Arthritis Rheum 1993;36:84-90

Drug Name: various   *Drug Category:* nonsteroidal antiinflammatory drugs (NSAIDs)   *Study Methodology:* case–control study, retrospective   *Population Selection Criteria:* case = hospitalization because of gastrointestinal hemorrhage   *Control:* patients in the acute-admission register   *Total Number of Subjects:* 1466   *Number of Cases:* 494   *Number of Controls:* 972   *Drug Event:* gastrointestinal abnormalities (peptic ulcer)   *Validation of Outcome:* medical/hospital records   *Results:* NSAID OR = 5.1 (95% CI 3.8 to 6.8), adjusted OR = 4.1 (95% CI 2.8 to 5.9); piroxicam OR = 6.3 (95% CI 3.3 to 12.0), adjusted OR = 6.4 (95% CI 2.8 to 15%); combination of diclofenac, ketoprofen, and sulindac OR = 2.9 (95% CI 2.0 to 4.2), adjusted OR = 3.3 (95% CI 2.0 to 5.5)

93:30   Scarabin PY, et al. Haemostatic variables and menopausal status: influence of hormone replacement therapy. Thromb Haemost 1993;70:584-7

Drug Name: estrogen replacement therapy   *Drug Category:* estrogen–progestins, estrogens   *Treatment Duration:* long term   *Validation of Exposure:* clinic records   *Study Methodology:* cohort study, prospective   *Population Selection Criteria:* healthy women 45–54 years old attending clinic   *Total Number of Subjects:* 293   *Drug Event:* thromboembolism   *Validation of Outcome:* clinic records   *Results:* coagulation variables changed in direction to protect against thrombosis

93:31   Shorr RI, et al. Concurrent use of nonsteroidal anti-inflammatory drugs and oral anti-coagulants places elderly persons at high risk for hemorrhagic peptic ulcer disease. Arch Intern Med 1993;153:1665-70

Drug Name: warfarin   *Drug Category:* nonsteroidal antiinflammatory drugs, anticoagulants   *Treatment Duration:* long term, not specified   *Validation of Exposure:* Tennessee

Medicaid computer data   *Study Methodology:* cohort study, retrospective   *Population Selection Criteria:* hospitalization for peptic ulcer disease and documented hemorrhage   *Total Number of Subjects:* 103 954 (209 066 person-years)   *Number of Cases:* 1371 peptic ulcer disease; 661 gastrointestinal bleeding   *Drug Event:* hemorrhage (gastrointestinal)   *Validation of Outcome:* Medicaid data only   *Rule Out Alternative Explanation:* some confounding groups excluded   *Results:* RR for users of both types of drugs = 12.7 (95% CI 6.3 to 25.7)

93:32   Stampfer MJ, et al. Vitamin E consumption and the risk of coronary disease in women. N Engl J Med 1993;328:1444-9

Drug Name: vitamin E   *Drug Category:* vitamins   *Treatment Duration:* 8 years   *Validation of Exposure:* personal questionnaires   *Study Methodology:* cohort study, prospective   *Population Selection Criteria:* middle-aged nurses free from cancer and cardiovascular disease   *Total Number of Subjects:* 87 245   *Number of Cases:* 97% of above   *Number of Controls:* vitamin E intake stratified   *Drug Event:* coronary heart disease   *Validation of Outcome:* mailed questionnaires   *Rule Out Alternative Explanation:* age, smoking   *Results:* top fifth based on vitamin E intake RR of coronary artery disease = 0.66 (95% CI 0.5–0.87); short-term use was of little benefit

93:33   Troyer WA, et al. Association of maternal lithium exposure and premature delivery. J Perinatol 1993;13:123-7

Drug Name: lithium carbonate   *Drug Category:* antimanics   *Treatment Duration:* during pregnancy   *Validation of Exposure:* medical records, International Registry of Lithium Babies   *Study Methodology:* cohort study, retrospective   *Population Selection Criteria:* pregnant women treated with lithium   *Number of Cases:* 84   *Drug Event:* delivery, premature   *Validation of Outcome:* medical records, registry   *Results:* 36% born prematurely, 37% of premature infants were large for gestational age, 15% of term babies large for age; RR of lithium-treated mothers to have premature baby = 2.5; only significant finding was association with premature birth

93:34   van der Klauw MM, et al. A population based case–control study of drug-induced anaphylaxis. Br J Clin Pharmacol 1993;35:400-8

Drug Name: glafenine, amoxicillin, diclofenac   *Drug Category:* nonsteroidal antiinflammatory drugs, penicillins   *Treatment Duration:* various   *Validation of Exposure:* prehospital medication histories   *Study Methodology:* case–control study, retrospective   *Population Selection Criteria:* admissions to Dutch hospitals in 1987–1988 with anaphylaxis as principal diagnosis   *Total Number of Subjects:* 934   *Number of Cases:* 727   *Number of Controls:* external cohort of persons sorted by sample of Dutch pharmacies   *Drug Event:* anaphylaxis   *Validation of Outcome:* hospital and pharmacy records   *Results:* compared with all other drugs, RR in 1988 = 129 for glafenine, 4.4 for amoxicillin, and 6.1 for diclofenac; some varied greatly in 1987 from 1988

93:35   Walker AM, et al. Determinants of serious liver disease among patients receiving low-dose methotrexate for rheumatoid arthritis. Arthritis Rheum 1993;36: 329-35

Drug Name: methotrexate   *Drug Category:* antineoplastic agents   *Drug Treatment Duration:* ≥5 or ≥10 years   *Validation of Drug Exposure:* physician's patient chart, interview with physician   *Study Methodology:* case–control study, retrospective   *Population Selection Criteria:* rheumatoid arthritis patients   *Total Number of Subjects:* 63   *Case Subjects:* 24 with cirrhosis and liver failure   *Control Subjects:* 39   *Drug Event:* gastrointestinal abnormalities (hepatic disease)   *Validation of Outcome:* review of pathology specimens, diagnostic testing, and clinical presentations   *Rule Out Alternative Explanation:* downward bias, confounding factors, small number of patients, others   *Results:* 5-year cumulative incidence of ~1/1000 treated patients; 6 of the 24 cases died, 4 of the initial liver disease; 2 patients continue to have active liver disease; later age at first use of drug and duration of drug therapy were independent predictors of serious liver disease

93:36 Werler MM, et al. Periconceptional folic acid exposure and risk of ocurrent neural tube defects. JAMA 1993;269:1257-61

Drug Name: folic acid *Drug Category:* vitamins *Treatment Duration:* before and during early pregnancy *Study Methodology:* case–control study, retrospective *Population Selection Criteria:* mothers of occurrent cases of neural tube defects (NTD) and other defects *Number of Cases:* 436 mothers with children with occurrent NTD *Number of Controls:* 2615 mothers with children with other defects *Drug Event:* neural tube defects, congenital malformations *Validation of Outcome:* hospital records *Results:* mothers taking multivitamins with folic acid (0.4 mg) RR = 0.4 (95% CI 0.2 to 0.6); high dietary folate intake reduces risk also

93:37 Yuen J, et al. Hormone replacement therapy and breast cancer mortality in Swedish women: results after adjustment for "healthy drug user" effect. Cancer Causes Control 1993;4:369-74

Drug Name: estrogen replacement therapy *Category:* estrogen–progestins *Treatment Duration:* long term (12-y follow-up) *Validation of Exposure:* pharmacy records *Study Methodology:* cohort study, retrospective *Population Selection Criteria:* Swedish women prescribed hormone replacement therapy *Total Number of Subjects:* 23 000 *Number of Cases:* 108 *Number of Controls:* external historical data *Drug Event:* cancer (breast) *Validation of Outcome:* cases of death registry in Sweden *Rule Out Alternative Explanation:* external data adjusted for healthy drug-user effect *Results:* mortality not increased despite increased incidence of breast cancer

93:38 Zito JM, et al. Pharmacoepidemiology of clozapine in 202 inpatients with schizophrenia. Ann Pharmacother 1993;27:1262-9

Drug Name: clozapine *Drug Category:* antipsychotic agents *Treatment Duration:* 1 year *Study Methodology:* cohort study, prospective *Population Selection Criteria:* state-operated public psychiatric system (227 enrolled in cohort, 202 remaining) *Drug Event:* leukopenia, seizures, cardiovascular changes, fever, neuroleptic malignant syndrome *Rule Out Alternative Explanation:* age, gender, length of current hospitalization, existing schizophrenia diagnosis, baseline Brief Psychiatric Rating Scale score *Results:* at 6 weeks 19% showed improvement, at 12 weeks 29%; of those 29% at 12 weeks showing improvement, 23% deteriorated; of the 71% showing no improvement at 12 weeks, 26% improved; 11% left cohort because of unintended drug effects: 5% with decreased white blood cell count, 1% because of seizures, 4% because of cardiovascular disease, fever, or possible neuroleptic malignant syndrome

93:39 Zubialde JP, et al. Estimated gains in life expectancy with use of post-menopausal therapy: a decision analysis. J Fam Pract 1993;36:271-80

Drug Name: estrogen replacement therapy *Drug Category:* estrogen–progestins, estrogens *Treatment Duration:* long-term postmenopausal *Study Methodology:* computer-simulated Markov analysis *Drug Event:* longevity *Results:* cohorts beginning combined estrogen–progestin therapy at age 50 years had a 2.3-year increase in life expectancy if at high risk for coronary artery disease; little additional benefit was found to justify use of unopposed estrogen therapy even given the potential added mortality from endometrial cancer

94:1 Bengt-Kallen AJ. Maternal carbamazepine and infant spina bifida. Reprod Toxicol 1994;8:203-5

Drug Name: carbamazepine, valproic acid   *Drug Category:* anticonvulsants   *Treatment Duration:* not specified   *Validation of Exposure:* maternal health center records (weeks 10–12 of pregnancy)   *Study Methodology:* nested case–control study   *Population Selection Criteria:* 3625 infants identified by record linkage of Swedish health registries; 9 identified cases matched for year of birth, maternal age, and parity with 18 controls   *Total Number of Subjects:* 27   *Number of Cases:* 9   *Number of Controls:* 18   *Drug Event:* spina bifida   *Validation of Outcome:* medical birth registry   *Results:* excess risk, but findings not statistically significant

94:2   Fagan SC, et al. Safety of combination aspirin and anticoagulation in acute ischemic stroke. Ann Pharmacother 1994;28:441-3

Drug Name: aspirin, warfarin, heparin   *Drug Category:* anticoagulants, nonsteroidal antiinflammatory drugs   *Treatment Duration:* 8 days (mean)   *Validation of Exposure:* review of hospital medical records   *Study Methodology:* cohort study, retrospective   *Population Selection Criteria:* stroke patients receiving anticoagulant   *Total Number of Subjects:* 75   *Number of Cases:* 42   *Number of Controls:* 33   *Drug Event:* hemorrhage (general)   *Results:* 23.8% of aspirin-treated and 24.2% of non-aspirin-treated patients hemorrhaged (p = 0.78, not significant)

94:3   Garcia Rodriguez LA, Jick H. Risk of gynaecomastia associated with cimeti-dine, omeprazole, and other antiulcer drugs. BMJ 1994;308:503-6

Drug Name: cimetidine, misoprostil, omeprazole, ranitidine   *Drug Category:* antiulcer agents, histamine$_2$-receptor blockers, proton pump inhibitors   *Treatment Duration:* one prescription or more   *Validation of Exposure:* general practitioner's computer records in the UK   *Study Methodology:* open cohort with nested case–control analysis   *Population Selection Criteria:* men prescribed above drugs   *Total Number of Subjects:* 81 535   *Number of Cases:* 153   *Number of Controls:* 1000 nested controls   *Drug Event:* gyneco-mastia   *Validation of Outcome:* unconditional logistic regression   *Results:* RR of cimeti-dine = 7.2, omeprazole = 0.6, ranitidine = 1.5, misoprostil = 2.0

94:4   Glazer WM, et al. Race and tardive dyskinesia among outpatients at a CMHC. Hosp Community Psychiatry 1994;45:38-42

Drug Category: neuroleptics, antipsychotic agents   *Treatment Duration:* long term   *Validation of Exposure:* mental health clinic records   *Study Methodology:* retrospective, case review   *Population Selection Criteria:* ambulatory mental patients at risk for tardive dyskinesia   *Total Number of Subjects:* 398   *Number of Cases:* 398   *Number of Controls:* none   *Drug Event:* tardive dyskinesia   *Validation of Outcome:* clinic record review   *Rule Out Alternative Explanation:* covariate analysis   *Results:* African-Americans received higher dosages of neuroleptics and had two times as frequent tardive dyskinesia

94:5   Hogberg U. Effect of introduction of sulphonamides on the incidence of and mortality from puerperal sepsis in a Swedish county hospital. Scand J Infect Dis 1994;26:233-8

Drug Category: sulfonamides, antibacterials   *Validation of Exposure:* hospital records   *Study Methodology:* cohort study, retrospective   *Population Selection Criteria:* live births registered at one county hospital's obstetric department in Sweden, 1930–1950   *Total Number of Subjects:* 20 903   *Number of Cases:* 7496 (births before introduction of sulfon-amides)   *Number of Controls:* 13 407 (after)   *Drug Event:* sepsis (puerperal)   *Validation of Outcome:* hospital records   *Rule Out Alternative Explanation:* age, parity, birth weight, delivery time   *Results:* risk of contracting puerperal sepsis decreased by 80% after the introduction of sulfonamides

94:6   Lafferty FW, Fiske ME. Postmenopausal estrogen replacement: a long term cohort study. Am J Med 1994;97:66-77

Drug Name: estrogen replacement therapy *Drug Category:* estrogens *Treatment Duration:* long term (1964–1989) *Validation of Exposure:* private practice medical records *Study Methodology:* cohort study, prospective *Population Selection Criteria:* postmenopausal women receiving estrogen replacement therapy *Total Number of Subjects:* 157 *Number of Cases:* 81 *Number of Controls:* 76 *Drug Event:* fracture, hypercholesterolemia *Results:* estrogen therapy decreased fractures (RR = 0.28), decreased low-density lipoprotein cholesterol 21%, increased high-density lipoprotein cholesterol 37%

94:7   Lange WR. No evidence for chloroquine-associated retinopathy among missionaries on long-term malaria chemoprophylaxis. Am J Trop Med Hyg 1994;51:389-92

Drug Name: chloroquine *Drug Category:* plasmodicides *Treatment Duration:* 6250 person-years of chloroquine exposure *Study Methodology:* patient follow-up study, partly retrospective and partly prospective *Population Selection Criteria:* career missionaries *Total Number of Subjects:* 588 *Number of Cases:* 588 *Number of Controls:* none *Drug Event:* retinopathy *Validation of Outcome:* medical chart review (validated by telephone survey) and prospective examinations *Results:* one case, because of inappropriate use

94:8   Major CA, et al. Tocolysis with indomethacin increases the incidence of necrotizing enterocolitis in the low-birth-weight neonate. Am J Obstet Gynecol 1994;170:102-6

Drug Name: indomethacin *Drug Category:* tocolytics, nonsteroidal antiinflammatory drugs *Treatment Duration:* any duration antenatally *Validation of Exposure:* review of hospital medical records *Study Methodology:* cohort study, retrospective *Population Selection Criteria:* preterm labor patients treated with tocolytic *Total Number of Subjects:* 759 *Number of Cases:* 56 *Number of Controls:* 703 *Drug Event:* gastrointestinal abnormalities (colitis) *Results:* delivery within 24 hours of exposure: 20% drug versus 9% control (p = 0.005); delivery >48 hours: 26.4% drug versus 4.1% controls (p = 0.04)

94:9   McDougall R, et al. Outcome in patients with rheumatoid arthritis receiving prednisone compared with matched controls. J Rheumatol 1994;21:1207-13

Drug Name: prednisone *Drug Category:* glucocorticoids *Treatment Duration:* 6.9 years (mean) *Study Methodology:* cohort study, prospective *Population Selection Criteria:* a cohort of mostly white patients with adult-onset rheumatoid arthritis; controls matched to prednisone-treated patients by age, gender, disease duration, and global assessment *Total Number of Subjects:* 244 *Number of Cases:* 122 (receiving prednisone) *Number of Controls:* 122 *Drug Event:* cataracts, fracture *Validation of Outcome:* annual examinations, single-physician global assessment, medical records *Results:* Lansbury and global assessment worse in the prednisone-treated group after 10 years; cataracts and fractures more common in the prednisone-treated group (29% vs. 18%, 25% vs. 15%, respectively)

94:10   Monane M, et al. Topical glaucoma medications and cardiovascular risk in the elderly. Clin Pharmacol Ther 1994;55:76-83

Drug Name: betaxolol, pilocarpine, epinephrine, levobunolol, timolol, dipivefrin *Drug Category:* glaucoma agents, beta-adrenoreceptor antagonists *Treatment Duration:* one or more prescriptions *Validation of Exposure:* computerized Medicaid data in New Jersey *Study Methodology:* case–control study, retrospective *Population Selection Criteria:* new prescription for digoxin, loop diuretic, or pacemaker placement *Total Number of Subjects:* 35 445 (congestive heart failure), 4278 (conduction disturbance) *Number of Controls:* 2585 hospitalized patients *Drug Event:* congestive heart failure, cardiac arrhythmia *Validation of Outcome:* computer record linkage only *Rule Out Alternative Explanation:* univariate analysis *Results:* topical glaucoma drugs not associated with adverse cardiovascular effects

94:11 Pinczowski D, et al. Risk factors for colorectal cancer in patients with ulcerative colitis: a case–control study. Gastroenterology 1994;107:117-20

Drug Name: sulfasalazine   *Drug Category:* sulfonamides   *Treatment Duration:* ≥3 months   *Validation of Exposure:* clinic records   *Study Methodology:* nested case–control study, retrospective   *Population Selection Criteria:* ulcerative colitis patients in Uppsala, Sweden   *Total Number of Subjects:* 3112   *Total Number of Cases:* 102   *Total Number of Controls:* 196   *Drug Event:* cancer (colorectal)   *Validation of Outcome:* clinic records, national Swedish cancer registry   *Results:* pharmacologic therapy, especially sulfasalazine, is protective; RR = 0.38 (95% CI 0.20 to 0.69)

94:12 Pratt CM, et al. Risk of developing life-threatening ventricular arrhythmia associated with terfenadine in comparison with over-the-counter antihistamines, ibuprofen and clemastine. Am J Cardiol 1994;73:346-52

Drug Name: terfenadine, clemastine, ibuprofen   *Drug Category:* antihistamines, analgesics, nonsteroidal antiinflammatory drugs   *Treatment Duration:* 30 days   *Validation of Exposure:* computerized medical records in four states   *Study Methodology:* cohort study, retrospective   *Population Selected Criteria:* prescription for antihistamine or ibuprofen   *Total Number of Subjects:* terfenadine, 181 672; clemastine, 83 156; nonprescription antihistamine, 150 689   *Number of Cases:* same as above   *Number of Controls:* 181 672 (ibuprofen users)   *Drug Event:* cardiac arrhythmia   *Validation of Outcome:* computer record linkage only   *Rule Out Alternative Explanation:* covariate regression analysis   *Results:* 317 events (244 cardiac arrests); terfenadine RR = 0.36 compared with nonprescription antihistamines, 0.62 compared with ibuprofen, 1.08 (nonsignificant) compared with clemastine

94:13 Risch HA, Howe GR. Menopausal hormone usage and breast cancer in Saskatchewan: a record-linkage cohort study. Am J Epidemiol 1994;139:670-83

Drug Name: estrogen replacement therapy   *Drug Category:* estrogen–progestins, estrogens   *Treatment Duration:* long term   *Validation of Exposure:* computerized health plan records   *Study Methodology:* cohort study, retrospective   *Population Selection Criteria:* women receiving above medications   *Total Number of Subjects:* 32 790   *Number of Cases:* 742   *Drug Event:* cancer (breast)   *Validation of Outcome:* computer record linkage   *Results:* estrogens increase risk 7% per year, no additional risk when estrogen opposed by progestin use, oral contraceptives increased risk 14% per year

94:14 Rookus MA, van Leeuwen FE. Oral contraceptives and risk of breast cancer in women aged 20–54. Lancet 1994;344:844-51

Drug Name: oral contraceptives   *Drug Category:* estrogen–progestins   *Treatment Duration:* none, 0–1, <4, 4–7, 8–11, ≥12 years   *Validation of Exposure:* personal interview, life events calendar, prescriber questionnaire   *Study Methodology:* population-based case–control study, retrospective   *Population Selection Criteria:* Dutch-speaking women, aged <55 years, with invasive breast cancer diagnosed in 1986–1989 living in a defined geographic area in the Netherlands; controls randomly selected from municipal population registries, matched to cases by age (±1 y) and area   *Total Number of Subjects:* 1836   *Number of Cases:* 918   *Number of Controls:* 918   *Drug Event:* cancer (breast)   *Validation of Outcome:* cancer registries, medical records   *Rule Out Alternative Explanation:* sociodemographic variables, parity, breastfeeding, age at menarche, menopausal status, age at menopause, family history of breast cancer, body mass index, smoking, alcohol use   *Results:* ≥4 years of oral contraceptive use associated with increased risk (p = 0.03)

94:15 Rossing MA, et al. Ovarian tumors in a cohort of infertile women. N Engl J Med 1994;331:771-6

Drug Name: clomiphene, chorionic gonadotropin, menotropins, bromocriptine *Drug Category:* ovulation inducers *Treatment Duration:* five of nine cases exposed to ≥12 cycles *Validation of Exposure:* Cancer Surveillance System records *Study Methodology:* case–control study, retrospective *Population Selection Criteria:* cohort selection: defined geographic areas covered by the Cancer Surveillance System, attempted conception for at least 1 year, made two visits to infertility clinic *Total Number of Subjects:* 3837 in total cohort *Number of Cases:* 11 *Number of Controls:* 135 women randomly selected for each age stratum *Drug Event:* cancer (ovarian) *Validation of Outcome:* Cancer Surveillance System records *Results:* standardized incidence density ratio = 2.5 (95% CI 1.3 to 4.5); for all ovulation-inducing agents, users' incidence density ratio = 2.3 (95% CI 0.5 to 11.4)

94:16 Schomburg A, et al. Hepatic and serologic toxicity of systemic interleukin-2 and/or interferon-alpha: evidence of a risk–benefit advantage of subcutaneous therapy. Am J Clin Oncol 1994;17:199-209

Drug Name: interleukin-2, interferon-alfa *Drug Category:* immunomodulators *Treatment Duration:* 6–8 weeks *Validation of Exposure:* clinic records *Study Methodology:* cohort study, retrospective *Population Selection Criteria:* ambulatory cancer patients *Total Number of Subjects:* 107 *Number of Cases:* 107, subcutaneous dosing *Number of Controls:* historical intravenous use of the drugs *Drug Event:* metabolic toxicity, gastrointestinal abnormalities (hepatic disease) *Validation of Outcome:* biochemical blood testing *Results:* subcutaneous dosing much safer than intravenous dosing

94:17 Siscovick DS, et al. Diuretic therapy for hypertension and the risk of primary cardiac arrest. N Engl J Med 1994;330:1852-7

Drug Category: diuretics *Treatment Duration:* receipt of prescription in 1-year time frame before index date *Validation of Exposure:* computerized health maintenance organization pharmacy records *Study Methodology:* population-based case–control study, retrospective *Population Selection Criteria:* Group Health Cooperative of Puget Sound; cases: hypertensive patients with primary cardiac arrest; controls: stratified sample of hypertensive patients *Total Number of Subjects:* 649 *Number of Cases:* 114 *Number of Controls:* 535 primary *Drug Event:* cardiac arrest *Validation of Outcome:* Medicaid record; primary cardiac event defined as sudden pulseless condition in the absence of a known or cardiac condition as the cause of cardiac arrest *Rule Out Alternative Explanation:* ambulatory care medical record *Review:* age, smoking, diabetes mellitus, multiple drugs, clinic list frequency *Results:* OR of primary cardiac arrest among patients receiving combined thiazide and potassium-sparing diuretic therapy was lower than with a thiazide without potassium-sparing therapy: OR = 0.3 (95% CI 0.1 to 0.7); hydrochlorothiazide 25 mg versus 50 mg daily, OR = 1.7 (95% CI 0.7 to 4.5); hydrochlorothiazide 10 mg versus 25 mg, OR = 3.6 (95% CI 1.2 to 10.8); potassium-sparing diuretic added to low-dose hydrochlorothiazide was associated with reduced risk of cardiac arrest, OR = 0.4 (95% CI 0.1 to 1.5)

94:18 Suissa S, et al. A cohort analysis of excess mortality in asthma and the use of inhaled β-agonists. Am J Respir Crit Care Med 1994;149:604-10

Drug Name: fenoterol, albuterol *Drug Category:* bronchodilators, beta-adrenoreceptor agonists *Treatment Duration:* 0, 1–12, 13–24, ≥25 canisters per year *Validation of Exposure:* pharmacy billing records *Study Methodology:* cohort study, retrospective *Population Selection Criteria:* cohort of 12 301 users of asthma drugs covered by Saskatchewan Health Plan, aged 5–54 years, filled >10 prescriptions for asthma drugs in 1978–1987 *Total Number of Subjects:* 47 842 person-years of follow-up *Number of Cases:* 46 asthma-related deaths *Number of Controls:* 134 non-asthma-related deaths

Drug Event: death (asthma)   *Validation of Outcome:* vital statistics, Saskatchewan Health Insurance Plan, death certificate, autopsy report, coroner's report, and hospital discharge summary   *Results:* strong association between the use of inhaled β-agonists and asthma mortality related to use in excess of recommended dose; nonasthma mortality shows no association with use of inhaled β-agonists

94:19   Suissa S, et al. Patterns of increasing beta-agonists use and the risk of fatal or near-fatal asthma. Eur Respir J 1994;7:1602-9

Drug Name: salbutamol, fenoterol, metaproterenol, terbutaline   *Category:* bronchodilators, beta-adrenoreceptor antagonists   *Treatment Duration:* use pattern for 1 year   *Validation of Exposure:* pharmacy dispensing records, established a profile score 0–11, with 0 indicating all canisters dispensed in first month, 11 all canisters dispensed in month 11, with 5.5 an even distribution of dispensing over time period   *Study Methodology:* nested case–control study, retrospective   *Population Selection Criteria:* >12 inhalers   *Total Number of Subjects:* 350   *Number of Cases:* 97   *Number of Controls:* 258   *Drug Event:* death, asthma   *Validation of Outcome:* Saskatchewan database   *Rule Out Alternative Explanation:* comorbidities   *Results:* RR = 15.2 (95% CI 2.4 to 96.2) per unit of increase on profile score in subjects with profile score ≥6.5

94:20   Travis LB, et al. Risk of leukemia following treatment for non-Hodgkin's lymphoma. J Natl Cancer Inst 1994;86:1450-7

Drug Name: prednimustine, mechlorethamine, procarbazine, chlorambucil, cyclophosphamide   *Drug Category:* antineoplastic agents   *Treatment Duration:* variable, in combination with radiation therapy to active bone narrow   *Validation of Exposure:* medical records; hospitals, radiotherapy facilities, offices of private physician   *Study Methodology:* case–control study, retrospective   *Population Selection Criteria:* cases and controls selected from cohort study of 11 386 patients with diagnosis of non-Hodgkin's lymphoma, ages 18–70 years, survival of 2 or more years without development of second invasive primary malignancy   *Total Number of Subjects:* 175   *Number of Cases:* 35   *Number of Controls:* 140   *Drug Event:* cancer (leukemia)   *Validation of Outcome:* cancer registry incidence data, vital records, and records of pathology and histology departments   *Results:* prednimustine RR = 13.4, 95% CI 1.1 to 156, dose–effect relationship, p < 0.05; mechlorethamine or procarbazine RR = 12.6, 95% CI 2.0 to 79, dose–effect relationship; p < 0.05; chlorambucil RR = 6.5, 95% CI 1.6 to 26; cyclophosphamide RR = 1.8, 95% CI 0.7 to 4.9

94:21   van Leeuwen FE, et al. Leukemia risk following Hodgkin's disease: relation to cumulative dose of alkylating agents, treatment with teniposide combinations, number of episodes of chemotherapy, and bone marrow damage. J Clin Oncol 1994;12:1063-73

Drug Name: teniposide, mechlorethamine, cyclophosphamide, procarbazine, lomustine   *Drug Category:* antineoplastic agents   *Treatment Duration:* ≤6 cycles; >6 cycles; ≥2 treatment episodes   *Validation of Exposure:* medical record abstraction   *Study Methodology:* case–control study, retrospective   *Population Selection Criteria:* cohort of 1939 patients treated for Hodgkin's disease in the Netherlands   *Total Number of Subjects:* 168   *Number of Cases:* 44   *Number of Controls:* 124   *Drug Event:* cancer (leukemia)   *Validation of Outcome:* medical records   *Rule Out Alternative Explanation:* low platelet count   *Results:* comparing patients with radiotherapy to those with the antineoplastic drugs: ≤6 cycles of combination of mechlorethamine and procarbazine, RR = 8 (p = 0.08); >6 cycles, RR = 40 (p < 0.001); ≥2 time periods of treatment, RR = 40

94:22   van Leeuwen FE, et al. Risk of endometrial cancer after tamoxifen treatment of breast cancer. Lancet 1994;343:448-52

Drug Name: tamoxifen   *Drug Category:* antineoplastic agents   *Treatment Duration:* various   *Validation of Exposure:* medical record; for each period of tamoxifen treatment starting date, stopping date, and dosage   *Study Methodology:* case–control study, retrospective   *Population Selection Criteria:* women with endometrial cancer diagnosed at least 3 months after diagnosis of previous breast cancer through the Netherlands Cancer Registry and two hospital-based registries   *Total Number of Subjects:* 383   *Number of Cases:* 98   *Number of Controls:* 285 matched for age (±3 y), year of breast cancer diagnosis (±2 y), and survival time with intact uterus   *Drug Event:* cancer (endometrial)   *Validation of Outcome:* histologically or cytologically confirmed diagnosis, using full medical records   *Rule Out Alternative Explanation:* new unusual status, stage of breast cancer, other treatments: radiotherapy, chemotherapy, other normal treatment   *Results:* RR = 1.3 (95% CI 0.7 to 2.4); >2 years' exposure RR = 2.3 (95% CI 0.9 to 5.9) increasing risk with duration of use (p = 0.049), increasing risk with increasing cumulative dose (p = 0.046)

94:23   Welage LS, et al. Risk factors for acute renal insufficiency in patients with suspected or documented bacterial pneumonia. Ann Pharmacother 1994;28:515-22

Drug Category: cephalosporins, penicillins, aminoglycosides, antibacterials   *Treatment Duration:* ≥3 days   *Validation of Exposure:* review of hospital medical records   *Study Methodology:* cohort study, prospective   *Population Selection Criteria:* bacterial pneumonia treated with above antibiotics   *Total Number of Subjects:* 1822   *Number of Cases:* 149 (8.2%)   *Drug Event:* renal failure   *Validation of Outcome:* univariate and multivariate analysis   *Results:* severity of underlying conditions and aminoglycosides (OR = 2.6) associated with acute renal failure; amphotericin B strongly associated (OR = 13.6) and clindamycin moderately associated (OR = 2.35) when aminoglycosides used also

95:1   Andrade SE, et al. Discontinuation of antihyperlipidemic drugs—Do rates reported in clinical trials reflect rates in primary care settings? N Engl J Med 1995;332:1125-31

Drug Name: cholestyramine, colestipol, niacin, lovastatin, gemfibrozil, probucol, dextrothyroxine, clofibrate   *Drug Category:* cholesterol-lipid-lowering agents   *Treatment Duration:* 1 year   *Validation of Exposure:* computerized pharmacy records   *Study Methodology:* cohort study, prospective   *Population Selection Criteria:* new users of antihyperlipidemic therapy at two health maintenance organizations, 1988–1990, who had prescription drug coverage throughout the study   *Total Number of Subjects:* 2369 (bile acid sequestrants n = 1335, niacin n = 729, lovastatin n = 537, gemfibrozil n = 453)   *Drug Event:* drug discontinuation   *Validation of Outcome:* computerized pharmacy records, medical charts   *Results:* 1-year probability of discontinuation, 41% for bile acid sequestrants (95% CI 38 to 44), 46% for niacin (95% CI 42 to 51), 15% for lovastatin (95% CI 11 to 19), and 37% for gemfibrozil (95% CI 31 to 43), which are higher than those observed in clinical trials

95:2   Bagwell MA, et al. Primary infertility and oral contraceptive steroid use. Fertil Steril 1995;63:161-6

Drug Name: oral contraceptives   *Drug Category:* estrogen–progestins   *Treatment Duration:* none, <3 consecutive months, ≥3 consecutive months   *Validation of Exposure:* personal interviews, life events calendar   *Study Methodology:* population-based case–control study, retrospective   *Population Selection Criteria:* women 19–40 years of age serving as controls in the Cancer and Steroid Hormone Study   *Total Number of Subjects:* 2539   *Number of Cases:* 419   *Number of Controls:* 2120   *Drug Event:* infertility   *Validation of Outcome:* infertility diagnosis after 24 consecutive months of unprotected intercourse, identified by life events calendar   *Rule Out Alternative Explanation:* race, age when smoking was initiated, Quetelet index at age 18 years, age at first conception or infertility diagnosis, barrier method use   *Results:* oral contraceptive use associated with decreased risk of primary infertility; crude OR = 0.60 (95% CI 0.42 to 0.86)

95:3   Barbour ML, et al. The impact of conjugate vaccine on carriage of *Haemophilus influenzae* type b. J Infect Dis 1995;171:93-8

Drug Name: H. influenzae type b (HIB) vaccine   *Drug Category:* vaccines   *Validation of Exposure:* parent-held records   *Study Methodology:* cohort study, prospective   *Population Selection Criteria:* healthy newborn infants, born 1991–1992 in Oxford and Buckinghamshire, England, who have a sibling aged 3–4 years   *Total Number of Subjects:* 371   *Number of Cases:* 205 (vaccinated at 2, 3, and 4 mo of age)   *Number of Controls:* 79 (controls), 87 (late vaccinees)   *Drug Event:* vaccine failure   *Validation of Outcome:* throat swabs   *Rule Out Alternative Explanation:* father's occupation, day care attendance, number of rooms in the home   *Results:* RR = 4.3 (95% CI 1.1 to 17.7) for carrying HIB at some time between ages 6 and 12 months in controls versus vaccinees; adjusted OR of the period prevalence of HIB carriage = 2.94 (95% CI 1.18 to 7.28)

95:4   Bendix G, et al. Cancer morbidity in rheumatoid arthritis patients treated with Proresid or parenteral gold. Scand J Rheumatol 1995;24:79-84

Drug Name: podophyllotoxin, gold sodium thiomylate   *Drug Category:* antirheumatic drugs, gold compounds   *Treatment Duration:* podophyllotoxin, 22 months (mean); parenteral gold, 19 months (mean)   *Validation of Exposure:* hospital outpatient register   *Study Methodology:* cohort study, prospective   *Population Selection Criteria:* patients exposed to Proresid and parenteral gold identified from the outpatient register of one hospital in Sweden   *Total Number of Subjects:* 710   *Number of Cases:* podophyllotoxin = 305, 2117 person-years; parenteral gold = 305, 2293 person-years   *Drug Event:* cancer   *Validation of Outcome:* regional cancer register, death certificates   *Results:* no increased risk for overall cancer morbidity for either drug; significantly increased risk of lymphoma and leukemia in the gold-treated group

95:5   Bernstein L, et al. Treatment with human chorionic gonadotropin and risk of breast cancer. Cancer Epidemiol Biomarkers Prev 1995;4:437-40

Drug Name: human chorionic gonadotropin   *Drug Category:* ovulation inducers   *Treatment Duration:* never, ever   *Validation of Exposure:* personal interviews   *Study Methodology:* population-based case–control study, retrospective   *Population Selection Criteria:* white women, residents of Los Angeles County, aged ≤40 years, diagnosed with primary breast cancer in 1983–1989; one neighborhood control matched to each case by birth date (±36 mo), race, and parity   *Total Number of Subjects:* 1488   *Number of Cases:* 744   *Number of Controls:* 744   Drug Event: cancer (breast)   *Rule Out Alternative Explanation:* age at menarche, family history of breast cancer, oral contraceptive use, parity, breast-feeding, exercise during reproductive years   *Results:* adjusted OR = 0.77 (95% CI 0.5 to 1.19); among women with maximum body mass index ≤27.5 kg/m², significant protective effect of human chorionic gonadotropin (adjusted OR = 0.42, 95% CI 0.20 to 0.88)

95:6   Bonnier P, et al. Clinical and biologic prognostic factors in breast cancer diagnosed during postmenopausal hormone replacement therapy. Obstet Gynecol 1995;85:11-7

Drug Name: estrogen replacement therapy   *Drug Category:* estrogens, estrogen–progestins   *Treatment Duration:* none, ≥6 months   *Study Methodology:* cohort study, prospective   *Population Selection Criteria:* postmenopausal women treated for breast cancer in one French hospital, 1976–1992   *Total Number of Subjects:* 340   *Number of Cases:* 68 (receiving hormone replacement therapy)   *Number of Controls:* 272   *Drug Event:* cancer (breast)   *Validation of Outcome:* clinical examination, histologic studies, immunoassays

Rule Out Alternative Explanation: age, date of onset of cancer treatment   *Results:* hormone replacement therapy did not affect the prognosis of breast cancer

95:7   Boumendil E, et al. Depression-induced absenteeism in relation to antihyperlipidemic treatment: a study using GAZEL cohort data. Epidemiology 1995;6:322-5

Drug Category: cholesterol-lipid-lowering agents   *Validation of Exposure:* mail questionnaires   *Study Methodology:* cross-sectional cohort study, prospective   *Population Selection Criteria:* middle-aged employees of a national company in France 1991   *Total Number of Subjects:* 17 244   *Number of Cases:* 289   *Drug Event:* depression   *Validation of Outcome:* diagnosed by company physician   *Rule Out Alternative Explanation:* gender, professional status   *Results:* prevalence ratio = 1.83 (95% CI 1.30 to 2.58) for antihyperlipidemic diet (including drugs); no increased risk during 1-year follow-up

95:8   Brinton LA, et al. Oral contraceptives and breast cancer risk among younger women. J Natl Cancer Inst 1995;87:827-35

Drug Name: oral contraceptives   *Drug Category:* estrogen–progestins   *Treatment Duration:* <6 months, 6 months to <5 years, 5–9 years, ≥10 years   *Validation of Exposure:* personal interviews, life event calendars   *Study Methodology:* population-based case–control study, retrospective   *Population Selection Criteria:* cases, aged 20–54 years, with newly diagnosed invasive or in situ breast cancer identified through population-based cancer registries in three areas of the US, 1990–1992   *Total Number of Subjects:* 3153   *Number of Cases:* 1648   *Number of Controls:* 1505   *Drug Event:* cancer (breast)   *Validation of Outcome:* hospital records   *Rule Out Alternative Explanation:* age, gender, race, number of births, age at first birth, study site   *Results:* among women aged <45 years, RR = 1.3 (95% CI 1.1 to 1.5) for oral contraceptive use ≥6 months; increasing risk with duration of use and early initiation

95:9   Bunduki V, et al. Maternal–fetal folate status and neural tube defects: a case–control study. Biol Neonate 1995;67:154-9

Drug Name: folic acid   *Drug Category:* vitamins   *Validation of Exposure:* fetal and maternal blood samples   *Study Methodology:* case–control study, prospective   *Population Selection Criteria:* elective terminations of abnormal pregnancies in a French hospital; cases with neural tube defects; controls with other malformations   *Total Number of Subjects:* 28   *Number of Cases:* 14   *Number of Controls:* 14   *Drug Event:* neural tube defects, congenital malformations   *Validation of Outcome:* pathologic examination   *Rule Out Alternative Explanation:* gestational age   *Results:* in mothers of neural tube defect fetuses, blood folate concentrations significantly lower than in controls; no difference in the fetal folate status

95:10   Carozza SE, et al. Maternal exposure to *N*-nitrosatable drugs as a risk factor for childhood tumours. Int J Epidemiol 1995;24:308-12

Drug Category: nitrosatable agents   *Treatment Duration:* various during pregnancy   *Validation of Exposure:* parent interviews   *Study Methodology:* case–control study, retrospective   *Population Selection Criteria:* patients, aged ≤18 years, with brain tumor identified from eight population-based registries in California, Georgia, Hawaii, Iowa, Michigan, New Mexico, Utah, Washington; controls selected through random-digit dialing, matched by age, gender, mother's race/ethnicity   *Total Number of Subjects:* 1444   *Number of Cases:* 361   *Number of Controls:* 1083   *Drug Event:* cancer (brain)   *Validation of Outcome:* National Cancer Institute's Surveillance, Epidemiology, and End Results Program   *Rule Out Alternative Explanation:* maternal age, history of fetal or infant death, use of anesthesia during delivery, maternal history of epilepsy, maternal education, birth order, birth weight, exposure to X-rays in utero, other sources of *N*-nitroso compounds   *Results:* no increased risk

95:11   Castelbaum AJ, et al. Endometrial integrin expression in women exposed to diethylstilbestrol in utero. Fertil Steril 1995;63:1217-21

Drug Name: diethylstilbestrol   *Drug Category:* estrogens   *Validation of Exposure:* personal interview, confirmed with mother's recall   *Study Methodology:* case–control study, retrospective   *Population Selection Criteria:* women exposed in utero to diethylstilbestrol; age and cycle-day matched controls   *Total Number of Subjects:* 30   *Number of Cases:* 13 (history of in utero exposure)   *Number of Controls:* 17   *Drug Event:* endometrial integrin expression   *Validation of Outcome:* endometrial biopsies, immunohistochemical staining   *Rule Out Alternative Explanation:* age, cycle-day   *Results:* markers of uterine receptivity similar in the endometrium of exposed and unexposed

95:12   Colditz GA, et al. The use of estrogens and progestins and the risk of breast cancer in postmenopausal women. N Engl J Med 1995;332:1589-93

Drug Name: estrogen replacement therapy   *Drug Category:* estrogen–progestins, estrogens   *Treatment Duration:* none, current, or past use; 1–23, 24–59, 60–119, ≥120 months   *Validation of Exposure:* mail questionnaire   *Study Methodology:* cohort study, prospective   *Population Selection Criteria:* women, postmenopausal ≥2 years, participating in the Nurses' Health Study, 1978–1992   *Total Number of Subjects:* 69 586 (725 550 person-years)   *Number of Cases:* 1935   *Drug Event:* cancer (breast)   *Validation of Outcome:* mail questionnaire, National Death Index, hospital records   *Rule Out Alternative Explanation:* age, type of menopause, age at menopause, parity, age at first delivery, age at menarche, family history of breast cancer, history of benign breast cancer   *Results:* RR = 1.32 (95% CI 1.14 to 1.54) for current use of estrogen alone and RR = 1.41 (95% CI 1.15 to 1.74) for use of estrogen plus progestin; adjusted RR = 1.46 for current users having received hormone therapy 5–9 years (95% CI 1.22 to 1.74) or ≥10 years (95% CI 1.20 to 1.76) compared with women having never received hormone therapy; addition of progestins to estrogen therapy does not decrease the risk of breast cancer in postmenopausal women

95:13   Czeizel AE, Kodaj I. A changing pattern in the association of oral contraceptives and the different groups of congenital limb deficiencies. Contraception 1995;51:19-24

Drug Name: oral contraceptives   *Drug Category:* estrogen–progestins   *Treatment Duration:* ≥3, <3 months before conception, during pregnancy   *Validation of Exposure:* mother interview   *Study Methodology:* population-based case–control study, retrospective   *Population Selection Criteria:* cases born with isolated congenital limb deficiency, 1975–1984, identified through the Hungarian Congenital Abnormality Registry, orthopedic surgery clinics, genetic counseling clinics, financial support services; controls selected from birth registries, matched by gender, birth year, area of residence   *Total Number of Subjects:* 1074   *Number of Cases:* 537   *Number of Controls:* 537   *Drug Event:* congenital malformations   *Validation of Outcome:* personal examination, autopsy reports   *Results:* use of high-dose combination of ethynodiol diacetate and ethinyloestradiol during the periconceptional period, OR = 1.9 (95% CI 1.1 to 3.4) for terminal transverse defect

95:14   Dieckmann RA, Vardis R. High-dose epinephrine in pediatric out-of-hospital cardiopulmonary arrest. Pediatrics 1995;95:901-13

Drug Name: epinephrine   *Drug Category:* adrenergic drugs   *Validation of Exposure:* hospital records, paramedic run records   *Study Methodology:* cohort study, retrospective   *Population Selection Criteria:* children aged <18 years who developed nontraumatic cardiopulmonary arrest treated by prehospital paramedic services in San Francisco, 1989–1993   *Total Number of Subjects:* 65   *Number of Cases:* 40 (epinephrine >0.1 mg/kg)   *Number of Controls:* 13 (epinephrine <0.1 mg/kg), 12 (no epinephrine)   *Drug Event:* resuscitation   *Validation of Outcome:* hospital records, ambulatory records   *Results:* high-dose epinephrine does not improve outcome compared with standard dose

95:15   Evans JMM, et al. Topical non-steroidal anti-inflammatory drugs and admission to hospital for upper gastrointestinal bleeding and perforation: a record linkage case–control study. BMJ 1995; 311:22-6

Drug Category: nonsteroidal antiinflammatory drugs   *Treatment Duration:* none, during 45 days prior to hospital admission, ever   *Validation of Exposure:* pharmacy records   *Study Methodology:* case–control study, retrospective   *Population Selection Criteria:* residents in Tayside, 1989–1994, admitted to hospital for gastrointestinal bleeding or perforation, 1990–1992; six community and two hospital controls matched for gender and age   *Total Number of Subjects:* 9880   *Number of Cases:* 1103   *Number of Controls:* 8777   *Drug Event:* hemorrhage (gastrointestinal)   *Validation of Outcome:* hospital records   *Rule Out Alternative Explanation:* concomitant use of oral antiinflammatory drugs, antiulcer drugs   *Results:* no increased risk

95:16   Fitch LL, et al. Effect of aspirin use on death and recurrent myocardial infarction in current and former cigarette smokers. Am Heart J 1995;129:656-62

Drug Name: aspirin   *Drug Category:* nonsteroidal antiinflammatory drugs   *Treatment Duration:* none, intermittent, regular use   *Validation of Exposure:* clinical trial records   *Study Methodology:* cohort study, prospective   *Population Selection Criteria:* former or current cigarette smokers participating in the Program on the Surgical Control of the Hyperlipidemias   *Total Number of Subjects:* 182 (90 current smokers, 48 of whom are aspirin users; 92 former smokers, 62 of whom are aspirin users)   *Drug Event:* death, myocardial infarction   *Validation of Outcome:* clinical trial records   *Rule Out Alternative Explanation:* age, gender, low-density lipoprotein cholesterol, high-density lipoprotein cholesterol, Quetelet index, ejection fraction, coronary disease, length of follow-up   *Results:* risk significantly reduced for any use of aspirin among current and former smokers

95:17   Gale CR, et al. Vitamin C and risk of death from stroke and coronary heart disease in a cohort of elderly people. BMJ 1995; 310:1563-6

Drug Name: vitamin C   *Drug Category:* vitamins   *Validation of Exposure:* 7-day dietary records, plasma ascorbic acid concentrations   *Study Methodology:* cohort study, prospective   *Population Selection Criteria:* a random sample of people aged ≥65 years living in eight areas of Britain, no history of stroke, cerebral arteriosclerosis, or coronary heart disease, followed 20 years   *Total Number of Subjects:* 730   *Drug Event:* death, stroke, coronary heart disease   *Validation of Outcome:* death certificates   *Rule Out Alternative Explanation:* age, gender   *Results:* mortality from stroke highest in those with the lowest vitamin C status; no association between mortality from coronary heart disease and vitamin C status

95:18   Gales BJ, Menard SM. Relationship between the administration of selected medications and falls in hospitalized elderly patients. Ann Pharmacother 1995;29:354-8

Drug Category: antidepressants, antihypertensive agents, antipsychotic agents, benzodiazepines, diuretics, opioid analgesics, sedatives, vasodilators, digitalis agents   *Validation of Exposure:* hospital records   *Study Methodology:* case–control study, retrospective   *Population Selection Criteria:* patients aged ≥70 years, hospitalized in a private acute care hospital, 1990–1991   *Total Number of Subjects:* 200   *Number of Cases:* 100   *Number of Controls:* 100   *Drug Event:* fall   *Validation of Outcome:* hospital incident reports   *Rule Out Alternative Explanation:* hospitalizations for syncope, falling, or orthopedic surgery and patients unable to ambulate during the hospitalization excluded   *Results:* administration of benzodiazepines and ≥3 concurrent psychoactive drugs more common in cases than in controls (40% vs. 20%, 17% vs. 4%, respectively)

95:19   Gardner TW, et al. Digoxin does not accelerate progression of diabetic retinopathy. Diabetes Care 1995;18:237-40

Drug Name: digoxin   *Drug Category:* digitalis agents   *Validation of Exposure:* patient report   *Study Methodology:* cohort study, prospective   *Population Selection Criteria:* participants with older-onset (≥30 y of age) type I diabetes in the Wisconsin Epidemiologic Study of Diabetic Retinopathy and participants with type II diabetes in the Early Treatment Diabetic Retinopathy Study   *Total Number of Subjects:* 2987   *Number of Cases:* 237 (digoxin users)   *Number of Controls:* 2750   *Drug Event:* retinopathy, diabetic retinopathy   *Validation of Outcome:* stereoscopic color photographs, the modified Airlie House classification scheme, a two-step difference in baseline retinopathy grade considered significant   *Rule Out Alternative Explanation:* baseline retinopathy, glycosylated hemoglobin, age, duration of diabetes   *Results:* no increased risk

95:20   Giles WH, et al. Serum folate and risk for ischemic stroke. First National Health and Nutrition Examination Survey Epidemiologic Follow-up Study. Stroke 1995;26:1166-70

Drug Name: folic acid   *Drug Category:* vitamins   *Validation of Exposure:* biochemical assays of blood samples   *Study Methodology:* cohort study, prospective   *Population Selection Criteria:* National Health and Nutrition Examination Survey I   *Total Number of Subjects:* 2006   *Number of Cases:* 356 (serum folate ≤9.2 nmol/L)   *Number of Controls:* 1650 (>9.2 nmol/L)   *Drug Event:* stroke (ischemic)   *Validation of Outcome:* hospital records or death certificate diagnosis   *Rule Out Alternative Explanation:* age, race, gender, education, diabetes, history of heart disease, low/high systolic blood pressure, body mass index, hemoglobin concentration, smoking, alcohol intake   *Results:* folate concentration ≤9.2 nmol/L, RR = 1.18 (95% CI 0.67 to 2.08) in whites and RR = 3.60 (95% CI 1.02 to 12.71) in African-Americans

95:21   Giovannucci E, et al. Aspirin and the risk of colorectal cancer in women. N Engl J Med 1995;333:609-14

Drug Name: aspirin   *Drug Category:* nonsteroidal antiinflammatory drugs   *Treatment Duration:* none, 1–4, 5–9, 10–19, ≥20 years   *Validation of Exposure:* mail questionnaires   *Study Methodology:* cohort study, prospective   *Population Selection Criteria:* Nurses' Health Study; cancer cases in 1986–1992   *Total Number of Subjects:* 89 446 (551 651 person-years)   *Number of Cases:* 331   *Drug Event:* cancer (colorectal)   *Validation of Outcome:* mail questionnaires, hospital records, pathology studies, National Death Index   *Rule Out Alternative Explanation:* age, family history of colorectal cancer, smoking, body mass index, physical activity, diet   *Results:* ≥2 tablets per week for ≥20 years, OR = 0.56 (95% CI 0.36 to 0.09) for colorectal cancer; no statistically significant reduction for shorter use

95:22   Grant CC, et al. Independent parental administration of prednisone in acute asthma: a double-blind, placebo-controlled, crossover study. Pediatrics 1995;96:224-9

Drug Name: prednisone   *Drug Category:* glucocorticoids   *Treatment Duration:* 6 months   *Validation of Exposure:* parent interviews   *Study Methodology:* randomized, double-blind, placebo-controlled, crossover trial   *Population Selection Criteria:* asthmatic children aged 2–14 years, ≥2 visits to emergency department/acute care clinic for asthma at Johns Hopkins Hospital   *Total Number of Subjects:* 78   *Drug Event:* asthma   *Validation of Outcome:* parent interviews, hospital records, chart reviews   *Results:* use of a single dose of prednisone for an asthma attack associated with an increase in outpatient visits for acute asthma

95:23   Hallas J, et al. Nonsteroidal anti-inflammatory drugs and upper gastrointestinal bleeding, identifying high-risk groups by excess risk estimates. Scand J Gastroenterol 1995;30:438-44

Drug Category: nonsteroidal antiinflammatory drugs (NSAIDs)   *Validation of Exposure:* prescription registry   *Treatment Duration:* 20 defined daily doses (median)   *Study Methodology:* cohort study, prospective   *Population Selection Criteria:* all NSAID users born before 1975 identified from the Odense University Pharmacoepidemiologic Database, 1990–1992; four randomly selected nonusers, matched to cases by gender and age   *Total Number of Subjects:* 138 700   *Number of Cases:* 31 503 (users), 107 197 (nonusers)   *Drug Event:* hemorrhage (gastrointestinal)   *Validation of Outcome:* hospital records, main or secondary discharge diagnosis   *Rule Out Alternative Explanation:* age, gender, peptic ulcer history   *Results:* excess risk 207/100 000 person-years for users

95:24   Hanharan JP, et al. Terfenadine-associated ventricular arrhythmias and QT$_c$ interval prolongation. A retrospective cohort comparison with other antihistamines among members of a health maintenance organization. Ann Epidemiol 1995;5:201-9

Drug Name: terfenadine   *Drug Category:* antihistamines   *Validation of Exposure:* pharmacy records   *Study Methodology:* cohort study, prospective   *Population Selection Criteria:* Harvard Community Health Plan members dispensed >1 antihistamine prescriptions, 1988–1990   *Total Number of Subjects:* 26 320   *Number of Cases:* 9008 (terfenadine-only users), 3968 (users of terfenadine and other antihistamines)   *Number of Controls:* 13 344 (nonterfenadine antihistamine users)   *Drug Event:* cardiac arrhythmia   *Validation of Outcome:* review of outpatient and inpatient records by an expert panel   *Rule Out Alternative Explanation:* age, gender, number of antihistamine courses, comorbidities   *Results:* no excess risk for terfenadine; joint courses of antihistamines and erythromycin associated with an increased risk of QTc prolongation

95:25   Harlow BL, Cramer DW. Self-reported use of antidepressants or benzodiazepine tranquilizers and risk of epithelial ovarian cancer: evidence from two combined case–control studies (Massachusetts, United States). Cancer Causes Control 1995;6:130-4

Drug Category: antidepressants, antianxiety agents, benzodiazepines   *Treatment Duration:* study I: >1 month; study II: ≥6 months   *Validation of Exposure:* personal interviews   *Study Methodology:* population-based case–control study, retrospective   *Population Selection Criteria:* English-speaking women, 18–80 years of age, diagnosed with epithelial ovarian malignancies in 10 hospitals in Boston metropolitan area, 1978–1981 (study I), 1984–1987 (study II); controls identified from Massachusetts town books, frequency matched to cases by age, race, precinct of residence   *Total Number of Subjects:* 904   *Number of Cases:* 450   *Number of Controls:* 454   *Drug Event:* cancer (ovarian)   *Validation of Outcome:* hospital records, pathology studies   *Rule Out Alternative Explanation:* parity, prior use of oral contraceptives, religion, body mass index, prior hysterectomy, therapeutic abortion   *Results:* adjusted OR = 2.1 (95% CI 0.9 to 4.8) for antidepressants, adjusted OR = 1.8 (95% CI 1.0 to 3.1) for benzodiazepines

95:26   Harris RE, et al. Breast cancer and NSAID use: heterogeneity of effect in a case control study. Prev Med 1995;24:119-20

Drug Category: nonsteroidal antiinflammatory drugs (NSAIDs)   *Treatment Duration:* 0, 1–4, ≥5 years   *Validation of Exposure:* personal interviews   *Study Methodology:* hospital-based case–control study, retrospective   *Population Selection Criteria:* women with newly diagnosed breast cancer presenting in hospitals in the northeastern US, 1988–1992; noncancer and cancer controls from the same hospitals, frequency matched to cases by age, month of diagnosis, hospital   *Total Number of Subjects:* 1511   *Number of Cases:* 744   *Number of Controls:* 767   *Drug Event:* cancer (breast)   *Validation of Outcome:* hospital records   *Rule Out Alternative Explanation:* age, menopausal status, parity, family history of breast cancer, body mass index   *Results:* adjusted OR = 0.63 (95% CI 0.5 to 0.9) when compared with combined control groups; heterogeneity of NSAID use among controls

95:27 Herings RMC, et al. Hypoglycaemia associated with use of inhibitors of angiotensin converting enzyme. Lancet 1995;345:1195-8

Drug Name: captopril, enalapril, lisinopril   *Drug Category:* antihypertensive agents, angiotensin-converting enzyme inhibitors   *Treatment Duration:* none, former use, current use   *Validation of Exposure:* drug-dispensing records   *Study Methodology:* nested case–control study, retrospective   *Population Selection Criteria:* patients treated with insulin or oral antidiabetic drugs for ≥1 year, 1986–1992, identified through the Dutch PHARMO record-linkage system   *Total Number of Subjects:* 748   *Number of Cases:* 94   *Number of Controls:* 654   *Drug Event:* hypoglycemia   *Validation of Outcome:* hospital admission diagnosis   *Rule Out Alternative Explanation:* age, gender, index year, city, diabetes treatment, admission for diabetes, history of glucagon use, use of other cardiovascular drugs   *Results:* current use of angiotensin-converting enzyme inhibitors, adjusted OR = 2.8 (95% CI 1.4 to 5.7)

95:28 Hornsby PP, et al. Onset of menopause in women exposed to diethylstilbestrol in utero. Am J Obstet Gynecol 1995;172:92-5

Drug Name: diethylstilbestrol   *Drug Category:* estrogens   *Treatment Duration:* starting before the 20th week of gestation   *Validation of Exposure:* clinical trial records   *Study Methodology:* cohort study, retrospective   *Population Selection Criteria:* women whose mothers participated in a clinical trial of use of diethylstilbestrol in pregnancy, aged 37–39 years   *Total Number of Subjects:* 542   *Number of Cases:* 296 (exposed to diethylstilbestrol)   *Number of Controls:* 246   *Drug Event:* menopause (premature)   *Validation of Outcome:* personal interview, medical records   *Results:* no increased risk

95:29 Jassal SK, et al. Low bioavailable testosterone levels predict future height loss in postmenopausal women. J Bone Miner Res 1995;10:650-4

Drug Name: testosterone   *Drug Category:* androgens   *Validation of Exposure:* radioimmunoassays   *Study Methodology:* cohort study, prospective   *Population Selection Criteria:* postmenopausal white women, aged 55–80 years, from an upper middle-class Southern California community   *Total Number of Subjects:* 170   *Drug Event:* osteoporosis   *Validation of Outcome:* measurements by trained observers   *Rule Out Alternative Explanation:* age, obesity, cigarette smoking, alcohol intake, exercise, use of thiazides and estrogen   *Results:* estimated and measured bioavailable testosterone predicted future height loss independently

95:30 Jick SS, et al. Antidepressants and suicide. BMJ 1995;310:215-18

Drug Name: dothiepin, amitriptyline, clomipramine, imipramine, flupentixol, lofepramine, mianserin, fluoxetine, doxepin, trazodone   *Drug Category:* antidepressants   *Validation of Exposure:* computerized medical records   *Study Methodology:* nested case–control study, retrospective   *Population Selection Criteria:* patients having received ≥1 prescriptions for antidepressants identified from the General Practice Research Database, 1988–1993   *Total Number of Subjects:* 1143   *Number of Cases:* 143   *Number of Controls:* 1000   *Drug Event:* suicide (within 6 mo of prescription)   *Validation of Outcome:* General Practice Research Database, physician records, death certificates   *Rule Out Alternative Explanation:* age, gender, calendar year   *Results:* RR = 2.8 (95% CI 1.8 to 4.3) for use of multiple antidepressants; adjusted rates similar for all 10 drugs

95:31 Kaldor JM, et al. Bladder tumours following chemotherapy and radiotherapy for ovarian cancer: a case–control study. Int J Cancer 1995;63:1-6

Drug Name: cyclophosphamide, melphalan, thiotepa   *Drug Category:* antineoplastic agents   *Validation of Exposure:* medical records   *Study Methodology:* case–control study, retrospective   *Population Selection Criteria:* patients diagnosed with primary bladder tumor ≥1 year after diagnosis of ovarian cancer identified in 10 cancer registries in Europe and Canada, and two oncology hospitals in Europe, 1960–1987; three controls with ovarian cancer selected for each case, matched by age, year of diagnosis, and survival time   *Total Number of Subjects:* 251   *Number of Cases:* 63   *Number of Controls:* 188   *Drug Event:* cancer (bladder)   *Validation of Outcome:* medical records, pathology reports   *Results:* compared with surgery only, RR = 3.2 (95% CI 0.97 to 10) for chemotherapy only, RR = 5.2 (95% CI 1.6 to 16) for chemotherapy and radiotherapy; for those treated with cyclophosphamide, RR = 4.2 (95% CI 1.2 to 14) without radiotherapy, RR = 3.2 (95% CI 0.86 to 12) with radiotherapy

95:32   Krumholz HM, et al. Aspirin in the treatment of acute myocardial infarction in elderly Medicare beneficiaries. Patterns and outcomes. Circulation 1995;92: 2841-7

Drug Name: aspirin   *Drug Category:* nonsteroidal antiinflammatory drugs (NSAIDs)   *Treatment Duration:* ≤2 days of hospitalization for acute myocardial infarction   *Validation of Exposure:* hospital medical record review   *Study Methodology:* cohort study, retrospective   *Population Selection Criteria:* Medicare beneficiaries hospitalized in Alabama, Connecticut, Iowa, and Wisconsin, June 1992–February 1993, aged ≥65 years, excluding those for whom aspirin therapy contraindicated   *Total Number of Subjects:* 10 018   *Number of Cases:* 6139 (received aspirin)   *Number of Controls:* 3879   *Drug Event:* death (30-day), myocardial infarction   *Validation of Outcome:* Medicare enrollment database   *Rule Out Alternative Explanations:* demographic, clinical, pharmacologic variables   *Results:* adjusted OR = 0.78 (95% CI 0.70 to 0.89)

95:33   Lalumandier JA, Rozier RG. The prevalence and risk factors of fluorosis among patients in a pediatric dental practice. Pediatr Dent 1995;17:19-25

Drug Name: fluoride   *Drug Category:* fluoride supplements   *Treatment Duration:* daily, <daily use; toothpaste use before 2 years of age, or later   *Validation of Exposure:* parent interviews, mail questionnaires, samples of drinking water   *Study Methodology:* case–control study, retrospective   *Population Selection Criteria:* cases identified among patients, aged 5–19 years, in one pediatric dental practice in North Carolina; controls randomly selected from patient records   *Total Number of Subjects:* 593   *Number of Cases:* 156   *Number of Controls:* 437   *Drug Event:* fluorosis   *Validation of Outcome:* dental examination by trained examiners, Tooth Surface Index of Fluorosis classification   *Results:* among subjects drinking fluoride-deficient water, OR = 6.5 for daily fluoride supplement use versus less frequent use, OR = 3.0 for initiating brushing at age <2 years versus ≥2 years; among subjects drinking fluoridated water, OR = 3.1 for initiating brushing at age <2 years

95:34   Lanza LE, et al. Peptic ulcer and gastrointestinal hemorrhage associated with nonsteroidal antiinflammatory drug use in patients younger than 65 years. Arch Intern Med 1995;155:1371-7

Drug Name: diclofenac, naproxen, piroxicam, sulindac   *Drug Category:* nonsteroidal antiinflammatory drugs (NSAIDs)   *Validation of Exposure:* pharmacy claims   *Study Methodology:* cohort study, prospective   *Population Selection Criteria:* enrollees of a network of health maintenance organizations dispensed study drugs, 1989–1991, aged <65 years   *Total Number of Subjects:* 68 028   *Drug Event:* gastrointestinal abnormalities (peptic ulcer), hemorrhage (gastrointestinal)   *Validation of Outcome:* insurance claims, medical records   *Results:* risk = 1.6 per 1000 people taking NSAIDs

95:35   Lapane KL, et al. Is the use of psychotropic drugs associated with increased risk of ischemic heart disease? Epidemiology 1995;6:376-81

Drug Category: antidepressants, benzodiazepines, antianxiety agents, hypnotics *Treatment Duration:* current use at baseline *Validation of Exposure:* personal interviews *Study Methodology:* cohort study, prospective *Population Selection Criteria:* participants in the Pawtucket Heart Health Program, aged 35–65 years *Total Number of Subjects:* 6039 *Number of Cases:* 471 (benzodiazepine users n = 339, antidepressant users n = 132) *Number of Controls:* 5568 (nonusers) *Drug Event:* cardiac ischemia *Validation of Outcome:* hospital discharge summaries, death certificates *Rule Out Alternative Explanation:* age, gender, other cardiovascular risk factors *Results:* adjusted RR = 2.0 (90% CI 1.1 to 3.9) for benzodiazepine use; adjusted RR = 5.7 (90% CI 2.6 to 12.8) for antidepressant use

95:36   La Vecchia AL, et al. Hormone replacement treatment and breast cancer risk: a cooperative Italian study. Br J Cancer 1995;72:244-8

Drug Name: estrogen replacement therapy *Drug Category:* estrogen–progestins, estrogens *Treatment Duration:* none, <1, 1–4, ≥5 years *Validation of Exposure:* personal structured interviews *Study Methodology:* hospital-based case–control study, retrospective *Population Selection Criteria:* cases, aged <75 years, with incident histologically confirmed breast cancer admitted to six Italian hospitals, 1991–1994; controls admitted for acute conditions *Total Number of Subjects:* 5157 *Number of Cases:* 2569 *Number of Controls:* 2588 *Drug Event:* cancer (breast) *Validation of Outcome:* histologic studies *Rule Out Alternative Explanation:* age, study center, marital status, education, body mass index, age at menarche, parity, age at first birth, menopausal status, age at menopause, type of menopause, history of benign breast cancer, family history of breast cancer *Results:* compared with nonusers, an increased risk (adjusted OR = 2.0, 95% CI 1.3 to 2.9) only for past users who stopped therapy <10 years ago

95:37   La Vecchia C, et al. Oral contraceptives and breast cancer: a cooperative Italian study. Int J Cancer 1995;60:163-7

Drug Name: oral contraceptives *Drug Category:* estrogen–progestins *Treatment Duration:* <1, 1–4, 5–8, >8 years *Validation of Exposure:* patient interviews *Study Methodology:* hospital-based case–control study, retrospective *Population Selection Criteria:* women <65 years of age with incident breast cancer admitted to major teaching and general hospitals in six areas in Italy; controls admitted for acute conditions to the same network of hospitals *Total Number of Subjects:* 3890 *Number of Cases:* 1991 *Number of Controls:* 1899 *Drug Event:* cancer (breast) *Validation of Outcome:* physician diagnosis, histologic studies *Rule Out Alternative Explanation:* age, study center, marital status, education, body mass index, age at menarche, parity, age at first birth, menopausal status, age at menopause, family history of breast cancer *Results:* no significant increase in risk

95:38   LeLorier J. Patterns of prescription of nonsteroidal antiinflammatory drugs and gastroprotective agents. J Rheumatol 1995;22(suppl 43):26-7

Drug Name: ibuprofen *Drug Category:* nonsteroidal antiinflammatory drugs (NSAIDs) *Validation of Exposure:* pharmacy records *Study Methodology:* cross-sectional cohort study, prospective *Population Selection Criteria:* all residents of the province of Quebec, aged ≥65 years, receiving nonaspirin NSAID identified from the Quebec Health Insurance Board database *Drug Event:* gastrointestinal abnormalities (gastric ulcer) *Validation of Outcome:* pharmacy records *Results:* patients using ibuprofen received antiulcer drugs less commonly than those using other nonaspirin NSAIDs; findings may result from prescribing based on risk perception

95:39   Li D-K, et al. Oral contraceptive use after conception in relation to the risk of congenital urinary tract anomalies. Teratology 1995;51:30-6

Drug Name: oral contraceptives *Drug Category:* estrogen–progestins *Treatment Duration:* none, ≤4 weeks, or >4 weeks after last menstruation *Validation of Exposure:*

mother interview   *Study Methodology:* case–control study, retrospective   *Population Selection Criteria:* singleton congenital urinary tract anomaly cases with no chromosomal abnormality from seven counties in Washington, 1990–1991; controls randomly selected from singleton births in five hospitals of King County, Washington   *Total Number of Subjects:* 487   *Number of Cases:* 118   *Number of Controls:* 369   *Drug Event:* congenital malformations, urinary tract anomaly   *Validation of Outcome:* Washington State Birth Defect Registry   *Rule Out Alternative Explanation:* birth year, county of maternal residence, sociodemographic factors, reproductive history, perinatal exposure to exogenous agents, past oral contraceptive use   *Results:* oral contraceptive use after conception, OR = 4.8 (95% CI 1.6 to 14.1)

95:40   Li D-K, et al. Periconceptional multivitamin use in relation to the risk of congenital urinary tract anomalies. Epidemiology 1995;6:212-8

Drug Category: vitamins   *Treatment Duration:* none, before, during, after first trimester   *Validation of Exposure:* mother interview   *Study Methodology:* case–control study, retrospective   *Population Selection Criteria:* singleton congenital urinary tract anomaly cases with no chromosomal abnormality from seven counties in Washington, 1990–1991; controls randomly selected from singleton births in five hospitals of King County, Washington   *Total Number of Subjects:* 487   *Number of Cases:* 118   *Number of Controls:* 369   *Drug Event:* congenital malformations, urinary tract anomaly   *Validation of Outcome:* Washington State Birth Defect Registry   *Rule Out Alternative Explanation:* maternal race, family income, county of residence, birth year   *Results:* adjusted OR = 0.17 (95% CI 0.05 to 0.43) for any periconceptional multivitamin use

95:41   Lidegaard Ø. Oral contraceptives, pregnancy, and the risk of cerebral thromboembolism: the influence of diabetes, hypertension, migraine, and previous thrombotic disease. Br J Obstet Gynaecol 1995;102:153-9

Drug Name: oral contraceptives   *Drug Category:* estrogen–progestins   *Validation of Exposure:* mail questionnaire   *Study Methodology:* case–control study, retrospective   *Population Selection Criteria:* cases, aged 15–44 years, hospitalized for cerebral thromboembolic attacks, 1985–1989, identified from the Danish National Patient Register; two randomly selected controls for each case from the National Personal Register, matched by age   *Total Number of Subjects:* 1867   *Number of Cases:* 497   *Number of Controls:* 1370   *Drug Event:* thromboembolism (cerebral)   *Validation of Outcome:* hospital records   *Results:* no increased risk for combined oral contraceptives

95:42   Linet M, et al. Analgesics and cancers of the renal pelvis and ureter. Int J Cancer 1995;62:15-8

Drug Category: nonsteroidal antiinflammatory drugs   *Treatment Duration:* no regular use, ≤4, 5–9, ≥10 years of use   *Validation of Exposure:* personal structured interviews   *Study Methodology:* population-based case–control study, retrospective   *Population Selection Criteria:* cases with renal pelvis and ureter cancer diagnosed in 1983–1986 from cancer registries in New Jersey, Iowa, and Los Angeles; controls through random-digit dialing and Medicare files, frequency matched to cases by age and gender   *Total Number of Subjects:* 998   *Number of Cases:* 502   *Number of Controls:* 496   *Drug Event:* cancer (renal)   *Validation of Outcome:* cancer registries, histologically confirmed   *Rule Out Alternative Explanation:* age, gender, geographic area, cigarette smoking   *Results:* no increased risk

95:43   Liu BA, et al. Falls among older people: relationship to medication use and orthostatic hypotension. J Am Geriatr Soc 1995;43:1141-5

Drug Category: antidepressants, antihypertensive agents, diuretics, hypnotics, sedatives   *Treatment Duration:* current use at baseline   *Validation of Exposure:* residence health office records, physician questionnaires   *Study Methodology:* cohort study, prospective *Population Selection Criteria:* older residents of two self-care residential facilities in Toronto, independent in activities of daily living and able to stand unaided   *Total Number of Subjects:* 96   *Number of Cases:* 59 (fallers)   *Drug Event:* fall   *Validation of Outcome:* weekly self-report by postcard for 1-year period   *Results:* RR = 1.6 (95% CI 1.24 to 2.06) for antidepressant use, no increased risk for use of other drugs

95:44   Magee LA, et al. Pregnancy outcome after gestational exposure to amiodarone in Canada. Am J Obstet Gynecol 1995;172:1307-11

Drug Name: amiodarone   *Drug Category:* antiarrhythmics   *Treatment Duration:* various, exposed at least from the 32nd week of gestation   *Validation of Exposure:* chart review, physician interview   *Study Methodology:* cohort study, retrospective   *Population Selection Criteria:* mothers treated with amiodarone during pregnancy, identified by the treating cardiologist   *Total Number of Subjects:* 12   *Drug Event:* thyroid dysfunction (perinatal)   *Validation of Outcome:* chart review, physician interview   *Results:* 9% incidence of neonatal hypothyroidism and hyperthyroidism (1 case each)

95:45   Nucci M, et al. Antibiotic regimen as an independent risk factor for disseminated fungal infections in neutropenic patients in Brazil. Trans R Soc Trop Med Hyg 1995;89:107-10

Drug Name: ceftazidime, imipenem, amikacin   *Drug Category:* antibacterials *Validation of Exposure:* treatment protocols   *Study Methodology:* nested case–control study, retrospective   *Population Selection Criteria:* a cohort of febrile episodes in 50 consecutive neutropenic patients in one hospital in Brazil, 1987–1991   *Total Number of Subjects:* 40 *Number of Cases:* 10   *Number of Controls:* 30   *Drug Event:* fungal infection   *Validation of Outcome:* histopathologic studies, blood or tissue cultures, clinical evaluation   *Results:* OR = 14.18 (95% CI 1.05 to 191.80) for use of the new antibiotic combination

95:46   Olsen JH, et al. Antiepileptic treatment and risk for hepatobiliary cancer and malignant lymphoma. Cancer Res 1995;55:294-7

Drug Name: phenobarbital, phenytoin   *Drug Category:* anticonvulsants   *Treatment Duration:* never (<5 g), ever used   *Validation of Exposure:* medical records   *Study Methodology:* nested case–control study, retrospective   *Population Selection Criteria:* an epileptic cohort treated at one epilepsy center in Denmark, 1932–1962, followed for cancer incidence through 1984; 2 controls matched to each hepatobiliary cancer case and 5 controls to each lymphoma case by age, gender, and survival time   *Total Number of Subjects:* 231   *Number of Cases:* 60   *Number of Controls:* 171   *Drug Event:* cancer (biliary, hepatic, malignant melanoma)   *Validation of Outcome:* histopathologic studies   *Rule Out Alternative Explanation:* Thorotrast exposure   *Results:* no increased risk

95:47   Paganini-Hill A. Aspirin and colorectal cancer: the Leisure World Cohort revisited. Prev Med 1995;24:113-5

Drug Name: aspirin   *Drug Category:* nonsteroidal antiinflammatory drugs   *Validation of Exposure:* mail questionnaire   *Study Methodology:* cohort study, prospective   *Population Selection Criteria:* residents in a retirement community in Leisure World, Laguna Hills, California, 1981–1991   *Total Number of Subjects:* 12 180   *Number of Cases:* 1738   *Drug Event:* cancer (colorectal)   *Validation of Outcome:* death certificates, hospital pathology and tumor registry files, the Cancer Surveillance Program   *Rule Out Alternative Explanation:* age, gender, rheumatoid arthritis, heart disease   *Results:* aspirin use not protective

95:48   Palmer JR, et al. Oral contraceptive use and breast cancer risk among African-American women. Cancer Causes Control 1995;6:321-31

Drug Name: oral contraceptives   *Drug Category:* estrogen–progestins   *Treatment Duration:* never, <1, 1–2, 3–4, 5–9, ≥10 years   *Validation of Exposure:* personal interviews

Study Methodology: hospital-based case–control study, retrospective   *Population Selection Criteria:* African-American women, aged 25–59 years, with primary invasive breast cancer admitted to hospitals in New York, Philadelphia, and Baltimore; controls hospitalized for nonmalignant conditions, frequency matched to cases by age and geography   *Total Number of Subjects:* 1545   *Number of Cases:* 524   *Number of Controls:* 1021   *Drug Event:* cancer (breast)   *Validation of Outcome:* hospital discharge summaries, pathology reports   *Rule Out Alternative Explanation:* age, geography, interview year, education, parity, age at first birth   *Results:* among women aged <45 years, adjusted RR = 2.2 (95% CI 1.5 to 3.2) for ≥3 years of use; among women aged 45–59 years, no significant increase in risk

95:49   Porkka KVK, et al. Influence of oral contraceptive use on lipoprotein (a) and other coronary heart disease risk factors. Ann Intern Med 1995;27:193-8

Drug Name: oral contraceptives   *Drug Category:* estrogen–progestins   *Treatment Duration:* none, constant use, former use, new use   *Validation of Exposure:* questionnaires   *Study Methodology:* cohort study, prospective   *Population Selection Criteria:* women aged 18, 21, and 24 years in 1986 participating in the Cardiovascular Risk in Young Finns Study   *Total Number of Subjects:* 559   *Number of Cases:* 210 (triphasic/levonorgestrel n = 127, monophasic/desogestrel n = 83)   *Number of Controls:* 349 (nonusers)   *Drug Event:* hypertension, hyperlipoproteinemia   *Validation of Outcome:* radioimmunoassay, blood pressure measurement   *Results:* use of triphasic/levonorgestrel associated with lower lipoprotein (a) compared with use of monophasic/desogestrel and no use (p = 0.005); oral contraceptive users had higher systolic blood pressure and triglyceride concentrations than did nonusers (p < 0.001)

95:50   Primic-Zakelj M, et al. Breast-cancer risk and oral contraceptive use in Slovenian women aged 25 to 54. Int J Cancer 1995;62:414-20

Drug Name: oral contraceptives   *Drug Category:* estrogen–progestins   *Treatment Duration:* none, <24, 25–48, 49–96, ≥97 months   *Validation of Exposure:* personal interview, life event calendar, prescriber inquiries   *Study Methodology:* case–control study, retrospective   *Population Selection Criteria:* Slovenian women, aged 25–54 years, with breast cancer diagnosed in five hospitals, 1988–1990; randomly selected controls from the population registry, matched to cases by age and area of residence   *Total Number of Subjects:* 1248   *Number of Cases:* 624   *Number of Controls:* 624   *Drug Event:* cancer (breast)   *Validation of Outcome:* physician diagnosis, histologic and/or cytologic studies   *Rule Out Alternative Explanation:* years of education, age at menarche, menopausal status, age at menopause, parity, age at first delivery, number of deliveries, family history of breast cancer   *Results:* no increased risk with duration of use; current users OR = 2.92 (95% CI 1.10 to 7.74) compared with nonusers

95:51   Psaty BM, et al. The risk of myocardial infarction associated with antihypertensive drug therapies. JAMA 1995;274:620-5

Drug Category: antihypertensives, beta-adrenoreceptor antagonists, calcium-channel blockers, diuretics   *Treatment Duration:* various   *Validation of Exposure:* pharmacy records   *Study Methodology:* population-based case–control study, retrospective   *Population Selection Criteria:* enrollees of the Group Health Cooperative of Puget Sound with pharmacologically treated hypertension; cases: first fatal or nonfatal myocardial infarction during 1986–1993 for women and 1989–1993 for men; controls: a stratified random sample, frequency matched to cases by age, gender, calendar year   *Total Number of Subjects:* 2655   *Number of Cases:* 623   *Number of Controls:* 2032   *Drug Event:* myocardial infarction   *Validation of Outcome:* medical records, telephone interviews of survivors   *Rule Out Alternative Explanation:* age, gender, calendar year, smoking, diabetes, pretreatment systolic blood pressure, duration of hypertension, physical activity, education   *Results:* for use of short-acting calcium-channel blockers, adjusted RR = 1.62

(95% CI 1.11 to 2.34) compared with use of diuretics alone and RR = 1.57 (95% CI 1.21 to 2.04) compared with use of beta-blockers; high doses of calcium-channel blockers are associated with increased risk (p < 0.01)

95:52   Radis CD, et al. Effects of cyclophosphamide on the development of malignancy and on long-term survival of patients with rheumatoid arthritis. Arthritis Rheum 1995;38:1120-7

Drug Name: cyclophosphamide   *Drug Category:* antineoplastic agents   *Validation of Exposure:* patient interviews   *Study Methodology:* cohort study, prospective   *Population Selection Criteria:* patients with refractory rheumatoid arthritis treated with oral cyclophosphamide in one rheumatology practice in Pittsburgh, 1968–1978; controls evaluated at the same time, matched by age, gender, disease duration, functional class   *Total Number of Subjects:* 238   *Number of Cases:* 119 (exposed to cyclophosphamide)   *Number of Controls:* 119   *Drug Event:* cancer   *Validation of Outcome:* patient interviews, office and hospital records, pathology reports, death certificates   *Results:* for cyclophosphamide exposure, RR = 1.5 (95% CI 0.93 to 5.5)

95:53   Reinisch JM, et al. In utero exposure to phenobarbital and intelligence deficits in adult men. JAMA 1995;274:1518-25

Drug Name: phenobarbital   *Drug Category:* anticonvulsants, sedatives   *Treatment Duration:* ≥5 days during third trimester and/or last month only, third trimester and earlier, prior to third trimester only   *Validation of Exposure:* medical records   *Study Methodology:* cohort study, retrospective   *Population Selection Criteria:* men born in 1959–1961 identified from the Danish Perinatal Cohort; cohort I: ≥2 periods of exposure to barbiturate; cohort II: ≥1 period of exposure to barbiturates, no maternal central nervous system disorders, no hormone exposure; controls matched to cases by numerous maternal variables   *Total Number of Subjects:* 267   *Number of Cases:* cohort I, 33 exposed; cohort II, 81 exposed   *Number of Controls:* cohort I: 52, cohort II: 101   *Drug Event:* intelligence deficit   *Validation of Outcome:* Wechsler Adult Intelligence Scale cohort (I), Danish Military Draft Board Intelligence Test (cohort II)   *Results:* men exposed to phenobarbital had lower (SD, 0.5) verbal intelligence scores than predicted; exposure in the last trimester had most effect

95:54   Rich JB, et al. Nonsteroidal anti-inflammatory drugs in Alzheimer's disease. Neurology 1995;45:51-5

Drug Category: nonsteroidal antiinflammatory drugs (NSAIDs)   *Validation of Exposure:* interviews with the patients' caregivers by physician   *Study Methodology:* cross-sectional cohort study, prospective   *Population Selection Criteria:* patients diagnosed with probable or possible Alzheimer disease entering the Johns Hopkins Alzheimer's Disease Research Center, 1984–1987   *Total Number of Subjects:* 209   *Number of Cases:* 32 (daily users of NSAIDs)   *Number of Controls:* 177   *Drug Event:* Alzheimer disease   *Rule Out Alternative Explanation:* duration of illness   *Results:* at baseline, daily users of NSAIDs performed better on the Mini-Mental State Examination, Boston Naming Test, and the delayed condition of the Benton Visual Retention Test than did nonusers; after 1 year, users had less decline on measures of verbal fluency, spatial recognition, and orientation than did nonusers

95:55   Risch HA, Howe GR. Menopausal hormone use and colorectal cancer in Saskatchewan: a record linkage cohort study. Cancer Epidemiol Biomarkers Prev 1995;4:21-8

Drug Name: estrogen replacement therapy   *Drug Category:* estrogen–progestins, estrogens   *Treatment Duration:* never, ever (>3.5 y)   *Validation of Exposure:* prescription claims   *Study Methodology:* cohort study, retrospective   *Population Selection Criteria:* women, aged

43–49 years, residing in Saskatchewan in 1976 *Total Number of Subjects:* 33 003 *Number of Cases:* 230 *Drug Event:* cancer (colorectal) *Validation of Outcome:* provincial cancer registry *Rule Out Alternative Explanation:* age *Results:* no significant association

95:56 Robinson DC, et al. A retrospective study of tamoxifen and endometrial cancer in breast cancer patients. Gynecol Oncol 1995;59:186-90

Drug Name: tamoxifen *Drug Category:* antineoplastic agents *Treatment Duration:* >1 year *Validation of Exposure:* patient records *Study Methodology:* case–control study, retrospective *Population Selection Criteria:* breast cancer patients treated at Wilford Hall Medical Center, 1978–1989; followed for 5–16 years (mean 9) *Total Number of Subjects:* 586 *Number of Cases:* 108 (exposed to tamoxifen) *Number of Controls:* 478 *Drug Event:* cancer (endometrial) *Validation of Outcome:* single pathologist using FIGO grading *Rule Out Alternative Explanation:* diabetes mellitus, hypertension, race, age, weight, tobacco use, family history of breast or gynecologic cancer *Results:* exposure to low-dose tamoxifen, RR = 15.2 (95% CI 2.8 to 84.4)

95:57 Rohan TE, et al. Dietary factors and risk of prostate cancer: a case–control study in Ontario, Canada. Cancer Causes Control 1995;6:145-54

Drug Name: vitamin A, vitamin C, vitamin E *Drug Category:* vitamins *Validation of Exposure:* personal interviews *Study Methodology:* population-based case–control study, retrospective *Population Selection Criteria:* English-speaking male residents of a defined area in Canada with recently confirmed adenocarcinoma of the prostate identified in the Ontario Cancer Registry, 1990–1992; randomly selected controls, frequency matched to cases by age *Total Number of Subjects:* 414 *Number of Cases:* 207 *Number of Controls:* 207 *Drug Event:* cancer (prostate) *Validation of Outcome:* histologic studies *Rule Out Alternative Explanation:* age, energy intake, family history of prostate cancer, history of benign prostatic hypertrophy *Results:* no significant associations

95:58 Shaw GM, et al. Periconceptional vitamin use, dietary folate, and the occurrence of neural tube defects. Epidemiology 1995;6:219-26

Drug Name: folic acid *Drug Category:* vitamins *Treatment Duration:* none, 3 months before conception, 3 months after conception *Validation of Exposure:* mothers' interviews *Study Methodology:* population-based case–control study, retrospective *Population Selection Criteria:* singleton fetuses and liveborn infants with neural tube defects delivered by California residents, 1989–1991; controls randomly selected from live singleton births *Total Number of Subjects:* 1164 *Number of Cases:* 624 *Number of Controls:* 540 *Drug Event:* neural tube defects *Validation of Outcome:* hospital records, ultrasound reports *Rule Out Alternative Explanation:* race, education, gravidity, oral contraceptive use, smoking *Results:* OR = 0.65 (95% CI 0.45 to 0.94) for any use 3 months before conception, OR = 0.60 (95% CI 0.46 to 0.79) for any use 3 months after conception

95:59 Shaw GM, et al. Risks of orofacial clefts in children born to women using multivitamins containing folic acid periconceptionally. Lancet 1995;346:393-6

Drug Name: folic acid *Drug Category:* vitamins *Treatment Duration:* 1 month before to 2 months after conception *Validation of Exposure:* mother interview by telephone *Study Methodology:* population-based case–control study, retrospective *Population Selection Criteria:* California Birth Defects Monitoring Program, 1987–1989; liveborn controls from California vital records, 1987–1989 *Total Number of Subjects:* 1465 *Number of Cases:* 731 *Number of Controls:* 734 *Drug Event:* cleft palate *Validation of Outcome:* medical records, necroscopy reports, surgical reports, classification by medical geneticist *Rule Out Alternative Explanation:* maternal race, education, age, gravidity, smoking, alcohol use *Results:* reduced risk of orofacial clefts for multivitamin use containing folic acid (OR = 0.5–0.73, depending on cleft phenotype)

95:60 Smalley WE, et al. Nonsteroidal anti-inflammatory drugs and the incidence of hospitalizations for peptic ulcer disease in elderly persons. Am J Epidemiol 1995;141:539-45

Drug Category: nonsteroidal antiinflammatory drugs   *Treatment Duration:* none, <30 days, 30–180 days, intermittent   *Validation of Exposure:* pharmacy claims   *Study Methodology:* cohort study, retrospective   *Population Selection Criteria:* Tennessee Medicaid enrollees, aged ≥65 years   *Total Number of Subjects:* 103 954 (209 068 person-years)   *Number of Cases:* 1371   *Drug Event:* gastrointestinal abnormalities (peptic ulcer)   *Validation of Outcome:* hospital claims, medical records   *Rule Out Alternative Explanation:* age, gender, nursing home status, hospitalizations in the previous year   *Results:* excess rate of 12.5 per 1000 person-years (95% CI 11.4 to 13.6) for current users; risk increased with increasing dose

95:61 Spinillo A, et al. The impact of oral contraception on vulvovaginal candidiasis. Contraception 1995;51:293-7

Drug Name: oral contraceptives   *Drug Category:* estrogen–progestins   *Treatment Duration:* nonusers, current users   *Validation of Exposure:* personal structured interview   *Study Methodology:* case–control study, retrospective   *Population Selection Criteria:* cases with ≥4 episodes of vulvovaginal candidiasis in the previous year seen in a vaginitis clinic; control group I, asymptomatic women; control group II, symptomatic women with nonrecurrent vulvovaginal candidiasis   *Total Number of Subjects:* 748   *Number of Cases:* 136   *Number of Controls:* group I, 306; group II, 306   *Drug Event:* candidiasis (vulvovaginal)   *Validation of Outcome:* vaginal cultures   *Rule Out Alternative Explanation:* age   *Results:* OR = 2.15 (95% CI 1.34 to 3.45) compared with group I; OR = 1.67 (95% CI 1.04 to 2.68) compared with group II

95:62 Stanford JL, et al. Combined estrogen and progestin hormone replacement therapy in relation to risk of breast cancer in middle-aged women. JAMA 1995;274:137-42

Drug Name: estrogen replacement therapy   *Drug Category:* estrogen–progestins, estrogens   *Treatment Duration:* various   *Validation of Exposure:* personal interviews, life event calendars   *Study Methodology:* population-based case–control study, retrospective   *Population Selection Criteria:* white women, aged 50–64 years, diagnosed with breast cancer, 1988–1990, residing in King County, Washington, having a telephone; randomly selected controls frequency matched to cases by age   *Total Number of Subjects:* 1029   *Number of Cases:* 537   *Number of Controls:* 492   *Drug Event:* cancer (breast)   *Validation of Outcome:* Seattle–Puget Sound Surveillance, Epidemiology, and End Results cancer registry   *Rule Out Alternative Explanation:* age, age at first full-term pregnancy, family history of breast cancer   *Results:* no increased risk

95:63 Stenius-Aarniala B, et al. Slow-release theophylline in pregnant asthmatics. Chest 1995;107:642-7

Drug Name: theophylline   *Drug Category:* bronchodilators, methylxanthines   *Treatment Duration:* none, throughout the pregnancy, second and third trimesters only   *Validation of Exposure:* serum drug measurement   *Study Methodology:* cohort study, prospective   *Population Selection Criteria:* pregnant women with asthma referred to pulmonary medicine and maternity clinics in Finland, 1982–1990; control group I, pregnant asthmatic patients without theophylline treatment; control group II, healthy controls matched by age and parity   *Total Number of Subjects:* 741   *Number of Cases:* 212 (theophylline users)   *Number of Controls:* 292 (asthmatic nonusers), 237 (healthy nonusers)   *Drug Event:* preeclampsia, gastrointestinal abnormalities (hepatic toxicity)   *Validation of Outcome:* hospital and outpatient records   *Results:* incidence of preeclampsia and jaundice in the newborn higher in the theophylline-treated group compared with healthy controls (15.6 % vs. 6.4% and 15.0 vs. 7.8%, respectively).

95:64 Thapa PB, et al. Psychotropic drugs and risk of recurrent falls in ambulatory nursing home residents. Am J Epidemiol 1995;142:202-11

Drug Category: antipsychotic agents, benzodiazepines, antidepressants, antianxiety agents, hypnotics   *Validation of Exposure:* medication administration records   *Study Methodology:* cohort study, prospective   *Population Selection Criteria:* ambulatory residents of 12 Tennessee nursing homes, 1991–1992, aged ≥65 years   *Total Number of Subjects:* 282 (178 regular users of psychotropic drugs, 104 nonusers)   *Drug Event:* fall   *Validation of Outcome:* review of nursing home incident reports and nursing home charts by trained nurses   *Rule Out Alternative Explanation:* symptoms of dementia, depression, other fall risk factors   *Results:* adjusted incidence density ratio = 1.97 (95% CI 1.28 to 3.05) for regular users compared with nonusers

95:65 Thomas DB, et al. Cervical carcinoma in situ and use of depot-medroxyprogesterone acetate (DMPA). Contraception 1995;51:25-31

Drug Name: medroxyprogesterone   *Drug Category:* progestins   *Treatment Duration:* none, 1–12, 13–60, ≥61 months   *Validation of Exposure:* personal interviews   *Study Methodology:* hospital-based case–control study, retrospective   *Population Selection Criteria:* new admissions for cervical carcinoma in three hospitals in Mexico and Thailand, aged 20–58 years   *Total Number of Subjects:* 10 173   *Number of Cases:* 1217   *Number of Controls:* 8956   *Drug Event:* cancer (cervical)   *Validation of Outcome:* pathology and outpatient records   *Rule Out Alternative Explanation:* hospital, age, parity, cervical smear frequency, use of oral contraceptives   *Results:* risk elevated for users and increased significantly with duration of use

95:66 Thomson JA, et al. Risk factors for the development of amoxicillin–clavulanic acid associated jaundice. Med J Aust 1995;162:638-40

Drug Name: amoxicillin/clavulanic acid   *Drug Category:* antibacterials   *Treatment Duration:* 5.7 days (mean)   *Validation of Exposure:* patient records   *Study Methodology:* case–control study, retrospective   *Population Selection Criteria:* jaundice cases diagnosed within 8 weeks of starting amoxicillin/clavulanic acid reported to the Australian Adverse Drug Reactions Advisory Committee, 1988–1993; four controls receiving amoxicillin/clavulanic acid randomly selected from the prescriber's patient register   *Total Number of Subjects:* 197   *Number of Cases:* 34   *Number of Controls:* 163   *Drug Event:* gastrointestinal abnormalities (hepatic disease)   *Validation of Outcome:* patient records   *Results:* older age and male gender associated with an increased risk of jaundice

95:67 Toniolo PG, et al. A prospective study of endogenous estrogens and breast cancer in postmenopausal women. J Natl Cancer Inst 1995;87:190-7

Drug Name: estrone, estradiol   *Drug Category:* estrogens   *Validation of Exposure:* biochemical and immunochemical analyses   *Study Methodology:* nested case–control study, retrospective   *Population Selection Criteria:* participants in a cohort study of New York City women, aged 35–64 years, free of breast cancer and postmenopausal at baseline   *Total Number of Subjects:* 381   *Number of Cases:* 130   *Number of Controls:* 251   *Drug Event:* cancer (breast)   *Validation of Outcome:* annual mammographic screening, mail questionnaires   *Rule Out Alternative Explanation:* Quetelet index   *Results:* adjusted OR = for increasing quartiles of total estradiol = 1.0, 0.9, 1.8, and 1.8 (trend, p = 0.06); OR = for increasing quartiles of estrone = 1.0, 2.2, 3.7, and 2.5 (trend, p = 0.56), respectively

95:68 Traversa G, et al. Gastroduodenal toxicity of different nonsteroidal antiinflammatory drugs. Epidemiology 1995;6:49-54

Drug Name: ketorolac, diclofenac, naproxen, piroxicam   *Drug Category:* nonsteroidal antiinflammatory drugs (NSAIDs)   *Treatment Duration:* none, past, recent, current use   *Validation of Exposure:* pharmacy claims   *Study Methodology:* population-based case–control study, retrospective *Population Selection Criteria:* residents of one province in Italy with confirmed endoscopic diagnosis of ulcer and erosion, 1991–1992; 10 controls for each case randomly selected from the National Health Service Beneficiaries, matched by age and gender *Total Number of Subjects:* 6600 *Number of Cases:* 600 *Number of Controls:* 6000 *Drug Event:* gastrointestinal abnormalities (duodenal ulcer) *Validation of Outcome:* endoscopy *Rule Out Alternative Explanation:* use of other drugs *Results:* OR = 1.3 (95% CI 0.98 to 1.18) for current use of NSAIDs; use of ketorolac associated with the greatest risk of gastrotoxicity

95:69   Vessey MP, Painter R. Endometrial and ovarian cancer and oral contraceptives—findings in a large cohort study. Br J Cancer 1995;71:1340-2
Drug Name: oral contraceptives *Drug Category:* estrogen–progestins *Treatment Duration:* none, ≥48, 49–96, >96 months *Validation of Exposure:* personal interviews *Study Methodology:* cohort study, prospective *Population Selection Criteria:* Oxford Family Planning Association Contraceptive Study *Total Number of Subjects:* 15 292 *Number of Cases:* 9411 (oral contraceptive users) *Number of Controls:* 5881 (nonusers) *Drug Event:* cancer (endometrial, ovarian) *Validation of Outcome:* hospital discharge summaries, pathology reports *Rule Out Alternative Explanation:* age, parity *Results:* ever users compared with never users, RR = 0.1 (95% CI 0.0 to 0.7) for endometrial cancer, RR = 0.4 (95% CI 0.2 to 0.8) for ovarian cancer

95:70   Weaver GA, et al. Nonsteroidal antiinflammatory drugs are associated with gastric outlet obstruction. J Clin Gastroenterol 1995;20:196-8
Drug Category: nonsteroidal antiinflammatory drugs (NSAIDs) *Treatment Duration:* various *Validation of Exposure:* chart review *Study Methodology:* case–control study, retrospective *Population Selection Criteria:* patients undergoing endoscopy at the Mary Imogene Basset Hospital, 1987–1990 *Total Number of Subjects:* 99 *Number of Cases:* 9 *Number of Controls:* 90 *Drug Event:* gastrointestinal abnormalities (gastric outlet obstruction) *Validation of Outcome:* chart review *Rule Out Alternative Explanation:* age, gender *Results:* higher proportion and longer duration of NSAID use in cases than in controls

95:71   Weil J, et al. Prophylactic aspirin and risk of peptic ulcer bleeding. BMJ 1995;310:827-30
Drug Name: aspirin *Drug Category:* nonsteroidal antiinflammatory drugs (NSAIDs) *Treatment Duration:* none, irregular use, daily use (≥5 d/wk) <1 mo, or daily use ≥1 month *Validation of Exposure:* patient interviews *Study Methodology:* case–control study, retrospective *Population Selection Criteria:* patients aged ≥60 years admitted to hospitals in the UK (Glasgow, Newcastle, Nottingham, Oxford, Portsmouth) *Total Number of Subjects:* 3236 *Number of Cases:* 1121 *Number of Controls:* 2115 *Drug Event:* gastrointestinal abnormalities (peptic ulcer), hemorrhage (gastrointestinal) *Validation of Outcome:* hospital admission diagnosis *Rule Out Alternative Explanation:* age, gender, prior ulcer history or dyspepsia, concurrent nonaspirin NSAID use, smoking, alcohol intake *Results:* OR raised for all doses of aspirin taken daily for ≥1 month; 75 mg, OR = 2.3 (95% CI 1.2 to 4.4); 150 mg, OR = 3.2 (95% CI 1.7 to 6.5); 300 mg, OR = 3.9 (95% CI 2.5 to 6.3)

95:72   Weir S, et al. Nonoxynol-9 use, genital ulcers, and HIV infection in a cohort of gender workers. Genitourin Med 1995;71:78-81
Drug Name: nonoxynol-9 *Drug Category:* spermicides *Validation of Exposure:* coital logs completed by women *Study Methodology:* cohort study, prospective *Population Selection Criteria:* seronegative female sex workers in Cameroon *Total Number of Subjects:* 273 *Number of Cases:* frequent users (n = 110), intermediate users (n = 117), infrequent users (n = 39) *Drug Event:* genital ulcer, HIV seroconversion *Validation of Outcome:* gyneco-

logic examinations, enzyme-linked immunosorbent assay tests, and Western blot for HIV
Results: no association between nonoxynol-9 use and ulcers nor between ulcers and HIV

95:73   Wejda B, et al. Hip fractures and the thyroid: a case–control study. J Intern Med 1995;237:241-7

Drug Name: levothyroxine   *Drug Category:* thyroid hormones   *Treatment Duration:* none, present, past use   *Validation of Exposure:* personal interviews, radioimmunoassays   *Study Methodology:* case–control study, retrospective   *Population Selection Criteria:* female patients with osteoporotic hip fracture presenting in two hospitals in Germany; ambulatory controls selected from homes for the aged and those attending day care centers   *Total Number of Subjects:* 518   *Number of Cases:* 116   *Number of Controls:* 402   *Drug Event:* fracture (bone)   *Validation of Outcome:* presenting diagnosis   *Results:* OR for hyperthyroidism = 2.5 (95% CI 1.2 to 5.3); OR for levothyroxine exposure = 0.67 (95% CI 0.32 to 1.41)

95:74   Wood R. Bronchospasm and cough as adverse reactions to the ACE inhibitors captopril, enalapril, and lisinopril. A controlled retrospective cohort study. Br J Clin Pharmacol 1995;39:265-70

Drug Name: captopril, enalapril, lisinopril   *Drug Category:* antihypertensive agents, angiotensin-converting enzyme (ACE) inhibitors   *Validation of Exposure:* physician questionnaire   *Study Methodology:* cohort study, retrospective   *Population Selection Criteria:* New Zealand Intensive Medicine Monitoring Programme prescription database   *Total Number of Subjects:* 2030   *Number of Cases:* 1013 (users of ACE inhibitors)   *Number of Controls:* 1017 (users of lipid-lowering drugs)   *Drug Event:* bronchospasm, cough   *Validation of Outcome:* physician questionnaire   *Results:* prevalence of bronchospasm and cough significantly greater among users of ACE inhibitors than among users of lipid lowering drugs (5.5% vs. 2.3%, 12.3% vs. 2.7%, respectively)

95:75   Ye Z, et al. Combined oral contraceptives and risk of cervical carcinoma in situ. Int J Epidemiol 1995;24:19-26

Drug Name: oral contraceptives   *Drug Category:* estrogen–progestins   *Treatment Duration:* none, 1–12, 13–60, ≥61 months   *Validation of Exposure:* personal structured interviews   *Study Methodology:* hospital-based case–control study, retrospective   *Population Selection Criteria:* new admissions for cervical cancer in hospitals in Mexico, Chili, and Thailand   *Total Number of Subjects:* 10 979   *Number of Cases:* 1365   *Number of Controls:* 9614   *Drug Event:* cancer (cervical)   *Validation of Outcome:* pathologist diagnosis, World Health Organization classification of tumors   *Rule Out Alternative Explanation:* hospital, age, marital status, number of pregnancies, history of induced abortion, number of cervical smears, use of injectable contraceptives, use of condom   *Results:* increased risk for use >60 months, especially in women who first used oral contraceptives in the past 5–10 years

96:1   Abenhaim L, et al. Appetite-suppressant drugs and the risk of primary pulmonary hypertension. N Engl J Med 1996;335:609-16

Drug Name: fenfluramine, dexfenfluramine, clobenzorex, fenproporex, mazindol, phenmetrazine   *Drug Category:* anorexics   *Validation of Exposure:* face-to-face interview using three methods: spontaneous reporting by the patient, presentation of list of drug increases, prompting with pictures of drug packages   *Study Methodology:* case–control study, prospective   *Population Selection Criteria:* 35 centers in France, Belgium, the UK, and the Netherlands, men and women 18–70 years of age between September 1992 and September 1994   *Number of Cases:* 95   *Number of Controls:* 355   *Comparability of Controls:* recruited from general practice and matched to patients' gender, age, and number of physician visits per year; same practices as cases randomly selected   *Drug*

Event: primary pulmonary hypertension   *Validation of Outcome:* primary pulmonary hypertension at time of right heart catherization   *Risk Factors:* family history of pulmonary hypertension, HIV infection, cirrhosis, use of cocaine, or iv drug use   *Results:* OR = 6.3 (95% CI 3.0 to 13.2); OR = 10.1 (95% CI 3.4 to 29.9) use in preceding year; OR = 23.1 (95% CI 6.9 to 77.7) used >3 months

96:2   Adesanya OO, Colie CF. Evaluating oral contraceptive use at 6 and 12 months. J Reprod Med 1996;41:431-4

Drug Name: oral contraceptives   *Drug Category:* estrogen–progestins   *Study Methodology:* patient fellowship study; 6 versus 12 months   *Population Selection Criteria:* chart review of 3100 patients attending obstetric–gynecologic clinic at Georgetown Medical Center; those starting low-dose oral contraceptives   *Number of Subjects:* 195   *Comparability of Controls:* cases served as own controls   *Drug Event:* blood pressure changes, breast or pelvic complications   *Validation of Outcome:* systolic >140 mm Hg, diastolic >90 mm Hg; breast mass, tenderness, nipple discharge, pelvic mass or tenderness   *Results:* allowing for Type I error of 80% and Type II error of 90%; no difference in incidence was found between 6 and 12 months

96:3   Writing committee headed by Poulter NR. Haemorrhagic stroke, overall stroke risk, and combined oral contraceptives: results of an international, multicentre, case–control study. WHO Collaborative Study of Cardiovascular Disease and Steroid Hormone Contraception. Lancet 1996;348:505-10

Drug Name: oral contraceptives   *Drug Category:* estrogen–progestins   *Dosing Criteria:* current users of oral contraceptives (any use in the previous 3 mo)   *Validation of Exposure:* cases and controls interviewed while in hospital   *Study Methodology:* case–control study   *Population Selection Criteria:* women aged 20–44 years in participating hospitals   *Number of Cases:* 1068 aged 20–44   *Number of Controls:* 2910   *Comparability of Controls:* age matched   *Drug Event:* stroke (hemorrhagic)   *Validation of Outcome:* reviewed hospital records   *Results:* in developing countries, significant OR = 1.76 (95% CI 1.34 to 2.3) but not in Europe, where OR = 1.38 (95% CI 0.84 to 2.25); age <35 years, no increased risk in any country; >35 years, OR >2; history of nonpregnancy-related hypertension OR increased 10- to 20-fold; ORs for any type of stroke with low-dose or high-dose oral contraceptive were 1.41 (95% CI 0.90 to 2.20) and 2.71 (95% CI 1.71 to 4.32), respectively, in Europe and 1.86 (95% CI 1.49 to 2.33) and 1.92 (95% CI 1.48 to 2.50) in developing countries; estimated that 13% and 8% of all strokes in women aged 20–44 years in Europe and developing countries, respectively, are due to oral contraceptive use

96:4   Anonymous. Ischaemic stroke and combined oral contraceptives: results of an international, multicentre, case–control study. WHO Collaborative Study of Cardiovascular Disease and Steroid Hormone Contraception. Lancet 1996;348: 498-505

Drug Name: oral contraceptives   *Drug Category:* estrogen–progestins   *Dosing Criteria:* current users of oral contraceptives (any use in previous 3 mo)   *Validation of Exposure:* cases and controls were interviewed while in hospital in regard to contraceptive use and blood pressure measurements   *Study Methodology:* hospital-based case–control study   *Population Selection Criteria:* 21 international hospital centers where diagnosis of stroke based on computed tomography, magnetic resonance imaging, or cerebral angiography within 3 weeks of event   *Number of Cases:* 697   *Number of Controls:* 1962   *Comparability of Controls:* matched by 5-year age band, hospital, and time of admission   *Drug Event:* stroke (ischemic)   *Validation of Outcome:* reviewed hospital records   *Results:* overall OR = 2.99 (95% CI 1.65 to 5.40) in Europe and 2.93 (95% CI 2.15 to 4.00) in non-European developing countries; although overall incidence is very low, ischemic stroke risk in oral contraceptive users can be lowered by normalizing blood pressure, users <35 years, and avoiding smoking

96:5   Beck RW, et al. Uveitis associated with topical beta-blockers. Arch Ophthalmol 1996;114:1181-2

Drug Name: metipranolol, timolol, betaxolol   *Drug Category:* beta-adrenoreceptor antagonists   *Dosing Criteria:* 0.3% solution of metipranolol   *Validation of Exposure:* pharmacy dispensing data   *Study Methodology:* prescription sequencing cohort study, retrospective   *Population Selection Criteria:* drug dispensing data from Humana Health Care Plan   *Number of Cases:* 1928 exposed to 0.3% metipranolol; 1972 person-years   *Number of Controls:* 3903 exposed to other beta-blockers; 2674 person-years   *Drug Event:* uveitis, identified by prescription of a topical corticosteroid and confined by chart review   *Validation of Outcome:* chart review   *Results:* no cases were detected

96:6   Botto LD, et al. Periconceptional multivitamin use and the occurrence of conotruncal heart defects: results from a population-based, case–control study. Pediatrics 1996;98:911-7

Drug Category: multivitamins   *Dosing Criteria:* use: regular use for 3 months before conception through third month of pregnancy   *Validation of Exposure:* telephone interview   *Study Methodology:* population-based case–control study   *Population Selection Criteria:* Atlanta Birth Defects Case–Control Study, born in 1968–1980 for mothers in metropolitan Atlanta   *Number of Cases:* 158   *Number of Controls:* 3026   *Comparability of Controls:* 1% random sample of infants without birth defects born in same period, matched by hospital of birth, calendar quarter of birth, and race   *Drug Event:* heart defects (conotruncal)   *Validation of Outcome:* registry records   *Confounders:* maternal age, education, race, smoking, alcohol use, chronic illness   *Results:* multivariate analysis: OR = 0.57 (95% CI 0.33 to 1.00) use versus no use for all conotruncal heart defects; OR = 0.41 (95% CI 0.20 to 0.84) use versus no use for isolated conotruncal defects compared with noncardiac defects

96:7   Braga C, et al. Fertility treatment and risk of breast cancer. Hum Reprod 1996;11:300-3

Drug Category: ovulation inducers   *Validation of Exposure:* hospital records   *Study Methodology:* case–control study   *Population Selection Criteria:* Italian women with histologically confirmed breast cancer   *Number of Cases:* 2569   *Number of Controls:* 2588   *Comparability of Controls:* women admitted to hospitals without neoplastic or hormonal gynecologic problems   *Drug Event:* cancer (breast)   *Validation of Outcome:* hospital records   *Results:* women with fertility drug treatment OR = 1.43; those without drug treatment OR = 0.85 (not significant)

96:8   Braun S, et al. Calcium antagonists and mortality in patients with coronary artery disease: a cohort study of 11,575 patients. J Am Coll Cardiol 1996;28:7-11

Drug Name: nifedipine, verapamil, diltiazem, amlodipine   *Drug Category:* calcium-channel blockers   *Validation of Exposure:* at screening, nifedipine, 38%; verapamil, 6%; diltiazem, 57%; combination, 3%   *Study Methodology:* cohort study   *Population Selection Criteria:* patients with coronary artery disease enrolled in "Bezafibrak Infarction Prevention," February 1990–October 1992, aged 45–74 years   *Number of Subjects:* 11 575   *Number of Cases:* 5843   *Number of Controls:* 5732   *Comparability of Controls:* adjustments for age, gender, prevalence of previous myocardial infarction, angina pectoris, hypertension, peripheral vascular disease, chronic obstructive pulmonary disease, diabetes mellitus, current smoking; further adjustments for concomitant medications, life status in Israel Population Registry   *Drug Event:* death   *Results:* age I adjusted RR ratio = 1.08 (95% CI 0.95 to 1.24); age II adjusted RR ratio = 0.97 (95% CI 0.84 to 1.11); and further age III adjusted RR ratio = 0.94 (95% CI 0.82 to 1.08)

**96:9   Chambers CD, et al. Birth outcomes in pregnant women taking fluoxetine.
N Engl J Med 1996;335:1010-5**

Drug Name: fluoxetine   *Drug Category:* antidepressants   *Dosing Criteria:* average exposure, fluoxetine 28 mg ± 15 mg   *Validation of Exposure:* questionnaire for historical exposure information and other risk factors; diary and phone survey for concurrent exposure and risk factors   *Study Methodology:* cohort study, prospective   *Population Selection Criteria:* from 1989 through 1995, California Teratogen Information Service and Clinical Research Program; cases: pregnant women using fluoxetine and currently taking drug; controls: pregnant women not taking drug   *Number of Cases:* 228   *Number of Controls:* 254   *Comparability of Controls:* control for age, gravity, parity, number of spontaneous abortions, number of therapeutic abortions   *Drug Event:* birth outcome   *Validation of Outcome:* telephone interview with mother, medical records, and survey of infants' physicians   *Results:* when exposed for first and second trimester: spontaneous pregnancy loss fluoxetine (10.5%), control (9.1%) (not significant); major structural anomalies with fluoxetine (5.5%), control (4.0%)(not significant); when exposed during third trimester: RR = 4.8 (95% CI 1.1 to 20.8); admission to special-care nursery RR = 2.6 (95% CI 1.1 to 6.9); poor neonatal adaptation RR = 8.7 (95% CI 2.9 to 26.6)

**96:10   Chan TY, et al. The relationship between upper gastrointestinal hemorrhage
and drug use: a case–control study. Int J Clin Pharmacol Therapeut 1996;34:304-8**

Drug Category: nonsteroidal antiinflammatory drugs (NSAIDs)   *Dosing Criteria:* any use   *Validation of Exposure:* medication history via structured questionnaire   *Study Methodology:* case–control study   *Population Selection Criteria:* patients admitted to Hong Kong hospital with diagnosed upper gastrointestinal hemorrhage   *Number of Cases:* 251   *Number of Controls:* 251   *Comparability of Controls:* matched for age, gender, and excluded if history of upper gastrointestinal hemorrhage   *Drug Event:* hemorrhage (gastrointestinal)   *Validation of Outcome:* hospital records, drug use questionnaire   *Results:* NSAID use in cases versus control OR = 14.0, p < 0.00001; ulcer-healing drugs OR = 12.5, p < 0.00001; acetaminophen OR = 2.5, p < 0.01

**96:11   Chasan-Taber L, et al. A prospective study of folate and vitamin B$_6$ and risk of
myocardial infaction in US physicians. J Am Coll Nutr 1996;15:136-43**

Drug Name: folic acid, vitamin B$_6$ *Validation of Exposure:* patient questionnaire at index in every 6 months for 7.5 years, plasma samples and each case–control followed for 7.5 years   *Study Methodology:* nested case–control study   *Population Selection Criteria:* participants in Physicians' Health Study, male physicians 40–84 years of age with no prior mycardial infarction or stroke who provided plasma samples   *Number of Subjects:* 14 916   *Number of Cases:* 333   *Number of Controls:* 333   *Comparability of Controls:* matched by age and smoking   *Drug Event:* myocardial infarction, death   *Confounders:* diabetes, angina, hypertension, Quetelet index, total high-density lipoprotein cholesterol   *Results:* men with lowest 20% of folate concentration (<2.0 ng/mL) had an RR = 1.4 (95% CI 0.9 to 2.3) compared with those in the top 80%; for the lowest 20% of B$_6$ values, RR = 1.5 compared with high levels of folate where RR = 1.3 (95% CI 0.8 to 2.1) and for B$_6$ where RR = 1.3 (95% CI 0.9 to 2.1); thus, low intakes of folate and vitamin B$_6$ are associated with increased incidence of myocardial infarction

96:12   Chasan-Taber L, et al. Prospective study of oral contraceptives and hypertension among women in the United States. Circulation 1996;94:483-9

Drug Name: oral contraceptives   *Drug Category:* estrogen–progestins   *Dosing Criteria:* oral contraceptive exposure duration <2 months; 2–10 months; >10 months to 2 years; progestational potency: low, medium, or high; estrogenic activity: low (<30 µg); medium (>30–<50 µg); high (>50 µg)   *Study Methodology:* cohort study, prospective (4-y follow-up)   *Population Selection Criteria:* US female nurses aged 25–42 years; excluded those with hypertension, diabetes, coronary heart disease, stroke, and cancer *Number of Subjects:* 68 297 *Number of Cases:* 1193 (past users), 167 236 person-years; 163 (current users), 28 437 person-years *Number of Controls:* 211 (35 333 person-years) *Comparability of Controls:* same population *Drug Event:* hypertension *Validation of Outcome:* self-reported by questionnaire, validated in subsample *Confounders:* age, body mass index, cigarette smoking, alcohol intake, family history of hypertension, ethnic group, parity, physical activity *Results:* adjusted RR = 1.8 (95% CI 1.5 to 2.3) current users versus never users; adjusted RR = 1.2 (95% CI 1.0 to 1.4) past users versus never users

96:13 Czeizel AE, et al. Population-based case–control study of folic acid supplementation during pregnancy. Teratology 1996;53:345-51

Drug Name: folic acid *Drug Category:* vitamins *Dosing Criteria:* 3 mg bid *Validation of Exposure:* mail questionnaire *Study Methodology:* nested case–control study *Population Selection Criteria:* Hungarian Case Control Surveillance of Congenital Abnormalities, 1980–1991 *Number of Cases:* 17 300 *Number of Controls:* 30 663 *Comparability of Controls:* matched for gender, birth week, district of parents' residence *Drug Event:* cardiovascular defects, neural tube defects, cleft lip, cleft palate *Validation of Outcome:* Hungarian Congenial Abnormality Registry *Confounders:* date of maternal age, birth order, proportion of threatened abortion and preterm births, maternal disorders *Results:* 54.9% of healthy infants used folic acid, 50.4% of cases used folic acid

96:14 Derby LE, Jick H. Acetaminophen and renal and bladder cancer. Epidemiology 1996;7:358-62

Drug Name: acetaminophen *Drug Category:* nonsteroidal antiinflammatory drugs *Dosing Criteria:* no use, low use (1 over-the-counter purchase or prescription [Rx]), incidental use (2–9 Rx), moderate use (10–19 Rx), regular use (20–39 Rx), heavy use (>40 Rx) *Validation of Exposure:* computerized prescription data from Group Health Cooperative of Puget Sound *Study Methodology:* matched case–control study *Population Selection Criteria:* all cases of renal or bladder cancer *Number of Subjects:* 380 000 health plan members *Number of Cases:* 222 renal, 504 bladder *Number of Controls:* 885 renal, 2009 bladder *Comparability of Controls:* matched for gender, age, duration of health plan membership *Drug Event:* cancer (renal, bladder) *Validation of Outcome:* health plan medical and pharmacy records *Results:* renal cancer >40 Rx RR = 2.6 (95% CI 1.1 to 6.0); bladder cancer >40 Rx RR = 1.3 (95% CI 0.6 to 2.8)

96:15 Dombrowski MP, et al. Preliminary experience with triamcinolone acetonide during pregnancy. J Matern-Fetal Med 1996;5:310-3

Drug Name: triamcinolone acetonide, beclomethasone, theophylline *Drug Category:* bronchodilators, glucocorticoids *Dosing Criteria:* any dose used during pregnancy (inhaled and/or systemic) *Validation of Exposure:* hospital and clinical records *Study Methodology:* cohort study, retrospective *Population Selection Criteria:* from computerized perinatal database in Detroit, pregnant women treated with above three drugs and hospitalized for exacerbation of asthma were identified in 1992–1995 *Number of Cases:* triamcinolone (n = 15), beclomethasone (n = 14), theophylline (n = 25) *Drug Event:* birth weight, hospitalization *Validation of Outcome:* review of medical records *Results:* birth weight of newborns of mothers receiving triamcinolone 502 g > beclomethaxone 316 g > theophylline (p = uc); hospitalization of mothers on triamcinolone was 33%; beclomethasone, 79% (p < 0.05); theophylline, 28% (p = uc)

96:16 Fernandez E, et al. Oral contraceptives, hormone replacement therapy, and the risk of colorectal cancer. Br J Cancer 1996;73:1431-5

Drug Name: oral contraceptives, estrogen replacement therapy *Drug Category:* estrogens, estrogen–progestins *Dosing Criteria:* never used/ever used; duration of use ≤2

years, >2 years; time since first use ≤15 years, >15 years; time since last use ≤10 years, >10 years   *Validation of Exposure:* trained interviewers using structured questionnaire   *Study Methodology:* case–control study   *Population Selection Criteria:* Northern Italy general hospitals, 1985–1992   *Number of Cases:* 709   *Number of Controls:* 992   *Comparability of Controls:* admitted to same hospitals, <75 years of age   *Drug Event:* cancer (colorectal)   *Validation of Outcome:* histologic confirmation   *Results:* OR = 0.58 (95% CI 0.36 to 0.92) ever used oral contraceptives; OR = 0.52 (95% CI 0.27 to 1.02) used >2 years; OR = 0.40 (95% CI 0.25 to 0.66) ever used hormone replacement therapy

96:17 Fourrier A, et al. Nonsteroidal antiinflammatory drug use and cognitive function in the elderly: inconclusive results from a population-based cohort study. J Clin Epidemiol 1996;49:1201

Drug Category: nonsteroidal antiinflammatory drugs (NSAIDs)   *Dosing Criteria:* must be taking NSAID at baseline and at 1 year   *Validation of Exposure:* NSAID users were defined as individuals who reported taking NSAID at baseline and 1 year later; all others excluded; self-reported in an interview   *Study Methodology:* cohort study (Paquid Research Program)   *Population Selection Criteria:* representative sample of people ≥65 years, living in their own homes in southwest France   *Number of Subjects:* 2792   *Number of Cases:* 1252 fulfilled conditions of being interviewed at 1 year and at 3 years, presented no dementia, and being exposed to or not to NSAID   *Comparability of Controls:* control for age, Mini-Mental State Examination (MMSE) scores, and time   *Drug Event:* dementia (Alzheimer disease)   *Results:* NSAID use was related to unfavorable variation of the MMSE scores RR = 2.84 (95% CI 0.99 to 8.1); these results do not indicate a protective effect of NSAID against dementia as measured by MMSE performance and alteration of cognitive functions

96:18 Garcia Rodriguez LA, et al. A cohort study of the ocular safety of anti-ulcer drugs. Br J Clin Pharmacol 1996;42:213-6

Drug Name: omeprazole, cimetidine, famotidine, nizatidine, ranitidine   *Drug Category:* antiulcer agents, proton pump inhibitors, histamine$_2$-receptor antagonists   *Dosing Criteria:* exposure: current use; past use (90 d after current use); nonuse   *Validation of Exposure:* copy of prescription written by general practitioner in medical record   *Study Methodology:* cohort study, retrospective   *Population Selection Criteria:* General Practitioners' Research Database (GPRD) in the UK; population base of 4 million residents, included all subjects aged 20–74 years who received at least one prescription for an antiulcer drug between January 1990–September 1994; exclusion of persons with previous eye disorders   *Exposure Cases:* cimetidine, 351 120; famotidine, 19 070; nizatidine, 11 714; omeprazole, 130 076; ranitidine, 516 852   *Nonexposed:* 2 280 234 person-years of follow-up   *Drug Event:* ophthalmic inflammation   *Validation of Outcome:* identified from computerized files, verified by medical record review by specialists   *Results:* RR = 1.8 (95% CI 0.5 to 6.0) omeprazole versus nonuse; RR = 1.9 (95% CI 1.1 to 3.4) current use of any antiulcer drug versus nonuse

96:19 Garrett JE, et al. Risk of severe life threatening asthma and beta agonist type: an example of confounding by severity. Thorax 1996;51:1093-9

Drug Name: fenoterol   *Drug Category:* beta-adrenoreceptor agonists   *Dosing Criteria:* fenoterol 200 µg/inhalation; 100 µg plus ipratropium 40 µg inhalation   *Validation of Exposure:* special form for asthma medications and severity filled out on admission to emergency department   *Study Methodology:* cohort study, retrospective   *Population Selection Criteria:* Auchland hospital, admitted for acute asthma between 1986 and 1987 and followed until May 31, 1989   *Number of Subjects:* 655   *Number of Cases:* 90 admitted to intensive care unit, 15 asthma deaths   *Drug Event:* death (asthma), intensive care admission   *Confounders:* severity (hospital admission in previous year); oral corticos-

624 Pharmacoepidemiology: An Introduction

teroids; continuous corticosteroids, severity of attacks, race   *Results:* RR = 2.1 (95% CI 1.4 to 3.1) fenoterol versus salbutamol; adjusted RR = 1.5 (95% CI 1.0 to 2.3); adjusted RR = 1.0 (95% CI 0.6 to 1.7)

96:20   Glesby MJ, et al. Use of antiherpes drugs and the risk of Kaposi's sarcoma: data from the Multicenter AIDS Cohort Study. J Infect Dis 1996;173:1477-80

Drug Name: acyclovir, ganciclovir, foscarnet   *Validation of Exposure:* self-reported use of acyclovir at any visit   *Study Methodology:* nested case–control study   *Population Selection Criteria:* homosexual men from Multicenter AIDS Cohort Study, with diagnosis of AIDS at sixth visit   *Number of Subjects:* 935   *Number of Cases:* 221   *Number of Controls:* 714   *Comparability of Controls:* control for confounders on race, age, study size, history of herpes, sexual practices, smoking   *Drug Event:* Kaposi's sarcoma   *Results:* OR = 1.02 (95% CI 0.76 to 1.38) for all drugs listed above

96:21   Godstein F, et al. Prospective study of exogenous hormones and risk of pulmonary embolism in women. Lancet 1996;348:983-7

Drug Name: estrogen replacement therapy, oral contraceptives   *Drug Category:* estrogens, estrogen–progestins   *Validation of Exposure:* mailed questionnaire   *Study Methodology:* cohort study, prospective; biannual survey to verify exposure status and outcome   *Population Selection Criteria:* Nurses' Health Study, includes 121 700 female registered nurses in 11 states   *Number of Subjects:* 112 593 women aged 30–55 years in 1976 and followed during 1976–1992   *Number of Cases:* 68   *Number of Controls:* 633 817 persons in years of follow-up   *Drug Event:* pulmonary embolism   *Validation of Outcome:* self-reports and medical records, controlled by height, weight, cigarette smoking, diabetes, hypertension, serum cholesterol, myocardial infarction, parity, menopause   *Results:* adjusted RR = 2.1 (95% CI 1.2 to 3.8) for current users of postmenopausal hormones; adjusted RR = 1.3 (95% CI 0.7 to 2.4) for past users; adjusted RR = 2.2 (95% CI 0.8 to 5.9) for current users of oral contraceptives; adjusted RR = 0.8 (95% CI 0.5 to 1.2) for past users of contraceptives

96:22   Goldstein RE, et al. Marked reduction in long-term cardiac deaths with aspirin after a coronary event. J Am Coll Cardiol 1996;28:326-30

Drug Name: aspirin   *Drug Category:* nonsteroidal antiinflammatory drugs   *Dosing Criteria:* any regular aspirin dose   *Validation of Exposure:* medical records of patients enrolled in Multicenter Study of Myocardial Ischemia   *Study Methodology:* case–control study, retrospective   *Population Selection Criteria:* patients with myocardial infarction (n = 651) or unstable angina (n = 285) enrolled in above study 1–6 months after hospitalization   *Number of Cases:* 751 (aspirin users)   *Number of Controls:* 185 (nonusers of aspirin)   *Comparability of Controls:* similar except aspirin use   *Drug Event:* death (cardiac)   *Validation of Outcome:* hospital records   *Results:* follow-up mean, 23 months; cardiac deaths in 1.6% of aspirin users and 5.4% of nonusers (p = 0.005); difference in mortality rate particularly prominent in patients treated with thrombolysis at initial hospitalization (0.9% aspirin users vs. 8.8% nonusers) (p = 0.004)

96:23   Hansen JM, et al. Non-steroidal anti-inflammatory drugs and ulcer complications: a risk factor analysis for clinical decision-making. Scand J Gastroenterol 1996;31:126-30

Drug Category: nonsteroidal antiinflammatory drugs (NSAIDs)   *Dosing Criteria:* any use   *Validation of Exposure:* medical records in Odense University Hospital, Denmark   *Study Methodology:* case–control study   *Population Selection Criteria:* cases were consecutive NSAID users admitted with ulcer complication, and controls were random sample of all NSAID users without ulcer complication   *Number of Cases:* 118   *Number of Controls:* 540   *Comparability of Controls:* random selection by computer from NSAID

users in Odense region   *Drug Event:* gastrointestinal abnormalities (peptic ulcer)
Validation of Outcome: medical and pharmacy records   *Results:* risk factors for ulcer
problems at start of NSAID therapy were age 60–75 years OR = 3.5 (95% CI 1.8 to 7.1),
>75 years OR = 8.9 (95% CI 4.3 to 18.3), male gender OR = 1.7 (95% CI 1.0 to 3.0), ulcer
history OR = 2.5 (95% CI 1.2 to 5.1), steroid use OR = 2.0 (95% CI 0.8 to 4.6), smoking
OR = 1.6 (95% CI 0.9 to 2.7), alcohol use OR = 1.8 (95% CI 0.9 to 3.6)

96:24   Hayes C, et al. Case–control study of periconceptional folic acid supplementation and oral clefts. Am J Epidemiol 1996;143:1229-34

Drug Name: folic acid   *Drug Category:* vitamins   *Dosing Criteria:* periconceptual dose
0.5 mg–10 mg daily: any use, months 1–4, month 3, month 4, less than daily   *Validation
of Exposure:* interview by trained nurse interviewer, use of calendar   *Population Selection
Criteria:* metropolitan Boston, Philadelphia, and southeastern Ontario, Canada,
1988–1991   *Number of Cases:* oral clefts (n = 303), cleft palate (n = 108), cleft lip (n = 195)
Number of Controls: 1167   *Comparability of Controls:* liveborn or stillborn infants who had
congenital abnormalities other than oral clefts, neural tube defects   *Drug Event:* oral
cleft   *Validation of Outcome:* review of discharge diagnosis, contact with newborn nursery, review of admission/discharge lists, review of clinical and surgical logs   *Results:*
adjusted RR = 1.1 (95% CI 0.8 to 2.1) oral clefts, adjusted RR = 0.9 (95% CI 0.5 to 1.6) cleft
palate, adjusted RR = 1.3 (95% CI 0.8 to 2.1) cleft lip

96:25   Herings RM, et al. Current use of thiazide diuretics and prevention of femur fractures. J Clin Epidemiol 1996;49:115-9

Drug Category: diuretics   *Dosing Criteria:* <1 year of use, ≥1 year of use, ever used
Validation of Exposure: computerized pharmacy records   *Study Methodology:* case–control
study   *Population Selection Criteria:* 386 patients hospitalized for femur fractures between
1986 and 1990, ≥45 years of age   *Number of Subjects:* 772   *Number of Cases:* 386   *Number
of Controls:* 386   *Comparability of Controls:* matched age within 3 years, gender, pharmacy,
and general practitioner   *Drug Event:* fracture (femur)   *Validation of Outcome:* automated
hospital record, medical record abstracted for sample   *Results:* adjusted OR = 0.5 (95% CI
0.3 to 0.9) ever used, adjusted OR = 0.3 (95% CI 0.1 to 0.9) >1 year of use

96:26   Johnson AG, et al. Histamine-2 receptor antagonists and gastric cancer. Epidemiology 1996;7:434-6

Drug Name: ranitidine, cimetidine   *Drug Category:* histamine$_2$ (H$_2$)-receptor antagonist
Validation of Exposure: computer hospital files and tumor registry files   *Study Methodology:* case–control study   *Population Selection Criteria:* members of Group Health Cooperative Puget Sound; all cases of gastric cancer from January 1, 1988, to December 31,
1992   *Number of Cases:* 113   *Number of Controls:* 452   *Comparability of Controls:* 4 controls for each case randomly selected and matched by year of birth, gender, and date of
first pharmacy use   *Drug Event:* cancer (gastric)   *Confounders:* history of other cancer,
first prescription present on records was filled <2 years before diagnosis   *Results:* RR
comparing users of H$_2$-antagonist with nonusers = 2.0 (95% CI 1.0 to 3.9); for gastric cancer at other site, the crude RR = 1.7 (95% CI 0.7 to 4.2); effect of time since first use, RR
= 6.5, 1.2, and 1.0 for 2–4 years of use, 5–9 years of use, and >10 years, respectively; long-
term H$_2$-antagonist use is not associated with gastric cancer

96:27   Jonas HA, et al. Current progestin and estrogen replacement therapy in elderly women: association with carotid atherosclerosis. Ann Epidemiol 1996;6:314-23

Drug Name: estrogen replacement therapy   *Drug Category:* estrogen–progestins, estrogens   *Dosing Criteria:* women with prescription for oral estrogen (E) or estrogen–progestins (EP) recorded by medication inventory   *Validation of Exposure:* medication inventory from pharmacies and hospitals   *Study Methodology:* cross-sectional cohort study

Population Selection Criteria: elderly women >65 years of age currently receiving estrogen replacement therapy; Cardiovascular Health Study patients were randomly recruited from a Medicare eligibility list   *Number of Subjects:* 2962 women participating in the Cardiovascular Health Study   *Number of Cases:* 1762 never used any replacement therapy, 787 used in past, 280 currently use E alone, 73 currently use EP   *Drug Event:* carotid stenosis   *Validation of Outcome:* anthropometric measurements, blood sampling, blood pressure measurements, echocardiography, spirometry, blood chemistries, electrocardiography, and carotid sonography   *Results:* both current E and EP had decreased carotid atherosclerosis; measures did not differ significantly between the two groups; mean age-adjusted internal carotid wall thickness using EP: 1.12 mm (95% CI 1.01 to 1.22), E: 1.27 mm (95% CI 1.20 to 1.35), nonusers of hormone replacement therapy: 1.41 mm (95% CI 1.38 to 1.45); adjustments were made for age, smoking, lipid-lowering medications, race, income, education, cognitive status, serum albumin concentrations, diabetes, hypertension, prevalent coronary heart disease, calcium supplements, exercise intensity, waist circumference, alcohol consumption, hysterectomy, and age at menopause; after these adjustments were made, the results were EP versus nonusers: –0.22 mm, p = 0.003; E versus nonusers: –0.09 mm; further adjustments for high- and low-density lipoprotein concentrations altered results by EP versus nonusers: –0.16 mm, p = 0.03, E versus nonusers: –0.03 mm, p = 0.5   *Common carotid arteries:* EP: 0.89 mm (95% CI 0.87 to 0.92), E: 0.95 mm (95% CI 0.93 to 0.96), and nonusers: 0.98 mm (95% CI 0.97 to 0.99); after above adjustments, EP versus nonusers: –0.05 mm, p = 0.03; E versus nonusers: –0.02 mm, p = 0.11; there were no significant changes in results for varying high- and low-density lipoprotein   *Prevalence of carotid stenosis:* stenosis of internal carotid arteries was less prevalent in EP and E users (p = not significant); adjusted OR: EP versus nonusers: 0.61 (95% CI 0.36 to 1.01), E versus nonusers: 0.91 (95% CI 0.67 to 1.24)

96:28   Jorgensen C, et al. Oral contraceptives, parity, breast feeding, and severity of rheumatoid arthritis. Ann Rheum Dis 1996;55:94-8

Drug Name: oral contraceptives   *Drug Category:* oral contraceptives, estrogen–progestins   *Dosing Criteria:* duration and dates of use: none, <5 years, >5 years   *Validation of Exposure:* mailed questionnaire, April 1994   *Study Methodology:* case–control study   *Population Selection Criteria:* Immuno-Rheumatology Department, Grin de Chauliac Hospital, Montpellier, France; women outpatients aged 25–28 years with at least one child   *Number of Cases:* 176 (82 = severe, 89 = mild rheumatoid arthritis)   *Number of Controls:* 145   *Comparability of Controls:* ≥one child, involved in systematic breast screening program in geographic area of hospital   *Drug Event:* rheumatoid arthritis   *Validation of Outcome:* joint evaluation, radiologic score, biologic inflammation, presence of HLA-DR1 or DR4 alleles; other explanatory factors: parity and breastfeeding   *Results:* RR = 0.1 (95% CI 0.01 to 0.6) oral contraceptive use >5 years versus none for developing severe rheumatoid arthritis after controlling for age, parity, and breastfeeding

96:29   Joseph KS, et al. Increased morbidity and mortality related to asthma among asthmatic patients who use major tranquillisers. BMJ 1996;312:79-82

Drug Name: chlorpromazine, chlorprothixene, fluphenazine, flupenthixol, haloperidol, mesoridazine, periciazine, perphenazine, pimozide   *Drug Category:* antipsychotic agents   *Dosing Criteria:* >1 prescription for major tranquilizer in the 12 months preceding the index date   *Validation of Exposure:* Saskatchewan prescription database   *Study Methodology:* nested case–control study   *Population Selection Criteria:* computerized health database of Saskatchewan; cohort of asthmatic patients in the Saskatchewan Asthma Epidemiology Project Cohort of 12 301 patients aged 5–54 years, with >10 prescriptions for antiasthmatic drugs between 1978 and 1987   *Number of Cases:* 131   *Number of Controls:* 3930   *Drug Event:* death or near-death related to asthma   *Validation of Outcome:* death certificate, coroner's reports, necropsy reports, hospital discharge summaries   *Results:* RR = 3.2 (95% CI 1.4 to 7.5) asthmatic patients who had used major tranquilizers in past 12 months versus nonusers; RR = 6.6 (95% CI 2.5 to 17.6) past users who had recently discontinued versus nonusers

96:30   Julian DG, et al. A comparison of aspirin and anticoagulation following throm-bolysis for myocardial infarction (the AFTER study): a multicentre unblinded clinical trial. BMJ 1996;313:1429-31

Drug Name: aspirin, heparin, warfarin   *Drug Category:* anticoagulants, nonsteroidal antiinflammatory drugs   *Dosing Criteria:* used after treatment of acute myocardial infarction (AMI) with anistreplase   *Validation of Exposure:* clinical trials in 38 hospitals in six countries   *Study Methodology:* randomized, unblinded study   *Population Selection Criteria:* AMI treated with anistreplase ≤6 hours   *Total Number of Subjects:* 1036   *Number of Cases:* aspirin treated = 519   *Number of Controls:* heparin/warfarin-treated = 519   *Comparability of Controls:* similar, randomized trial   *Drug Event:* hemorrhage, stroke, death, reinfarction   *Validation of Outcome:* 30-day and 90-day hospital and clinic follow-up after treatment of AMI   *Results:* OR death or reinfarction = 1.02 (95% CI 0.69 to 1.50); 11.0% with anticoagulants versus 11.2% with aspirin; patients receiving anticoagulants more likely than aspirin patients to have bleeding or stroke by 90 days (39.0% vs. 1.7%); OR = 0.44 (95% CI 0.20 to 0.97, p = 0.04)

96:31   Kelly JP, et al. Risk of aspirin-associated major upper-gastrointestinal bleeding with enteric-coated or buffered product. Lancet 1996;348:1413-6

Drug Name: aspirin   *Drug Category:* nonsteroidal antiinflammatory drugs   *Dosing Criteria:* daily doses of ≤325 mg, >325 mg   *Validation of Exposure:* phone interview or interview for use 7 days prior to onset use of standard questionnaire   *Study Methodology:* population-based case–control study   *Population Selection Criteria:* multicenter US study, 1987–1994, incident cases identified in 28 Massachusetts hospitals among individuals aged 18–79 years; exclusion of previous episode or history of peptic ulcer disease, gastric intestinal symptoms >30 days, cancer, history of gastric cancer, cirrhosis of the liver   *Number of Cases:* 550   *Number of Controls:* 1202   *Comparability of Controls:* match for residence, gender, 5 years of age   *Drug Event:* upper gastrointestinal bleeding   *Validation of Outcome:* confirmed by endoscopy; controlled for age, gender, marital status, date, education, cigarette smoking, alcohol use, and use of aspirin   *Results:* plain aspirin <325 mg/day RR = 2.6 (95% CI 1.7 to 4.0); plain aspirin >325 mg/day RR = 5.8 (95% CI 3.9 to 8.6); enteric-coated <325 mg/day RR = 2.7 (95% CI 1.4 to 5.3); buffered <325 mg/day RR = 3.1 (95% CI 1.3 to 7.6); buffered >325 mg/day RR = 7.0 (95% CI 3.0 to 16.0)

96:32   Kroman N, et al. Oestrogen-related cancer risk in mothers of testicular-cancer patients. Int J Cancer 1996;66:438-40

Drug Name: estrogen replacement therapy   *Drug Category:* estrogens, estrogen–progestins   *Study Methodology:* population-based cohort study, retrospective   *Population Selection Criteria:* Danish Cancer Registry, all testicular cancer patients born in Denmark and diagnosed between 1950 and 1993, their mothers were reviewed from date of birth of son until death, immigration, or December 31, 1991   *Number of Cases:* 2204   *Comparability of Controls:* expected incidence of cancer in the cohort was calculated by means of multiplication of age- and calendar period-specific (5-y intervals) national cancer incidence rates in women with the appropriate person-years in the cohort   *Drug Event:* cancer (breast, endometrial, ovarian)   *Validation of Outcome:* Danish Cancer Registry   *Results:* RR = 0.8 (95% CI 0.6 to 1.1) observed breast cancer in cohort versus population incidence; RR = 0.6 (95% CI 0.3 to 1.0) observed endometrial cancer in cohort versus population incidence; RR = 1.0 (95% CI 0.6 to 1.6) observed ovarian cancer in cohort over population

96:33   Lewis MA, et al. Third generation oral contraceptives and risk of myocardial infaction: an international case–control study. BMJ 1996;312:88-90

Drug Name: oral contraceptives   *Drug Category:* estrogen–progestins   *Dosing Criteria:* current use: ≤3 months of event, and for controls ≤3 months of hospital admission or interview   *Validation of Exposure:* interview and inspection of oral contraceptive packages   *Study Methodology:* case–control study   *Population Selection Criteria:* 16 centers in Austria, France, Germany, Switzerland, and the UK: women aged 16–44 years   *Number of Cases:* 153   *Number of Controls:* 498   *Comparability of Controls:* matched for age ≤5 years and for hospital and community setting ≤4 months of index date   *Drug Event:* myocardial infarction   *Validation of Outcome:* clinical data verified with medical records, panel of clinic specialists   *Results:* adjusted OR = 0.36 (95% CI 0.1 to 1.2) third generation versus second generation; adjusted OR = 3.1 (95% CI 1.5 to 6.3) second generation versus no current use; adjusted OR = 1.1 (95% CI 0.4 to 3.4) second-generation products versus no current use; adjusted OR = 10.1 (95% CI 5.7 to 17.9) independent contribution of smoking

96:34   Magee LA, et al. The safety of calcium channel blockers in human pregnancy: a prospective, multicenter cohort study. Am J Obstet Gynecol 1996;174:823-8

Drug Name: diltiazem, felodipine, nicardipine, nifedipine   *Drug Category:* calcium-channel blockers   *Dosing Criteria:* first trimester exposure   *Validation of Exposure:* telephone or clinic interview; calcium-channel blocker, dose, timing, toxicity, indication for therapy   *Study Methodology:* cohort study, prospective   *Population Selection Criteria:* six teratogen information services, patients contracting exposure centers with risks of exposure to calcium-channel blockers   *Number of Cases:* 81   *Number of Controls:* 81   *Comparability of Controls:* matched for maternal age; randomly selected from same database   *Drug Event:* malformations   *Validation of Outcome:* phone interview after expected date of delivery   *Results:* live births, calcium-channel blockers 79%, controls 89% (p = 0.09); birth defects, calcium-channel blockers 3.0%, controls 0% (p = 0.2)

96:35   Mary JY, et al. Drug use and aplastic anaemia: the French experience. French Cooperative Group for the Epidemiological Study of Aplastic Anaemia. Eur J Haematol 1996;60:35-41

Drug Name: gold salts, D-penicillamine, colchicine, allopurinol, acetaminophen, aspirin   *Drug Category:* gold salts, nonsteroidal antiinflammatory drugs   *Validation of Exposure:* case and control interviewed by same person   *Study Methodology:* case–control study   *Population Selection Criteria:* population-based registry of aplastic anemia was used by clinicians to recruit cases; cases must have two depressed blood cell lineages at the time of diagnosis and a bone marrow biopsy specimen with decreased cellularity   *Number of Cases:* 147   *Number of Controls:* 294   *Comparability of Controls:* matched for age and gender   *Drug Event:* aplastic anemia   *Validation of Outcome:* medical records   *Results:* association between aplastic anemia and the following: gold salts, OR = 11.7 (95% CI 1.3 to 108; p = 0.04); D-penicilliamine, OR = 11.3 (95% CI 11.2 to 109; p = 0.04); colchicine, OR = 15 (95% CI 1.8 to 128; p = 0.01); allopurinol, OR = 5.9 (95% CI 1.5 to 24; p = 0.02); salicylates, OR = 1.9 (95% CI 1.1 to 3.2; p = 0.04); acetaminophen, OR = 2.0 (95% CI 1.0 to 3.8; p = 0.05)

96:36   Matikainen M, Kangas E. Is there a relationship between the use of analgesics and non-steroidal anti-inflammatory drugs and acute upper gastrointestinal bleeding? A Finnish case–control prospective study. Scand J Gastroenterol 1996;31:912-6

Drug Category: nonsteroidal antiinflammatory drugs (NSAIDs)   *Dosing Criteria:* duration of use <1 month, 1–3 months, >3 months   *Validation of Exposure:* interview, hospital records   *Study Methodology:* case–control study   *Population Selection Criteria:* patients collected among those admitted to two surgical departments for acute upper gastrointestinal bleeding between October 1992 and May 1993   *Number of Cases:* 48 *Number of Controls:* 156   *Comparability of Controls:* matched for age within 5 years, gender, same emergency unit, and admission within 2 months   *Drug Event:* hemorrhage (gastrointestinal)   *Validation of Outcome:* gastroscopy records   *Results:* 24 patients (50%) and 90 controls (57.6%) had no previous upper abdominal symptoms; there were more heavy smokers among patients (n = 9, 18.8%) than controls (n = 7, 4.5%); 5 patients (10.4%) and 1 control (0.6%) had taken more than 20 drinks during the week before admission (p < 0.001); 29 patients (62.5%) and 81 controls (51.9%) had used some analgesics during the week before admission; there was no difference in the duration of the use of analgesics in the patients and controls; the results do not support the concept that NSAID use is a major factor associated with serious upper gastrointestinal bleeding

96:37   Neal KR, et al. Omeprazole as a risk factor for *Campylobacter* gastroenteritis: case–control study. BMJ 1996;312:414-5

Drug Name: omeprazole   *Drug Category:* proton pump inhibitors, histamine$_2$ (H$_2$)-receptor antagonists, antibiotics   *Validation of Exposure:* general practice records   *Study Methodology:* case–control study   *Population Selection Criteria:* individuals aged >45 years in two local district councils within Nottingham Health Authority   *Number of Cases:* 211   *Number of Controls:* 422   *Comparability of Controls:* next two patients in computerized records matched for gender and age within 2 years   *Drug Event: Campylobacter* gastroenteritis   *Validation of Outcome:* fecal culture, general practice records   *Confounders:* surgical operations, prescriptions for H$_2$-antagonists, antibiotics, hydroxocobalamin, glucocorticoids, and other drugs   *Results:* adjusted OR = 10.0 (95% CI 2.2 to 46) omeprazole 1 month before infection; adjusted OR = 1.8 (95% CI 0.8 to 3.9) H$_2$-receptor antagonists 1 month before infection; adjusted OR = 0.9 (95% CI 0.4 to 1.9) antibiotics 1 month before infection; omeprazole leads to a significant risk of *Campylobacter* infections in people aged ≥45 years

96:38   Nevitt MC, et al. Association of estrogen replacement therapy with the risk of osteoarthritis of the hip in elderly white women. Arch Intern Med 1996;156:2073-80

Drug Name: estrogen replacement therapy   *Drug Category:* estrogens, estrogen–progestins   *Dosing Criteria:* length of exposure   *Validation of Exposure:* interview   *Study Methodology:* cross-sectional study   *Population Selection Criteria:* white women participating in a cohort study of osteoporotic fracture (n = 4366, >65 y)   *Number of Cases:* current users of oral estrogen ≥1 year, 16.5%   *Number of Controls:* past use of oral estrogens ≥24.3%   *Drug Event:* osteoarthritis of the hip   *Validation of Outcome:* radiographic assessment scale from 0 (none) to 4 (severe osteoarthritis)   *Confounders:* height, weight, body mass index, and so on   *Results:* 12.3% mild or greater findings of osteoporosis; 4.9% moderate to severe; women currently using oral estrogens OR = 0.62 (95% CI 0.49 to 0.86); current users for ≥10 years OR = 0.57 (95% CI 0.40 to 0.82) compared with users <10 years

96:39   Oliveria SA, et al. Estrogen replacement therapy and the development of esteoarthritis. Epidemiology 1996;7:415-9

Drug Name: estrogen replacement therapy   *Drug Category:* estrogens, estrogen–progestins   *Dosing Criteria:* new users, past users, ongoing users (past and new), and never users of estrogen replacement therapy   *Validation of Exposure:* pharmacy records *Study Methodology:* nested case–control study   *Population Selection Criteria:* all incident cases of hand, hip, and knee osteoarthritis in women members of the Fallon Community Health Plan, aged 20–89 years, from January 1, 1990, to December 31, 1993   *Number of Cases:* 60   *Number of Controls:* 60   *Comparability of Controls:* controls matched to closest date of birth and controlled for obesity and healthcare utilization   *Drug Event:*

osteoarthritis *Validation of Outcome:* computerized research file, medical records, pharmacy files *Confounders:* height, weight, menopausal status, type of menopause, smoking status *Results:* after controlling for obesity and healthcare use, study found that new use of estrogen replacement therapy was a predictor of new osteoarthritis diagnosis; past use was inversely associated with risk of osteoarthritis; adjusted OR = 0.7 (95% CI 0.3 to 1.9); for ongoing use and osteoarthritis, adjusted OR = 1.4 (95% CI 0.6 to 3.3); for long-term users, adjusted OR = 1.0 (95% CI 0.4 to 2.8) risk for osteoarthritis

96:40   O'Sullivan DP, et al. Postmarketing surveillance of oral terbinafine in the UK: report of a large cohort study. Br J Clin Pharmacol 1996;42:559-65

Drug Name: terbinafine   *Drug Category:* fungicides   *Dosing Criteria:* daily dose, 250 mg; median therapy, 65 days   *Study Methodology:* patient follow-up study, prospective *Population Selection Criteria:* hospital-based dermatology outpatient and general practice centers (+ 5% of exposed population in Great Britain, no exclusion criteria)   *Number of Subjects:* 9879   *Drug Event:* nausea and vomiting, diarrhea, constipation, abdominal discomfort, indigestion, colitis   *Validation of Outcome:* patient assessment at beginning and completion of care; data verification on 13% randomly selected from cohort *Results:* 14.5% reported medical events and, of these, 49% possibly or probably related to terbinafine; 74 (<1%) classified as serious with only 5 possibly or probably related to terbinafine; 0.6% of patients experienced taste disturbances

96:41   Paganini-Hill A, Henderson VW. Estrogen replacement therapy and risk of Alzheimer disease. Arch Intern Med 1996;156:2213-7

Drug Name: estrogen replacement therapy   *Drug Category:* estrogens, estrogen–progestins   *Dosing Criteria:* dose <0.625 mg ≤3 years of use; 4–14; ≥15 years; dose >1.25 mg ≤3 years of use; 4–14; ≥15 years   *Validation of Exposure:* periodic surveys, review of hospital admission records   *Study Methodology:* nested case–control study   *Population Selection Criteria:* postmenopausal women cohort of retirees of Leisure World, Laguna Hills, California; of the 8877-women cohort, 3760 died   *Number of Cases:* 248 women died with Alzheimer disease among 3760 deaths   *Number of Controls:* 1193   *Comparability of Controls:* matched to age and year of death   *Drug Event:* Alzheimer disease, senile dementia, dementia, senility   *Validation of Outcome:* National Death Index: death certificates *Results:* OR = 0.65 (95% CI 0.49 to 0.88) for Alzheimer disease estrogen users versus no users; risks decreased with increasing dosages and increased duration of oral therapy with conjugated equine estrogen; long-term and high-dose use OR = 0.48 (95% CI 0.19 to 1.17)

96:42   Palareti G, et al. Bleeding complications of oral anticoagulant treatment: an inception-cohort, prospective collaborative study (ISCOAT). Lancet 1996;348:423-8

Drug Name: warfarin, acenocoumarol   *Drug Category:* anticoagulants   *Dosing Criteria:* target anticoagulation (international normalized ratio [INR] system for prothrombin time) ≤2.8 in 71% of patients and >2.8 in 29% of patients   *Validation of Exposure:* INR   *Study Methodology:* inception cohort mean length follow-up, 267 days from May 1993 to October 1994, prospective   *Population Selection Criteria:* 34 Italian anticoagulant clinics; new patients start anticoagulation therapy, exclusion for pregnancy and expected difficulty in follow-up visit   *Number of Subjects:* 2745 (43% women)   *Drug Event:* bleeding, thrombosis, cerebral hemorrhage   *Results:* age >70 RR = 1.75 (95% CI 1.29 to 2.39; p < 0.001)

96:43   Penttinen J, Valonen P. Use of psychotropic drugs and risk of myocardial infarction: a case–control study in Finnish farmers. Int J Epidemiol 1996;25:760-2

Drug Category: antidepressants, antipsychotic agents   *Dosing Criteria:* amount of drug, no starting and stopping dates were entered   *Validation of Exposure:* questionnaire, verified in patient records of local health community healthcare unit   *Study Methodology:* nested case–control study   *Population Selection Criteria:* population-based cohort of

3172 Finnish farmers followed from February 1, 1980, to December 31, 1992   *Number of Cases:* 158   *Number of Controls:* 3062   *Comparability of Controls:* 1% random sample of infants without birth defects born in same period, matched by hospital of birth, calendar quarter of birth, and race   *Drug Event:* heart defects (conotruncal)   *Validation of Outcome:* registry records   *Results:* OR = 2.5 (95% CI 1.2 to 5.2) risk for myocardial infarction; antipsychotropic drug users versus nonusers; OR = 5.4 (95% CI 1.8 to 16.1) risk for myocardial infarction, antidepressant users versus nonusers

96:44   Perez Gutthann S, et al. Nonsteroidal anti-inflammatory drugs and the risk of hospitalization for acute renal failure. Arch Intern Med 1996;156:2433-9

Drug Name: diclofenac, diflunisal, fenoprofen, calcium, ibuprofen, indomethacin, ketoprofen, mefenamic acid, naproxen, phenylbutazone, piroxicam, tolmetin, aspirin   *Drug Category:* nonsteroidal antiinflammatory drugs (NSAIDs)   *Dosing Criteria:* current use (prescription filled 0–30 d before incident); recent users (most recent prescription filled 31–60 d before index date); past users (61–150 d before index date); nonusers did not fill prescription in 150 days   *Validation of Exposure:* computerized files from prescription drug plan database   *Study Methodology:* population-based case–control study   *Population Selection Criteria:* residents of Saskatchewan receiving at least one NSAID prescription between January 1, 1982, and December 31, 1986   *Number of Cases:* 28   *Number of Controls:* 467 000 person-years of experience for nonusers of NSAID   *Comparability of Controls:* random selection of eligible controls, excluding individuals with idiopathic acute renal failure, malignant neoplasm, or any type of renal disease   *Drug Event:* acute renal failure   *Validation of Outcome:* Saskatchewan Hospital Services Plan computerized records; record review by trained nurses; risk factors: age, gender, recent hospitalization for disorders other than renal, prescription for defined comorbidity   *Results:* OR = 4.1 (95% CI 1.5 to 10.8)

96:45   Petitti DB, et al. Stroke in users of low-dose oral contraceptives. N Engl J Med 1996;335:8-15

Drug Name: oral contraceptives   *Drug Category:* estrogen–progestins   *Dosing Criteria:* daily dose of estrogen <50 μg   *Validation of Exposure:* interview using standardized questionnaire of patient or proxy; major life events and calendar to obtain information on contraceptive methods; prompting devices were used to help in recall of the oral contraceptive brand   *Study Methodology:* population-based case–control study   *Population Selection Criteria:* California Kaiser Permanente Medical Care Program, women 15–44 years of age, May 1991 to August 1994, from hospital admission and discharge records, emergency department, and out-of-plan hospitalizations   *Number of Cases:* 408; 295 cases included in study (144 ischemic infarction; 151 hemorrhagic infarction)   *Number of Controls:* 774   *Comparability of Controls:* matched for year of birth, location of healthcare facility, randomly selected from female members of program   *Drug Event:* fatal and nonfatal stroke; stroke defined as the new onset of rapidly developing symptoms and signs of loss of cerebral function that lasted at least 24 hours with apparent nonmuscular cause   *Control:* cigarette smoking, hypertension, diabetes, and race   *Results:* adjusted RR = 1.18 (95% CI 0.54 to 2.59) for ischemic stroke; adjusted RR = 1.14 (95% CI 0.60 to 2.16) for hemorrhagic stroke; adjusted RR = 3.64 (95% CI 0.95 to 13.87) for contraceptive use and smoking

96:46   Potter JD, et al. Hormone replacement therapy is associated with lower risk of adenomatous polyps of the large bowel: the Minnesota Cancer Prevention Research Unit Case–Control Study. Cancer Epidemiol Biomarkers Prev 1996;5:779-84

Drug Name: estrogen replacement therapy   *Drug Category:* estrogens, estrogen–progestins   *Dosing Criteria:* hormone replacement therapy (HRT) <5 years compared with no use   *Validation of Exposure:* patient interviews   *Study Methodology:* case–control study   *Population Selection Criteria:* women at digestive clinic in Minneapolis with colonoscopy-proven, pathology-confirmed adenomatous polyps of colon and rectum   *Number of Cases:* 219   *Number of Controls:* 438 women without polyps seen at clinics; 247 women matched from community   *Comparability of Controls:* parity, age of first live birth, oral contraceptive use   *Drug Event:* polyps (colorectal adenomatous)   *Validation of Outcome:* medical records   *Results:* multivariate, adjusted OR = 0.52 (95% CI 0.32 to 0.85) versus colonoscopy-negative controls and 0.74 (95% CI 0.44 to 1.26) versus community controls; reduction in risk of colorectal neoplasia is an additional benefit of postmenopausal HRT

96:47   Pritchard RS, et al. Dietary calcium, vitamin D, and the risk of colorectal cancer in Stockholm, Sweden. Cancer Epidemiol Biomarkers Prev 1996;5:867-72

Drug Name: vitamin D, calcium   *Drug Category:* vitamins   *Validation of Exposure:* dietary history for the past 5 years (quantitative food frequency questionnaire; supplemental intake not ascertained)   *Study Methodology:* population-based case–control study, retrospective   *Population Selection Criteria:* colon and rectal cancer cases identified by Cancer Surveillance Network in Stockholm, Sweden   *Number of Cases:* 352 colon cancer; 217 rectal cancer   *Number of Controls:* 512   *Comparability of Controls:* similar demographics but without cancer   *Drug Event:* cancer (colorectal)   *Validation of Outcome:* patient interviews and medical records   *Results:* increasing concentrations of dietary vitamin D inversely associated with rectal cancer (OR = 0.5 [95% CI 0.3 to 0.9] between highest and lowest quartiles) and colon cancer (OR = 0.6 [95% CI 0.4 to 1.0] same quartiles); dietary calcium not associated with either cancer

96:48   Rea HH, et al. The association between asthma drugs and severe life-threatening attacks. Chest 1996;110:1446-51

Drug Name: fenoterol, theophylline, cromolyn   *Drug Category:* bronchodilators, glucocorticoids, beta-adrenoreceptor agonists   *Dosing Criteria:* any use at time of emergency admission   *Validation of Exposure:* clinic and hospital records   *Study Methodology:* cohort study, restrospective   *Population Selection Criteria:* asthmatic patients attending a New Zealand emergency department, 1986–1987, followed until death or May 1989; cases died or were admitted to intensive care unit (ICU) due to severe asthma   *Total Number of Subjects:* 655   *Number of Cases:* 105   *Drug Event:* death (asthma), ICU admission   *Validation of Outcome:* hospital records   *Results:* confounding is substantial due to nonrandomized use of asthma drugs; previous hospital admission and glucocorticoid use are confounders; some drugs are used primarily in more severe cases and, therefore, more likely to be associated with death or ICU admission

96:49   Reeves MJ, et al. Nonsteroidal anti-inflammatory drug use and protection against colorectal cancer in women. Cancer Epidemiol Biomarkers Prev 1996;5:955-60

Drug Name: aspirin   *Drug Category:* nonsteroidal antiinflammatory drugs (NSAIDs)   *Dosing Criteria:* >twice weekly use >12 months   *Validation of Exposure:* telephone interview   *Study Methodology:* population-based case–control study   *Population Selection Criteria:* colorectal cancer in women aged 40–74 years identified in Wisconsin cancer registry   *Number of Cases:* 184   *Number of Controls:* 243   *Comparability of Controls:* controlled for age, prior sigmoidoscopy, family history of cancer, body mass index, and NSAID use   *Drug Event:* cancer (colorectal)   *Validation of Outcome:* patient interviews, medical records   *Results:* controls more likely than cases to report regular NSAID use (38% vs. 27%, OR = 0.65 [95% CI 0.40 to 1.03]); nonaspirin NSAID more effective than aspirin in reducing colorectal cancer

96:50   Rosenberg L, et al. Case–control study of oral contraceptive use and risk of breast cancer. Am J Epidemiol 1996;143:25-37

Drug Name: oral contraceptives   *Drug Category:* estrogen–progestins   *Dosing Criteria:* duration of use <1 year; 1–4 years; 5–9 years; ≥10 years   *Validation of Exposure:* nurse interviews using standardized questionnaires prompted for indication: contraception, regulation of periods, menstrual problems, endometriosis; episode of use; date use started; duration of use   *Study Methodology:* case–control study   *Population Selection Criteria:* hospitals in Boston, New York, and Philadelphia, 1977–1992, white women aged 25–59 years   *Number of Cases:* 3540   *Number of Controls:* 4488   *Comparability of Controls:* nonmalignant, nongynecologic conditions unrelated to oral contraceptive use, within 5 years of age, geographic region   *Drug Event:* cancer (breast)   *Validation of Outcome:* discharge summaries, pathology reports   *Results:* >1 year of use to <1 year of use: OR = 1.7 (95% CI 1.3 to 2.3) for women aged 25–34 years; 0.9 (95% CI 0.7 to 1.0) 35–44 years; 1.2 (95% CI 1.0 to 1.4) 45–59 years; p < 0.01 for difference across age

96:51   Sasco AJ. Tamoxifen and menopausal status: risks and benefits. Lancet 1996;347:761

Drug Name: tamoxifen   *Drug Category:* estrogen blockers   *Dosing Criteria:* no use, ≤5 years of use, >5 years of use   *Validation of Exposure:* hospital and clinic records   *Study Methodology:* case–control study   *Population Selection Criteria:* cases of endometrial cancer following breast cancer in the Rhone and Cote d'Or regions of France   *Number of Cases:* 43   *Number of Controls:* 177   *Comparability of Controls:* matched for age, region, year of breast cancer diagnosis, survival time with intact uterus   *Drug Event:* cancer (endometrial)   *Results:* of women treated >5 years, those exposed to tamoxifen when pre- or perimenopausal were at higher risk of endometrial cancer; RR with ever use of drug = 4.9 (95% CI 0.8 to 29.9) for women <50 years of age and 1.8 (95% CI 1.1 to 3.0) for women >50 years of age

96:52   Sasco AJ, et al. Endometrial cancer following breast cancer: effect of tamoxifen and castration by radiotherapy. Epidemiology 1996;7:9-13

Drug Name: tamoxifen   *Drug Category:* estrogen blocker   *Dosing Criteria:* any treatment before diagnosis of endometrial cancer   *Validation of Exposure:* review of medical records   *Study Methodology:* case–control study   *Population Selection Criteria:* women in French regions of the Rhone and Cote d'Or with endometrial cancer >1 year after breast cancer; hospital reported   *Number of Cases:* 43   *Number of Controls:* 177   *Comparability of Controls:* matched for age, region, year of diagnosis of breast cancer, and survival from breast cancer   *Drug Event:* cancer (endometrial)   *Validation of Outcome:* review of hospital records   *Results:* tamoxifen used in 67% of cases and 60% of controls; OR = 1.4 (95% CI 0.60 to 3.5); RR increased with duration of tamoxifen use: >5 years OR = 3.5 (95% CI 0.94 to 12.7); radiotherapeutic castration OR = 7.7 (95% CI 1.8 to 32.8)

96:53   Schaefer C, et al. Pregnancy outcome after prenatal quinolone exposure. Evaluation of a case registry of the European Network of Teratology Information Services. Eur J Obstet Gynecol Reprod Biol 1996;69:83-9

Drug Name: ciprofloxacin, norfloxacin, ofloxacin, perfloxacin, enoxacin, cinoxacin   *Drug Category:* quinolones   *Dosing Criteria:* prenatal exposure   *Validation of Exposure:* prospectively by phone interview   *Study Methodology:* follow-up study, prospective   *Population Selection Criteria:* case registry of the European Network for Teratology Information Services (ENTIS); pregnant women who contacted ENTIS between 1986 and 1994   *Number of Subjects:* 549 pregnancies   *Drug Event:* pregnancy outcomes, malformation rate among the liveborn   *Validation of Outcome:* mailed questionnaire or phone interview of mother or physician   *Results:* malformation rate, 4.8%

96:54   Sidney S, et al. Myocardial infarction in users of low-dose oral contraceptives. Obstet Gynecol 1996;88:939-44

Drug Name: oral contraceptives   *Drug Category:* estrogen–progestins   *Dosing Criteria:* estrogen <50 µg   *Validation of Exposure:* hospital administration records, hospital discharge records, emergency department logs, requests for payment for out-of-plan hospitalizations; all cases and controls were interviewed using a standardized instrument *Study Methodology:* population-based case–control study   *Population Selection Criteria:* all incident myocardial infarctions in women, 15–44 years, who were members of Kaiser Permanente Medical Care Program, in northern and southern California regions from July 1991 to August 1994   *Number of Cases:* 187   *Number of Controls:* up to 3 per case *Comparability of Controls:* randomly chosen from same group of women and matched for year of birth and location of family   *Drug Event:* myocardial infarction   *Confounders:* age, body mass index, months of oral contraceptive use, parity, current or occasional smoker, alcohol use, treated hypertension, treated diabetes, treated high cholesterol, current use of oral contraceptive, college education, annual income, race, marital status *Results:* OR for myocardial infarction in current oral contraceptive users versus noncurrent users = 1.65 (95% CI 0.45 to 6.06); OR for past users was not relevant

96:55   Spinillo A, et al. The impact of oral contraception on chlamydial infection among patients with pelvic inflammatory disease. Contraception 1996;54:163-8

Drug Name: oral contraceptives   *Drug Category:* estrogen–progestins   *Dosing Criteria:* previous or current oral contraceptive users   *Validation of Exposure:* drug history of hospitalized or outpatient women with pelvic inflammatory disease (PID)   *Study Methodology:* recruitment of women with PID, prospective   *Population Selection Criteria:* women 17–40 years of age with PID, Italian hospital and clinic   *Number of Cases:* 144 *Drug Event:* PID   *Validation of Outcome:* medical and laboratory records   *Results:* the rates of chlamydial infection (15.0%) or of detection of antichlamydial immunoglobulins G and A (13.9%) were determined for all cases; in patients with chlamydial documentation, the rate of use of oral contraceptives is lower than in patients with nonchlamydial PID; other studies confirm this association

96:56   Spitzer WO, et al. Third generation oral contraceptives and risk of venous thromboembolic disorders: an international case–control study. BMJ 1996;312:83-8

Drug Name: oral contraceptives   *Drug Category:* estrogen–progestins   *Dosing Criteria:* current use: ≤3 months before the event (case) or before date of interview (control); first generation, any preparation containing ethinylestradiol ≥50 µg; second generation, containing ethinylestradiol ≤35 mg and a progestogen other than gestodene or desogestral; third generation, containing low doses of ethinylestradiol (20 or 30 µg) and either gestodene or desogestral   *Validation of Exposure:* interview and inspection of oral contraception packages at home in subsample   *Study Methodology:* case–control study *Population Selection Criteria:* 10 centers in Germany and the UK, women aged 16–44 years *Number of Cases:* 471   *Number of Controls:* 1772   *Comparability of Controls:* matched for age, hospital, and community setting (for each case, there are at least 1 community and hospital control)   *Drug Event:* thromboembolism (venous)   *Validation of Outcome:* clinical data verified with medical records by a panel of clinical specialists   *Confounders:* alcohol consumption, body mass index, hypertension, diabetes, any pregnancy, rheumatic heart disease, any family history of stroke or myocardial infarction, educational level   *Results:* adjusted OR = 4.0 (95% CI 3.1 to 5.3) any oral contraceptive versus no use; adjusted OR = 3.2 (95% CI 2.3 to 4.3) low-dose ethinylestradiol versus no use; adjusted OR = 4.8 (95% CI 3.4 to 6.7) low-dose ethinylestradiol, gestodene, or desogestral versus no use; adjusted OR = 1.5 (95% CI 1.1 to 2.1) third generation versus second generation; adjusted OR = 1.5 (95% CI 1.0 to 2.2) gestodene versus second generation; adjusted OR = 1.5 (95% CI 1.1 to 2.2) desogestral versus second generation

96:57 Suissa S, et al. Bronchodilators and acute cardiac death. Am J Respir Crit Care Med 1996;154:1598-602

Drug Name: theophylline, albuterol, fenoterol, metaproterenol, terbutaline *Drug Category:* bronchodilators, beta-adrenoreceptor agonists *Dosing Criteria:* at least 10 separate prescriptions dispensed for asthma drugs *Validation of Exposure:* pharmacy records *Study Methodology:* population-based cohort study *Population Selection Criteria:* Saskatchewan community health insurance plan, subjects 5–54 years of age for the period of 1978–1987 *Number of Cases:* 30 *Number of Controls:* 4080 *Drug Event:* cardiac arrest *Validation of Outcome:* pulmonologist and pediatrician classified each death as asthma related or cardiovascular; hospital death records, discharge records, and autopsy reports were used *Risk Factors:* age, prior use of cardiac drugs *Results:* RR = 2.7 (95% CI 1.2 to 6.1) of cardiac arrest in users of theophylline; RR = 2.4 (95% CI 1.0 to 5.4) for users of beta-agonists taken orally or as nebulizers; RR = 1.2 (95% CI 0.5 to 2.7) for users of beta-agonists given by metered-dose inhalers

96:58 Tomasson H, Tomasson K. Oral contraceptives and risk of breast cancer. Acta Obstet Gynecol Scand 1996;75:157-61

Drug Name: oral contraceptives *Drug Category:* estrogen–progestins *Validation of Exposure:* data collected at screening clinics *Study Methodology:* historic, prospective cohort study *Population Selection Criteria:* cancer detection clinic, 25 years of follow-up data for women aged 25–69 years; mothers and sisters of cases are identified through a national genealogy registry *Number of Cases:* 1062 *Number of Controls:* 5662 *Comparability of Controls:* matched with six controls, born closest to the cases' birthday *Drug Event:* cancer (breast) *Validation of Outcome:* national cancer registry *Risk Factors:* age at first delivery, number of children, family history of breast cancer *Results:* OR = 2.38 (95% CI 1.62 to 3.46) for developing breast cancer for women with mother with breast cancer; OR = 0.92 (95% CI) for those never using oral contraceptives; OR = 1.84 (95% CI 1.45 to 2.9) for those having a sister with breast cancer; OR = 0.92 (95% CI 0.73 to 1.16) for those using oral contraceptives for 1–4 months compared with 0; OR = 0.89 (95% CI 0.64 to 1.24) for those with 49–96 months of use compared with 0; OR = 0.96 (95% CI 0.69 to 1.33) for those with ≥96 months of oral contraceptive use

96:59 van der Meer FJ, et al. Assessment of a bleeding risk index in two cohorts of patients treated with oral anticoagulants. Thromb Haemost 1996;76:12-6

Drug Name: phenprocoumon, acenocoumarol *Drug Category:* anticoagulants *Dosing Criteria:* target international normalized ratio (INR) specific for each indication *Validation of Exposure:* patient medical records of the centralized Leiden Thrombosis Service (Netherlands) *Study Methodology:* Poisson regression analysis of the influence of bleeding risk factors *Population Selection Criteria:* two cohorts: all patients in service in years 1988 and 1991 *Total Number of Subjects:* 460 000 population in Leiden area *Number of Cases:* cohort 1: 6814; cohort 2: 6512 (4121 also in cohort 1); these are patients in service *Number of Controls:* none *Drug Event:* hemorrhage (general) *Validation of Outcome:* patient reports, clinic observation, clinic–hospital records *Risk Factors:* age, INR, specific anticoagulant, gender *Results:* combined results of consistent risk factors for both cohorts: incidence = $-5.64 + 0.42 \times$ age $+ 0.36 \times$ INR

96:60 Van Marter LJ, et al. Persistent pulmonary hypertension of the newborn and smoking and aspirin and nonsteroidal antiinflammatory drug consumption during pregnancy. Pediatrics 1996;97:658-63

Drug Name: aspirin, ibuprofen, indomethacin, naproxen *Drug Category:* nonsteroidal antiinflammatory drugs (NSAIDs) *Validation of Exposure:* self-report, interview by trained interviewers *Study Methodology:* case–control study *Population Selection*

Criteria: two Harvard-affiliated newborn intensive care units, newborn infants, July 1, 1985, to March 31, 1989, >2500 g at birth, no congenital anomalies   *Number of Cases:* 103   *Number of Controls:* 298; control newborn using random-number table using medical record numbers, born within 1 month of case   *Comparability of Controls:* confounding variables, maternal education, Medicaid health insurance, maternal urinary tract infection, diabetes mellitus, gender of newborn   *Drug Event:* pulmonary hypertension (persistent)   *Validation of Outcome:* newborn screened and meets case criteria: PaO_2 <100 when breathing 100% oxygen, a ductal or atrial right-to-left hemodynamic shunt demonstrated by echocardiography or a transductal PaO_2 gradient of 20% or more, in the presence of a preductal PaO_2 <100 mm   *Results:* aspirin adjusted OR = 4.9 (95% CI 1.6 to 15.3); NSAID adjusted OR − 6.2 (95% CI 1.8 to 21.8)

96:61   Visser LE, et al. Cough due to ACE inhibitors: a case–control study using automated general practice data. Eur J Clin Pharmacol 1996;49:439-44

Drug Name: captopril, enalapril, lisinopril   *Drug Category:* angiotensin-converting enzyme (ACE) inhibitors   *Validation of Exposure:* records of 14 general practitioners in the Netherlands   *Study Methodology:* population-based case–control study   *Population Selection Criteria:* any patient reporting coughing incidents from September 1992 to March 1994   *Number of Subjects:* 44 787   *Number of Cases:* 1458   *Number of Controls:* 4182 (4 per case)   *Comparability of Controls:* similar age and lack of typical diseases causing coughing   *Drug Event:* cough   *Validation of Outcome:* medical records   *Results:* adjusted OR of ACE inhibitor use = 1.4 (95% CI 0.9 to 2.1); adjusted OR for captopril = 0.9 (95% CI 0.4 to 1.7), for enalapril = 1.7 (95% CI 1.03 to 2.8), for lisinopril = 1.7 (95% CI 0.4 to 7.9); risk declined with length of prescription

96:62   Wide K, et al. Antiepileptic drug treatment during pregnancy and neonatal screening results. Acta Paediatr 1996;85:870-1

Drug Name: carbamazepine, phenytoin   *Drug Category:* anticonvulsants   *Dosing Criteria:* doses adequate to maintain therapeutic serum concentrations of anticonvulsants   *Validation of Exposure:* clinic records   *Study Methodology:* case–control study   *Population Selection Criteria:* newborns of mothers treated with one or more anticonvulsants   *Number of Subjects:* 68   *Number of Cases:* 34   *Number of Controls:* 34   *Comparability of Controls:* newborns of untreated mothers matched for gender, gestational age, mode of delivery, place and date of birth   *Drug Event:* hypothyroidism, adrenal hypoplasia (congenital)   *Validation of Outcome:* measurement of blood thyroid-stimulating hormone (TSH) and 17-hydroxyprogesterone (17-OHP)   *Results:* no differences in cases versus controls in newborns of mother on single drug therapy; in 6 newborns of mothers on two-drug therapies, there was a nonsignificant tendency to lower TSH and 17-OHP blood concentrations

96:63   Zondervan KT, et al. Oral contraceptives and cervical cancer—further findings from the Oxford Family Planning Association contraceptive study. Br J Cancer 1996;73:1291-7

Drug Name: oral contraceptives   *Drug Category:* estrogen–progestins   *Dosing Criteria:* total duration of use; time since last use; time since first use; age at first use; calendar year of first use   *Validation of Exposure:* annual interview by physician or nurse at time of clinic visit   *Study Methodology:* nested case–control study   *Population Selection Criteria:* Oxford Family Planning Association inclusion criteria at date of enrollment: (1) aged 25–39 years; (2) married; (3) white and British; (4) current user of oral contraceptive 7.5 months or current user of diaphragm or an intrauterine device   *Number of Cases:* 310   *Number of Controls:* 3091   *Comparability of Controls:* same year of birth and attending same clinic   *Drug Event:* invasive carcinoma (n = 33), carcinoma in situ (n = 121), dysplasia (n = 159)   *Confounders:* social class of husband, current cigarette smoking, age at first marriage   *Results:* OR = 1.4 (95% CI 1.00 to 1.96) ever users for all types of cervical neoplasia; OR = 4.44 (95% CI 1.04 to 31.6) ever users for invasive carcinoma; OR = 1.73 (95% CI 1.00 to 3.00) ever users for cacinoma in situ; OR = 1.07 (95% CI 0.69 to 1.66) ever users for dysplasia; OR = 3.34 (95% CI 1.96 to 5.67) current or recent users, 49–72 months, for all types of cervical neoplasia; OR = 1.69 (95% CI 0.97 to 2.95), 73–96 months of use, for all types of cervical neoplasia; OR = 2.04 (95% CI 1.34 to 3.11), 97 months or more of use for all types of cervical neoplasia

97:1   Beresford S, et al. Risk of endometrial cancer in relation to use of oestrogen combined with cyclic progestagen therapy in postmenopausal women. Lancet 1997;349:458-61

Drug Name: estrogen replacement therapy   *Drug Category:* estrogen–progestins   *Validation of Exposure:* face-to-face interview, prompting with pictures   *Study Methodology:* population-based case–control study   *Population Selection Criteria:* women aged 45–74 years in western Washington State; cases identified in cancer registry with histologically confirmed endometrial cancer 1985–1991   *Number of Cases:* 832   *Number of Controls:* 1114   *Comparability of Controls:* identified by random-digit dialing, screened for intact uterus, frequency matched for age and county   *Drug Event:* cancer (endometrial)   *Validation of Outcome:* validation by independent and pathology review   *Results:* OR = 4.0 (95% CI 3.1 to 5.1) for unopposed estrogen versus nonusers; OR = 1.4 (95% CI 1.0 to 1.9) for estrogen with cyclic progestogen; OR = 3.1 (95% CI 1.7 to 5.7) for estrogen with <10 days of progestogen; OR = 1.3 (95% CI 0.8 to 2.2) for estrogen with 10–21 days of progestogen; OR = 3.7 (95% CI 1.7 to 8.2) for estrogen with <10 days for >5 years; OR = 2.5 (95% CI 1.1 to 5.5) for estrogen with progestogen 10–21 days for >5 years

97:2   Cumming RG, Mitchell P. Hormone replacement therapy, reproductive factors, and cataract. Am J Epidemiol 1997;145:242-9

Drug Name: estrogen replacement therapy   *Drug Category:* estrogens, estrogen–progestins   *Dosing Criteria:* usage: ever users, never users, exusers, current users; duration of use: <5, 5–9, ≥10 years of use   *Validation of Exposure:* interview-administered questionnaire data   *Study Methodology:* population-based cross-sectional study   *Population Selection Criteria:* Blue Mountain Eye Study, Australia, 1992–1993   *Number of Subjects:* 2072 women aged 49–97 years   *Number of Cases:* critical cataracts (n = 1939); nuclear cataracts (n = 1395); posterior subcapsular (n = 1944)   *Exposed:* hormone replacement therapy (n = 555): 312 current, 243 exusers   *Drug Event:* cataracts   *Validation of Outcome:* complete eye examination at local clinic   *Confounders:* age at menopause, age at menarche, number of children, use of oral contraceptives, surgical versus natural menopause   *Results:* for critical cataract: adjusted OR = 0.4 (95% CI 0.2 to 0.8) for current users, aged 65 years versus never users; posterior subcapsular cataract: adjusted OR = 2.1 (95% CI 1.1 to 4.1) for current users with nonsurgical menopause

97:3   El-Serag HB, Sonnerberg A. Association of esophagitis and esophageal strictures with diseases treated with nonsteroidal anti-inflammatory drugs. Am J Gastroenterol 1997;92:52-6

Drug Category: nonsteroidal antiinflammatory drugs (NSAIDs)   *Validation of Exposure:* computer files   *Study Methodology:* case–control study   *Population Selection Criteria:* all patients with esophagitis or esophageal stricture who were discharged from a Veterans Affairs hospital 1981–1994   *Number of Cases:* 101 366 (92 860 esophagitis, 14 201 stricture)   *Number of Controls:* 101 366 (random subjects without gastroesophageal reflux disease)   *Drug Event:* esophagitis, esophageal stricture   *Validation of Outcome:* hospital records   *Confounders:* age, gender, ethnicity, comorbid occurrence of NSAID-related diagnosis   *Results:* a variety of NSAID-related diseases were found to be associated with esophagitis; increased risk association with the diseases ranged from 34% to 57%;

old age, male gender, and white ethnicity as well as NSAID diseases contributed to an increase in esophagitis; multivariate esophageal stricture occurred more readily as a result of old age and ethnicity and with NSAID diseases; esophagitis and stricture were associated with dental erosion OR = 1.76 (95% CI 1.35 to 2.30); gastric outlet obstruction OR = 4.54 (95% CI 4.01 to 5.14); Zollinger–Ellison syndrome OR = 5.41 (95% CI 3.40 to 8.62); laryngitis OR = 1.64 (95% CI 1.29 to 2.09); asthma OR = 1.45 (95% CI 1.38 to 1.53); chronic obstructive pulmonary disease OR = 1.14 (95% CI 1.09 to 1.20)

97:4   Farmer RD, et al. Population-based study of risk of venous thromboembolism associated with various oral contraceptives. Lancet 1997;349:83-8

Drug Name: oral contraceptives (OCs)   *Drug Category:* estrogen–progestins   *Dosing Criteria:* women, years of exposure, duration of the prescription for each type of contraceptive   *Validation of Exposure:* computerized medical records   *Study Methodology:* population-based nested case–control study   *Population Selection Criteria:* computer records of patients from 143 general practices in the UK: 540 000 women born between 1941 and 1981   *Number of Cases:* 85   *Number of Controls:* 313   *Comparability of Controls:* matched year of birth, practice of current use of OCs   *Drug Event:* deep-vein thrombosis, venous thrombosis, pulmonary embolus, and treated with an anticoagulant   *Validation of Outcome:* medical records printed out and reviewed by two physicians; controlled for body mass index (BMI), number of cycles, change in type of OC prescribed within 3 months of event, previous pregnancy, and concurrent diseases   *Results:* venous thromboembolism adjusted age OR = 1.68 (95% CI 1.04 to 2.75) third generation to second generation, controlling for BMI, number of cycles, change in type of OC prescribed within 3 months of event, previous pregnancy, and concurrent diseases by logistic regression and no difference was found; OR = 3.49 (95% CI 1.21 to 10.12) desogestral with 20 mg of ethinylestradiol versus all second generation; OR = 1.18 (95% CI 0.66 to 2.17) second generation to other two-generation OCs

97:5   Garbe E, et al. Inhaled and nasal glucocorticoids and the risks of ocular hypertension or open-angle glaucoma. JAMA 1997;277:722-7

Drug Name: beclomethasone, budesonide, triamcinolone   *Drug Category:* glucocorticoids   *Dosing Criteria:* patients categorized into low to medium exposure (<1600 µg/d beclomethasone equivalent); high-dose exposure (>1600 µg/d); and long-term exposure, use for ≥3 months   *Validation of Exposure:* all prescriptions that had been filled were identified for cases and controls   *Study Methodology:* case–control study   *Population Selection Criteria:* enrollees with Regie de l'assurance maladie du Quebec (RAMQ) database aged ≥66 years; all patients were ophthalmology patients with a new diagnosis for borderline glaucoma, open-angle glaucoma, or were newly started on treatment for ocular hypertension or glaucoma between 1988 and 1994   *Number of Subjects:* 48 118   *Number of Cases:* 9793   *Number of Controls:* 38 325 (randomly selected among noncases with ophthalmology visits in the same month and year as the case event)   *Comparability of Controls:* OR was adjusted for age, gender, diabetes mellitus, systemic hypertension, use of ophthalmic and oral glucocorticoids, and characteristics of healthcare system use in the year before the index   *Drug Event:* ocular hypertension, open-angle glaucoma   *Validation of Outcome:* OR calculated by conditional logistic regression using the Statistical Analysis System (SAS) PHREG program in which validation occurred using models that accounted for all variables   *Results:* use of inhaled and nasal glucocorticoid was not associated with an increased risk of ocular hypertension or open-angle glaucoma; current users of high doses of inhaled steroids prescribed regularly for ≥3 months were at an increased risk with an OR = 1.44 (95% CI 1.01 to 2.06)

97:6   Grodstein F, et al. Postmenopausal hormone therapy and mortality. N Engl J Med 1997;336:1764-75

Drug Name: estrogen replacement therapy   *Drug Category:* estrogens, estrogen–progestins   *Dosing Criteria:* any use at last questionnaire before death or before diagnosis of fatal disease   *Validation of Exposure:* biennial questionnaire since 1976   *Study Methodology:* case–control study   *Population Selection Criteria:* nurses participating in the Nurses' Health Study aged 30–55 years at the time of study start in 1976   *Number of Subjects:* original number in 1976 = 121 700   *Number of Cases:* 3637   *Number of Controls:* 10 per case (36 370)   *Comparability of Controls:* each death matched to 10 live controls at time of death   *Drug Event:* death, cancer (breast), cardiovascular mortality   *Validation of Outcome:* deaths reported by families or National Death Index; death certificates examined and, when possible, medical records   *Results:* current estrogen users' death adjusted RR = 0.63 (95% CI 0.56 to 0.70) versus nonusers; after >10 years of use RR = 0.80 (95% CI 0.67 to 0.96) due to increase in mortality from breast cancer; current estrogen users with cardiac risk factors (69% of women) had largest decrease in death RR = 0.51 (95% CI 0.45 to 0.57)

97:7   Heath CW, et al. Hypertension, diuretics, and antihypertensive medications as possible risk factors for renal cell cancer. Am J Epidemiol 1997;145:607-13

Drug Category: diuretics, antihypertensives   *Dosing Criteria:* nonusers; pills per month: occasional, 1–29, 30, ≥31; duration of use: ≤5 years, 6–10 years, ≥11 years   *Validation of Exposure:* questionnaire   *Study Methodology:* cohort study, prospective   *Population Selection Criteria:* Cancer Prevention Study II, under auspices of the American Cancer Society, 1982   *Number of Subjects:* 998 904 followed for 7 years (1982–1989)   *Number of Cases:* 335   *Drug Event:* cancer (renal), death   *Validation of Outcome:* mortality follow-up every 2 years   *Confounders:* high blood pressure, kidney disease, kidney stones, bladder disease, cancer, family history of renal cancer, smoking history, body mass, exposure to asbestos   *Results:* adjusted OR = 2.2 (95% CI 1.4 to 3.5) hypertension use versus nonuse; adjusted OR = 2.5 (95% CI 1.5 to 4.3) diurectic use versus nonuse

97:8   Monane M, et al. The impact of thiazide diuretics on the initiation of lipid-reducing agents in older people: a population-based analysis. J Am Geriatr Soc 1997;45:71-5

Drug Category: diuretics, antihypertensive agents, cholesterol-lipid-lowering agents   *Dosing Criteria:* low dose: 1–24 hydrochlorothiazide (HCTZ) mg-equivalents; median dose: 25–49 HCTZ mg-equivalents; and high dose ≥50 HCTZ mg-equivalents   *Validation of Exposure:* prescription dosing database; duration of therapy by multiplying the number of days' supply by a factor of 1.5   *Study Methodology:* prescription sequence study, inception cohort   *Population Selection Criteria:* patients enrolled in New Jersey Medicaid and Medicare programs between 1981 and 1989 who are on new antihypertensives; patients were followed for 2 years after the start of the antihypertensive therapy   *Number of Subjects:* 9274 (aged 65–79 y)   *Number of Cases:* 226 received lipid-reducing agent   *Drug Event:* lipid-reducing agent (niacin, 39%; gemfibrozil, 29%; lovastatin, 10%; cholestyramine, 10%; clofibrate, 7%; probucol, 5%)   *Validation of Outcome:* claims databases; risk-adjusted covariables: age, race, nursing home residency   *Results:* adjusted RR = 1.4 (95% CI .89 to 2.40) for overall thiazide users or other antihypertensive users; adjusted RR = 1.97 (95% CI 1.12 to 3.45) for high-dose thiazides

97:9   Newton KM, et al. Estrogen replacement therapy and prognosis after first myocardial infarction. Am J Epidemiol 1997;145:269-77

Drug Name: estrogen replacement therapy   *Drug Category:* estrogens, estrogen–progestins   *Dosing Criteria:* current use: >2 prescriptions for estrogens and second prescription filled <6 months of first prescription and at or after hospital discharge   *Validation of Exposure:* computerized pharmacy records   *Study Methodology:* cohort study, retrospective   *Population Selection Criteria:* Group Health Cooperation of Puget Sound, women who survived their first myocardial infarction to hospital discharge, from 1980 to 1991 *Number of Subjects:* 726 (who survived first myocardial infarction) *Number of Cases:* reinfarction (n = 135), deaths (n = 183) *Exposed:* hormone replacement therapy (n = 122) *Drug Event:* death *Validation of Outcome:* outpatient record review, hospital database, death file *Covariables:* age, race, marital status, smoking, body mass index, serum cholesterol, diabetes, blood pressure, angina pectoris, congestive heart failure, peripheral vascular disease prior to first myocardial infarction *Results:* adjusted RR = 0.64 (95% CI 0.32 to 1.30) for reinfarction current estrogen use versus no use, adjusted for age and time since infarction; adjusted RR = 0.90 (95% CI 0.62 to 1.31) for reinfarction past estrogen use versus no use; adjusted RR = 0.50 (95% CI 0.25 to 1.00) all-cause mortality current estrogen use versus no use; adjusted RR = 0.79 (95% CI 0.56 to 1.09) all-cause mortality past estrogen use versus no use

97:10 O'Keefe JH Jr, et al. Estrogen replacement therapy after coronary angioplasty in women. J Am Coll Cardiol 1997;29:1-5

Drug Name: estrogen replacement therapy *Drug Category:* estrogens, estrogen–progestins *Dosing Criteria:* current long-term therapy *Validation of Exposure:* medical records of Mid America Heart Institute *Study Methodology:* case analysis, retrospective *Population Selection Criteria:* all women undergoing elective percutaneous transluminal coronary angioplasty (PTCA) between 1982 and 1994 *Number of Subjects:* 337 *Number of Cases:* 137 *Number of Controls:* 200 *Comparability of Controls:* patients with acute or recent myocardial infarction excluded, computer-matched demographics similar *Drug Event:* death *Validation of Outcome:* follow-up mean of 65 ± 35 months *Results:* 7-year survival rate 93% for estrogen users and 75% for controls (p = 0.001); estrogen use was associated with improved long-term outcome after PTCA

97:11 Tavani A, et al. Hormone replacement treatment and breast cancer risk: an age-specific analysis. Cancer Epidemiol Biomarkers Prev 1997;6:11-4

Drug Name: estrogen replacement therapy *Drug Category:* estrogens, estrogen–progestins *Dosing Criteria:* use of hormone replacement therapy (HRT): new versus ever; duration: ≤60 months, >60 months; age at start: ≤50 years, >50 years; time since start: ≤15 years, >15 years; time since stopped: ≤10 years, >10 years *Validation of Exposure:* structured questionnaires, interviews conducted in the hospital *Study Methodology:* case–control study *Population Selection Criteria:* six Italian major teaching and general hospitals, women <75 years of age *Number of Cases:* 5984 *Number of Controls:* 5504 *Comparability of Controls:* admitted to same hospital *Drug Event:* cancer (breast) *Validation of Outcome:* histologically confirmed cases *Confounders:* smoking, alcohol use, coffee consumption, gynecologic data, use of oral contraceptives, hormone preparations for other indications *Results:* adjusted OR = 1.2 (95% CI 1.0 to 1.4) ever used HRT versus never used; adjusted OR = 1.2 (95% CI 0.9 to 1.5) for women 55–64 years of age; adjusted OR = 1.6 (95% CI 1.2 to 2.3) for those 65–74 years of age; adjusted OR = 1.6 (95% CI 1.1 to 2.3) 65–74 years old and ≤60 months of use; adjusted OR = 2.2 (95% CI 1.1 to 4.7) 65–74 years old and >60 months of use

97:12 Townsend MF, et al. Bone fractures associated with luteinizing hormone–releasing hormone agonists used in the treatment of prostate carcinoma. Cancer 1997;79:545-50

Drug Category: luteinizing hormone–releasing hormone agonist (LHRH-a) *Dosing Criteria:* any dose or duration *Validation of Exposure:* review of medical records of patients with prostatic cancer in three Atlanta hospitals *Study Methodology:* medical review, retrospective *Population Selection Criteria:* patients treated with LHRH-a between 1988 and 1995 *Number of Subjects:* 224 *Number of Cases:* 20 *Drug Event:* fracture (bone) *Validation of Outcome:* medical record documentation *Results:* 20 of 224 patients (9%) had at least one fracture during LHRH-a treatment (mean treatment 22.2 mo); seven fractures (32%) were osteoporotic (vertebral or hip); others due to trauma or mixed etiology; 5% of cases had osteoporotic fractures

97:13 Tryggvadottir L, et al. Oral contraceptive use at a young age and the risk of breast cancer: an Icelandic, population-based cohort study of the effect of birth year. Br J Cancer 1997;75:139-43

Drug Name: oral contraceptives   *Drug Category:* estrogen–progestins   *Dosing Criteria:* use <20 years of age and born after 1944   *Validation of Exposure:* data from Icelandic Cancer Registry and the Cancer Detection Clinic of the Icelandic Cancer Society   *Study Methodology:* nested case–control study with cohort   *Population Selection Criteria:* women in cancer registry   *Total Number of Subjects:* 90 000   *Number of Cases:* 236   *Drug Event:* cancer (breast)   *Validation of Outcome:* clinic records   *Results:* for women born in 1951–1967 (81 cases), the RR for use >4 years = 2.0 (95% CI 1.1 to 3.7); when women born in 1945–1950 were included, RR = 1.1 (95% CI 0.8 to 1.6), adding 123 cases; for women born after 1950, RR = 0.9, 1.7, and 3.0 for <4 years, 4–8 years, and >8 years of use, respectively

24

Pharmacoepidemiology: The Future

Hugh H Tilson
Abraham G Hartzema
Miquel Porta

Abstract

The future of pharmacoepidemiology as a field of scientific inquiry and its application to therapeutic decision-making, like all other futures, are not entirely clear. However, major societal forces
exist that are driving the agenda for pharmacoepidemiology. This chapter reviews and weighs
"factors" such as changes in drug development, technology, developments in data sources,
methodologic innovations, the move toward managed care, and an increasing public aversion for
risks. The evolving roles of the major related "actors" (particularly physicians, pharmacists,
patients, government, academia, industry) are also analyzed. Pharmacoepidemiology's immediate future must build on its past successes in the progressive reduction of uncertainty in the
making of therapeutic decisions at the individual level; the move to evidence-based medicine,
practice guidelines, and disease state management programs at the organizational level; and the
development of public policies regarding acceptable uncertainty and risk, as well as the cost-
effectiveness requirements for pharmaceuticals at the sector level. Like all health futures, the
future of pharmacoepidemiology can be influenced positively by responsible contributions,
particularly by the pharmaceutical community.

Outline

P redicting the future in any scientific field is hazardous work, given the complexities of human endeavor, the apparent randomness of technologic progress, and the weaknesses of our predictive tools. In epidemiology, predicting the future is all in a day's work as the epidemiologist searches for predictive models within various components of the living equation—models that are leading or contributing to better patient outcomes. One could call the variables in the model risk factors, confounders, or causes and their effects; inputs and their related outputs; or, the current favorite term appearing extensively in this book, "outcomes."

Predicting the future of the field of pharmacoepidemiology is equally challenging, perhaps even more so because the data supporting therapeutic reasoning are mostly lacking or soft. These data are increasingly needed where society's tolerance for risk is diminishing and, more and more, clinicians are held accountable for producing optimal outcomes for the least costs. This chapter looks at trends in pharmacoepidemiology and addresses the extent to which they rely on future trends in the environment—"the factors," that is, technology, methodology, organization, and delivery of health care. It also addresses the impact of changes among "the actors," that is, changes in the behaviors and competencies of the participants or stakeholders in the impact of medications and the responsiveness of pharmacoepidemiology to society's needs in meeting its demand for valid, reliable, and relevant clinical information.

The trends seem to be convergent, relatively powerful, and, on balance, quite positive for a bright and exciting future for pharmacoepidemiology. The technology is burgeoning; the capacity is expanding; the public and private expectations, even demands, seem unrelenting; and the commitments of those critical actors in the field appear progressively positive. Pharmacoepidemiology is already accepted as a fundamental clinical discipline and, as a major contributor to evidence-based medicine, the future will bring increased focus and opportunity to the field.

The Evolving Factors

What changes in the factors in the healthcare environment can be predicted and what influence will they have on pharmacoepidemiology?

DRUG DEVELOPMENT PARADIGM

Political, economic, and scientific challenges and opportunities are creating dramatic changes in the way drugs are developed in the US and internationally. With these changes, pharmacoepidemiology will experience unprecedented prominence.

Pharmacoepidemiology found its origin in epidemiologic intelligence, the identification and quantification of rare unintended drug effects (UDEs) in larger populations. In Europe, this area is commonly referred to as pharmacovigilance.

Through pharmacovigilance, truly rare events can currently be, and perhaps always will need to be, detected only through a global "hands-on" monitoring and signaling system. This is the pharmacologic equivalent of the epidemiologic intelligence network for detecting communicable disease epidemics. Although toxicologic screening methodologies, such as tissue cultures and other animal and nonanimal models, and cell solutions have become increasingly sophisticated in identifying toxicities in the drug development process, they still fall short of prediction of UDEs in humans; likewise, the variability and incomplete understanding of human pharmacogenetic markers (e.g., cytochrome P450 isoenzymes) make it impossible to predict and prevent UDEs by patient-based screening. Our limited preclinical and laboratory sciences will, predictably, continue to warrant population-based surveillance systems. Under these systems, physicians, pharmacists, and nurses will continue to be asked to report voluntarily to the manufacturer or the regulatory authority (e.g., the Food and Drug Administration [FDA], European Medicine Evaluation Agency) any adverse medical experiences in association with the use of pharmacologic agents. Such voluntary reporting will remain at once the strongest and weakest of such systems: strongest because it uses as its denominator the entire population of treated people and weakest because it uses as its numerator reports generated by busy practitioners with little experience with the system and little incentive to provide reports, even, on occasion, as they fear that these reports will incriminate them. Pharmacovigilance will continue to be an important part of pharmacoepidemiology.

However, the role of pharmacoepidemiology in the drug development process will greatly expand. Pharmacoepidemiologic or formal observational methods will play an important role in achieving additional efficiencies in the drug development process. In preparation for Phase II and Phase III clinical trials, observational studies are already being used to establish power and sample size estimations. Pharmacoepidemiology has amply demonstrated its ability to assist in the development of disease severity indices and risk adjustment procedures.

Early approvals of drugs on the basis of the most elegant and focused efficacy studies will be facilitated by the ability to continue to monitor the impact of these agents—both beneficial and undesirable—in large populations following approvals. The shift in regulatory emphasis will witness a corollary, burgeoning demand for continuing Phase IV observational outcomes research.

Pharmacoepidemiology will assume a leading role in the development of tools for outcomes assessment and health-related quality-of-life instrumentation. Pharmacoepidemiology already forms the basis for cost-of-illness studies and can establish outcome probabilities for cost–effectiveness calculations where the randomized, controlled trial efficacy data leave off. These will become the rule in drug development programs as society progressively acquires documentation of the value of its new therapies.

Finally, after evidence-based medicine takes hold, managed care reduces practice variability by adopting practice guidelines or implementing disease management programs, and the demands to move medicine into a continuous-improvement mode occur, pharmacoepidemiology will play an increasingly important role in practice guideline development and maintenance. Drug therapy will be recognized as the most common, effective, and cost-effective form of medical care and, increasingly, pharmacoepidemiology will significantly contribute to that insight.

TECHNOLOGY

Perhaps the strongest single trend in the development of the new paradigm will be the evolving capacity to monitor society's healthcare transactions through large computerized databases. As the costs of processing time, computer memory, and other hardware decrease, as software becomes more user-friendly, as voice recognition becomes more accurate, and as the contributions of computerized systems to cost containment and service effectiveness become progressively better understood and clearly proven, the computer will be as central to the healthcare transaction as are the stethoscope, ballpoint pen, and pill-counting trays of today.

Part of the compelling trend will be the advance of studies of drug effects through evolving systems of automated medical record-keeping, permitting record linkage. How simple and ancient in concept is the methodology, and yet how complex and revolutionary in practice! Introduction of automation into medical practice will progressively permit, first, the establishment of a "marker" (e.g., a unique identification number or code for each patient) that can be attached to each transaction for each patient. Second, the technology will permit the actors (all of those involved in advancing the health of patients, including pharmacoepidemiologists) to capture information on all healthcare transactions. Record linkage can be achieved by linking pharmacy and healthcare activity for each individual and combining those with similar exposure into cohorts. Of course, not all systems will have developed fully automated healthcare information systems, but even for those less advanced, if computer-assisted listing of patients' medical and pharmacy records is not a possibility, several sophisticated linking algorithms have been established that may provide high-probability linkings for incompletely automated systems. If linking pharmacy and medical care data at the inpatient level is a first step, a following logical step will be progressively sophisticated ways of linking these data at the outpatient visit level or at the level of the disease episode. The final step is the development of linking diagnosis (i.e., the indications for the prescription) to actual drug exposure at the level of each patient encounter. Progress has already been made in this area through automation of hospital outpatient pharmacies and computerized hospital tracking systems, but linkage of indication to prescription will greatly expand the research capabilities of pharmacoepidemiology and facilitate its move in the realm of pharmaceutical outcomes research.

Soon, more healthcare plans and systems will have introduced automation into accounting, patient tracking, and quality assurance on the way to comprehensive automation of medical records. The miracle of automation will drastically shorten the multiyear tedium of more traditional approaches to population-based research for countless clerks and student research associates to a few hours of programming data that have been downloaded from automated pharmacies and linking these data via a patient identification marker to the coded computerized hospital discharge file. Manual reviewing of medical records to find all the events or health problems associated with exposure to the drug in question will be replaced by careful programming, permitting rates of large numbers of events to be compared quickly with those experienced by one or more comparable nonexposed, similarly linked cohorts or groups. Today's computer technology already allows us to scan computerized medical records. Tomorrow's text-processing software with string searching capabilities will identify even better any occurrences of any manifestation of even subtle events. Then rates of events will be compared with one or more comparable nonexposed, similarly linked cohorts or groups automatically selected by the computer fully matching the exposed group with a control group, as a matter of routine.

The large, multispecialty healthcare and health maintenance organization (HMO) will not be the only data source of such linkages. Third-party payment programs and reimbursement schemes will continue to evolve; their evolving computer support will also contain medical and prescription data with potential for record linkage, already in evidence through provincial health plan data from Saskatchewan and US data from state-level Medicaid programs. An increasing proportion of the US population will be covered under these health plans, and increasing automation of data regarding medical transactions will occur in other countries, particularly throughout Europe. Special computerized patient registries, such as the Medicare End-Stage Renal Disease Program, will also provide powerful tools for pharmacoepidemiologic analysis. Cross-plan and cross-system links will permit automated downloading of data to regional public health bodies, maintaining population-based registries (e.g., birth defects, tumor monitoring). On the other hand, medical information will also become more portable. Microchip technology probably will be extended so that we will carry vital medical information encoded in a "smart card" in our wallet, allowing us to plug in each time there is a new transaction and to have the chip updated.

Many new and different technologies are emerging, some based on decentralized data collection systems as represented by the smart card and others based on centralized systems such as the larger claims databases and automated medical records found in managed care. The future of both will provide powerful tools for automated support of population-based formal study. The pharmacoepidemiologist must demand a seat at the automation table to ensure that these tools develop and that society's benefit is clearly achieved.

CONCEPTUALIZATION

The changing environment will precipitate changes in the way pharmacoepidemiology is approached. Because of the need of large group practices, managed healthcare organizations, and indemnity plans to constrain costs in an increasingly competitive healthcare market, the sophistication of the questions being asked of clinical data is increasing; in the decade ahead, this trend will demand increasing and increasingly diverse contributions by the pharmacoepidemiologist. The capture of clinical data follows the need to better manage both patient care and patient outcomes. Considerable practice variations will still exist, combined with considerable variation in patient outcomes. Increasingly, it will become clear that practice variation is not always justified by patient needs, and that some of these practice variations may not produce optimal patient outcomes or may even contribute to reduced efficiencies. Conversely, the clinical world will rebel against rigid, inflexible "universal guidelines" and embrace the more dynamic approach to continuous learning from the data at hand.

These considerations will drive the move to collecting more and better patient information. The trend will be to capture even richer clinical information, such as patient lifestyle and behavioral data. More detailed medical data will also be gathered regarding allergies, clinical procedures performed, comorbidities, test results, and laboratory values. Direct computerized data capture of clinical pathology, laboratory tests, and intervention data will be accompanied by multisite data linkage to provide easy availability of these data to the clinicians.

Advanced vector computers with string searching capabilities will help to identify any occurrence of any clinical observation or event in the computerized medical record, transferring the challenge to the pharmacoepidemiologist from being a traditional primary data collector to being a sophisticated data manager and organizer. Such sophistication widely enhances the domain of research questions asked, but it also adds to the complexity of the research endeavor. The accessibility of more clinical data and a better quality of data will enhance the explanatory power of pharmacoepidemiology. It will also increase the likelihood of finding small but "statistically significant" differences and increase the challenge to understand the difference between statistical and medical significance!

Methodologic innovations in biostatistics and the development of new statistical procedures will be urgently needed. Already sophisticated statistical procedures, logistic regression, log–linear models, and time-to-event procedures for censored data referred to as grouped survival data or categorical survival data have greatly benefited the development of the field during the past two decades. These statistical procedures also depend on increased computational capabilities supporting pharmacoepidemiologic research to address more sophisticated and complex questions, while increasing the reliability and validity of the estimates by controlling for confounders and other covariates. New rules, however, will need to be conceived to assist the artificial intelligence and systematic data "dredging" comparisons.

Econometric modeling and decision-tree software will evolve to support the pharmacoepidemiologist's ability to develop sophisticated decision models. The increase in processing speed and power will allow the researcher to use larger populations and more clinical information through advanced statistical procedures. These will allow the pharmacoepidemiologist to answer the more complex research questions that are put forward by the healthcare system.

Methodologies that take into account the complex dimensions of cost–benefit and cost-effectiveness analyses and routinely provide computer-assisted risk/benefit comparisons using all the available data against all the available alternative scenarios will be common in our society. In a practice application, a physician will be able to key individual patient risk factors and desired outcomes into an online computer system at the office workstation; the physician will then have these matched against the benefit-to-risk algorithms tempered for (stratified by) the patient's specific risk category for computer-assisted therapeutic decision-making. The policymaker will likewise use the same simulation methodologies at the population level to assess relative merits and proper indications (placement) and to balance these against the risks of various therapeutic modalities. However, one should recognize that all these trends are data driven. The availability, accessibility, accuracy, completeness, and timeliness of data are essential ingredients in supporting these developments.

The next logical step is to identify the variables that are important in our decision analysis and consequently to quantify these by assigning a probability score to them. By the year 2000, pharmacoepidemiology will have introduced computer-assisted decision algorithms, not to replace thinking but to help us quantify the extent to which our concentrated thinking is in fact governed by information that may reduce our level of uncertainty. Translated into the positive, the future of epidemiology lies in progressive incremental reduction of uncertainty in both the making of therapeutic decisions at the individual level and developing public policy regarding application therapeutics in practice guidelines at the population level.

HEALTHCARE DELIVERY

A fourth variable of change to factor into the equation predicting the future of pharmacoepidemiology is reflected in the movement of Western cultures into organization-based delivery of health services, for example, in medicine, the marriage of the profession and business, or at least the change from individual entrepreneurship to an organized management structure as the means of healthcare delivery. In the US, where healthcare reform at the national legislative level failed to materialize, a self-correcting managed care revolution will succeed. Paradoxically, in the nations of Europe, a similar trend will be from the national monolithic systems of organization and financing of care to smaller medical management, fund-holding, risk-sharing organizations much like an HMO in the US. Within these emerging large healthcare organizations, innovative means of financing healthcare are characteristic.

These financial innovations will include cost reductions by budgeting at the department level. However, reducing cost in one department may increase to a larger proportion the cost in another department. If, for example, the pharmacist is being instructed to cut costs, the pharmacist may actually increase overall costs by substitution of a more costly surgical or medical alternative for a cost-effective pharmaceutical product, effectively shifting the pharmacy cost to the medical department. The classic example of this cost-shifting occurs when the formulary committee turns down an innovative drug because it is "too expensive," without considering the cost of the emergency department visit that could have been shortened, the intense monitoring that could have been offset, or the earlier discharge that the marginally better innovative product could have made possible.

The HMO concept means efficiency; efficiency means computers; and computers may mean yet another population that can be added to the denominator of potential users of a new pharmaceutical product, thus expanding the power for such linkage efforts to detect rare events. Indeed, one of the great challenges to the pharmacoepidemiologic community will be to make ourselves actively involved in the design of these databases and systems to ensure that, when health plans' data become automated, the systems that develop are compatible with the public policy imperatives of data linkage and are suitable for pharmacoepidemiologic research. When working together, the various elements of the structured system can keep costs down and can, in fact, obtain the synergy inherent in any managed care system.

The pharmacoepidemiologist will benefit from the evolution of large healthcare organizations that will inevitably bring not only more computerization, but also the application of the technology and methodology described above to more enrolled populations. The greater the population covered by the databases, the greater the power to detect important associations through linkage methodology.

New issues about proprietary rights to data will arise. In times of cost containment and increasing revenue shares, managed care corporations increasingly will see their databases as a source for additional revenue. Access to these databases will need to be ensured also to answer those pharmacoepidemiologic questions that are not directly of interest to the database owner, and cross-sector collaboration will be an essential skill.

PUBLIC EXPECTATION

One of the major forces driving the pharmacoepidemiology movement will be an evolving public intolerance in North America, Western Europe, and Japan to any risk, including that of injury from UDEs, and this intolerance will promote consumer advocacy programs that respond to public demand for monitoring and responsible corporate action. The emerging technology and healthcare reforms will reinforce this for prevention of UDEs. As more data sets become available and affordably accessible, we will all know more, sooner. It seems highly unlikely that a new chemical entity would escape vigorous monitoring in structured data sets, in as large a population as available, simply to reduce the time required between the generation of a signal of a potential problem, for example, through voluntary, spontaneous UDE reports, and the making of public policy decisions. The availability of large population-based data sets will create the expectation of their being used.

Among other challenges, healthcare organizations will emphasize prevention not solely as a method of cost containment, but also as a value in itself, the benefits of which are probably better documented than are the benefits of many therapeutic interventions now covered by traditional medical insurance plans. With this change will come greater demand for more preventive medicines, that is, drugs used by healthy people to promote health or counteract risk factors. The healthier the patient, the less acceptable are risks of severe, although rare complications of treatment, the greater the demand to find any such problems early in the drug regimen, and the greater the need for large populations under continuous surveillance and sophisticated methodologies to detect rare but unacceptable risks.

This cybernetic age will also require a reconceptualization of the nature and dimensions of patient privacy, as already in evidence in the hot debates regarding privacy in Europe and North America in the mid-1990s. Concerns about confidentiality that have limited our progress are being successfully addressed. New techniques must and will be used to ensure that we protect against conspiracies that misuse confidential information and compromise our ability to get the most from the power of the computer. The computer can identify important details about us that our physicians, pharmacists, and we ourselves never even understood, much less remembered, and we must be mindful of the sensitivities of people who have the right to demand their privacy. Balancing the need for individual privacy with the public health need for access to population-based information will require continuing priority attention in the decade ahead.

LIABILITY

Important factors increasing the interest in and commitment to rigorous structured monitoring of drug safety following approval are two current major public policy crises: burgeoning malpractice costs and crumbling liability insurance systems. As a symptom of society's unwillingness to tolerate risks, coupled with major dysfunctions in the tort liability system, injury settlements for people with drug- and vaccine-associated UDEs have become major threats to the ability of drug companies to obtain insurance protection. Both have driven up the cost of doing business: in 1985, AH Robins, a major US drug manufacturer, was forced to file for reorganization under the bankruptcy laws because of litigation surrounding UDEs associated with one of its contraceptive products, the Dalkon Shield; and Merrell Dow Pharmaceuticals was forced to remove from the market Bendectin, a product used to treat the incapacitating nausea of pregnancy, because it could no longer afford defense against litigation, despite the lack of evidence for causal association between that product and any of the congenital defects involved in the litigation. More recently, American Home Products became involved in allegations that the Teflon coating used for its Norplant drug may result in an autoimmunologic response.

This trend will precipitate, in the decade ahead, a major push for tort liability reform, including limitation of settlements, limitation of punitive damages, and a reevaluation of contingency fees for the plaintiff's lawyers. Although difficult to predict, recent congressional debate suggests that it will lead to some form of "workmen's compensation model" to support claims of injured parties. The need for development of an actuarial base for such a fund will surely lead to the development of still greater demand for better epidemiologic information regarding the likelihood and extent of injury and for estimates of the contributions of coexisting factors. Corporate programs to reduce legal exposure will require proactive population-based monitoring to ensure the earliest possible detection, clarification, and warning.

The Evolving Actors

Paralleling and reinforcing these institutional trends during the pharmacoepidemiologic future will be enabling changes in the perspective and performance of the participants in the enterprise.

THE PHYSICIAN

Every medical educator in epidemiology/preventive medicine hopes that the 21st century will present an educational atmosphere that demands rather than tolerates rigorous epidemiologic content in curricula and expects rather than accepts rigorous epidemiologic competence among graduates. Epidemiology will have attained the clear status of fundamental science in undergraduate medical curricula. The physician's ability to understand and apply the lessons of pharmacoepidemiology to the therapeutic choice of finding the proper balance between risk and benefit in the individual patient's treatment will be understood to represent an essential end product of undergraduate education in pharmacoepidemiology (perhaps every bit as important as the public policy outcome of society's ability to review, approve, and regulate such products). Every medical school will have a recognized curriculum in evidence-based and preventive medicine. Every emerging physician will understand decision theory and the application of the principles of population risk to the individual, including medication-associated benefits. In the last analysis, the intelligent use of medicines must lie in the hands of intelligent users, not at the inflexible ends of computer-assisted decision trees.

Prediction. Physicians in the era of pharmacoepidemiology will understand and apply the findings of pharmacoepidemiologic studies. Warning: They won't if we don't teach them.

THE PHARMACIST

Pharmacoepidemiology will emerge as a dominant requisite skill for the clinical pharmacist. Clinical pharmacists in managed care, hospitals, and community practice are already becoming more involved in assessing the effectiveness of drug therapy in their practice settings. This trend will continue. Pharmacy education programs in the US and abroad will have implemented pharmacoepidemiology course work at the undergraduate level. Undergraduates will need to understand pharmacoepidemiologic study methodologies to be able to interpret the literature and to stay abreast of advances in pharmacotherapy.

In many of the large HMOs and managed care organizations, the pharmacist will be at the center of the new technology. Almost all community pharmacies will be computerized and linked into treatment networks. The evolution of the computer-supported pharmacy holds great promise in the pharmacoepidemiology sector. The development of computer-supported patient drug profiles, direct computer links between the physician's office and the pharmacy, and a resurgent patient demand for better drug information will continue. This will provide enormous potential for developing an ambulatory-care database. Pharmacy networking for economic reasons (e.g., buying groups) may be an impetus to use the same broad-based data for epidemiology purposes. Several countries have already established community pharmacy networks to create large prescription data files, for example, the Netherlands, Portugal, and others. These data files are especially suited as they miss the link to diagnostic outcome data for prescription-sequencing studies (e.g., prescriptions for antidepressant medications after initiation of beta-blocker therapy, prescriptions for antidiabetic medications after initiation of antihypertension treatment).

Community pharmacy software will be more sophisticated in the future. All pharmacy computer programs can screen for drug–drug interactions, drug compatibilities, and dosing ranges. However, these systems currently can neither estimate probabilities accurately nor predict the probability of the clinical significance of the event. In the future, such information may allow pharmacists to determine patient-monitoring intensity for potential UDEs or focus pharmaceutical care interventions; advances in pharmacogenetics may provide this necessary information. As more clinical pharmacists and drug information specialists participate in direct patient care, there will be an increased demand for better risk/benefit data to complement their consultation on the pharmacokinetic and pharmacodynamic properties of drugs.

Prediction. Pharmacoepidemiology will provide a major tool to pharmacists to contribute as affirmative partners in the Treatment Team. Warning: If they won't accept and train for this challenge, others will!

THE PATIENT

The person who benefits from the medication is the primary reason for our pharmacoepidemiologic efforts. As the population of the developed and developing worlds achieves better economic and healthcare success, it is becoming progressively older; the projected growth in the US population older than 65 years is from 25 million today to 55 million by the year 2030. With age will come more chronic illnesses, more need for potent medicines, and more demand than ever for responsible safety monitoring of medicines. The population will change, and its needs and expectations will change, as will the role the patient can play in systems designed to address drug safety concerns.

The patient will also increasingly demand to be treated as an individual. Pharmacogenetics and a better understanding of the effects of cytochromes P450 on human variability in drug metabolism will require in the future individually tailored therapeutic active compounds. As our understanding of pharmacogenetics is increasing, we come to realize more the large individual variation in pharmacodynamics and kinetics that not only explains the variation in responses to therapy, but also the individual differences in probabilities of UDE occurrences. As combinational chemistry further simplifies the synthesis of chemical entities, and as we learn more about the pharmacogenetic makeup of humans that predicts variability in drug kinetics and dynamics, it may well be that, in the future, pharmaceutical products will be customized for each individual patient based on diagnosis and the patient's pharmacogenetic makeup. This may be the future, but the future is almost here.

Moreover, in evaluating the outcomes of therapy, we have moved from biologic markers and clinical manifestations as outcome measures to the use of health-related quality-of-life measures. Patients and patient focus groups have had a great influence in developing the domains that make up the quality-of-life instrumentation. Patients have also been the source for the items making up each of these domains. The patient preferential state has become an important area of scientific endeavor, and different economic theory such as utility theory guides this research paradigm. What is your preference: a better quality of life or a longer life? How differently do these relate at the beginning of life and at the conclusion of life? Patients' preferences for treatment options will increasingly drive the delivery of medical services.

Finally, the patient will progressively demand being treated as a partner in decision-making. The cybernetic revolution that will provide us with powerful population risk data will also generate a population far more sophisticated in informatics and far more demanding of full disclosure of the latest and most sophisticated data to empower them in making their own decisions about the balance and risks of competing alternative therapeutic interventions.

Prediction. Patients in the era of pharmacoepidemiology will better understand concepts of acceptable risk and acceptable uncertainty and demand the use of both. Warning: They won't if we don't simplify our message and understand the concepts better ourselves!

THE GOVERNMENT

In America, public policy follows public expectation and capacity in its mandates, but may lead both in its incentives. Thus, in the next millennium, in the face of all these trends, we will see first incentives and then mandates for pharmacoepidemiologic monitoring of known and potential drug-associated events, outcomes, and problems. Incentives will fall into three broad categories: (1) system- and capacity-building efforts; (2) incorporation of epidemiologic planning into discussions with the FDA during investigational stages of product development (Phase II and III) and into consideration governing approval of new drug applications (NDAs); and (3) FDA receptiveness to epidemiologic data for ongoing assessments of postmarketing drug safety and secondary indications, particularly in labeling negotiations.

There is much discussion of postapproval epidemiologic studies as part of the drug development process, not as substitutes for the best achievable and acceptable safety assurance at the time of approval, but as catalysts for speeding the transition following NDA submission to approval. This postsubmission preapproval hiatus reflects a period of residual anxiety in which no further structured drug development studies are to be expected, yet the level of assurance from the data on hand may be too low for comfort. Extending or adding more trials in the late phases of preapproval drug development (Phase III) or creating a "Phase II 1/2" study seems to be a less acceptable option than does adding more affordably the structured assurance of good science and even larger numbers after approval.

Evolving approaches to product labeling represent the third incentive to good drug epidemiology. FDA Advisory Committee debates about the nonsteroidal antiinflammatory drugs have set the tone for acceptance of properly conducted, large-scale, nonexperimental, observational studies to determine more exact frequencies that can be incorporated into the education of health professionals and their patient partners and into the approved labeling itself.

The exact timing and nature of any specific mandate for inclusion of pharmacoepidemiologic studies as part of the approval of an NDA are difficult to predict. In the mid-1990s, several products were approved conditional on the manufacturer's willingness to complete studies that include major programs in pharmacoepidemiology, and major debates about "FDA reform" in the mid-1990s suggested that the power to ensure proper studies following approval may not require any legislation.

The emergence of dramatic collaborative efforts among government, industry, and practice to develop and distribute new drugs for life-threatening conditions, particularly in the face of the epidemic of AIDS during the 1990s, has increased emphasis on epidemiologic, observational studies in the preapproval phases. For a "fast-track" review, a treatment investigational new drug and expanded access system requires epidemiologic monitoring of open treatment for broader availability of a drug during the period of preapproval, final reporting of clinical trials, and FDA review. Furthermore, an extensive program of postapproval epidemiologic studies often is offered to help to "fill in the gaps" left by the urgency of rapid development and shortened NDA review time. The next decade will see efforts expand as further therapies for AIDS are developed and new applications of fast-track and enhanced availability approaches are brought to bear on other life-threatening illnesses.

On the international level, there is strong emerging consensus that postapproval epidemiology must include more than spontaneous voluntary UDE report monitoring. The development of record linkage capacity similar to that in North America is a high priority for nations comprising the European market, starting with important efforts in the UK with automated medical records supporting outpatient medical practice (e.g., the General Practice Research Database formerly known as VAMP; and the Medi-Plus IMS System) and a record-linkage scheme bridging prescription pricing authority-documented dispensing and automated hospital discharge information (e.g., the medication events monitoring program [MEMO] in Dundee, Scotland).

Prediction. A follow-through effort built upon the promising efforts of a decade's work on international harmonization by the International Conferences on Harmonization, in collaboration with the pharmaceutical industry and regulatory agencies of North America, Europe, and Japan, will provide the momentum for developing the contributions of observational epidemiologic research and support for the capacity to ensure it. Warning: If nations do not maintain this dialog, wasteful, duplicative, and potentially even contradictory approaches will emerge.

THE ACADEMIA

The 1990s witnessed the emergence of academic university-based research programs in pharmacoepidemiology. This trend will continue as three inevitable forces continue to influence the sector: progressive erosion of "core" funds and "hard money" in academia, and, with it, a progressive dependence of academic units on ad hoc and project-specific funding for their survival; a progressive realization on the part of the factors in the sector that freedom of intellect and independence of thought are most likely to result in epidemiologic projects that are scientifically credible and independent of proprietary or vested interests; and emerging recognition within academia itself that the specialized field of epidemiology is not simply important, but also scientifically meritorious in comparison with other scholarly pursuits. Over the next decade, pharmacoepidemiologic teaching, advice, and research will be recognized as credible and applicable by promotion and tenure committees; more than a dozen academic centers of excellence for teaching and research will be actively pursuing pharmaco-epidemiology.

The development of trained professionals in the field, however, will take concerted effort over the next decade. Several summer institutes are successfully offering short pharmacoepidemiology courses; several other universities, notably, the University of North Carolina at Chapel Hill, the University of Washington, and others, encourage PhD students to special-ize in pharmacoepidemiology. Funding for postgraduate training (residen-cy and fellowships) will be needed, and curriculum time will be necessary to ensure that no physician, nurse, or pharmacist can graduate without ori-entation to the fundamental principles of pharmacoepidemiology, and that the capacity is present in academia to which the sector can turn for learned and scholarly research.

Prediction. Academic departments with special expertise in pharmaco-epidemiology, pharmacoeconomics, and pharmaceutical outcomes research will thrive over the next decade. Warning: They won't thrive without prop-er academic influence as well as strong demand and financial support from the other actors.

THE INDUSTRY

Perhaps the most extensive and encouraging trend among the actors in this field is the assumption of responsibility by the pharmaceutical manu-facturer for rigorous scientific monitoring in the postapproval period. This explosion of interest is reflected in the creation of a strong body of indus-try scientists who meet regularly under the aegis of the Pharmaceutical Research and Manufacturers of America (the Clinical Safety Surveillance Committee), which involves more than 40 research-based pharmaceutical companies. In Europe, industry associations and independent counsels, extending the excellent work of the Risk Assessment Detection Analysis and Response (RADAR) working groups in many nations, are providing leadership for development of the sector. Over the next decade, there will be no question about the need for and desirability of pre- and postapproval epidemiology as a complement to ongoing programs of clinical research. Departments of pharmacoepidemiology in the major drug companies will couple traditional (passive) surveillance techniques (e.g., collection of UDE reports) with the epidemiologic quasi-experimental design observational study. Decisions regarding exactly which approach to use, and at what time in the life of the drug, will be based on rational criteria, possibly even algo-rithm application, balancing the need to know more than can be known at the time of preapproval experimentation with the costs of obtaining that knowledge. These decisions will be made according to need, feasibility, and return on investment. Here again, prompting this trend toward industry responsibility are the pressures of society's unwillingness to accept risks and uncertainty as well as industry's need to manage liabilities and risks, coupled with the opportunity posed by decreasing costs of obtaining data occasioned by large automated data sets.

Prediction. Pharmacoepidemiology will have become generally recognized as a highly cost-effective contributor to the armamentarium of industry-based drug research. Warning: It won't if we allow bad science and bad policy-making to prevail.

Summary

The fundamental goal for the future of the field must be to provide society with the evidence base to strike the dynamic balance between the early and aggressive use of needed new medications and the prevention of preventable drug injury (i.e., the optimization of therapeutic intervention).

The fundamental strategic question to be confronted by future decision-makers regarding the conduct of pharmacoepidemiologic studies will be how far they can justify the costs of knowing what is potentially knowable (so that we may do what is potentially "doable" to protect the public against unforeseen risks) against the cost of not knowing. The availability of large automated databases, with their stores of drug exposure and medical outcomes information, coupled with the growing demand to prevent human suffering by early detection, will likely lead to progressively more complicated and extensive studies undertaken collaboratively by the key actors in government, academia, and industry, and to progressively more focused answers applied in more sophisticated ways by all the key actors in the helping professions.

Perhaps the best point with which to end this glimpse into the future is the prediction of a continuing truth in this field: the occurrence of UDEs will continue to be an undesirable aspect of the practice of medicine, including pharmaceutical medicine; society will continue to demand and responsible partners will continue to strive to ensure that this adverse aspect be reduced to an irreducible minimum in the pursuit of benefit. In the area of drug safety, then, the interests and concerns of industry will be no different from the interests and concerns of practice, of academia, and of regulation: to know as much as possible as soon as possible and as accurately as possible, to help bring about the best possible therapeutic decision-making for humanity at all levels of policy-making—individual, institutional, and national. This is the commitment of the future. The new era of pharmacoepidemiology brings this promise substantially closer to today's reality.

Appendix

Guidelines for Good Epidemiology Practices for Drug, Device, and Vaccine Research in the United States

E pidemiologic studies provide valuable information about the relationship between human health and therapeutic agents. However, because of the nonexperimental nature of many epidemiologic studies, scientific controversy often surrounds their interpretation. In addition, controversy frequently concerns the quality of the data used, the appropriateness of the study design, and the process used to conduct the study. The Guidelines for Good Epidemiology Practices (GEPs) address those issues — data quality, study design, and study conduct — that are under the control of the investigator.

These GEPs have been adapted from a document prepared by the Chemical Manufacturer's Association's Epidemiology Task Group.[1] Wherever appropriate, we have (with permission) retained the exact text of that document. The GEPs propose practices and procedures in the following areas:

- Protocol
- Organization and personnel
- Facilities, resource commitment, and contractors
- Study conduct
- Communication
- Archiving

The following ISPE members helped draft these guidelines: Elizabeth B Andrews PhD MPH, Jerry Avorn MD, Edward A Bortnichak PhD MPH, Robert Chen MD MA, Wanju S Dai MD DrPH, Gretchen S Dieck PhD MPH, Stanley Edlavitch PhD MA, Joel Freiman MD MPH, Allen A Mitchell MD, Robert C Nelson PhD, C Ineke Neutel PhD FACE, Andrew Stergachis PhD, Brian L Strom MD MPH, Alexander M Walker MD DrPH. Reprinted with permission of the International Society for Pharmacoepidemiology. Revised: March 27, 1996.

Goals for the Guidelines for Good Epidemiology Practices

The GEPs propose minimum practices and procedures that should be considered to help ensure the quality and integrity of data used in epidemiologic research and to provide adequate documentation of the research methods. The GEPs and analyses do not prescribe specific research methods.

The guidelines have the following goals:

1. to provide a framework to assist researchers in adhering to good epidemiologic research principles;

2. to promote sound epidemiologic research by encouraging rigorous data collection and analysis;

3. to provide a framework for evaluating epidemiologic studies;

4. to improve the acceptance of studies that use sound scientific methods;

5. to facilitate the appropriate utilization of technical resources by promoting careful study design and planning of study conduct.

Guidelines do not guarantee good research, but adherence to these guidelines will facilitate the conduct, interpretation, documentation, and acceptance of epidemiologic studies.

Scope and Application

The GEPs can be applied to all types of epidemiologic research. Epidemiologic studies often evolve through a number of stages that precede the development of a protocol. These include, for example, proposals, feasibility studies, and measurement instrument validation studies.

Clearly, large complex studies will benefit from the careful planning and thorough documentation implicit in these guidelines. Adherence to the spirit of the guidelines will be beneficial for those activities preceding protocol development as well as more informal investigations such as health hazard assessments/evaluations or small cluster investigations. Particularly in circumstances of immediate public health concern, the guidelines will provide a useful framework to ensure that all research issues are adequately addressed.

These guidelines should evolve based on the experiences gained through their application to studies.

PROTOCOL

Each study shall have a written protocol.

The protocol should include the following:

A. A descriptive title, including original date of approval.

B. The names, titles, degrees, addresses, and affiliations of all responsible parties, including at least the principal investigator and all coinvestigators, and a list of all collaborating primary and other relevant institutions and study sites.

C. The name(s) and address(es) of the sponsor(s).

D. An abstract of the protocol.

E. The proposed study tasks, milestones, and timeline.

F. A statement of research objectives, specific aims, and rationale. Research objectives describe the kinds of knowledge or information to be gained from the study. Specific aims list the measurements to be made, and any hypotheses to be tested. The protocol must distinguish between a priori research hypotheses and ones that have been based on knowledge of the data. The rationale explains how achievement of the specific aims will further the research objectives.

G. A critical review of the literature to evaluate relevant variables and gaps in knowledge. For example, the literature review should be of sufficient depth to identify potential confounders and effect modifiers and to determine areas where new knowledge is needed. The literature review might encompass relevant animal and human experiments, clinical studies, vital statistics, and previous epidemiologic studies.

H. A description of the research methods, including:

1. The overall research design and strategy and reasons for choosing the proposed study design. Research designs include, for example, case–control, cohort, cross-sectional, nested case–control, or other hybrid designs. The rationale for the selection of the proposed design over others should be presented.

2. The population and sample to be studied. The population is defined in terms of persons, place, time period, and exclusions. The protocol should identify any changes in population or sample that were implemented after the beginning of the study.

3. The data sources for exposure, health status, and risk factors. For example, questionnaires, hospital discharge files, abstracts of primary clinical records, automated records such as prescription drug files, biological measurements, exposure/work history record reviews, or exposure/disease registries.

4. Clear operational definitions of health outcomes, exposure, and other measured risk factors as well as selection criteria, as appropriate, for exposed and nonexposed persons, morbidity or mortality cases, and referent groups. An operational definition is one that can be implemented using the data available in the proposed study. For example, "PCP episode" is not an operational definition, whereas "hospitalization with a primary diagnosis of ICD-9-CM code 136.3" is.

5. Projected study size, statistical precision, and the basis for their determination. Present the relation between the study size and the specific aims of the study.

6. The methods to be used in assembling the study data. This should include a description of, or reference to, methods used to control, measure, or reduce various forms of error — e.g., bias due to selection, misclassification, interviewer, or confounding — and their impact on the study. Pretesting procedures for research instruments and any manuals and formal training to be provided to interviewers, abstractors, coders, or data entry personnel should be described or referenced.

7. Procedures for data management. This should include data management programs and hardware to be used in the study.

8. Methods for data analysis. Data analysis includes all the major steps that lead from raw data to a final result. It comprises comparisons and methods for analyzing and presenting results, categorizations, as well as procedures to control, if possible, sources of bias and their influence on results. The statistical tests to be applied to the data and procedures for obtaining point estimates and confidence intervals of measures of occurrence or association should also be presented.

9. A description of quality assurance and quality control procedures for all phases of the study. Mechanisms to ensure data quality and integrity should be described, including, for example, reabstraction of original documents. As appropriate, include certification and/or qualifications of any supporting laboratory or research groups.

10. Major limitations of the study design, data sources, and analytic methods. At a minimum, issues relating to confounding, bias, generalizability, and random error should be considered. The likely success of efforts to reduce errors, presented in section H6, should be discussed.

I. A description of plans for protecting human subjects. This should include information about whether study subjects will be placed at risk as a result of the study, under what circumstances informed consent will be required, provisions for maintaining confidentiality of information on study subjects, and circumstances, if any, under which personally identifiable information may be provided to entities outside the study.

J. A description of plans for disseminating and communicating study results, including the presence or absence of any restrictions on the extent and timing of publication. There is an ethical obligation to disseminate findings of public health importance.

K. Resources required to conduct the study. Describe, for example, time, personnel, and equipment required to conduct the study, including a brief description of the role of each of the personnel assigned to the research project.

L. The bibliographic references.

M. Dated amendments to the protocol.

Significant deviationsfrom the protocol should be documented in writing.

ORGANIZATION AND PERSONNEL

A. Organizational structure. The organization or individual conducting the research shall be fully responsible for the research. The relationship, roles, and responsibilities of the organizations and/or individuals sponsoring or conducting the study should be carefully defined in writing. For example, this should include delineating the roles and responsibilities to be assumed by the study sponsor and the contractor(s) in communicating various aspects of the study as well as data ownership, archiving.

B. Personnel. Personnel engaged in epidemiologic research and related activities shall have the education, training, and/or experience necessary to perform the assigned functions competently. The organization shall maintain a current summary of training and experience of these personnel. A list of individuals engaged in or supervising activities shall be maintained and updated periodically, with complete job titles.

FACILITIES, RESOURCE COMMITMENT, AND CONTRACTORS

A. Facilities. Adequate physical facilities shall be provided to all those engaged in epidemiologic research and related activities. Sufficient resources, e.g., office space, relevant equipment, and office/professional supplies, shall be available to ensure timely and proper completion of all studies. Suitable storage facilities shall be available to maintain research materials in a safe and secure environment.

B. Resource commitment. Sufficient commitment shall be made at the beginning of each study to ensure its timely and proper completion (see Protocol K).

C. Contractors. For the purposes of ensuring and documenting the contractor's conformance with the GEPs, it is recommended that the study sponsor have the right during the course of the study, and for a reasonable period following completion of the study, to inspect the contractor's facilities, including equipment, technical record, and record relating to the work conducted under the sponsor's contract. The nature of the audit, including procedures that guarantee patient confidentiality, will be agreed upon at the outset of any contract.

STUDY CONDUCT

The principal investigator shall be responsible for the overall content of the individual research project, including the day-to-day conduct of the study, interpretation of the study data, and preparation of a final report.

These responsibilities extend to all aspects of the study, including periodic reporting of study progress as well as quality assurance.

The unusual decision to terminate a study prematurely should be taken with great caution, and should be based on good scientific and ethical reasons and documented in writing. There may be rare instances in which administrative reasons require study termination. Such decisions must be made independent of any study results. Investigators and sponsors should specify and agree in advance about the circumstances under which the study could be terminated early. Included should be a mechanism for resolution of any disagreement.

A. Protection of human subjects. Institutional review board approval should be obtained or, if not, applicable regulations specifying the reason for exemption should be referred to in the protocol. Investigators will ensure that personal identifiers will be removed from any study files that are accessible to non-study personnel. All personnel with access to data containing personal identifiers will sign a pledge to maintain the confidentiality of study subjects. They will maintain an ability to verify the origin and integrity of data sets from which personal identifiers will have been removed.

B. Data collection and verification. All data collected for the study should be recorded directly, accurately, promptly, and legibly. The individual(s) responsible for the integrity of the data, computerized and hard copy, shall be identified. All procedures used to verify and promote the quality and integrity of the data shall be outlined in writing. A historical file of these procedures shall be maintained, including all revisions and the dates of such revisions. Any changes in data entries shall be documented.

C. Analysis. All data management and statistical analysis programs and packages used in the analyses should be documented. Reasonable effort should be made to validate interim steps in the analysis.

D. Study report. Completed studies shall be summarized in a final report that accurately and completely presents the study objectives, methods, results, and the principal investigator's interpretation of the findings.

The final report shall include at a minimum:

1. a descriptive title;
2. an abstract;
3. purpose (objectives) of the research as stated in the protocol;
4. the names, titles, degrees, addresses, and affiliations of the principal investigator and all coinvestigators;
5. name(s) and address(es) of sponsor(s);
6. dates on which the study was initiated and completed;
7. introduction with background, purpose, and specific aims of the study;
8. a description of the research methods, including:
   a. the selection of study subjects and controls,

    b. the data collection methods used,
    c. the transformations, calculations, or operations on the data, and
    d. statistical methods used in data analyses;
9. a description of circumstances that may have affected the quality or integrity of the data. Describe also the initially identified limitations of study approach and the methods used to address them (e.g., response rates, or missing data)(See Protocol, Sections H6 and H9);
10. a summary and analyses of the data. Include sufficient tables, graphs, and illustrations to present the pertinent data and to reflect the analyses performed;
11. a statement of the conclusions drawn from the analyses of the data;
12. a discussion of the implication of study results. Cite prior research in support of and in contrast to present findings. Discuss possible biases and limitations in present research;
13. references.

COMMUNICATION

Each organization and its advisory board, if there is one, shall predetermine procedures under which communications of the intent, conduct, results, and interpretations of an epidemiologic study will occur, including what function individuals associated with the research must fulfill. These individuals should include the principal investigator, study director, and/or the sponsor. This procedure may be documented in the form of a company standard operating procedure, in the study protocol, or through contractual agreement.

Government agencies and all sponsors shall be informed of study results in a manner that complies with applicable regulatory requirements.

There is an ethical obligation to disseminate findings of public health importance. Scientific peers shall be informed of study results by publication in the scientific literature or presentations at scientific conferences, workshops, or symposia.

Potential conflicts of interest should be disclosed.

ARCHIVING

There shall be secure archives for the orderly storage and expedient retrieval of all study-related material. An index shall be prepared to identify the archived contents, to identify their location, and to identify by name and location any materials that by their general nature are not retained in the study archive.

Access to the archives shall be controlled and limited to authorized personnel only. Special procedures may be necessary to ensure that access to confidential information is limited and that the confidentiality of information about study subjects is protected (see Protocol, Section I).

The archive should be maintained for at least 5 years after final report or first publication of study results, whichever comes later. At a minimum, the study archive should contain, or refer to, the following:

A. Study protocol and copies of all approved modifications.

B. A final report of the study.

C. All source data and, where feasible, specimens. A printed sample of the master computer data file(s) with reference to the location of the machine readable master. All "source data" should comprise the raw data that provided the basis for the final analysis of the study. The archival material should be sufficiently detailed to permit re-editing and re-analysis.

D. Documentation adequate to identify and locate all computer programs and statistical procedures used, including version numbers where appropriate (see Study Conduct C).

E. Copies of computer printouts, including relevant execution code, that form the basis of any tables, graphs, discussions, or interpretations in the final report. Any manually developed calculations shall be documented on a work sheet and similarly retained.

F. Correspondence pertaining to the study, standard operating procedures, informed consent releases, copies of all relevant representative material, copies of signed institutional review board and other external reviewer reports, and copies of all quality assurance reports and audits. Include, for example, questionnaires, name, make and model numbers of relevant measurement instruments, calibration information and procedures.

G. Documentation relating to the collection and processing of study data, including laboratory/research notebooks, training and reference documents for abstracts, interviews, and coders.

Reference

1. Chemical Manufacturer's Association's Epidemiology Task Group. Guidelines for good epidemiology practices for occupational environmental epidemiologic research. JOM 1991;33:1221-9.

Index

Academia, 656
Accelerated drug approval, 31, 53
Acetylation, 171
Activity of daily living scales, 351
Acute myocardial infarction, 13, 525, 535
Ad hoc data collection, 17, 393
Adverse drug event, 49, 219, 390; see also,
  Adverse drug reaction, Adverse event,
  Unintended drug effect
Adverse drug reaction, 72; see also, Adverse
  drug event, Adverse event, Unintended
  drug effect
Adverse event, 218, 422; see also, Adverse
  drug event, Adverse drug reaction,
  Unintended drug effect
Adverse Event Reporting System, 426; see
  also, Food and Drug Administration,
  Prescription-event monitoring, Spontaneous
  reporting system
Agency for Health Care Policy and
  Research, 191
Algorithms, 462; see also, Attribution,
  Causality assessment, Standardized assess-
  ment method, Unintended drug effect
American Hospital Formulary Service, 137
Analytic studies, 73, 85
Anatomical-Therapeutic Chemical
  Classification, 137, 408
Anticonvulsant hypersensitivity, 174
Association of the British Pharmaceutical
  Industry, 468
Asthma, 474
Attributable risk, 289
Attribution, 287; see also, Algorithms,
  Causality assessment, Standardized assess-
  ment method, Unintended drug effect
Automated databases, 16, 369
Average new drugs, 66
Bias, 100; diagnostic suspicion, 16; informa-
  tion, 100, 241, 269; measurement, 100; proce-
  dure selection, 14; recall, 100, 268; selection,
  15, 93, 100, 242, 269, 398; sources, 187, 241;
  susceptibility, 14
Biologic markers, 162
Biotechnology, 18
Birth defects, 86
Blinding, 102, 237
Breakthrough drugs, 64
British Committee on the Safety of
  Medicines, 434
Case reports, 77
Case series, 78

Case–control studies, 8, 91, 239, 249;
  matched, 95, 251; see also, Cohort studies,
  Cross-sectional studies, Observational stud-
  ies
Case–crossover studies, 99
Causal model, 14
Causality assessment, 461; see also,
  Algorithms, Attribution, Standardized
  assessment method, Unintended drug effect
Causation, 74; see also, Attribution, Causal
  model, Causality assessment
Center for Drug Evaluation and Research,
  32, 426; see also, Food and Drug
  Administration
Centers for Disease Control and Prevention,
  78, 80
Clinical appropriateness, 502
Clinical trials, controlled, 101; double-blind,
  102; limitation, 70; prospective, 85; quality,
  328; quality of life, 357; randomized, 101;
  triple-blind, 102; see also, Experimental
  studies
Cohort studies, 239, 246; case, 99, 416; histori-
  cal, 85; prospective, 85; retrospective, 87; see
  also, Case–control studies, Cross-sectional
  studies, Observational studies
Compliance, causality assessment, 461;
  patient, 282
Conceptualization, 72
Confidence interval, 245, 326, 337, 339
Confidentiality, 222
Confounders, 12
Confounding, 243; by indication, 100, 244;
  variable, 12, 243
Coronary heart disease, 525
Cost containment, 72, 645
Cost data, 133
Cost-benefit analysis, 648
Cross-sectional studies, 8, 81; see also,
  Case–control studies, Cohort studies,
  Observational studies
Crossover design, 99
Crude analysis, 245
Database, exposure, 370; multipurpose, 369;
  specialized, 370
Databases, Boston Collaborative Drug
  Surveillance Network, 139, 374, 397, 432,
  510; Computerized Online Medicaid
  Pharmaceutical Analysis and Surveillance
  System, 139; Harvard Pilgrim Health Care,
  374; Medicaid Management Information
  System, 139; Mental Health Package of the